Rob & Smith's
Operative Surgery

Vascular Surgery

Fifth edition

General Editors

David C. Carter MD, FRCS(Ed), FRCS(Glas)
Regius Professor of Clinical Surgery, Royal Infirmary,
Edinburgh, UK

R. C. G. Russell MS, FRCS
Consultant Surgeon, Middlesex Hospital and Royal National
Throat, Nose and Ear Hospital, London, UK

Consulting Editor

Hugh Dudley CBE, ChM, FRCS(Ed), FRACS, FRCS
Emeritus Professor, St Mary's Hospital, London, UK

Art Editor

Gillian Lee FMAA, HonFIMI, AMI, RMIP
15 Little Plucketts Way, Buckhurst Hill, Essex, UK

Rob & Smith's
Operative Surgery

Vascular Surgery

Fifth edition

Edited by

Crawford W. Jamieson MS, FRCS
Consultant Surgeon, St Thomas' Hospital, London, UK

James S. T. Yao MD, PhD
Magerstadt Professor of Surgery, Division of Vascular Surgery, Northwestern University Medical School, Chicago, Illinois, USA

CHAPMAN & HALL MEDICAL
London · Glasgow · New York · Tokyo · Melbourne · Madras

Published by Chapman & Hall, 2–6 Boundary Row, London SE1 8HN

Chapman & Hall, 2–6 Boundary Row, London SE1 8HN, UK

Blackie Academic & Professional, Wester Cleddens Road,
Bishopbriggs, Glasgow G64 2NZ, UK

Chapman & Hall Inc., One Penn Plaza, 41st Floor,
New York, NY 10119, USA

Chapman & Hall Japan, Thomson Publishing Japan, Hirakawacho
Nemoto Building, 7F, 1-7-11 Hirakawa-cho, Chiyoda-ku, Tokyo 102,
Japan

Chapman & Hall Australia, Thomas Nelson Australia,
102 Dodds Street, South Melbourne, Victoria 3205, Australia

Chapman & Hall India, R. Seshadri, 32 Second Main Road, CIT East,
Madras 600 035, India

First edition 1957
Second edition 1968
Third edition 1976
Fourth edition 1985
Fifth edition 1994

© 1994 Chapman & Hall

Typeset in 10/11 Garamond ITC by Genesis Typesetting, Laser Quay, Rochester, Kent

Printed at The Bath Press, England

ISBN 0 412 58630 4

A catalogue record for this book is available from the British Library

Library of Congress Cataloging-in-Publication Data available

Contributors

S. S. Ahn MD
Assistant Professor, Department of Surgery, UCLA School of Medicine, 10833 Le Conte Avenue, Los Angeles, California 90024, USA

D. J. Allison BSc, MD, MRCP, FRCR
Professor and Director, Department of Diagnostic Radiology, Royal Postgraduate Medical School, Hammersmith Hospital, Du Cane Road, London W12 0NN, UK

G. Andros MD, FRCS(Glas)
Vascular Laboratory, Saint Joseph Medical Center, 501 South Buena Vista Street, Burbank, California 91505, USA

C. H. Andrus MD
Clinical Associate Professor of Surgery, University of Rochester Medical Center, Rochester, New York 14620, USA

A. B. Ayers MD, FRCR
Consultant Radiologist, St Thomas' Hospital, London SE1 7EH, UK

D. F. Bandyk MD
Professor of Surgery, Director, Division of Vascular Surgery, University of South Florida College of Medicine, Tampa, Florida 33606, USA

P. R. F. Bell MD, FRCS
Professor of Surgery, Clinical Sciences Building, Leicester Royal Infirmary, Leicester LE2 7LX, UK

D. Bergqvist MD, PhD
Professor, Department of Surgery, University Hospital, Uppsala, Sweden

K. G. Burnand MS, FRCS
Professor of Vascular Surgery, St Thomas' Hospital, London SE1 7EH, UK

B. B. Chang MD
Albany Medical College, Vascular Surgery Section A61, 47 New Scotland Avenue, Albany, New York 12208, USA

S. W. K. Cheng MD, FRCS
Visiting Assistant Professor, Vascular Division, University of California, 505 Parnassus Avenue, San Francisco, California 94143-0222, USA

K. J. Cherry Jr MD
Consultant and Head, Division of Vascular Surgery, Department of Surgery and Associate Professor of Surgery, Mayo Medical School, Mayo Clinic, 200 First Street SW, Rochester, Minnesota 55905, USA

M. D. Colburn MD
Resident, Department of General Surgery, UCLA School of Medicine, 10833 Le Conte Avenue, Los Angeles, California 90024, USA

E. Criado MD, RVT
Assistant Professor of Surgery, Vascular Surgery Section, University of North Carolina at Chapel Hill, 210 Burnett-Womack Building, CB No. 7210, Chapel Hill, North Carolina 27599-7210, USA

H. Dardik MD
Clinical Professor of Surgery, Mount Sinai Medical Center, New York and Chief, Department of General and Vascular Surgery, Englewood Hospital, Englewood, New Jersey 07631, USA

R. C. Darling III MD
Albany Medical College, Vascular Surgery Section A61, 47 New Scotland Avenue, Albany, New York 12208, USA

R. G. DePalma MD
Lewis B. Saltz Professor of Surgery, George Washington University School of Medicine, 2150 Pennsylvania Avenue NW, Washington, District of Columbia 20037, USA

J. A. DeWeese MD
Professor of Surgery and Chief Emeritus of Cardiothoracic and Vascular Surgery, University of Rochester Medical Center, 601 Elmwood Avenue, Rochester, New York 14642-8410, USA

R. H. Dean MD
Director, Division of Surgical Sciences and Professor and Chairman, Department of General Surgery, Bowman Gray School of Medicine, Winston-Salem, North Carolina 27103, USA

B. C. Eikelboom MD
Professor of Vascular Surgery, Department of Surgery, Section of Vascular Surgery, Utrecht University Hospital, PO Box 85500, 3508 GA Utrecht, The Netherlands

W. V. Ellis MD
Department of Neurosurgery, University of California, San Francisco, USA

C. B. Ernst MD
Clinical Professor of Surgery, University of Michigan Medical School and Head, Division of Vascular Surgery, Henry Ford Hospital, Detroit, Michigan 48202, USA

I. Faris MD, FRACS
Chairman, Department of Surgery, University of Adelaide and Head of Unit, Vascular Surgery, Royal Adelaide Hospital, Adelaide, South Australia 5000, Australia

P. Fiorani MD
Chief, Department of Vascular Surgery, University of Rome 'La Sapienza', Rome, Italy

W. R. Flinn MD
Associate Professor of Surgery, Division of Vascular Surgery, Department of Surgery, Northwestern University Medical School, Chicago, Illinois 60611, USA

P. Gloviczki MD
Associate Professor of Surgery, Mayo Medical School and Consultant, Division of Vascular Surgery, Mayo Clinic and Foundation, 200 First Street SW, Rochester, Minnesota 55905, USA

R. M. Green MD, FACS
Associate Professor of Surgery and Chief, Section of Vascular Surgery, University of Rochester School of Medicine, Rochester, New York 14620-4199, USA

J. W. Hallett Jr MD
Associate Professor, Section of Vascular Surgery, Mayo Clinic and Mayo Foundation, 200 First Street SW, Rochester, Minnesota 55905, USA

K. J. Hansen MD
Assistant Professor, Department of General Surgery, Bowman Gray School of Medicine, Winston-Salem, North Carolina 27103, USA

P. L. Harris MD, FRCS
Consultant Vascular Surgeon, Royal Liverpool University Hospital, Liverpool L7 8XP, UK

R. W. Harris MD
Vascular Laboratory, Saint Joseph Medical Center, 501 South Buena Vista Street, Burbank, California 91505, USA

W. P. Hederman MCh, FRCSI, FRCPS(Glas), FRCS(Ed)
Consultant Surgeon, Mater Misericordiae Hospital, Dublin, Eire

W. S. Helton MD
Assistant Professor, Department of Surgery, University of Washington School of Medicine, Harborview Medical Centre, Seattle, Washington 98104, USA

J. T. Hobbs MD, FRCS
Honorary Senior Lecturer in Surgery, University of London, London, UK

L. H. Hollier MD, FACS
Department of Surgery, Ochsner Clinic, 1514 Jefferson Highway, New Orleans, Louisiana 70121, USA

A. M. Imparato MD
Professor of Surgery, New York University Medical Center, 550 First Avenue, New York 10016, USA

J. E. Jackson MRCP, FRCR
Consultant Radiologist, Department of Diagnostic Radiology, Royal Postgraduate Medical School, Hammersmith Hospital, Du Cane Road, London W12 0NN, UK

C. W. Jamieson MS, FRCS
Consultant Surgeon, St Thomas' Hospital, London SE1 7UT, UK

K. Johansen MD, PhD
Professor, Department of Surgery, University of Washington School of Medicine, Harborview Medical Center, Seattle, Washington 98104, USA

G. Johnson Jr MD
Roscoe B. G. Cowper Professor of Surgery, University of North Carolina at Chapel Hill, 210 Burnett-Womack Building, CB No. 7210, Chapel Hill, North Carolina 27599-7210, USA

D. M. Justins FRCA
Consultant Anaesthetist and Director, Pain Management Centre, St Thomas' Hospital, London SE1 7EH, UK

R. L. Kistner MD
Clinical Professor of Surgery, University of Hawaii, Department of Vascular Surgery, Straub Clinic and Hospital, Honolulu, Hawaii 96813, USA

The late M. Lea Thomas MA, PhD, FRCP, FRCS, FRCR
Vascular Radiologist, St Thomas' Hospital, London SE1 7EH, UK

R. P. Leather MD
Albany Medical College, Vascular Surgery Section A61, 47 New Scotland Avenue, Albany, New York 12208, USA

R. J. Lusby MD, FRCS, FRACS
Professor of Surgery, Department of Surgery, Sydney University, Clinical Sciences Building, Concord Hospital, Concord 2139, Australia

H. I. Machleder MD
Professor, Department of Surgery, UCLA School of Medicine, 10833 Le Conte Avenue, Los Angeles, California 90024, USA

A. O. Mansfield ChM, FRCS
Consultant Vascular Surgeon, St Mary's Hospital, London W2 1NY, UK

T. Mätzsch MD, PhD
Associate Professor, Department of Surgery, Lund University, Malmö General Hospital, S-214 01 Malmö, Sweden

W. J. McCarthy MD
Assistant Professor of Surgery, Division of Vascular Surgery, Department of Surgery, Northwestern University Medical School, Chicago, Illinois 60611, USA

P. M. McFadden MD
Cardiovascular and Thoracic Surgeon, Department of Surgery, Ochsner Clinic, 1514 Jefferson Highway, New Orleans, Louisiana 70121, USA

J. L. Mills MD
Associate Professor of Surgery, University of South Florida College of Medicine, Tampa, Florida 33606, USA

Y. Mishima MD
Professor, IInd Department of Surgery, Tokyo Medical and Dental University, 1-5-45 Yushima, Bunkyoku, Tokyo 113, Japan

S. R. Money MD
Department of Surgery, Ochsner Clinic, 1514 Jefferson Highway, New Orleans, Louisiana 70121, USA

W. S. Moore MD
Professor of Surgery and Chief, Section of Vascular Surgery, UCLA School of Medicine, Los Angeles, California 90024, USA

B. H. Nachbur MD
Professor of Surgery, Department for Thoracic and Cardiovascular Surgery, University of Berne, 3010 Berne, Switzerland

K. D. Nolan MD, MPH
Instructor of Surgery, Division of Vascular Surgery, Department of Surgery, Northwestern University Medical School, Chicago, Illinois 60611, USA

J. L. Ochsner MD
Chairman Emeritus, Department of Surgery and Chief, Division of Thoracic and Cardiovascular Surgery, Ochsner Clinic, 1514 Jefferson Highway, New Orleans, Louisiana 70121, USA

K. Ouriel MD
Associate Professor of Surgery, University of Rochester School of Medicine and Dentistry, 601 Elmwood Avenue, Rochester, New York, 14642-8410, USA

J. C. Parodi MD
Chief, Department of Vascular Surgery, Instituto Cardiovascular de Buenos Aires, Blanco Encalad 1543/47, (1428) Capital Federal, Argentina

W. H. Pearce MD
Associate Professor of Surgery, Division of Vascular Surgery, Department of Surgery, Northwestern University Medical School, Chicago, Illinois 60611, USA

M. O. Perry MD
Professor and Chief of Vascular Surgery, Texas Tech University Health Sciences Center, 3601 4th Street, Lubbock, Texas 79430, USA

F. Quigley MS, FRACS
Staff Specialist, Vascular Surgery, Royal Adelaide Hospital, North Terrace, Adelaide, South Australia 5000, Australia

D. J. Reddy MD
Clinical Associate Professor of Surgery, University of Michigan Medical School and Senior Staff Vascular Surgeon, Henry Ford Hospital, Detroit, Michigan 48202, USA

I. P. Renzi MD
Resident, Department of Vascular Surgery, University of Rome 'La Sapienza', Rome, Italy

J. J. Ricotta MD
Professor of Surgery and Director, Division of Vascular Surgery, State University of New York at Buffalo, 3 Gates Circle, Buffalo, New York 14209, USA

T. S. Riles MD
New York University Medical Center, 550 First Avenue, New York, New York 10016, USA

C. G. Rob MChir, FRCS, FACS
Professor of Surgery, Uniformed Services University of the Health Sciences, F. Edward Hebert School of Medicine, Bethesda, Maryland 20816, USA

C. V. Ruckley MB, ChM, FRCS(Ed), FRCPE
Professor of Vascular Surgery, University of Edinburgh and Consultant Surgeon, Vascular Surgery Unit, Royal Infirmary, Edinburgh EH3 9YW, UK

P. A. Schneider MD
Vascular Laboratory, Saint Joseph Medical Center, 501 South Buena Vista Street, Burbank, California 91505, USA

J. H. Scurr BSc, FRCS
Senior Lecturer and Honorary Consultant Surgeon, Department of Surgical Studies, University College and Middlesex School of Medicine, Mortimer Street, London W1N 8AA, UK

D. M. Shah MD
Albany Medical College, Vascular Surgery Section A61, 47 New Scotland Avenue, Albany, New York 12208, USA

F. Speziale MD
Resident, Department of Vascular Surgery, University of Rome 'La Sapienza', Rome, Italy

R. J. Stoney MD
Professor of Surgery, Vascular Division, University of California, 350 Parnassus Avenue, San Francisco, California 94143-0222, USA

M. Taurino MD
Resident, Department of Vascular Surgery, University of Rome 'La Sapienza', Rome, Italy

R. W. H. van Reedt Dortland MD
Consultant Vascular Surgeon, Department of Surgery, Section of Vascular Surgery, Utrecht University Hospital, PO Box 85500, 3508 GA Utrecht, The Netherlands

F. J. Veith MD, FACS
Professor of Surgery, Division of Vascular Surgery, Montefiore Medical Center, 111 East 210th Street, Bronx, New York 10467, USA

J. H. H. Webster MA, MChir, FRCS
Consultant Surgeon, Southampton University Hospitals Trust, Tremona Road, Southampton SO9 4XY, UK

R. A. White MD
Chief, Vascular Surgery, Harbor-UCLA Medical Center, 1000 West Carson Street, Torrance, California 90509, USA

J. H. N. Wolfe MS, FRCS
Consultant Vascular Surgeon, St Mary's Hospital, London W2 1NY, UK

J. S. T. Yao MD, PhD
Magerstadt Professor of Surgery, Division of Vascular Surgery, Department of Surgery, Northwestern University Medical School, Chicago, Illinois 60611, USA

Contributing Medical Artists

Joanna Cameron BA(Hons), MMAA
11 Pine Trees, Portsmouth Road,
Esher, Surrey KT10 9JF, UK

Peter Cox RDD, MMAA, AIMI
2 Frome Villas, Frenchay,
Bristol BS16 1LT, UK

Marc Donon
45 Avenue Felix Faure,
75015 Paris, France

Patrick Elliott BA(Hons), ATC, MMAA, AIMI
46 Stone Delf,
Sheffield S10 3QX, UK

Raymond Evans BA(Hons), MMAA
Unit of Art in Medicine,
Department of Cell and Structural Biology,
University of Manchester, Manchester M13 9PT, UK

Diane Kinton BA(Hons)
Gillian Lee Illustrations,
15 Little Plucketts Way, Buckhurst Hill,
Essex IG9 5QU, UK

The late Robert Lane MMAA
Studio 19A, Edith Grove,
London SW10, UK

Mark Iley BA(Hons)
12 High Street, Great Missenden,
Buckinghamshire HP16 9AB, UK

Gillian Lee FMAA, HonFIMI, AMI, RMIP
Gillian Lee Illustrations,
15 Little Plucketts Way, Buckhurst Hill,
Essex IG9 5QU, UK

Gillian Oliver MMAA, AIMI
15 Bramble Road, Hatfield,
Hertfordshire AL10 9RZ, UK

Richard Neave FMAA, AIMI
Unit of Art in Medicine,
Department of Cell and Structural Biology,
University of Manchester, Manchester M13 9PT, UK

Paul Richardson BA(Hons)
54 Wellington Road,
Orpington, Kent BR5 4AQ, UK

Denise Smith BA(Hons), MMAA
Unit of Art in Medicine,
Department of Cell and Structural Biology,
University of Manchester, Manchester M13 9PT, UK

Ann Statham MMAA
Department of Medical Photography and Illustration,
Queen Elizabeth Hospital, Edgbaston, Birmingham B15 2TH, UK

Contents

Preface

We are honoured to have been invited to edit the 5th edition of the Vascular Surgery volume of Rob and Smith's Operative Surgery, as this is still considered the definitive atlas of surgical technique. With the support of the series editors we have made every effort to place the reader at the shoulder of an expert in the assessment of the preoperative status of the patient. During the operation each author has attempted to guide the reader through the details of the procedure, with particular attention to the danger points in the operation and the pitfalls, checks and balances which must be observed. Similarly, in the postoperative period advice is given on the likely complications and methods of their prevention. Surgery is a rapidly evolving specialty, particularly its relatively young offshoots such as surgery of arterial and venous disease, and the editors have faced a considerable dilemma in deciding which relatively untried and experimental new operations should be included in a standard textbook of this nature.

There is a current trend in textbooks to strive for the topical and fashionable. We feel that this vogue can be unfortunate as it confers the status of an accepted procedure which should be part of the armamentarium of every specialist surgeon on techniques which have yet to prove their value in the cut and thrust of clinical surgery. For this reason we have compromised and only included those new operations which we have guessed will find some place in the future of vascular surgery; indeed, we have omitted some operations from this edition which we feel have not proved their worth. We hope to have an opportunity to revise this judgement in the next edition.

C. W. Jamieson
J. S. T. Yao

Illustrations by Richard Neave

Intraoperative angiography

Herbert Dardik MD
Clinical Professor of Surgery, Mount Sinai School of Medicine, New York, and Chief, Department of General Surgery and Vascular Surgical Section, Englewood Hospital, Englewood, New Jersey, USA

Intraoperative angiography performed for the purpose of obtaining information regarding suitability for revascularization is usually referred to as prereconstruction arteriography. Arteriography performed intraoperatively after revascularization (completion arteriography) is used to assess the distal segment of the reconstruction as well as the run-off circulation. Both types of intraoperative angiography provide useful information that is clinically relevant: for example, the optimal site for distal anastomosis if this could not be determined before surgery, the potential for durable patency and possible alternative procedures should the primary procedure fail.

Prereconstruction arteriography

Prereconstruction arteriography is seldom necessary; in fact, there is an inverse relationship with the quality of and commitment to the performance of standard angiography in an angiographic suite. Where adequate visualization is not obtained, intraoperative prereconstruction arteriography can be performed with ease to define run-off anatomy and potential for revascularization[1-3].

1 Cannulation of the femoral artery is one means of performing prereconstruction arteriography and avoids open distal wounds if, in fact, the likelihood for revascularization is minimal. A butterfly needle is placed into the femoral artery and contrast medium injected with timed exposure to X-rays in the area of interest at the knee, leg or foot.

In some cases, distal placement of a needle or catheter may indeed be required if visualization is not possible due to extensive obliterative disease. These problems have in large measure been significantly reduced by using digital angiographic techniques as an adjunct to standard arteriography and complementary Doppler flow studies. The former can increase the likelihood of identifying crural vessels capable of sustaining a bypass in an additional 20% of cases where run-off could not be visualized by standard techniques[4]. The latter has been demonstrated to successfully localize distal vessels that can then be confirmed by prereconstruction arteriography or direct surgical exploration[5].

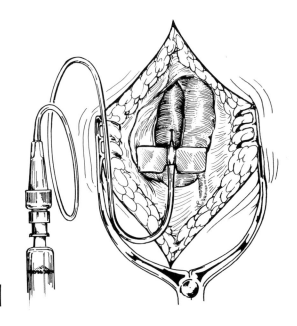

1

Completion arteriography

Intraoperative arteriography performed immediately after arterial reconstruction provides valuable information as to technical adequacy of the operation and prognosis for the durability of graft function[6-8]. The derived information is, in fact, usually more accurate than that provided by the preoperative arteriogram and may thus alter the prognosis for the particular reconstruction performed. Despite these favourable aspects, including the advantage of simplicity of performance, completion arteriography is not a universal routine. It is tempting at the conclusion of a long and tedious operation to get the patient 'off the table'. In fact, completion arteriography requires but a fraction of the overall surgical time, is easy to perform and is inexpensive. Surgeons must adjust their attitudes to this procedure which, with critical analysis of the findings, will improve results and ultimately the fate of their patients. Other monitoring techniques, though useful and providing additional physiological information, cannot supplant the important anatomical information so readily available with completion arteriography, particularly in demonstrating the run-off circulation. Furthermore, the 'hard copy' of the operation becomes the basis for directing the patient's course in the future, should secondary procedures become necessary.

The primary reason for performing a completion arteriogram is to visualize any potential mechanism for graft closure that would then enable either prophylactic correction or prompt revision after graft closure, depending upon individual clinical circumstances. Other benefits that have accrued from the routine performance of completion arteriography include refinements in technique which, in turn, have significantly decreased the incidence of surgical errors. Many of these technical faults would not otherwise have been appreciated, even by sophisticated non-invasive methods. In cases of severe distal atherosclerosis, the discovery of run-off vessels not previously appreciated or visualized by preoperative arteriography is reassuring. If necessary, a synchronous sequential bypass can be constructed or considered for a later date.

2 A completion arteriogram depicting a bypass constructed to an isolated popliteal segment is performed (*Illustration 2a*) and a distal anterior tibial artery is visualized on a second exposure (*Illustration 2b*). Subsequent closure of the femoropopliteal bypass enables a thrombectomy to be performed and a sequential jump to the anterior tibial artery (*Illustration 2c*).

Routine intraoperative completion arteriography for revascularization procedures of the lower extremity has enabled classification of the run-off and correlation of these findings with subsequent graft patency. In instances of the most advanced obliterative disease, fruitless and potentially harmful reoperative vascular procedures may be obviated. Delayed graft closure due to progressive atherosclerosis in the distal circulation occurs frequently in patients showing poor run-off by completion arteriography. This group, in particular, needs to undergo periodic surveillance to enable thoughtful consideration of prophylactic or therapeutic correction.

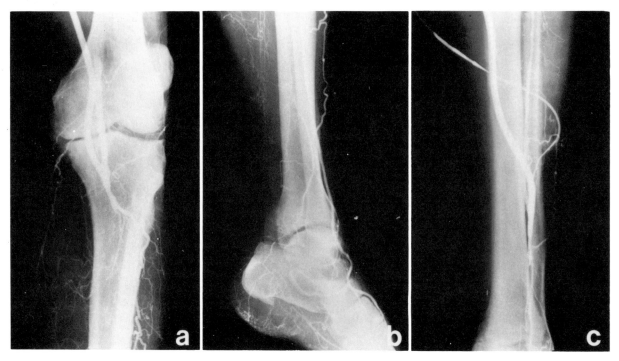

Intraoperative injecting methods

Several methods are available to the surgeon for the performance of prereconstruction or completion arteriography. It is important in all instances to avoid exposure to radiation, particularly since operating room personnel can otherwise suffer frequent exposure. The use of lead aprons and shields is helpful but, in addition to being burdensome and, to some extent, time consuming, complete protection from radiation is not afforded. For more than 15 years the author has used a simple, inexpensive apparatus that enables injection of contrast medium remote from the area of actual radiation exposure.

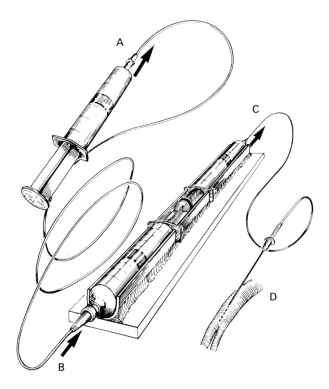

Apparatus for intraoperative arteriography

3 The injection device consists of two 50-ml disposable plastic syringes (A and B) coupled with plastic tubing approximately 9 m in length. The system is filled with water and purged of air. The volume of the fluid is such that it allows one syringe to be extended to its normal capacity (50 ml) when the other syringe is fully depressed. The second component of the device consists of a holding fixture constructed of metal, plastic or wood, the cross-section of which forms a U with straight, perpendicular sides. This holder is 50 cm in length and has two slots located in the vertical sides of the U at distances of 15 and 22.5 cm from either end. These slots accept the 'wings' of the syringes, holding them in place. The empty syringe of the coupled component is held in place by the holder which allows it to be aligned with a third syringe filled with contrast medium (C) that is delivered to the vascular system at D. This third syringe is attached to the patient via standard tubing and a 19-gauge butterfly needle. The remaining hydraulic syringe can then be positioned outside the operating room and, via the hydraulic link, remotely operate the injectate syringe.

3

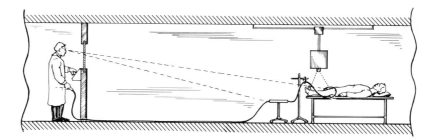

4

4 The surgeon has a full view of the holding fixture attached to a stand or intravenous pole just outside the sterile field and good tactile feel of the injectate syringe as the radiographer is directed to proceed with the exposure.

Radiographic film in a standard 14 × 17 inch (35 × 45 cm) cassette is used; the cassette, placed in a sterile plastic cover, is positioned directly under the area of interest. Most intraoperative arteriograms at the author's institution are performed for lower limb studies which include visualization of the mid-thigh and downwards, including the foot. For popliteal reconstructions, two or more radiographs are taken. One may be all that is required for tibial or peroneal reconstructions. Single radiographs are also taken after carotid endarterectomy.

Arteriography in the lower limb is usually preceded by direct injection of 20–30 mg of papaverine hydrochloride followed by a flush of dilute heparin solution. Patients with a history of cardiac disease or who are hypovolaemic must be observed closely for a possible decrease in blood pressure due to vasodilatation. This can be easily corrected with the rapid infusion of fluids. In some instances it may be prudent to omit the infusion of papaverine. A 19-gauge butterfly needle placed just proximal to the area of interest, either into a native artery or a graft, may be used. After completing the procedure and removing the needle, haemostasis is secured by direct pressure or placing a figure of eight 6/0 polypropylene suture.

When using the remote hydraulic syringe actuator, timing of radiographic exposure depends on the location of the cassette and the field to be visualized with respect to the site of the butterfly needle in the artery or graft. Normally exposure will be made 4–6 s after the start of the injection, when the contrast-filled syringe is one-half to two-thirds depressed.

Non-visualization of a completion arteriogram is ominous and suggests high resistance to flow that may result in early failure of the vascular reconstruction. In most instances proximal clamping of the graft or artery proximal to the site where the butterfly needle is placed is not performed. Arteriograms of excellent quality can be obtained with the native and graft circulations open, thus obviating the potential danger of repetitive clamping.

References

1. Dardik I, Ibrahim IM, Sprayregen S, Veith F, Dardik H. Routine intraoperative angiography: an essential adjunct in vascular surgery. *Arch Surg* 1975; 110: 184–90.

2. Flanigan DP, Williams LR, Keifer T, Schuler JJ, Behrend AJ. Prebypass operative arteriography. *Surgery* 1982; 92: 627–33.

3. Scarpato R, Gembarowicz R, Farber S *et al.* Intraoperative prereconstruction arteriography. *Arch Surg* 1981; 116: 1053–5.

4. Dardik H, Miller N, Adler J *et al.* Primary and adjunctive intra-arterial digital subtraction arteriography of the lower extremities. *J Vasc Surg* 1986; 3: 599–604.

5. King TA, Yao JST, Flinn WR, Bergan JJ. Extending operability by prebypass intraoperative arteriography. In: Bergan JJ, Yao JST, eds. *Evaluation and Treatment of Upper and Lower Extremity Circulatory Disorders.* Orlando: Grune and Stratton, 1984: 61–74.

6. Dardik H, Ibrahim IM, Koslow A, Dardik I. Evaluation of intraoperative arteriography as a routine for vascular reconstructions. *Surg Gynecol Obstet* 1978; 147: 853–8.

7. Liebman PR, Menzoian JO, Mannick JA, Lowney BW, LoGerfo FW. Intraoperative arteriography in femoropopliteal and femorotibial bypass grafts. *Arch Surg* 1981; 116: 1019–21.

8. O'Mara CS, Flinn WR, Neiman HL, Bergan JJ, Yao JST. Correlation of foot arterial anatomy with early tibial bypass patency. *Surgery* 1981; 89: 743–52.

Intraoperative use of ultrasound

J. L. Mills MD
Associate Professor of Surgery, University of South Florida College of Medicine, Tampa, Florida, USA

D. F. Bandyk MD
Professor of Surgery, Director, Division of Vascular Surgery, University of South Florida College of Medicine, Tampa, Florida, USA

History

During the past decade, explosive developments in the field of diagnostic ultrasound have occurred. Numerous investigators have recommended the use of some form of this technology to assess the anatomical, technical and haemodynamic adequacy of vascular reconstructions during operation. Currently available alternatives include continuous wave Doppler monitoring, pulsed-wave Doppler spectral analysis, ultrasonic B-mode imaging, duplex ultrasonography and, most recently, colour flow imaging.

The technique and relative efficacy of each method of intraoperative diagnostic ultrasound will be summarized here, and recommendations made for their application.

Principles and justification

Despite meticulous operative technique, technical and haemodynamic defects can occur which compromise patency of a vascular reconstruction. Such defects include not only technical problems such as clamp injury, intimal flap, and suture stenosis, but also platelet aggregation and atherosclerotic plaque dissection, luminal thrombus and inadequate outflow. Such defects are frequently not detectable by mere visual inspection or pulse palpation of the repair.

Objective assessment of the technical adequacy and haemodynamic performance of an arterial reconstruction is a fundamental principle of vascular surgery. When routine intraoperative arteriography has been used to assess arterial reconstructions, vascular defects warranting immediate revision have been identified in 5–10% of reported cases[1,2]. While generally accurate and readily available to the vascular surgeon, arteriography is not without risk. The technique is also cumbersome to apply in certain instances, such as complex renal and visceral reconstructions, as well as long bypasses requiring multiple exposures to assess the entire reconstruction. In addition, while providing anatomical information, arteriography does not assess haemodynamic performance, a factor of critical importance in outcome after bypasses to limited tibioperoneal or pedal outflow tracts. The ideal method of intraoperative assessment would thus provide both anatomical and haemodynamic data. The method chosen and the diligence with which it is pursued are also dependent upon the nature and difficulty of the reconstruction as well as the clinical consequences of failure. These factors should be considered in the application of ultrasound instrumentation at operation.

Instrumentation and technique

Diagnostic ultrasound units suitable for intraoperative use include Doppler ultrasonic flow velocity detectors (continuous and pulsed wave), ultrasonic B-mode imaging, and duplex scanning (including colour flow imaging). *Table 1* compares the relative advantages and disadvantages of each technique.

Table 1 Comparison of available methods of intraoperative ultrasound

Technique	Advantages	Disadvantages	Recommended use
Continuous wave Doppler	Inexpensive Simple Versatile	Less sensitive No anatomical data	Large artery reconstructions: aortic, axillo-femoral, femoro-femoral bypasses Confirm flow: distal to reconstruction
Pulsed Doppler	Relatively simple Sensitive Predicts outcome	No anatomical data Moderately expensive	Difficult reconstructions
Duplex scanning	Anatomical and haemodynamic data Sensitive Predicts outcome	Expensive Complex	Difficult reconstructions
Colour flow imaging	Anatomical and haemodynamic data Sensitive Predicts outcome	Most expensive Requires most expertise	Difficult reconstructions

Doppler flow analysis

The continuous wave Doppler flow detector remains the most readily available, inexpensive and prevalent method of intraoperative monitoring. A sterile Doppler probe with a transmission frequency of 7.5–10 MHz is acoustically coupled to surgically exposed vessels with saline and used to assess blood flow velocity signals. Abnormal flow patterns can be distinguished from normal ones by audible interpretation of the frequency shift and phasicity components of the Doppler signal during the cardiac cycle. The target arteries below the anastomosis should be examined, as well as the perianastomotic region, and the native artery in the vicinity of clamp applications. Flow at and just beyond a stenosis will characteristically be associated with an increased pitch of the Doppler signal. In addition to increased pitch, turbulent flow may also be manifested by a fluttering or 'bubbling' signal, usually indicative of a haemodynamically significant stenosis. Severe vasospasm, by reducing vessel diameter, may mimic the Doppler characteristics of a true stenosis. Stenoses which are not haemodynamically significant (less than 50% diameter reduction) do not usually produce an obvious detectable change in the Doppler signal. An occlusion at or distal to the recording site resulting from thrombus or intimal flap will produce a characteristic systolic thumping signal, with no diastolic component because of absence of outflow.

The continuous wave Doppler detector has been used to exclude residual stenosis after carotid endarterectomy, to monitor *in situ* saphenous vein conduits for residual competent valve leaflets and arteriovenous fistulae, to confirm flow in carotid shunts, and to assess the pattern of blood flow in vessels remote from the reconstruction (such as the mesenteric vessels after aortic reconstruction or the pedal vessels after femoro-popliteal bypass). When an abnormal signal is identified, intraoperative arteriography should be performed to confirm and characterize the lesion before re-exploration.

The continuous wave Doppler instruments are relatively inexpensive and easy to use. Routine intraoperative use of the continuous wave Doppler is an extremely useful teaching device to expose surgical trainees to the expected flow patterns in peripheral arteries, as well as the characteristic signal abnormalities associated with stenosis, outflow occlusion and technical defects. Audible interpretation of the blood flow data provided by this instrument requires experience, but the basic physiological and haemodynamic principles necessary for its use should be an integral part of every vascular surgeon's database.

The pulsed wave Doppler velocimeter allows greater precision and accuracy in the analysis of blood flow patterns than a continuous wave Doppler probe. A high frequency (20 MHz) pulsed Doppler probe can be used to interrogate in detail the blood flow characteristics in surgically exposed vessels or bypass conduits. The higher transmitting frequency allows the use of small sample volumes, that is, points within the vessel in which flow is detected.

1 Computer processing (using fast Fourier spectral analysis) of the pulsed Doppler signal permits detailed categorization of flow disturbances and measurement of angle-corrected blood flow velocities. Blood flow patterns can thus be classified into three clinically relevant categories: (a) normal or 'laminar' flow; (b) mild to moderate flow disturbance; and (c) severe flow disturbance or 'turbulence', based on flow velocity, waveform analysis and spectral criteria. The spectral width (content) of the Doppler signal represents the range of blood flow velocities identified within the sample volume. Laminar or non-disturbed flow is characterized by widening of the spectral width (so-called spectral broadening) only in late systole and a peak systolic velocity of under 125 cm/s. Mild to moderate non-haemodynamic stenoses result in spectral broadening throughout systole or into early diastole, but peak systolic velocity changes are minimal (velocity ratio of proximal *versus* distal to stenosis less than 1.5). Spectral width and subsequently blood flow velocity progressively increase as the severity of stenosis worsens. Severe, haemodynamically significant lesions, which reduce pressure and flow, show spectral broadening throughout the pulse cycle with simultaneous reverse flow components and an elevated systolic flow velocity in excess of 150 cm/s.

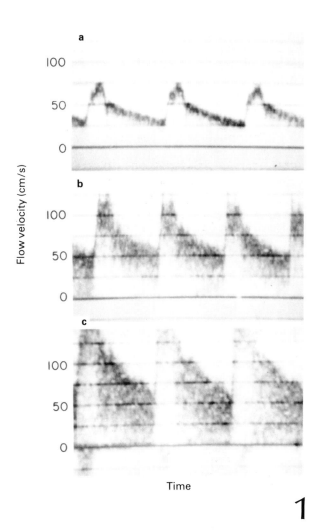

1

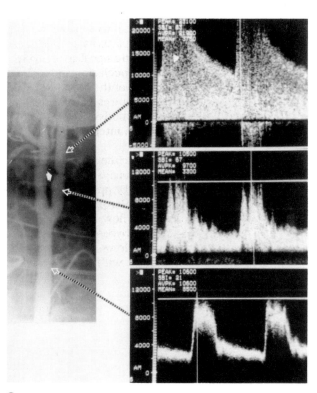

2

2 The presence of a severe flow disturbance correlates with a major vascular defect (white arrow) and should not be ignored. Immediate revision should be considered. If there is any uncertainty, intraoperative arteriography should be performed, and will confirm the presence of a major defect in over 90% of such cases. The detection of moderate flow disturbances requires careful judgement and experience. Such defects may occasionally serve as sites for platelet deposition and cause early graft thrombosis. These lesions may also predispose to the development of myointimal hyperplasia during the intermediate postoperative period.

Pulsed wave Doppler spectral analysis is suitable for assessing carotid endarterectomy sites, *in situ* saphenous vein bypasses, and renal and mesenteric reconstructions. Routine intraoperative use of this modality during carotid endarterectomy has documented its utility in the identification of important defects in 5% of cases which have the potential of leading to perioperative thrombosis and stroke[3].

Defects readily identifiable by B-mode imaging or altered haemodynamics include intimal flaps, suture stenosis, intraluminal platelet aggregation within the endarterectomy site, and distal internal carotid artery kinking (*Table 2*). Perioperative thrombosis virtually

Table 2   Characteristics of technical defects detectable with intraoperative ultrasound

Type of defect	B-mode image	Flow disturbance	Low flow
Stenosis	+	+	−
Intimal flap	+/−	+	+/−
Retained valve	+/−	+	+/−
Luminal clot	+	+	+
Platelet aggregation	+/−	+	+/−

never occurs if normal arterial flow patterns are demonstrated during operation at the endarterectomy site. This modality can also be used to examine the entire *in situ* bypass conduit. Previous experience documents a 5% incidence of residual competent valve cusps at valvulotomy sites, and a 6% incidence of anastomotic stenosis[4]. The presence of severe flow disturbances is always associated with a major defect on confirmatory arteriography. The flow pattern detected by pulsed Doppler spectral analysis is also of prognostic significance after distal lower extremity bypass. In patients with critical limb ischaemia, a hyperaemic flow pattern with antegrade flow throughout the pulse cycle should be present, as well as a peak systolic velocity in excess of 40 cm/s. The absence of these two findings indicates high outflow resistance; if no technical error or distal thrombosis is present, consideration should be given to the addition of a sequential bypass to another outflow vessel. In this setting, such a 'jump' or sequential bypass will increase graft flow and improve patency.

Pulsed Doppler instruments with spectral analysers require more experience to use properly than continuous wave Doppler probes, and are more expensive. The high-frequency pulsed Doppler probe offers considerably more information, however, and may be especially applicable for use during procedures in which technical precision is critical, such as femorodistal saphenous vein bypasses and mesenteric and renal reconstructions.

Ultrasonic B-mode imaging

Real-time B-mode scanners for intraoperative use generally use a 7.5-MHz or 10-MHz probe. This transmitting frequency allows good resolution, and defects as small as 1 mm are detectable. Sterile saline is instilled in the wound, and acoustic coupling is maintained by filling the end of a sterile sleeve containing the transducer with acoustic gel. The probe is hand-held by the operator and positioned directly over the vessels at the depth of the surgical wound. The real-time image is viewed on a video monitor and critical portions of the examination can be stored on videotape.

This modality has been used clinically to examine carotid endarterectomy sites, aortofemoral and infrainguinal bypasses, and portocaval shunts. The high-resolution imaging is extremely sensitive, and defects have been identified in 30–40% of patients after vascular reconstruction. Many of these defects are of no clinical consequence, however, and do not adversely affect either short- or long-term results. The haemodynamic significance of any apparent defect identified is also not provided by this technique. In addition to these limitations, the degree of technical expertise required to use this technique properly, and the high cost of such instrumentation, have limited the widespread use of intraoperative B-mode imaging for vascular reconstruction.

Duplex scanning

The duplex technique couples high-resolution B-mode imaging and pulsed wave Doppler spectral analysis to provide a theoretically attractive non-invasive method of assessing vascular reconstructions. The technology is especially useful because it provides both anatomical and haemodynamic information. Duplex ultrasound systems are expensive, but the same instruments available in vascular laboratories providing comprehensive testing can also be used in the operating room.

Duplex scanners consist of a high-resolution imaging transducer (7.5–10 MHz) combined with a pulse-gated Doppler velocimeter (5.0–7.5 MHz). The Doppler signals are analysed by fast Fourier spectral analysis. The addition of imaging capability allows precise placement of a single pulsed wave sample volume and accurate assessment of the flow disturbance caused by any defect identified on the B-mode image.

This modality has been successfully used during operation for carotid, renal and mesenteric reconstructions. The velocity spectra recorded by this modality and their interpretation are identical to those outlined above for the pulsed wave velocimeter.

Duplex scanning requires a higher level of expertise than either continuous wave or pulsed Doppler detectors. The team approach, with a vascular technologist in the operating room to assist the surgical team, is helpful. The technologist can make adjustments to optimize the image and velocity spectra while the surgeon positions and manipulates the scan head in the wound.

Colour flow imaging

Colour flow imaging represents a further development and refinement of duplex scanning. Colour Doppler flow mapping displays real-time images representing red blood cell velocities throughout the entire blood vessel lumen in contrast to standard duplex scanners which present the velocity spectra of a single intraluminal sample volume. Each digitized sample volume is assigned a colour based on velocity and direction of flow. The assignment of colour to flow direction expedites vessel localization and allows more rapid scanning of long vessel or bypass segments for haemodynamic abnormalities. Colour hue or saturation is proportional to the Doppler shift, which in turn depends on the red blood cell velocity and the angle of Doppler beam insonation. The degree of colour saturation is thus indicative of the relative red blood cell velocities. Less saturation of colour-coded pixels correlates with areas of increased red blood cell velocity.

We currently use a 7.5–10-MHz linear array colour flow imager. Studies are performed with a fluid-filled plastic wedge-shaped stand-off attached to the end of the transducer. Acoustic coupling is maintained with sterile saline and acoustic gel instilled into the end of a disposable plastic sleeve, as outlined previously. The probe is positioned over the exposed vessel or bypass conduit and manipulated by the surgeon to image the vascular repair in both sagittal and transverse planes.

Imaged arteries or bypass conduits are assessed for alterations in diameter, intraluminal defects and colour flow changes with each pulse cycle. Localized areas of decreased colour saturation are associated with increased red cell velocity and therefore stenosis. An abrupt change in colour flow during the pulse cycle is abnormal, and the so-called 'mosaic' pattern of red and blue colours indicates sites of turbulence. A great deal of experience is necessary to interpret colour flow data properly. Characteristic variations in flow during the pulse cycle must be understood. Blood flow may be absent or reversed during the diastolic component of the cardiac cycle in distal lower extremity bypasses and native arteries. In addition, Doppler angle is of critical importance since all colour assignments are angle-dependent. In addition to the colour flow data, the system can simultaneously display the Doppler velocity waveform obtained by spectral analysis of the range-gated pulsed Doppler. Inspection of this Doppler display during the examination facilitates placement of the sample volume and assignment of the Doppler angle.

With experience, colour imaging can be performed more rapidly than standard duplex scanning. Carotid endarterectomy sites and *in situ* saphenous vein bypasses can ordinarily be examined in 5–10 min.

Recommendations for application of intraoperative ultrasound

A proper vascular reconstruction is free from major technical defects, restores or improves haemodynamics, and is durable. To accomplish these ends, the reconstructed arterial segment or bypass conduit must be objectively assessed for its anatomical and haemodynamic integrity. Ultrasound techniques for imaging and/or flow detection are of great potential use in this regard. The technique selected depends upon the type of reconstruction performed, its degree of difficulty, and the consequences of failure. *Table 3* outlines important technical points fundamental to all methods of intraoperative ultrasound.

Table 3 Important technical considerations in using intraoperative ultrasound

Proper *acoustic coupling* (saline, gel, gel within plastic sleeve)

60° Doppler angle of insonation

Centre stream localization of the pulsed Doppler sample volume

Use of *highest frequency* probe possible for both imaging and flow assessment

Analysis of *waveform* characteristics, systolic and diastolic components of the flow cycle

Measurement of *peak systolic flow velocity*

Performance of *augmentation manoeuvres* (flow should increase in response to pharmacological vasodilatation with papaverine)

Continuous wave Doppler is inexpensive, simple and versatile. Audible interpretation of the continuous wave Doppler signal is probably sufficient to exclude major technical error and document flow after operations on large arteries with inherently low frequencies of technical error and early failure. Such procedures would include aortic reconstructions, axillofemoral and femorofemoral bypasses. The continuous wave Doppler probe is also useful for documenting bowel viability after aortic reconstruction by the presence of phasic arterial flow along the mesenteric border of the intestine. Arterial flow distal to the reconstructive site (i.e. the foot after aortofemoral reconstruction) can also be documented, and major intraoperative distal thromboembolization excluded. Continuous wave Doppler is also a useful teaching technique. For example, the characteristic signals audible in the high-resistance external carotid artery and the low-resistance internal carotid artery can be demonstrated after carotid endarterectomy. However, for technically demanding procedures such as carotid endarterectomy, infrainguinal bypass, and renal/visceral reconstruction, continuous wave Doppler alone is not sufficiently sensitive.

For the latter technically demanding procedures, in which technical imperfection can result in catastrophic morbidity (stroke, limb loss, mesenteric or renal infarction), continuous wave Doppler assessment alone is insufficient. In difficult vascular repairs and bypasses to small (less than 3 mm) vessels, high-frequency pulsed wave Doppler spectral analysis is preferred. This technique lends itself to examination of the carotid endarterectomy site; in addition, *in situ* vein conduits can be completely examined. The technique is also applicable to reversed and non-reversed vein bypasses. Even though the entire graft is not examined after its placement deep in an anatomical tunnel of the leg, interrogation of the juxta-anastomotic regions, the exposed portions of the bypass, and the distal target vessels allows analysis of the magnitude and configuration of the blood flow velocity waveforms. Absent diastolic flow, low peak systolic velocity, and failure of flow augmentation after pharmacological vasodilatation, for example, would prompt arteriography to assess patency of the outflow vessels. Pulsed Doppler is also ideally suited to investigate renal and mesenteric arterial reconstructions. This technique, when properly applied and interpreted, gives reliable and useful haemodynamic data and, by inference, anatomical data.

B-mode ultrasound imaging provides anatomical, but no haemodynamic, information. It is cumbersome to use, requires great expertise, and is sensitive but non-specific. It is our opinion that the technique is of little clinical use unless coupled with haemodynamic information.

Standard duplex scanning and, more recently, colour-flow imaging both hold great promise for intraoperative use. Although expensive, the instruments available in most vascular laboratories can also be used during operation. Both techniques provide anatomical and haemodynamic information, and, like the pulsed Doppler, have special application after 'difficult' reconstructions. If no major defects are identified and flow patterns are normal, the surgeon can be confident of the reconstruction. Vascular reconstructions in which moderate flow disturbances are identified should be carefully scrutinized in their entirety. Intraoperative arteriography should be performed if the significance of a defect is in question, or if major flow disturbances are present with no identifiable anatomical defects. A

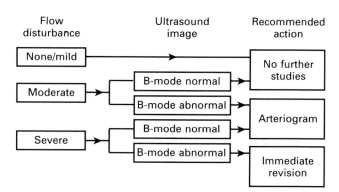

Figure 1 Diagnostic algorithm for surgical decision making based on intraoperative duplex imaging of arterial reconstructions

scheme depicting a clinically useful decision tree to be applied with the use of intraoperative ultrasound assessment is illustrated in *Figure 1*. Anatomical defects associated with severe flow disturbances should be re-explored; confirmatory arteriography is unnecessary in these instances.

Ultrasound in one of its various forms is of critical importance in the routine intraoperative assessment of vascular reconstructions. The continuous wave Doppler probe is the mainstay, but new improved techniques using pulsed Doppler, duplex scanning and, most recently, colour flow imaging[5], are becoming the standard of care for selected, difficult reconstructions.

References

1. Blaisdell RW, Lim R, Hall AD. Technical result of carotid endarterectomy: arteriographic assessment. *Am J Surg* 1967; 114: 239–46.

2. Mills JL, Fujitani RM, Taylor SM. Contribution of routine intraoperative completion arteriography to early infrainguinal bypass patency. *Am J Surg* 1992; 164: 506–11.

3. Bandyk DF, Kaebnick HW, Adams MB, Towne JB. Turbulence occurring after carotid bifurcation endarterectomy: a harbinger of residual and recurrent carotid stenosis. *J Vasc Surg* 1988; 7: 261–74.

4. Bandyk DF, Jorgensen RA, Towne JB. Intraoperative assessment of *in-situ* saphenous vein arterial grafts using pulsed Doppler spectral analysis. *Arch Surg* 1986; 121: 292–9.

5. Bandyk DF, Govostis DM. Intraoperative color flow imaging of 'difficult' arterial reconstructions. *Video J Color Flow Imaging* 1991; 1: 13–20.

Illustrations by Gillian Oliver

Exposure of major blood vessels

P. R. F. Bell MD, FRCS
Professor of Surgery, Leicester Royal Infirmary, Leicester, UK

The work of the peripheral vascular surgeon ranges widely through the anatomy of the whole body and he is required to command a wide range of anatomical knowledge. This chapter outlines the standard technique for exposure of the major arteries.

Both diseased and healthy arteries may be surprisingly friable, and rough dissection may cause severe damage and be sufficient to jeopardize the result of the vascular reconstruction. Gentleness must be observed at all times and, in general, it is desirable to dissect a little way from the exterior surface of the vessel so that the inadvertent division of a branch can be treated by ligation rather than requiring a suture flush with the vessel wall. Good angiography is essential to forewarn the surgeon of the presence of anatomical variations and to minimize the need for fruitless exposure of vessels which are not appropriate for the proposed operation. In some cases the role of angiography has now been replaced by duplex ultrasonography and shortly, possibly, by magnetic resonance imaging.

Exposure of the carotid artery

1 The patient is placed on the back with the head extended and placed on a rubber ring. The head is then turned away from the side to be operated on. The incision is placed along the anterior part of the sternocleidomastoid muscle as far as the angle of the jaw and passes slightly backwards.

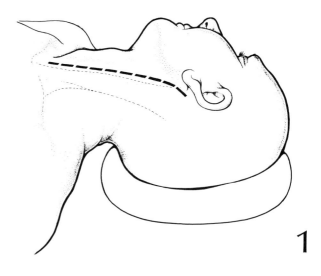

1

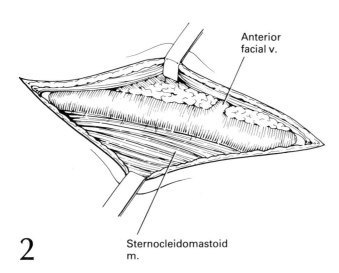

2

2 After incising the skin and platysma, the sterno-cleidomastoid muscle is displaced posteriorly and the internal jugular vein comes into view. The anterior facial vein can be seen passing forwards.

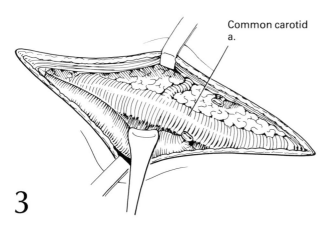

3

3 The anterior facial vein is divided and the internal jugular vein is retracted posteriorly exposing the internal carotid artery covered with a layer of areolar tissue.

4 By dissecting along the medial border of the common carotid artery the superior thyroid artery will be seen and can be encircled with a sling. The external carotid artery can also be controlled in the same way, care being taken to locate the hypoglossal nerve as it crosses the vessels high up in the wound. The internal jugular vein is retracted backwards and the vagus nerve will be seen between these two vessels. The descending hypoglossal nerve runs down the front of the common carotid artery. The slings around the superior thyroid and external carotid arteries can be used for retraction to expose the internal carotid artery more fully.

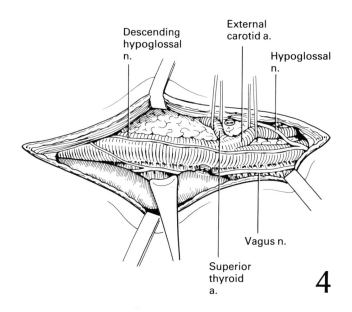

Descending hypoglossal n.

External carotid a.

Hypoglossal n.

Vagus n.

Superior thyroid a.

4

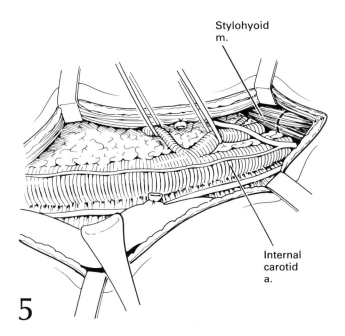

Stylohyoid m.

Internal carotid a.

5

5 If it proves necessary for more of the internal carotid artery to be exposed then the stylohyoid muscle should be divided as shown. More of the internal carotid artery can be exposed by division of the digastric tendon or subluxation of the jaw in a forward direction.

Exposure of the vertebral artery

6 For exposure of the vertebral artery an incision is made obliquely just lateral to the sternocleido-mastoid muscle.

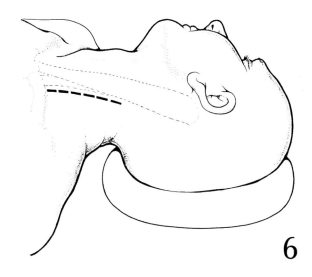

6

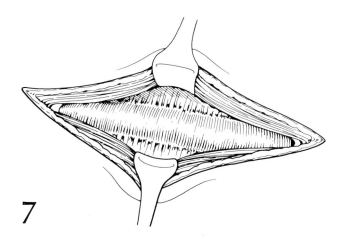

7

7 The internal jugular vein is exposed after dividing the lateral part of the muscle.

8 The internal jugular vein is retracted laterally to expose the vagus nerve which is also retracted laterally. The carotid artery will be seen medially and this should be dissected sufficiently to allow medial retraction. Dissection in the angle between the artery and the vein reveals the vertebral vein and behind it the vertebral artery crisscrossed by branches of the cervical sympathetic chain.

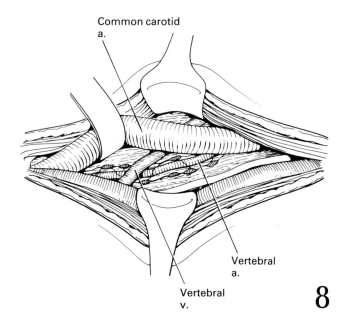

Common carotid a.

Vertebral a.

Vertebral v.

8

9 The vertebral vein and some elements of the sympathetic trunk are divided with downward extension of the incision to expose the whole of the lower part of the vertebral artery before it passes towards the vertebral bodies and also to expose the subclavian artery from which it arises.

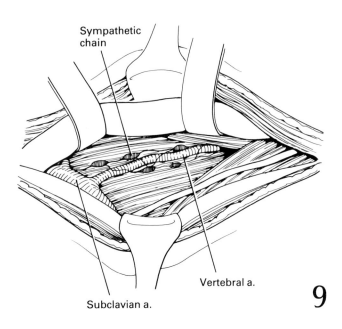

9

10 For exposure of the distal vertebral artery an incision should also be made along the line of the sternocleidomastoid muscle which, after exposure, is retracted medially. The dissection should proceed posteriorly, the carotid artery and vein being retracted medially if necessary. The accessory nerve will be found crossing the levator scapulae muscle and should be protected. The upper end of the levator scapulae should be divided with a scalpel passing an appropriate instrument behind it to protect the structures lying there.

10

11 When the levator scapulae muscle has been divided the anterior primary ramus of C2 will be seen crossing the cervical part of the artery. Further access to the artery can be obtained by dividing C2.

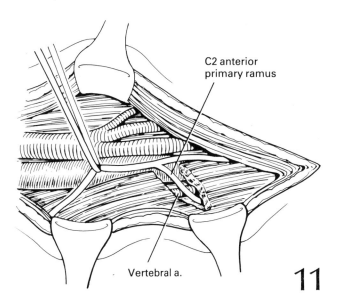

11

Exposure of the subclavian artery

12 An incision is made above the scapula, lateral to the insertion of the sternocleidomastoid muscle.

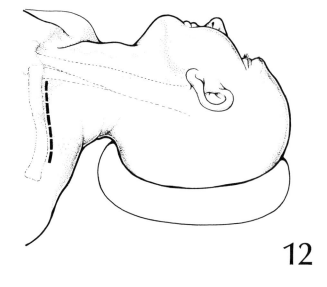

12

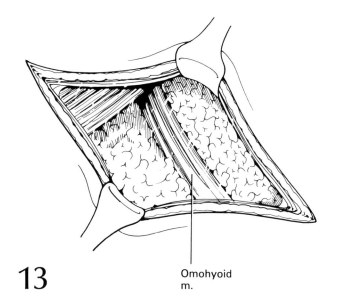

13

Omohyoid m.

13 The platysma and fascia are dissected to reveal the omohyoid muscle, lymph nodes and fat. The lymph nodes and fat should be displaced upwards.

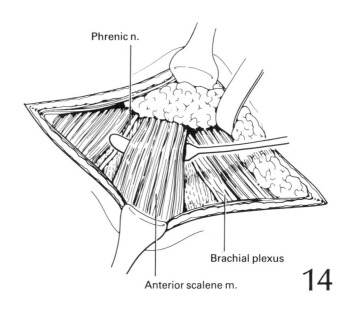

14 The phrenic nerve will be seen beneath the deep fascia overlying the anterior scalene muscle which can be felt as a band passing downwards and medially. The brachial plexus will easily be seen or felt laterally. A curved blunt instrument is passed behind the anterior scalene muscle.

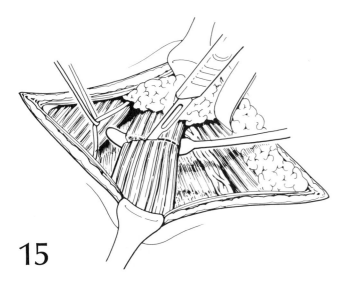

15 The anterior scalene muscle is divided carefully, protecting the phrenic nerve which is best performed by passing a sling around it.

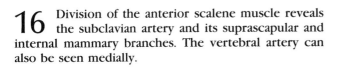

16 Division of the anterior scalene muscle reveals the subclavian artery and its suprascapular and internal mammary branches. The vertebral artery can also be seen medially.

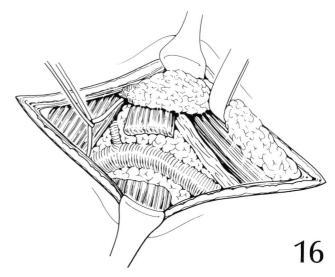

Exposure of the distal subclavian and proximal axillary artery

17 The subclavian artery should be exposed as already described, the incision being taken across the clavicle. This can be divided as shown.

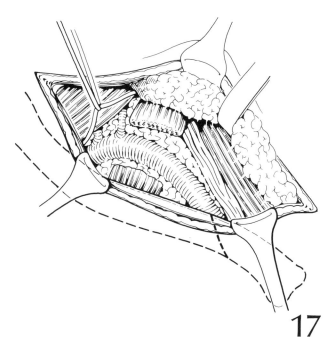

17

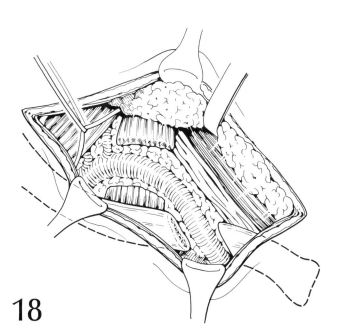

18

18 After division of the clavicle downward retraction reveals the distal part of the subclavian artery as it crosses the first rib and the upper part of the axillary artery beyond this.

19 The middle part of the axillary artery is exposed by making an incision below the middle third of the clavicle.

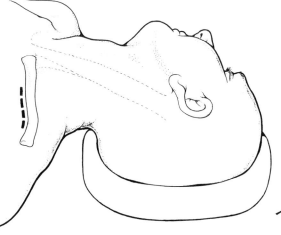

19

20 The skin and deep fascia are incised and branches of the acromioclavicular artery can be seen coming through the clavipectoral fascia. The pectoralis major muscle lies above and below these branches.

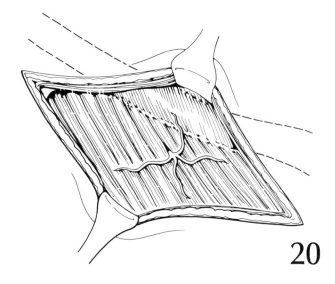

20

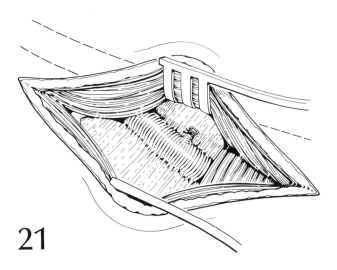

21

21 The muscle fibres of the pectoralis major are divided after tying off the branches of the acromioclavicular artery. The axillary artery can be felt in the depths of the wound and exposed by sharp dissection. One or two branches need to be tied to expose it fully.

22 For more distal exposure the pectoralis minor muscle in the lateral part of the wound needs to be divided completely. Retraction is required to access the artery.

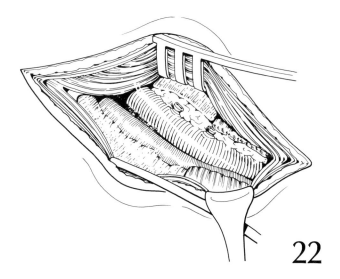

22

Exposure of the brachial artery

23 This can be exposed throughout the upper arm by an incision placed along its medial border just behind the biceps muscle.

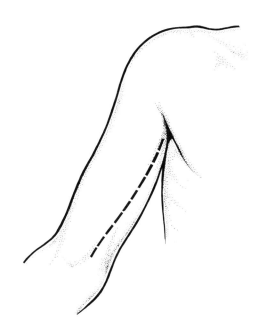

23

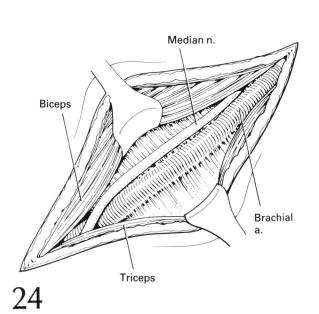

Median n.

Biceps

Brachial a.

Triceps

24

24 After incising the skin and deep fascia the biceps muscle is retracted anteriorly and the triceps posteriorly. The median nerve can be seen lying superior to the brachial artery.

25 Further dissection will reveal the brachial vein which can be retracted posteriorly to expose the ulnar nerve.

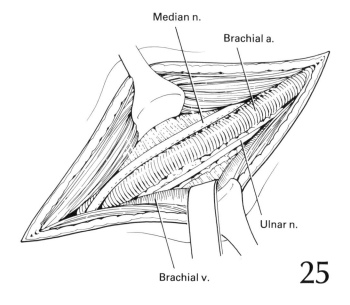

Median n.

Brachial a.

Ulnar n.

Brachial v.

25

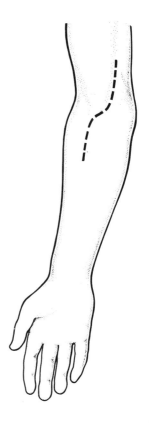

26 For exposure of the bifurcation of the brachial artery an S-shaped incision should be made in the antecubital fossa.

26

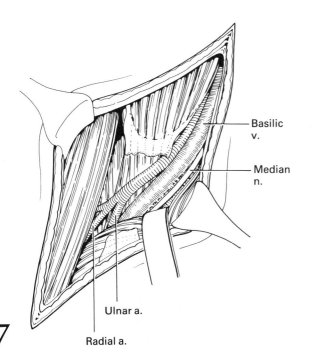

Basilic v.

Median n.

Ulnar a.

Radial a.

27

27 After division of the bicipital aponeurosis the brachial artery and its bifurcation into the radial and ulnar arteries will be seen where they pass between the brachioradialis and flexor muscles. The median nerve and basilic vein can be seen posteriomedial to the artery.

28 The ulnar and the radial arteries are exposed through incisions on the anterior surface of the forearm.

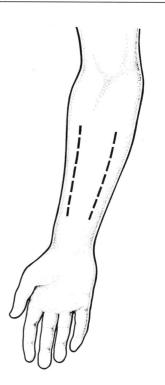

28

Radial
a.

Brachio-
radialis
m.

Flexor
carpi
radialis m.

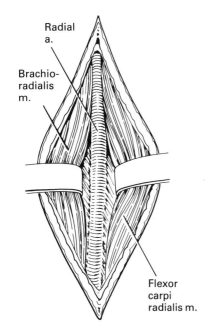

29

29 By dissection between the brachioradialis muscle medially and the flexor carpi radialis muscle laterally the radial artery will be exposed along with its associated veins.

30 By dissection of the pronator teres and brachioradialis muscles laterally and the flexor digitorum sublimus muscle medially the ulnar artery will be seen.

Pronator teres
and brachio-
radialis m.

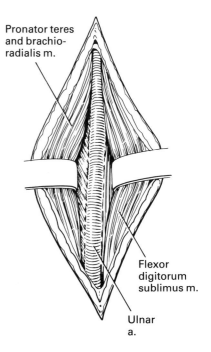

Flexor
digitorum
sublimus m.

Ulnar
a.

30

31 For exposure of the ulnar and radial artery at the wrist the incisions should be made as indicated.

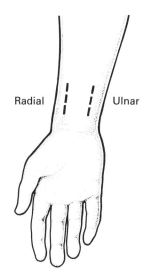

31

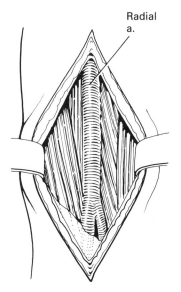

32

32 The radial artery is very superficial and may be palpated and exposed easily.

33 The ulnar artery is a little deeper but again is relatively superficial and can be exposed before it enters the deep aspect of the hypothenar eminence.

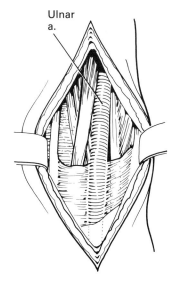

33

Exposure of the ascending aorta and arch branches

34 Various incisions are made to expose the ascending aorta and its branches in the neck. The most commonly used is a vertical incision.

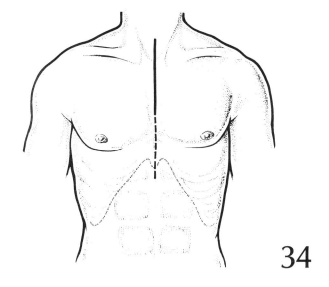

34

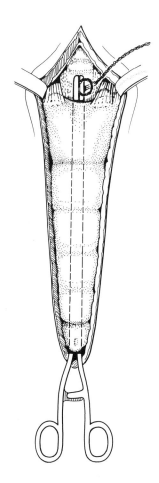

35

35 The incision is deepened to the sternum from the manubrium sternum to the xiphisternum. An appropriate clamp such as a Roberts is passed behind the sternum and a Gigli saw pulled through the tunnel. This is then used to divide the sternum. An electric saw can, as an alternative, be used to divide the sternum from the front.

36 After the sternum has been divided it is held apart by self-retaining retractors.

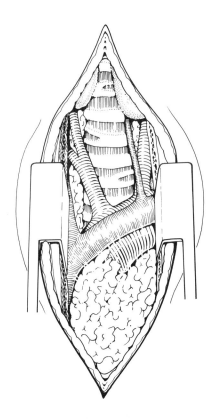

36

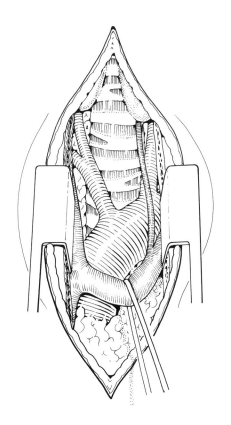

37

37 The brachiocephalic vein will be seen and should be retracted downwards to expose the aortic arch and the roots of the brachiocephalic, left carotid and subclavian arteries.

38 In order to expose the branches of the aortic arch in the neck a transverse limb is added to the vertical incision.

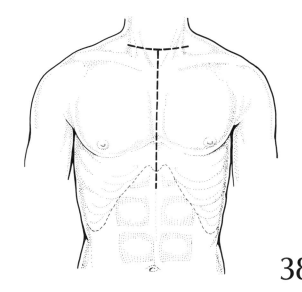

38

39

Phrenic
n.

Subclavian
a.

39 By division of the sternocleidomastoid and anterior scalene muscles, the subclavian artery can be seen and the phrenic nerve protected. This allows various types of graft to be inserted between the ascending aorta and its branches in the neck.

Exposure of the descending thoracic aorta

40 This is exposed through an incision in the fifth or eighth intercostal space, depending upon which level is to be exposed.

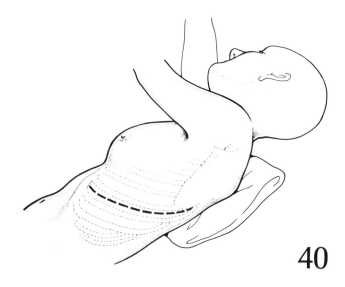

40

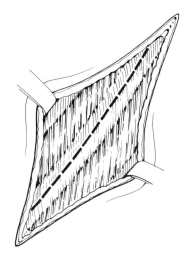

41a

41a, b The thoracic cavity is entered by removing the rib and the lung is displaced forwards. The descending aorta will be seen posteriorly.

Lung displaced forward

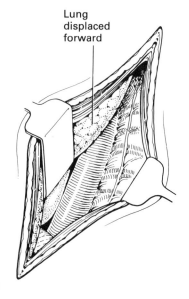

41b

Exposure of the lower thoracic and upper abdominal aorta

42 For exposure of the descending thoracic and upper abdominal aorta a midline incision is made in the abdomen with an extension through the costal margin along the seventh rib for exposure of the lower thoracic aorta and the fifth for exposure of the upper thoracic aorta.

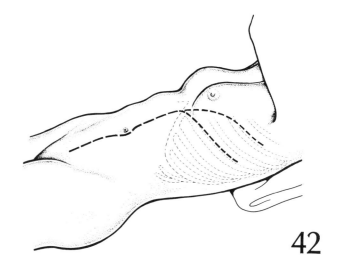

42

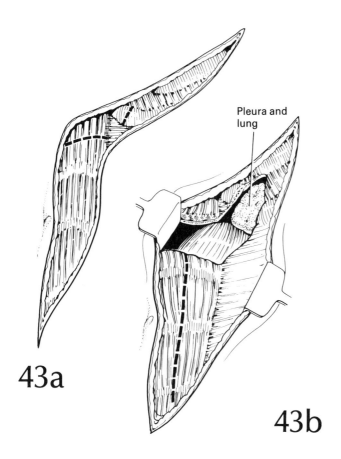

Pleura and lung

43a

43b

43a, b The rectus muscle and costal margin are divided to allow exposure of the pleura which is then opened.

44 The diaphragm can be divided either transversely close to the costal margin which avoids damage to the phrenic nerve, or vertically which damages the phrenic nerve but gives much better exposure.

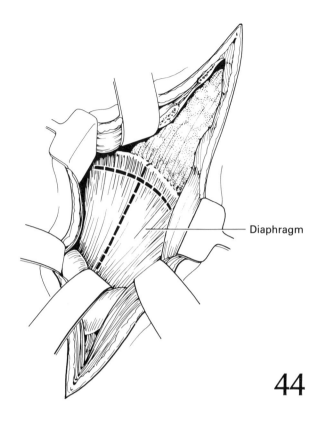

Diaphragm

44

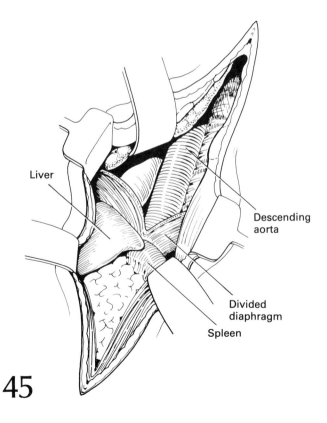

Liver

Descending aorta

Divided diaphragm

Spleen

45

45 After division of the diaphragm the thoracic aorta, liver, abdominal contents and spleen can be seen.

46 An incision is made in the peritoneum along the lateral border of the spleen and colon.

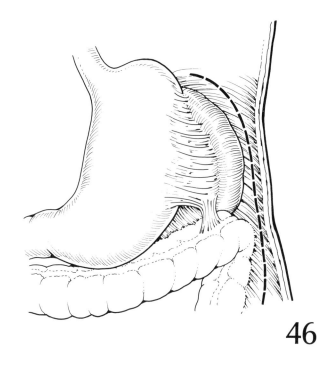

46

47 The colon, spleen and pancreas are mobilized to the right which exposes the abdominal aorta and its main branches, the coeliac axis, the superior mesenteric artery and the renal vessels. The left renal vein can be seen crossing the abdominal aorta.

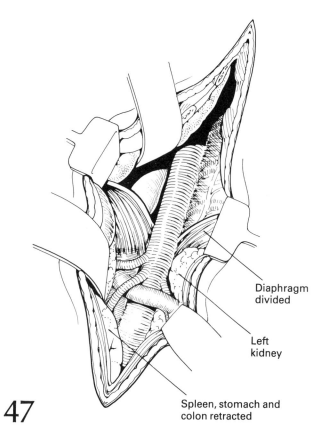

Diaphragm divided

Left kidney

47

Spleen, stomach and colon retracted

Exposure of the abdominal aorta and its branches

48 This is accomplished through a number of transverse incisions (A), a midline incision (B), or an oblique incision (C).

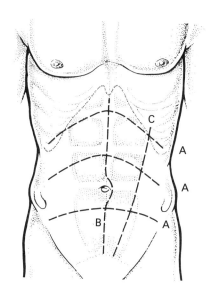

48

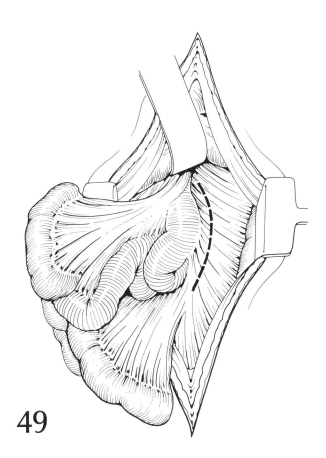

49

Superior mesenteric artery

49 The peritoneum on the left side of the duodeno-jejunal flexure is incised carefully and the bowel pushed to the right. This will expose the aorta.

50 Alternatively a transverse abdominal incision can be used with the same incision in the peritoneum close to the duodenojejunal flexure in order to expose the aorta.

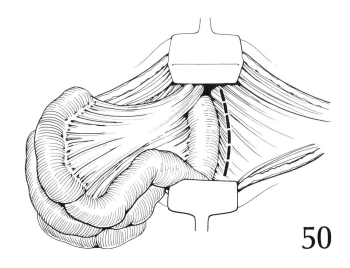

50

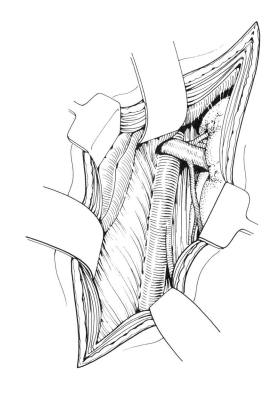

51 For a retroperitoneal exposure the abdominal muscles are divided as shown in *Illustration 48* (line C) and the peritoneum displaced to the right. This will expose the aorta and the kidney.

51

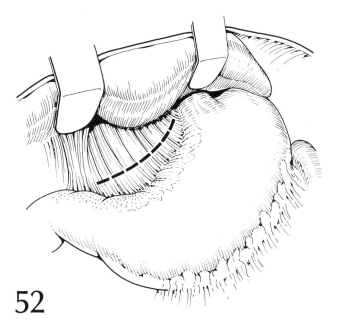

Coeliac axis

52 The coeliac axis is exposed after opening the abdomen through a transverse or vertical incision and opening the lesser omentum.

52

53 After ligating the vessels in the greater omentum the pancreas can be seen at the back of the lesser sac and the aorta felt just above the level where the crura cross it.

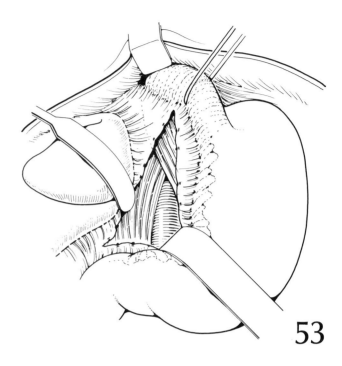

53

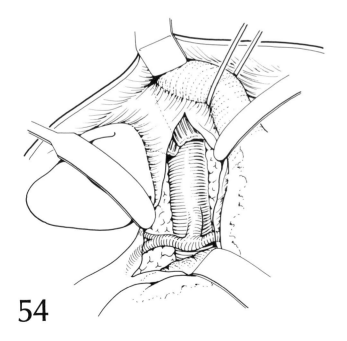

54

54 The crura are divided to expose the aorta and just above the stomach the origin of the coeliac axis will be seen.

Splenic artery

55 The splenic artery is exposed by dividing the greater omentum along the lower border of the stomach and displacing that organ proximally.

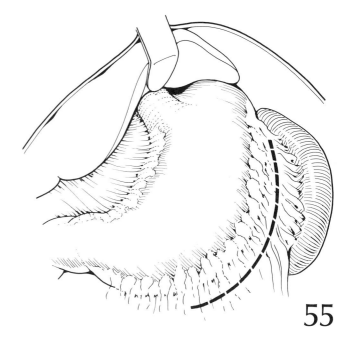

55

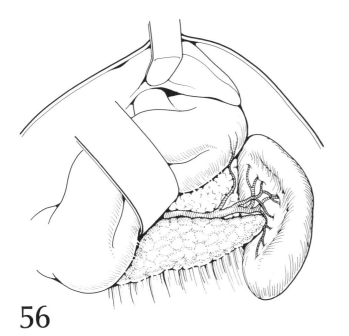

56

56 The artery will be seen running along the upper part of the pancreas.

Superior mesenteric artery origin

57 The origin of the superior mesenteric artery can be exposed through a transverse or vertical incision in the peritoneum lateral to the spleen and colon.

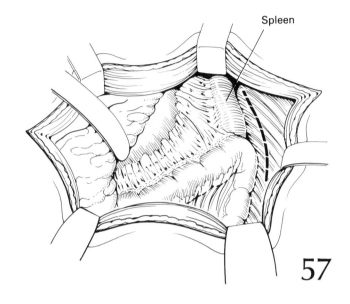

57

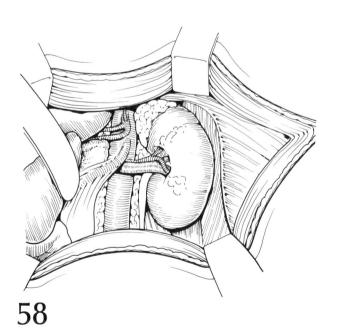

58

58 The spleen, pancreas and stomach are mobilized to the right exposing the kidney, the aorta, its major branches and the renal veins. The origins of the coeliac and superior mesenteric artery and other branches can be accessed in this way.

59 For exposure of the superior mesenteric artery lower down the intestine is mobilized to the right and the artery, along with the superior mesenteric vein, palpated in the free edge of the mesentery above the jejunum. Incising the peritoneum will expose the artery here.

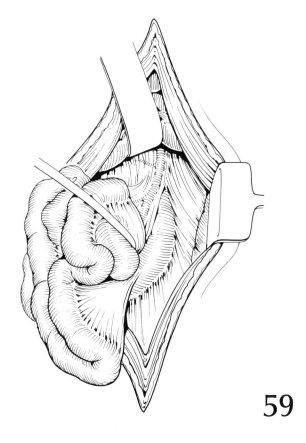

59

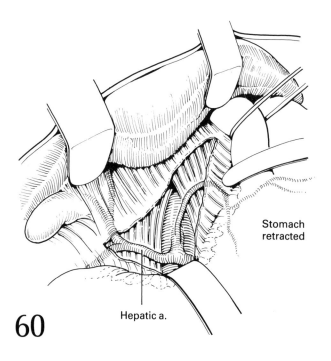

Stomach retracted

60

Hepatic a.

Hepatic artery

60 Division of the lesser omentum allows exposure of the hepatic artery as it crosses from the coeliac artery.

Renal arteries

61 The renal arteries are exposed using a transverse or vertical incision after passing a sling around the left renal vein which is pulled downwards.

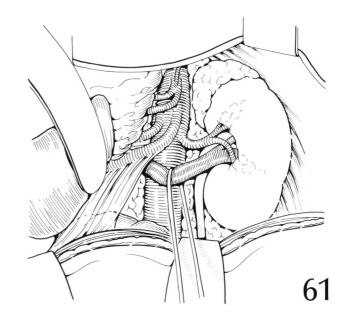

61

62, 63 The right renal artery is exposed by incising the peritoneum lateral to the duodenal loop and displacing it medially.

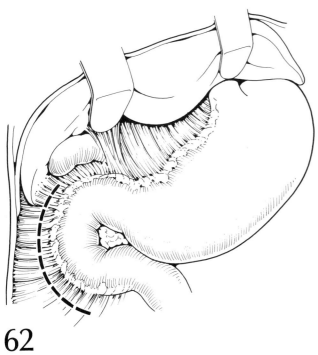

62

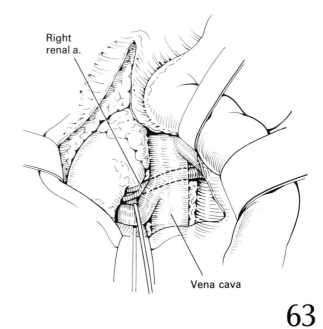

Right renal a.

Vena cava

63

Exposure of the iliac artery

64 An oblique incision is made in the left iliac fossa.

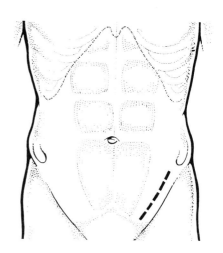

64

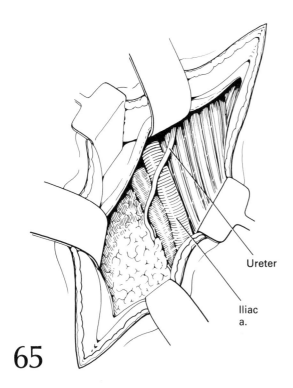

Ureter

Iliac
a.

65

65 To expose the iliac artery and vein the muscles are divided and the peritoneum mobilized medially, taking care to avoid the ureter which crosses the bifurcation of the common iliac artery.

Exposure of the internal iliac artery

66 In order to expose this vessel, the common and external iliac arteries are encircled with slings and pulled laterally. This allows exposure of the origin of the internal iliac artery which can be dissected free with scissors.

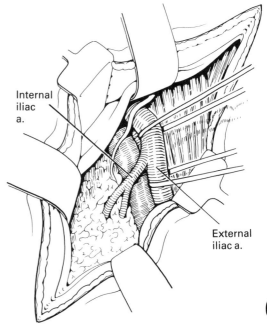

Internal
iliac
a.

External
iliac a.

66

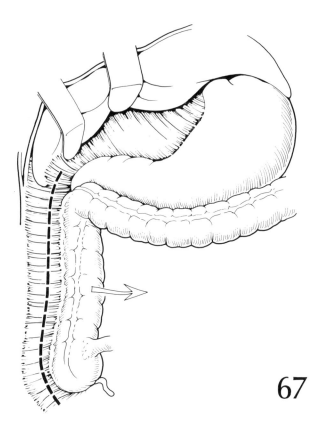

67

Exposure of the inferior vena cava

67, 68 The vena cava is exposed by opening the patient's abdomen through a transverse or vertical incision, incising the peritoneum lateral to the duodenal loop and ascending colon, and displacing these structures medially to expose the entire vena cava retroperitoneally.

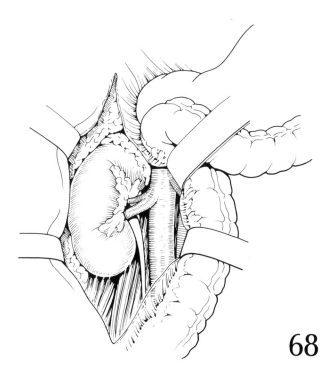

68

Exposure of the portal vein

69 This is exposed in the free edge of the porta hepatis. The hepatic artery is mobilized medially and the bile duct likewise. The portal vein lies behind these vessels.

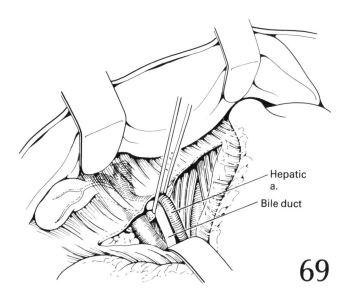

Hepatic
a.

Bile duct

69

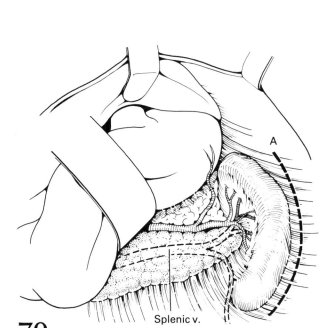

Splenic v.

70

Exposure of the splenic vein

70 As this structure lies behind the pancreas it is best exposed by incising the peritoneum lateral to the spleen as shown at A.

71 The spleen is then mobilized medially and the vein will be seen running along the back of the pancreas where it can be isolated if necessary.

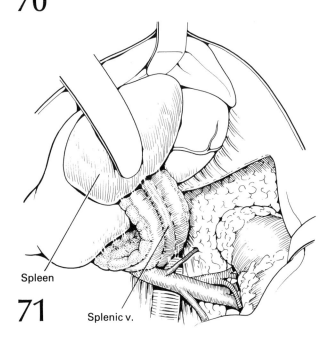

Spleen

71

Splenic v.

Exposure of the superficial and deep femoral arteries

72 A vertical or oblique incision is made in the groin.

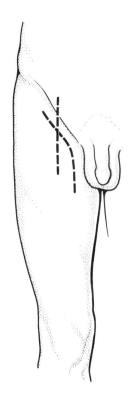

72

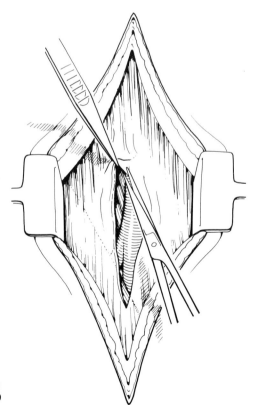

73 The fascia overlying the vessels is cut with a pair of scissors.

73

74 A pair of Lahey forceps is passed behind the artery and a sling passed around it.

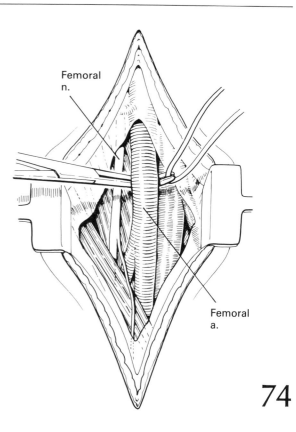

Femoral n.

Femoral a.

74

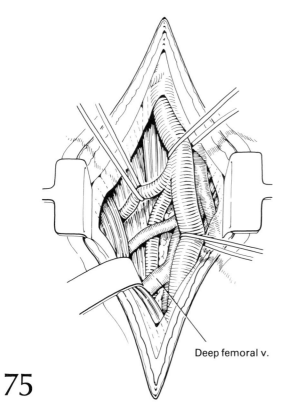

Deep femoral v.

75

75 Slings are similarly passed around the common and superficial femoral arteries and the upper branches of the deep femoral artery.

76 For extensive exposure of the deep femoral artery the small veins which often cross its origin and lower down the circumflex femoral vein are divided and the vessel fully exposed.

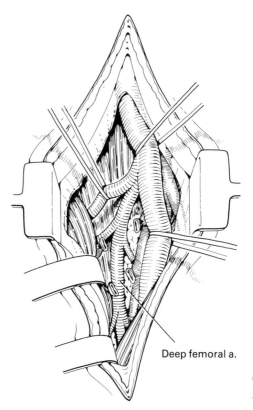

Deep femoral a.

76

Exposure of the femoral artery

77 For exposure of the femoral artery in the mid thigh a vertical incision is made.

78 The vastus medialis and adductor longus muscles are separated and the artery exposed.

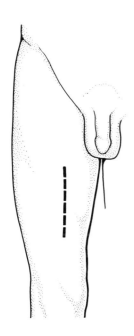

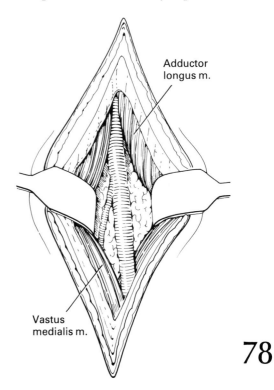

Adductor longus m.

Vastus medialis m.

77   **78**

Exposure of the popliteal artery

79 Using a posterior approach an S-shaped incision is made.

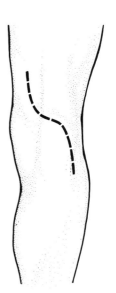

79

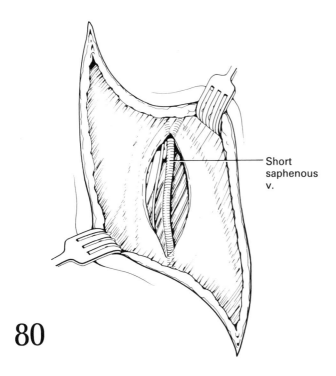

Short saphenous v.

80

80 When the fascia and fat have been divided the short saphenous vein will be seen. This has to be divided to gain access to the popliteal fossa.

81 The medial popliteal nerve and vessels will be seen passing between the two heads of the gastrocnemius muscle and are suprisingly superficial.

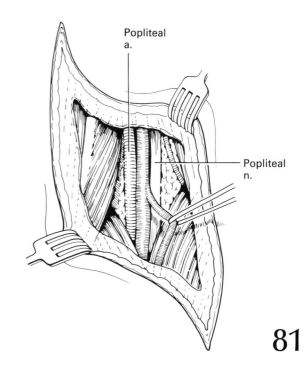

Popliteal a.

Popliteal n.

81

82 For exposure of the above knee popliteal artery an incision is made in the lower medial part of the thigh along the anterior border of the sartorius muscle.

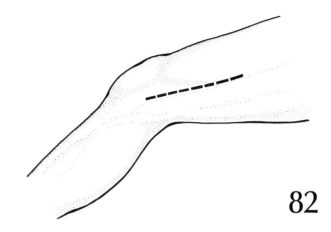

82

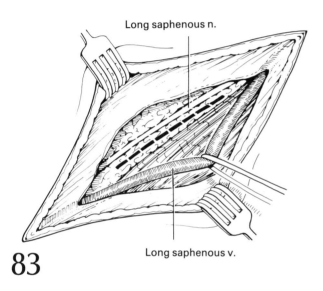

Long saphenous n.

Long saphenous v.

83

83 The incision is deepened until the long saphenous vein can be seen and should be protected. An incision is made in the deep fascia behind the nerve and the sartorius muscle retracted posteriorly.

84 Using finger dissection the popliteal artery is felt in the popliteal fossa lying anteriorly medial to the vein.

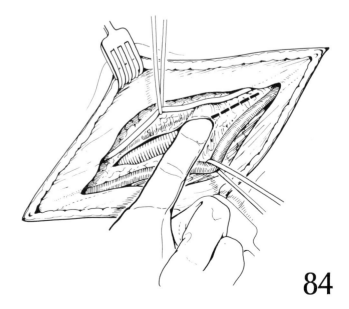

84

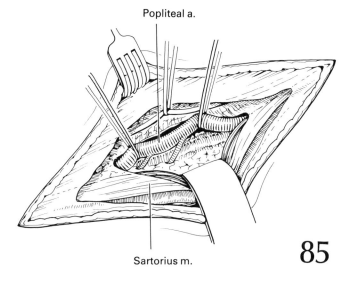

85 Appropriate retraction allows a sling to be passed around it to provide access.

86 The below knee popliteal artery is exposed by using an incision just behind the tibia, passing backwards slightly near to the knee joint.

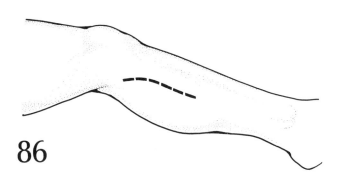

87 An incision is made in the deep fascia anterior to the gastrocnemius muscle.

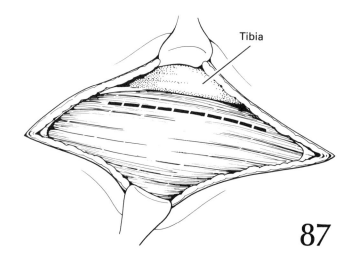

88 The gastrocnemius muscle is retracted posteriorly and the soleus muscle can be seen attached to the tibia. The vessels passing behind it can be felt above in the popliteal fossa.

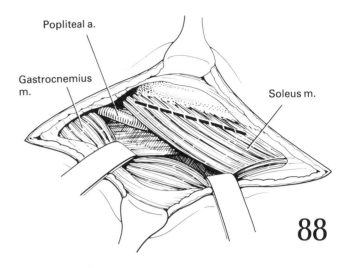

89 By dividing the tendon of the soleus muscle where it is attached to the tibia, the artery and vein can be followed downwards. The artery in particular is crossed by many small venous branches which require careful ligation.

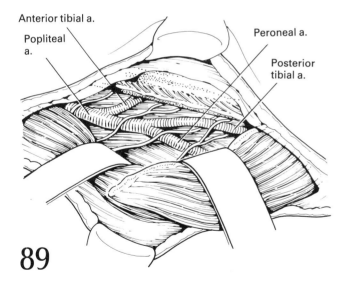

Exposure of the long saphenous vein

90 In order to remove the long saphenous vein multiple incisions are made along it and the vein exposed.

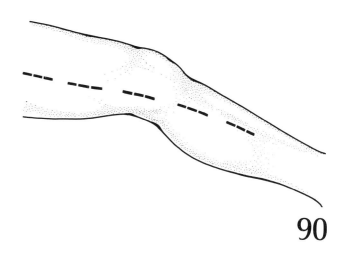

90

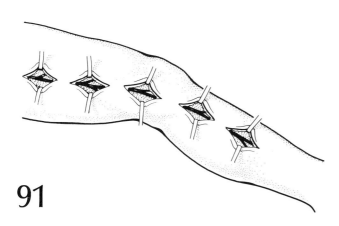

91

91 It is then removed by undermining the skin bridges. The upper end of the vein can be found first where it joins the saphenofemoral junction from where it can be traced by duplex ultrasonography and marked before surgery.

92 The vein is then removed through a continuous incision. This is probably better as it does less damage to the vein.

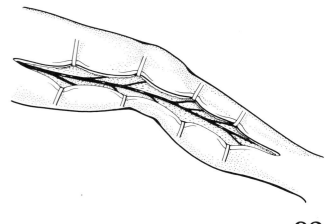

92

Exposure of the crural vessels

93 The posterior tibial and peroneal arteries are exposed by further detachment of the soleus muscle from the tibia until the peroneal artery disappears through the interosseous membrane half way down the leg.

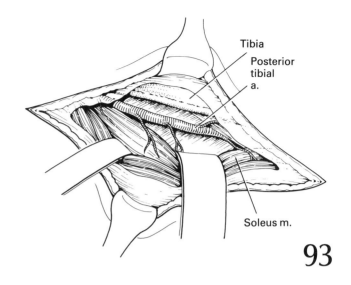

93

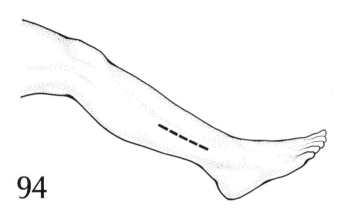

94

94 The peroneal artery is exposed in the lower half of the leg by an incision on the lateral side.

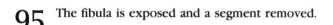

95 The fibula is exposed and a segment removed.

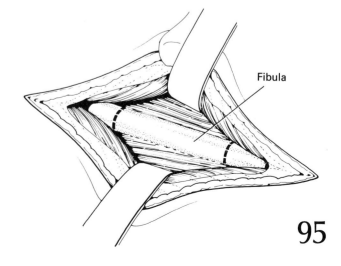

95

96 Once the fibula is removed the artery can be seen behind it.

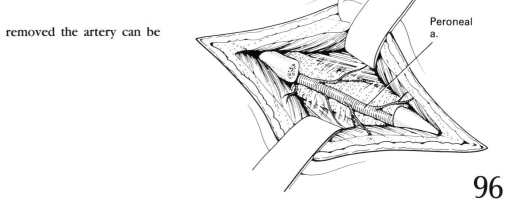

96

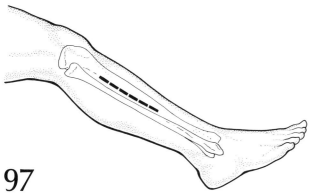

97

97 The anterior tibial artery is exposed by an incision over the anterior tibial muscles.

98 By dissection between the muscles the artery is found deep on the interosseous membrane. It can usually be located quite easily by finding a branch and following this backwards.

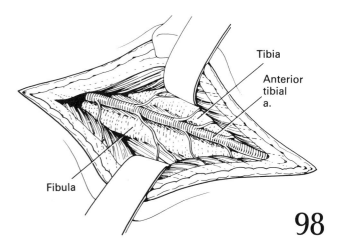

98

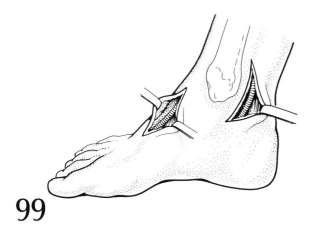

99

99 The anterior tibial and posterior tibial arteries are exposed at the foot or ankle by incisions over the posterior tibial artery behind the medial malleolus or anterior tibial artery on the dorsum of the foot.

Illustrations by Mark Iley

Arterial suture and anastomosis

P. L. Harris MD, FRCS
Consultant Vascular Surgeon, Royal Liverpool University Hospital, Liverpool, UK

History

The principles of vascular repair with sutures were established in the first decade of the 20th century by Alexis Carrel, who in 1912 was awarded the Nobel Prize for Medicine for this work. Since then, technical refinements of suture materials have made possible surgical reconstruction of most arteries, from the root of the aorta to microvascular anastomosis or repair of the smallest vessels, e.g. digital arteries or those on the surface of the brain. Fine sutures on atraumatic needles are best for arterial anastomosis. Silk was used for many years, but it has now been replaced by synthetic fibres, which are less traumatic to the vessel walls.

Principles and justification

Indications

There are three principal indications for operating on an artery: injury, aneurysmal dilatation and occlusion. Injury may result from sharp or blunt trauma and may be associated with damage to other structures, e.g. fractures of long bones. Iatrogenic injuries are increasingly common, arising from arterial access either for investigation or treatment. Another growing problem is that of self-induced arterial injury in main-line drug abusers. Occasionally, radical surgery for malignant disease may necessitate arterial repair. In most circumstances reconstruction of a damaged major artery is preferable to tying its ends, and this is particularly true in the lower limb.

Although elective and emergency treatment of aneurysmal and occlusive arterial lesions is mostly within the province of vascular specialists, the need for vascular repair may be encountered in all branches of surgery and it is therefore essential that all surgeons are familiar with the principles of arterial suture and anastomosis.

Contraindications

Total ischaemia of a limb for several hours resulting in massive muscle death is an absolute contraindication to vascular repair, because not only will the limb not be salvaged but fatal metabolic disturbance may ensue. Severe compound or crushing injury with gross tissue loss may also be an indication for amputation rather than vascular repair.

Arterial repair is superfluous where there is an adequate collateral circulation, as for example in the case of an injury to the radial artery at the wrist with an intact palmar arch.

Wherever possible, arterial suture should be avoided in the presence of infection.

Instruments

Clamps, needle holders and suture clamps

A wide selection of vascular clamps is essential. For large intra-abdominal and thoracic vessels the DeBakey Atraugrip range is effective, while for smaller arteries, for example femoral, popliteal, subclavian, brachial and carotid arteries, paediatric clamps of the Castaneda type are suitable. A range of small bulldog clamps is useful for controlling back bleeding from side branches, and for delicate vessels the Schofield–Lewis type is safe and effective.

Small peripheral arteries, including those distal to the popliteal and brachial arteries, should never be clamped as they are very sensitive to clamp damage. These vessels should be controlled with fine atraumatic plastic loops and by smooth round-ended atraumatic intraluminal catheters. Plastic loops may be colour-coded for easy identification.

Arteries must be handled gently and only with atraumatic non-toothed forceps.

Needle holders for vascular work must have fine points in order to facilitate accurate placement of sutures, and the jaws should be constructed from high-quality materials such as tungsten in order to ensure a firm grip of the needle. The range of sizes available should take account of the fact that arteries may be close to the surface or at considerable depth.

Rubber-shod clamps fashioned from small haemostats with the jaws cushioned by fine rubber or plastic tubing should be attached to the loose end of the suture in order to keep it out of the way. Unprotected metal instruments must never be applied to monofilamental sutures, which are relatively brittle and easily damaged.

Suture materials

Non-absorbable sutures on atraumatic needles are essential for arteries and there are three types in common usage.

1. Monofilamental material, such as polypropylene (Prolene), is very smooth and slips easily through the tissues. This property allows the anastomosis to be tightened easily by applying longitudinal tension on the suture. Its main disadvantage is a tendency to brittleness, and sutures of this type also tend to have a 'memory' causing twist (kink). It is essential to use several throws in each knot to ensure security.
2. The second type of suture is braided material coated with an outer layer of polyester to make it smooth. These sutures are less brittle and have no 'memory', but do not slide so easily through tissues.
3. Polytetrafluoroethylene (PTFE) sutures are available specifically for use with PTFE grafts. They are swaged onto very fine needles in order to overcome the problem of needle-hole bleeding from these grafts. The suture material itself is very strong and has excellent handling properties, but the needles are comparatively fragile and are unsuitable for suturing tough or calcified vessels and knots slip easily.

Arterial sutures may be single-ended with one needle or double-ended with two. They are available in varying sizes from 2/0 to 10/0. In general, the finest suture that is strong enough for the job should be used. As a rough guide, the following sizes are appropriate: 3/0 for the aorta; 4/0 for the iliac arteries; 5/0 for the femoral artery; 6/0 for the popliteal and brachial arteries; and 7/0 for tibial arteries.

For very fine work, a monofilament stitch is always necessary, and magnifying loops should be used.

Preoperative

Heparin

In non-traumatic situations, it is usual to give systemic heparin before application of the clamps. A standard dose of 5000 IU may be given. Alternatively, the dose may be related to the weight of the patient, for example 1000 IU/kg body weight. It is not always necessary to reverse the heparin, but one common practice is to reverse half of the dose of heparin originally used with the appropriate amount of protamine sulphate. (Protamine sulphate, 2 mg, neutralizes heparin, 1000 IU.)

For all arterial operations, a solution of heparinized saline should be prepared for irrigation of open vessels and instillation into vessels distal to a clamp. This is made up from heparin, 5000 IU in 500 ml normal saline.

Operation

SIMPLE SUTURE

Arteries are best opened longitudinally rather than transversely for three reasons. First, a longitudinal arteriotomy is easier to close; secondly, any thrombus that accumulates on the suture has less tendency to narrow the lumen; thirdly, it can easily be extended. A transverse arteriotomy is difficult to close because the intima retracts away from the outer layers and there is a greater risk of intimal dissection and flap formation.

1 Longitudinal arteriotomies in large or medium-sized arteries can usually be closed by simple lateral suture. The needle must pass through all layers of the arterial wall with every stitch, and care should be taken to ensure that the intima turns outwards. It is important to maintain a firm, even, tension on the suture line and optimal spacing and size of each bite, which can only be learned by experience. Even, regular spacing is usually best, but occasionally irregular stitches may be required to take account of calcified atheromatous plaques.

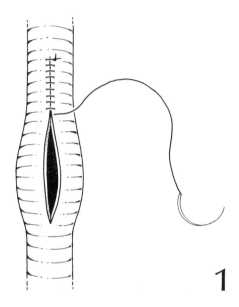

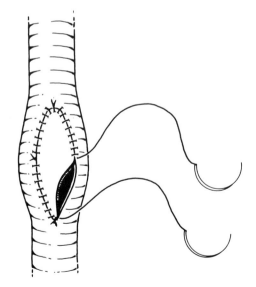

CLOSURE WITH A PATCH

2 For vessels of less than 4 mm in diameter (which usually includes the brachial artery) and where there is loss of substance of the arterial wall that would cause linear closure to narrow the lumen too greatly, it is preferable to close the artery with a patch. This technique can also be used to widen the lumen of a vessel that has become stenosed by disease, for example the deep femoral artery. For small vessels, a patch of autologous vein should be used (the long saphenous vein should not be sacrificed for this purpose). In larger vessels, prosthetic material (either Dacron or PTFE) may be used. An oval or rectangular patch is better than an elliptical one with sharp points which tends to narrow the vessel at each end.

END-TO-END ANASTOMOSIS

This is most easily accomplished by the triangulation technique, as described originally by Carrel.

Stay sutures

3   The transected ends of the vessels are first carefully cleared of excess adventitia, because if this should intrude on the lumen it will promote thrombosis. Three stay sutures are inserted, the first being placed in the centre of the back or deepest aspect of the anastomosis, with the other two positioned so as to divide the circumference of the vessels equally into three. Any disparity in calibre can be compensated for at this stage. Everting horizontal mattress or simple sutures may be used. Sometimes it may be simpler to use just two stay sutures placed either at the anterior and posterior points or at each side, but this is not recommended as a routine.

Interrupted sutures

4   Interrupted sutures should always be used for small or medium-sized vessels. By applying gentle traction to the stay sutures, each of the three segments of the anastomosis is completed in turn commencing with the two at the deepest aspects.

Continuous sutures

5   For larger vessels a continuous suture may be used, commencing on each side of the deepest part of the anastomosis. Care must be taken not to pull the suture too tight and cause a purse-string effect.

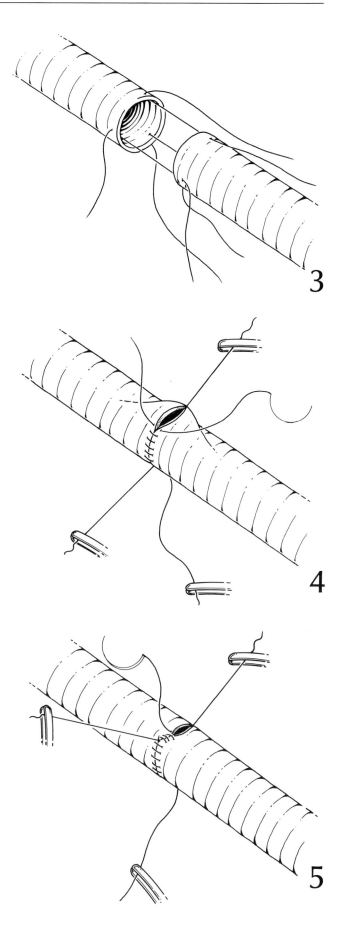

Single-stitch method

6 If there is difficulty in rotating the vessels, for example at a large bifurcation, a single stitch may be used. Commencing on the side nearest the operator, the sutures are inserted from within the lumen to complete the deep or posterior aspect and then continued across the anterior aspect to the starting point. Alternatively, a double-ended suture may be commenced at the midpoint posteriorly and each side completed in turn.

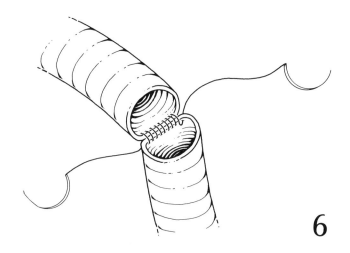

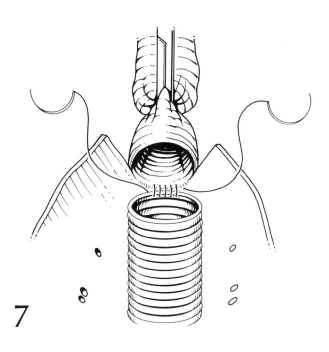

Inlay technique

7 This is the method used for abdominal aortic aneurysms. A horizontal mattress stitch using a double-ended suture is started in the middle of the back of the graft, picking up a double layer of the aortic wall at the neck of the aneurysm and inserting the needles from inside the lumen.

The suture may then be tied and each side of the anastomosis completed in turn. The needle should pass from graft to aorta, and it is essential to take large bites of the aorta to include all layers.

Parachute technique

8 Alternatively, the double-ended suture may be left untied in order to allow a number of stitches to be placed on each side before the graft is pulled down onto the artery.

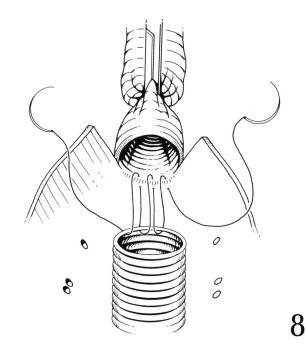

END-TO-SIDE ANASTOMOSIS

This is the usual method of anastomosis for bypass operations. The anastomosis should be oblique, and its length should be approximately twice the diameter of the lumen of the graft. The end of the graft should be fashioned into a spatulate shape, so that on completion of the anastomosis it adopts a 'cobra head' appearance.

Four-quadrant technique

9 A double-ended suture is placed at the 'heel' of the anastomosis and stitching is completed along each side of the anastomosis to the mid-point. If the 'toe' is left free at this stage, the inside of the anastomosis can be inspected to ensure apposition of the intima.

The 'toe' of the graft is then trimmed accurately to size and secured with a double-ended suture to the apex of the anastomosis. The procedure is completed by closing the two remaining quadrants. The 'toe' and 'heel' are the most crucial points of an end-to-side anastomosis, where there is the greatest risk of vessels becoming narrowed. To avoid this risk at the toe, the starting point should be offset to one side or other of the apex. Alternatively, a number of interrupted sutures can be placed around the toe.

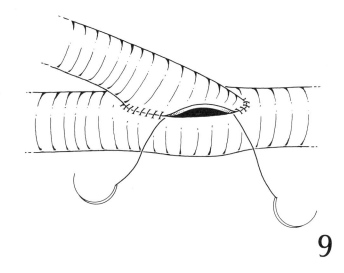

9

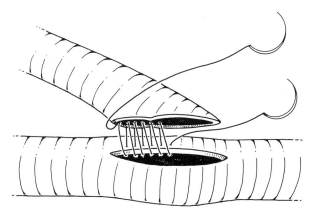

10

Parachute technique

10 Where access is difficult or good visualization of the anastomosis is impaired, this technique may be advantageous. Using a double-ended monofilament suture, a series of running stitches is placed at what will become the 'heel' of the anastomosis, with the graft and artery separated. These sutures are then pulled tight as the vessels are approximated.

SUTURING THE DISEASED ARTERY

Stronger material may be used for suturing densely sclerotic or calcified vessels. Wherever possible the needle should be passed from within the lumen to the outside of the arterial wall in order to 'pin back' loose plaques, and this requires the suture to pass from graft to artery rather than vice versa. In the presence of calcification it may be necessary to insert a large suture around the whole plaque, in which case additional fine adventitial stitches may be required for complete haemostasis. Care must be taken that sutures are not cut or frayed by calcified plaques. Caution must be exercised in removing plaques or performing local endarterectomy when suturing arteries.

Kunlin suture

11 If an endarterectomy has been performed, there is a risk of intimal flap dissection at the downstream edge. To eliminate this risk, sutures are inserted to secure the intima. The needle passes from outside to inside through an endarterectomized part of the wall and back from inside to outside through the atheroma to be finally tied on the outside.

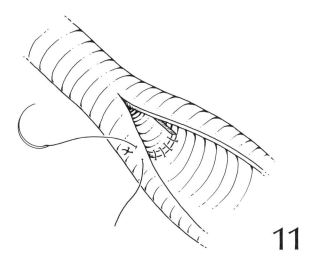

11

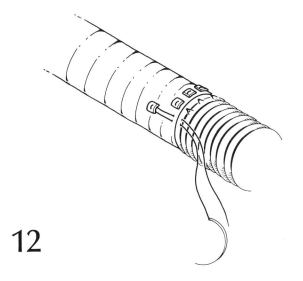

12

Buttressing sutures

12 Disease may sometimes cause the arterial wall to be friable so that it will not hold sutures, which then cut out. This can be a cause of serious haemorrhage. In these circumstances, the sutures should be buttressed with pads of Dacron for large arteries or small pieces of muscle for small arteries.

NON-SUTURED ANASTOMOSIS

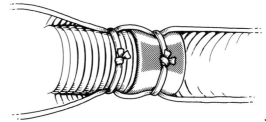

13 This technique has a limited application for the treatment of dissecting aneurysms and some atherosclerotic aneurysms involving the thoracic aorta, where it may confer some advantages over conventional suturing[1]. A rigid, Dacron-covered polypropylene ring attached to the end of the graft is inserted on an applicator within the lumen and held in place by tapes ligated around the outside of the aorta.

13

References

1. Harris PL, Moody AP, Edwards PR, Cave-Bigley DJ. Technical advantages of a ringed intraluminal graft in the management of difficult aortic aneurysms. *Eur J Vasc Surg* 1990; 4: 355–9.

Technique of endarterectomy

C. W. Jamieson MS, FRCS
Consultant Surgeon, St Thomas' Hospital, London, UK

Principles and justification

Indications

Endarterectomy of an artery is indicated in the presence of a short stenotic lesion (open endarterectomy) or, less frequently, in longer occlusions, particularly when the insertion of a synthetic bypass is contraindicated because of the risk of infection.

Preoperative

Good quality angiograms are more important in patients selected for endarterectomy than in those selected for bypass because the exact nature of the stenotic process must be evaluated with great care to make sure the correct segment is treated surgically. In bypass it is only really necessary for surgeons to know that the area selected for the origin of the bypass and that selected for the outflow tract are adequate.

Operations

OPEN ENDARTERECTOMY

Incision

1 The diseased segment is isolated between arterial clamps after full systemic heparinization of the patient. A small incision is made longitudinally in the artery, using a size 15 blade. The incision is deepened very carefully and the knife is withdrawn as soon as fresh blood is encountered, indicating that the arterial lumen has been opened.

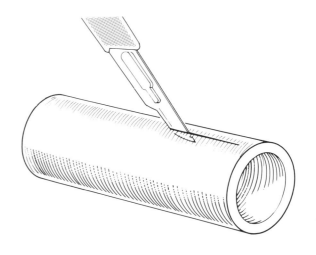

2 The incision is extended proximally and distally with a pair of Pott's scissors to cover the extent of the stenotic lesion.

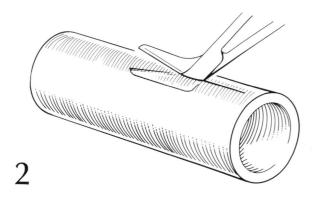

3 One side of the arteriotomy is lifted by the surgeon and the other by the assistant. The surgeon seeks to enter a plane of endarterectomy in the arterial wall using a Watson–Cheyne dissector.

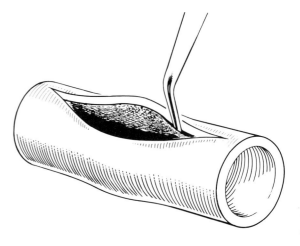

4 When a good plane is located the dissector is passed around the apex of the arteriotomy to ensure that the plane remains constant on both sides of the artery. The dissector is only passed around the proximal extremity of the arteriotomy. The inner layers of the vessel distal to the site of endarterectomy are carefully left adherent to their attachments to the remainder of the arterial wall.

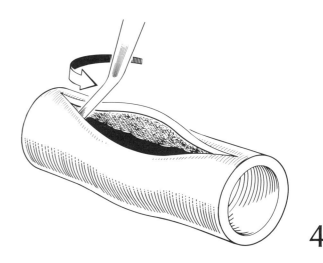

4

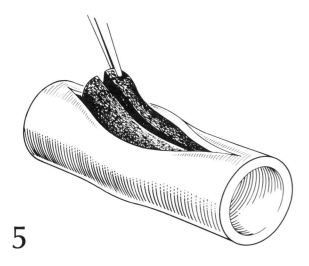

5

Removal of plaque

5 Using the dissector, the plane of endarterectomy is extended around the whole circumference of the vessel in the proximal part of the arteriotomy, totally freeing the plaque, which is then divided at the proximal end of the arteriotomy and lifted out of the vessel.

6 The distal extremity of the stenosing plaque is then carefully divided with Pott's scissors, exactly at the point at which it remains attached to the arterial wall, so that no loose free flap remains which might lift in the restored blood flow and cause occlusion of the artery.

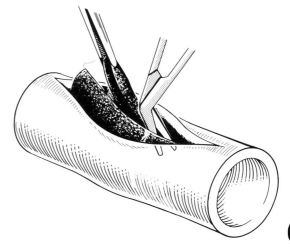

6

7 If there is any suggestion that this distal extremity of the endarterectomized segment may be loose, two anchoring sutures are passed through the arterial wall, through the endarterectomized segment and out through the unendarterectomized intima, to anchor it in place.

It is sometimes possible to divide the most distal extremity of the plaque first, with sharp dissection, and then to extend the plane of endarterectomy proximally, dividing the endarterectomized core at the proximal extremity of the arteriotomy; this is particularly useful in carotid endarterectomy, where the plaque tails off distally into thin, healthy artery.

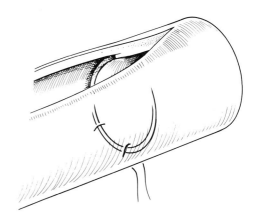

7

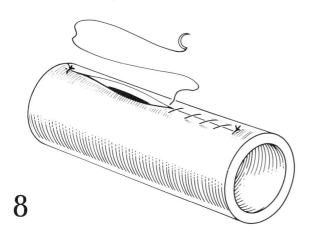

8

Closure

Downflow and backflow are tested by momentary release of each clamp. The arteriotomy is closed with appropriate calibre polypropylene sutures, using 3/0 polypropylene for large vessels such as the aorta and 4/0 or 5/0 for smaller arteries. It is best not to close arteries smaller than 5 mm in diameter directly but to use a patch to avoid the inevitable slight stenosis associated with direct closure.

8 An interrupted suture is placed in the proximal extremity of the arteriotomy and tied. A continuous suture then starts at the distal extremity of the arteriotomy and is advanced to meet the proximal suture. After completion of the suture line the proximal clamp is removed to drive air from the isolated arterial segment before the distal clamp is removed.

After removal of the clamps the vessel is palpated distal to the reconstruction to ensure that a palpable pulse has returned, and the vessel distal to the arteriotomy is observed closely for a few minutes to ensure that dissection has not taken place in the newly endarterectomized segment; this is immediately visible as a blue discoloration of the arterial wall, as blood is forced into it as the flap of intima lifts, and is associated with a loss of the distal pulse, though a strong pulse may persist in the dissection itself.

SEMI-CLOSED ENDARTERECTOMY

Incision

This technique is suitable for longer occlusions and may be performed through one or two arteriotomies. After systemic heparinization the occluded segment of vessel is exposed and clamps are applied above and below the occluded area.

9 An arteriotomy is made distal to the area of occlusion, extending into the occluded segment to permit exposure of the distal extremity of the stenosing plaque.

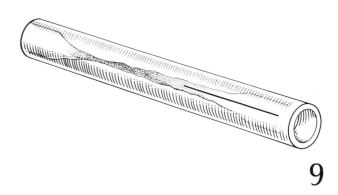

9

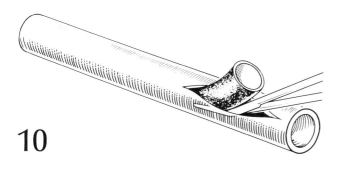

10

Removal of plaque

10 Using the same technique as for open endarterectomy, the arteriotomy is opened and the distal extremity of the plaque is dissected free using a Watson–Cheyne dissector, with a combination of sharp dissection and Pott's scissors.

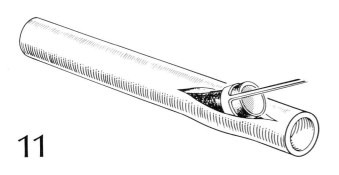

11

11 A loop or arc stripper is then passed up in the plane of endarterectomy to the proximal extremity of the occluding lesion. A loop stripper is relatively safe but, unfortunately, will not easily traverse an artery of varying lumen. An arc stripper will traverse such a vessel, but there is a danger that it may be caught in the wall if it is twisted as it is passed up and down the vessel.

12 After passage of the stripper proximally, arterial forceps are gently closed on the arterial wall with sufficient force to break the inner plaque but not the outer layer of the wall. The artery is held in the finger and thumb of the other hand while the clamp is applied and the plaque can be felt to break, with adequate pressure. The plaque is then milked distally from the vessel by a combination of traction with a pair of forceps and pressure of the finger and thumb of the other hand.

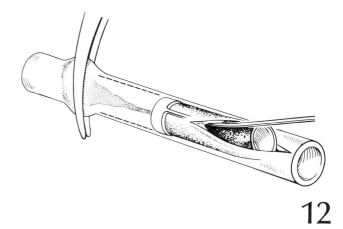

12

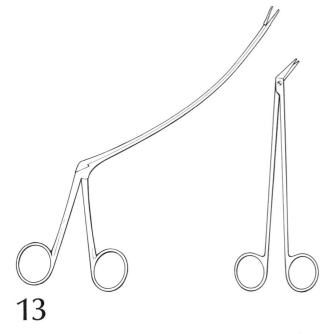

13

13 The plaque may not rupture satisfactorily, or fragments of atheroma may be left in the vessel lumen; these may be removed using a pair of Martin's thrombectomy forceps.

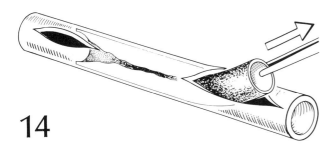

14

14 If the plaque will not rupture it is important that excessive pressure is not applied as this may destroy the arterial wall. A second arteriotomy is then made at the proximal extremity of the occlusion and the plaque is divided under direct vision, to be withdrawn distally.

Closure

The proximal arteriotomy is sutured first, as downflow may then be tested to assess the adequacy of clearance of the obstructed segment. The distal arteriotomy is then closed, again ensuring that there is no evidence of a dissection of the distal end of the intima which may have to be anchored.

EVERSION ENDARTERECTOMY

This elegant variation on the closed endarterectomy technique was described by Wiley.

15 After systemic heparinization the occluded segment of the vessel is clamped proximally and distally and divided transversely at the distal extremity of the occlusion.

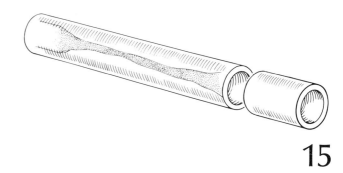

15

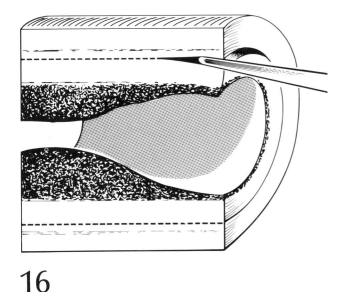

16

16 A Watson–Cheyne dissector is inserted into the plane of endarterectomy in the arterial wall and the adventitia and outer layer of the media are everted, allowing precise division of the adherent bands between the core and the outer wall. After division of the core the eversion is reduced.

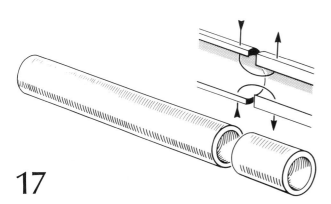

17

17 The divided artery is then resutured, using interrupted sutures to avoid stenosis. This effectively anchors the distal, undivided intima. The sutures should pass from the outer wall of the endarterectomized vessel into the lumen of the unendarterectomized vessel and out again, thereby anchoring the distal intima.

Outcome

Endarterectomy is technically more demanding than a bypass procedure and for this reason it has been practised less frequently in recent years, but it does have the advantage that sepsis is not so disastrous as is infection of a synthetic graft, and the long-term results of endarterectomy in most sites are comparable with those of bypass.

Angioscopy in vascular reconstructions

W. H. Pearce MD
Associate Professor of Surgery, Division of Vascular Surgery, Department of Surgery, Northwestern University Medical School, Chicago, Illinois, USA

K. D. Nolan MD, MPH
Instructor of Surgery, Division of Vascular Surgery, Department of Surgery, Northwestern University Medical School, Chicago, Illinois, USA

J. S. T. Yao MD, PhD
Magerstadt Professor of Surgery, Division of Vascular Surgery, Department of Surgery, Northwestern University Medical School, Chicago, Illinois, USA

History

Early attempts to perform endoscopy of the cardiovascular system were limited to the heart. Rigid endoscopes were used to visualize intracardiac pathology. While successful, these systems were too large to be used in peripheral vessels. In addition, displacement of the blood for clear visualization was difficult and was based on a transparent balloon. Using rigid choledochoscopes, Greenstone was able to visualize the lumens of large vessels in dogs and human cadavers in a blood-free field[1]. In 1974 Vollmar and Storz reported clinical success using a flexible choledochoscope[2]. Crispin (1973)[3] and, later, Towne (1977)[4] concurred that angioscopy was a safe technique which minimally prolonged the operative procedure, and was a potential alternative to completion arteriography. Modern technology has produced high-resolution, small-diameter angioscopes which provide high-quality images of even small-calibre vessels. Coupled with efficient irrigating systems, the lumens of many arteries and veins can now be inspected.

Principles and justification

Angioscopy is a new technique whose precise role in the care of patients with vascular disease is evolving. In preliminary studies, angioscopy appears to be useful in detecting technical errors, monitoring valve lysis during the *in situ* bypass, and determining the adequacy of a thromboembolectomy[5]. Completion arteriography is the most common method used to evaluate the anastomosis and run-off of a femorodistal bypass. Completion arteriography also provides detailed anatomy of the run-off vessels. Visualization of run-off is essential in making decisions such as whether to reoperate or to anticoagulate. Completion arteriography is also useful in evaluating options with late graft failures. Patent distal vessels may be used for subsequent reoperation. While completion arteriography is highly specific, it is only a moderately sensitive test[5]. Other intraoperative methods used to detect technical defects include electromagnetic flow probes, B-mode scans and Doppler spectral analysis.

Angioscopy offers another method of assessing the technical quality of an infrainguinal bypass. In 112 lower extremity bypasses Miller *et al.* reported that, in 48% of the cases, surgical decisions were made on the basis of angioscopy alone[6]. The angioscopic findings which prompted a change in the surgical procedure included incompletely cut venous valve leaflets and missed arteriovenous fistulae in *in situ* grafts. Unfortunately, comparative intraoperative arteriograms were performed in only 16% of patients. In studies which compared both techniques, angioscopy was more accurate than arteriography in detecting technical errors[5]. In one prospective study of 49 femorodistal bypasses, Baxter *et al.* found that completion arteriography was highly specific (95%) but not sensitive (67%) when compared with angioscopy[5]. The angioscopic findings in three grafts with normal arteriograms (false negatives) revealed intimal flaps (two) and intraluminal thrombus (one). In 10% of the procedures, angioscopy revealed a technical problem which required an unanticipated alteration in the surgical procedure.

Angioscopic monitoring of the *in situ* bypass is used to limit the length of the skin incision and to ensure valvular incompetence. For the first time since the original description of the *in situ* bypass by Hall in 1962, angioscopy permits the visualization of the venous valvulotomy[7]. Valve incision performed during an *in situ* bypass relies upon retrograde pressure (either arterial or from an irrigation catheter) to close the valve mechanism. A valvulotome is inserted and the venous leaflet is torn blindly. Vein wall injury may occur at any point but particularly when the leaflet is adjacent to a small side branch. The use of angioscopy to monitor the valvulotomy was introduced by Fleisher *et al.* in 1986[8]. Damage to venous conduit could be avoided and arteriovenous fistulae could be identified using the angioscope. In this preliminary report, angioscopy did not prolong the operative procedure and was not associated with fluid overload. Later reports by Matsumoto and Mehigan[9] confirmed the utility of angioscopy in performing *in situ* bypasses. The also recommended using the angioscope to 'prepare' translocated vein bypasses. Residual intact valve leaflets and persistent arteriovenous fistulae were avoided using this method. Miller *et al.* performed routine angioscopy following all infrainguinal bypasses and found a 17% incidence of retained valve leaflets and a 60% incidence of residual arteriovenous fistula[6]. These partially torn valves may create turbulent blood flow and be the site of later vein graft stenosis. In our own experience, angioscopy detected mid-vein graft abnormalities in only 4% of patients, all of which were unrelated to an incomplete valvulotomy. The lesions identified were sclerotic vein segments. Recently, there has been enthusiasm to perform pre-bypass angioscopy in all vein bypass cases to identify vein abnormalities. Since the incidence of undetected vein abnormalities in our experience is low (4%), routine pre-bypass angioscopy is not performed. These abnormalities were found with completion angioscopy and were corrected. Similar results have been noted by Mehigan who found only one functional valve leaflet in 55 patients and 3 patent side branches[9].

An additional benefit of angioscopy is that the operation may be performed without a long leg incision to expose the full length of the vein. A high wound complication rate has been associated with long leg incisions. Since it is possible to identify major side branches with the angioscope, only small cut downs are required for ligation. However, the below-the-knee incision for tibial artery bypasses is still required and this area is the site of the majority of wound problems.

The treatment of lower extremity arterial emboli has not changed significantly since the introduction of the Fogarty catheter in 1963. In combination with systemic heparinization, the Fogarty catheter has greatly increased the rates of limb salvage from 70% to 99%. Thromboembolectomy using the Fogarty catheter is a blind procedure. The catheter is placed in the distal arterial system and is withdrawn, using a subjective estimation of arterial drag. It is often difficult to selectively cannulate each of the tibial vessels. On occasion, it is necessary to cut down upon the infrapopliteal vessels and manually guide the catheter into the appropriate tibial vessels. Rarely, the artery is opened for passage of the catheter into each tibial vessel. Commonly, a distal clot and debris remain after what has been felt to be an adequate blind thromboembolectomy.

Angioscopy offers the ability to direct the Fogarty catheter into the tibial vessels without the use of fluoroscopy or distal popliteal artery exposure. Under direct vision, the Fogarty catheter is guided into the appropriate tibial vessel and the clot is extracted[10]. Angioscopy-assisted thromboembolectomy may also diminish catheter-related injuries by allowing visualization of the thromboembolectomy while the procedure is being performed. Under direct vision, only sufficient distension of the balloon catheter is needed to remove the thrombus.

Since prosthetic grafts do not have an intimal lining, damage to the intima does not occur. However, the pseudointima may be disrupted by the Fogarty catheter producing free floating debris. Removal of this debris is essential to ensure adequate prograde flow and prevent distal embolization. Angioscopy is invaluable in identifying mid-graft debris and inspecting the proximal and distal anastomoses. Loose debris can be extracted with brushes or biopsy forceps.

The development of lasers and other endovascular procedures has created new indications for angioscopy. Angioscopy allows the surgeon to guide such instruments under direct vision and theoretically limit laser ablation or atherectomy to the diseased arterial segment.

Indications

Angioscopy is indicated (1) to detect technical imperfection; (2) to monitor valve lysis during the *in situ* bypass; (3) to inspect thrombectomized grafts and arteries; and (4) to guide endovascular procedures.

Equipment

1 A complete system including angioscopes, cameras, monitors and other video components should be dedicated to the vascular operating room. The operating room nurses as well as the operating surgeon should be familiar with all pieces of the equipment. Angioscopes of different calibre should be available. At Northwestern University three sizes are used: a 1.4-mm solid non-steerable angioscope without an irrigating channel, a 2.2-mm steerable solid angioscope without an irrigation channel which allows a deflection of 120°, and a 2.8-mm non-steerable angioscope with a 1-mm irrigation channel. A 300-watt xenon light source is used. The angioscope is coupled with a camera, video monitor and 0.5-inch video cassette recorder. Still photography may be obtained with special additional equipment.

A dedicated system for irrigation capable of clearing the lumen of blood is necessary. Our system provides for high (150 ml/min) and low (50 ml/min) flow rates with a continuous digital read-out of the volume of fluid infused. The irrigation fluid is 0.9% sodium chloride with 2000 units/l heparin. Since inadvertent fluid overload is a potential complication, the digital read-out feature is particularly helpful for the surgeon and anaesthetist. Excessive pressures may develop in closed arterial or venous segments producing overdistension and damage to the vessel. Careful attention must be paid to both the volume infused and pressure build-up.

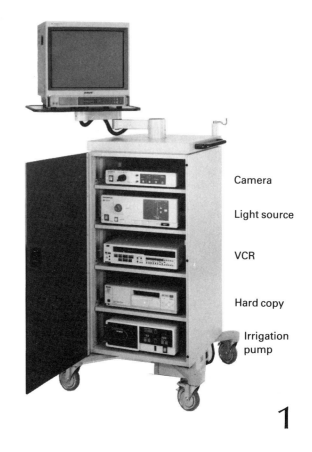

Camera

Light source

VCR

Hard copy

Irrigation pump

1

Operations

ANGIOSCOPY-ASSISTED *IN SITU* BYPASS

2, 3 Incision of the venous valves with the aid of the angioscope is performed following routine exposure of the saphenous vein, femoral vessels, and recipient popliteal/tibial vessels. The proximal venous valves are incised under direct vision. The angioscope and irrigating system are introduced either through the cut end of the saphenous vein or through large side branches.

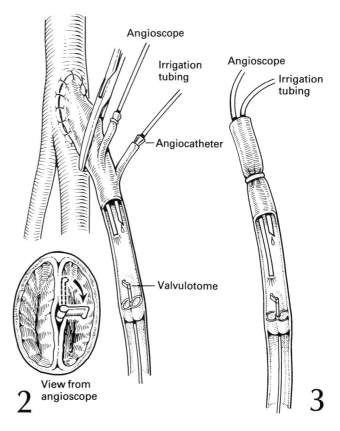

Angioscope

Irrigation tubing

Angioscope

Irrigation tubing

Angiocatheter

Valvulotome

View from angioscope

2

3

4a, b

A special flexible valvulotome, 100 cm in length with a detachable cutting blade (2.5 mm) is used. The instrument is passed from below using a blunt tip. The cutting blade is placed for valve incision. The angioscope and irrigating system are introduced through the open end of the saphenous vein with an encircling vessel loop. Occasionally, it is difficult to maintain a water seal with the vessel loop alone and may require additional digital pressure. An alternative method is to complete the proximal anastomosis preserving several large side branches. One branch is for the introduction of the irrigation system while the second is used for the angioscope. Once the angioscope is inserted, the vein is gently distended. With gentle irrigation, blood entering from tributaries is removed and the valve leaflets and the cutting instrument can be seen. The cutting instrument is placed at the leading edge of the closed valve and the valve leaflet torn. Occasionally the valve mechanism is adjacent to a side branch and with the angioscope it becomes apparent how vein injury may occur during the valvulotomy. The cutting edge of the valvulotome will inadvertently lodge in the orifice of a tributary. With the angioscope it is possible to redirect the valvulotome for accurate valve incision. Once both valve leaflets have been cut, the valve mechanism is irrigated to confirm free flow.

Large venous tributaries are identified by either passing the angioscope into their lumens or by placing the cutting instrument into their orifice. The light of the angioscope directs the dissection. This technique is particularly useful when a long skin incision is not used to expose the vein. Instead, several small skin incisions are made to ligate arteriovenous fistulae.

The angioscope and valvulotome are passed down the vein, sequentially disrupting each valve mechanism encountered. Once all of the valvulotomies have been performed, the angioscope is withdrawn, checking each valve for function. The distal anastomosis is completed in a standard fashion.

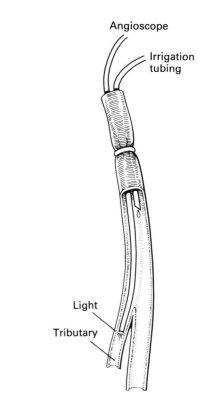

Angioscope

Irrigation tubing

Light

Tributary

4a

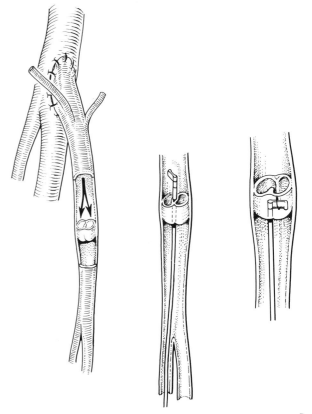

4b

ANGIOSCOPY-ASSISTED THROMBOEMBOLECTOMY

5   The surgical technique for lower extremity angio-scopy-assisted thromboembolectomy does not differ from the standard procedure. Indications for the operation and the need for preoperative arteriography are not different. The common femoral artery is opened transversely and a Fogarty catheter is passed for the retrieval of distal emboli and debris. The angioscope is inserted through the transverse arteriotomy along with an irrigating catheter. Using pump-driven perfusion, the distal arterial circulation is cleared of blood. The volume of infusion is carefully monitored by the anaesthetist and the operating surgeon. The length of the superficial femoral and popliteal arteries is inspected. Since the tibial peroneal trunk and peroneal arteries are the most direct route for the Fogarty catheter, careful inspection is made of the orifices of the posterior and anterior arteries. If embolic debris remains, the angioscope is left in a viewing position and the Fogarty catheter is guided under direct vision into the obstructed lumen. A gentle curve in the distal portion of the Fogarty catheter is useful for guidance. Steerable balloon catheters for thromboembolectomies are being developed but are not currently available. The angioscope and the Fogarty catheter are removed simultaneously. In some instances where there is a firm adherent intraluminal thrombus, biopsy forceps or brushes have been used to dislodge the material. The authors have not selected this approach but have used repeated irrigations and catheter passage in an attempt to remove these thrombi. It appears that the brush technique is associated with significant intimal injury. With the recent addition of intraoperative thrombolytic therapy, angioscopy allows for an objective appraisal of the efficacy of this mode of therapy. The authors have limited experience with the modality. With the complete removal of any visual thrombus, the arteriotomy is closed and an intraoperative completion arteriogram is performed.

When it is necessary to perform a proximal iliac embolectomy, proximal occlusion can be obtained by inserting a balloon catheter No. 4 or 5 in the aorta and withdrawing it to a position at the origin of the iliac vessels. This allows for proximal inflow control. If there is not significant back-bleeding from the hypogastric

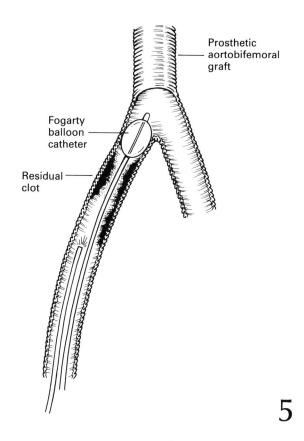

Prosthetic aortobifemoral graft

Fogarty balloon catheter

Residual clot

5

vessels, it is possible to examine the lumen of the external iliac and common iliac vessels. In selected cases the authors have found occlusive disease in the iliac artery which was responsible for initiation of the thrombus with distal embolus.

With graft thromboembolectomies, completion angioscopy is performed to ensure complete removal of intraluminal thrombus and any loosened pseudointima. When the graft is exposed distally, a Fogarty catheter is used for proximal control. In prosthetic grafts a large angioscope is used. The proximal and distal anastomoses are inspected for evidence of neointimal hyperplasia. Flaps of pseudointima are removed with a pair of flexible biopsy forceps if necessary. Graft revision is performed as needed.

ANGIOSCOPY AS A TECHNIQUE FOR DETECTING TECHNICAL ERRORS

6 Successful arterial reconstruction of the lower extremity is dependent upon a number of factors. These include adequate inflow, a suitable conduit, sufficient run-off, and meticulous surgical technique. At the end of the surgical procedure the angioscope is inserted into the graft, either through side branches, a large-bore angiocatheter or through open portions of the anastomosis. The smallest diameter angioscope is used. An irrigation catheter is inserted to provide a blood-free field. The angioscope is passed into the distal portion of the graft proximal to the anastomosis. The anastomosis is inspected for loose intimal debris, flaps or anastomatic narrowing produced by improperly placed sutures. Depending upon the size of the distal run-off vessel, it may be possible to pass the angioscope into the distal arterial tree. In patients with *in situ* bypasses the angioscope is withdrawn with irrigation to ensure incompetence of all valves. Residual arterial venous fistulae are detected by blood entering via their orifice. Free floating intima and fronds of tissue are of little consequence. Significant narrowing of the anastomosis requires revision.

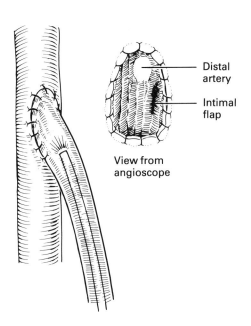

Distal artery

Intimal flap

View from angioscope

6

Outcome

Until recently there have been no prospective randomized studies comparing routine angioscopy with standard operative methods to improve infrainguinal graft patency. Recently, Miller and colleagues found no statistical difference in early patency (30 days) between bypass grafts having either completion angioscopy or arteriography (n = 250)[11]. There was, however, a clear trend in favour of angioscopy. Twelve grafts failed (4.8%); four (3.1%) in the angioscopy group and eight (6.6%) in the control group. In addition, clinically relevant decisions were made in 39 patients in the angioscopy group compared with seven in the angiography group. Overall it appears that angioscopy was more sensitive to mid-graft and anastomotic problems than arteriography. However, angioscopy was less sensitive to lesions distal to the anastomosis. Thus angioscopy and intraoperative arteriography are needed to assess the body of the graft and the run-off vessels.

Acknowledgements

Illustration 1 is reproduced with the permission of the Olympus Corporation, Lake Success, New York, USA.

References

1. Greenstone SM, Shore JM, Heringman EC, Massell TB. Arterial endoscopy (arterioscopy). *Arch Surg* 1966; 93: 811–12.

2. Vollmar JF, Storz LW. Vascular endoscopy: possibilities and limit of its clinical application. *Surg Clin North Am* 1974; 54: 111–22.

3. Crispin HA, Van Baarle AF. Intravascular observation and surgery using the flexible fibrescope. *Lancet* 1973; i: 750–1.

4. Towne JB, Berhard VM. Vascular endoscopy: useful tool or interesting toy. *Surgery* 1977; 82: 415–19.

5. Baxter BT, Rizzo RJ, Flinn WR *et al*. A comparative study of intraoperative angioscopy and completion arteriography following femorodistal bypass. *Arch Surg* 1990; 125: 997–1002.

6. Miller A, Campbell DR, Gibbons GW *et al*. Routine intraoperative angioscopy in lower extremity revascularization. *Arch Surg* 1989; 124: 604–8.

7. Hall KV. The great saphenous vein used in situ as an arterial shunt after extirpation of the vein valves: a preliminary report. *Surgery* 1962; 51: 492–5.

8. Fleisher HL, Tompson BW, McGowan TC *et al*. Angioscopically monitored saphenous vein valvulotomy. *J Vasc Surg* 1986; 4: 360–4.

9. Mehigan JT, Schell WW. Angioscopic control of in-situ saphenous vein arterial bypass. In: Moore WS, Ahn SS, eds. *Endovascular Surgery*. Philadelphia: WB Saunders, 1989: 82–6.

10. White GH, White RA, Kopchok GE, Wilson SE. Angioscopic thromboembolectomy: preliminary observations with a recent technique. *J Vasc Surg* 1988; 7: 318–25.

11. Miller A, Marcaccio E, Tannenbaum G *et al*. Comparison of angioscopy and angiography for monitoring infrainguinal bypass vein grafts: results of a prospective randomized trial. *J Vasc Surg* 1992; 15: 1078.

Arteriography

A. B. Ayers MD, FRCR
Consultant Radiologist, St Thomas' Hospital, London, UK

History

Although there was early recognition that the vascular system could be visualized by X-rays, it was not until the 1920s that radiologists were able to impress the medical and surgical fraternity that arteriography was clinically useful and important. Subsequent development was slow while the search for a safe intravascular contrast medium was pursued. Percutaneous needle puncture of the aorta, the carotid artery and other major arteries was developed and catheterization invariably required open access to an artery – usually the brachial or femoral. In 1953 Seldinger pioneered the percutaneous method of catheter introduction, and selective arteriography without the need for general anaesthesia became a reality. During the 1960s and 1970s demand for arteriography was at its height and there has been continuous development of catheters, guidewires, introduction sheaths and non-ionic low osmolar contrast media over the last decade. These developments have made arteriography a much safer and more freely available procedure throughout the world. Ironically, the demand for catheter arteriography is now diminishing with the introduction of new techniques such as digital subtraction, ultrasonography, dynamic computed tomographic scanning and magnetic resonance angiography.

This chapter describes the technical details of arteriography and outlines the new techniques for comparison and to indicate future potential.

Principles and justification

Indications

Although the risks are low, modern arteriography puts the patient at risk from ionizing radiation, iodine hypersensitivity, procedural discomfort and complications. The indication for investigation should be clear and the operator should understand what resulting information is required. The procedure to be undertaken and the radiographic exposures to be recorded are varied accordingly. There are two major categories: (1) organ arteriography, where definition of the circulation through a specific organ is required; and (2) 'anatomical' arteriography, where the 'plumbing' arrangements in the presence of arterial disease need to be defined. *Table 1* on pp. 81–83 gives an indication of the range and variation of the procedures.

Contraindications

There are no absolute contraindications to arteriography but there are many situations where it is wise to be resistant and to balance carefully need against risk and discomfort.

Wherever possible arteriography should be avoided in the pregnant patient. Sepsis or disease at the puncture site will increase risks of local complications. Bleeding disorders and anticoagulant therapy will increase the risk of haematoma formation and longer care after the procedure may be necessary. Systemic hypertension (diastolic pressure >100 mmHg) will similarly increase the local risks. There is much debate about the increased local risk of inserting needles and catheters into arterial grafts and, on the whole, this is best avoided if possible.

Equipment

Needles/cannulae

The original method of introducing contrast medium into the arterial system was by direct puncture of the artery, for which special needles were designed. For many years aortography was performed by translumbar needle puncture. Similarly, cerebral angiography was performed by direct puncture of carotid and vertebral arteries. In many instances general anaesthesia was needed and significant complications occurred. These areas are now usually studied by catheter procedures and direct needle injection is limited to the femoral and brachial arteries.

Today's needles are designed to gain atraumatic access to arteries for the introduction of wires, sheaths and catheters. Most have a basic design of an outer needle or cannula and an inner removable stylet. The stylet may be pointed or bevelled and is usually solid. The outer portion is usually metal and blunt ended so that it will not cause damage to the internal wall of the vessel.

The dimensions of these needles vary but are usually 7–12 cm in length and about 1 mm in outer diameter. The important selection is to choose the right needle for the purpose in hand. Clearly, smaller needles are used for children and small arteries. Cannulae usually have a metallic bevelled inner needle over which a thin polytetrafluoroethylene cannula fits snugly and can be advanced over the needle once the tip lies in the arterial lumen.

Wires

Wires are used through the puncture needle to gain access to the arterial system, and again there is a wide selection designed for different purposes. Most wires are made of steel with an inner straight wire and an outer wire which is tightly coiled. The main length of the wire is rigid but the tip which is introduced into the artery should be soft and flexible. For the majority of patients a simple straight wire will suffice but J wires are needed to pass through tortuous segments. J wires need to be straightened before introduction through the needle but take up their curve once in the artery.

In most cases the inner wire is fixed, but wires are available with a movable inner core which allows variation of the length of the flexible tip of the wire while it is in the artery and avoids the need for an exchange. A variety of diameters is available. The outer metal coil is coated with polytetrafluoroethylene to give a smooth surface. The inclusion of heparin in the coating to reduce the risk of thrombus formation has been popular, but this does not appear to have affected the incidence of this complication. Complex wire instruments are available which enable the operator to deflect the tip of the wire, but these are cumbersome and need considerable experience and expertise.

More recently, non-metallic hydrophilic wires have been introduced which become extremely slippery when wet. Their advantage is that they will pass stenoses and difficult curves more easily than the metallic wires, but they require considerable care as they can readily slide out of the artery and out of the operator's hands during use.

The wire to be used has to be selected in conjunction with catheter selection but in most adult cases a 0.035-in (8.89-mm) diameter wire, 100–150 cm long, is used. Very long wires (250 cm) are available when it is necessary to exchange a selective catheter for one of a different shape without losing access to the origin of the artery involved.

Dilators/sheaths

Dilators are rigid tubes with tapered tips which fit snugly over a guidewire and stretch the puncture hole through the soft tissues and arterial wall so that a softer catheter can subsequently be introduced without damage to its tip. Short, flexible connecting tubes with good locking connections are used for injection through needles, sheaths or dilators.

Sheaths are more rigid than cannulae and are used when multiple exchanges of wires and catheters are anticipated. They can be introduced either as part of a needle set or over a guidewire. The proximal end is fitted with a haemostatic valve through which wires and catheters can be passed without trauma to the arterial wall at the puncture site. The lumen of the sheath understandably has to be slightly larger (0.5 Fr) than the outer diameter of the largest catheter to be used, and therefore many sheath sets have a flexible side arm through which the sheath can be flushed with heparinized saline to prevent local thrombus formation while the catheter is in position.

Initially sheaths were not popular because of the need to use a size larger than the catheter needed to do the study, but as the use of small catheters has become more widespread the use of sheaths has become more acceptable. There is a good case for always using a sheath where selective catheterization is contemplated.

Catheters

1 There are many different catheters available to the angiographer, some of which are designed for specific procedures. A few of the basic shapes are illustrated. The shape and size of the catheter tip is chosen to suit the study anticipated and the shape and size of the patient. There are no rigid rules and practice varies considerably.

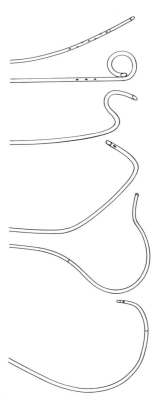

1

Catheters used for high-flow injections require multiple (12–16) side holes; catheters for selective studies should have 2–3 side holes to allow local exit of contrast without causing either a jet effect or recoil of the catheter tip during injection; catheters for small, highly selective injections or for embolization require a single end hole.

The pigtail catheter is used in preference to the straight flush catheter in situations where the vessels are tortuous and the walls considerably diseased with atheroma. It is the catheter of choice for traversing aneurysms and segments involved in dissection or other trauma.

Some of the selective catheters have to be straightened for introduction and their shape reconstructed within the aorta by using the opposite iliac vessels or branches of the aortic arch. In the latter case the operator should remember that extra length is required to reach the arch of the aorta even if the arteriography is limited to the abdomen.

Catheters are made of non-thrombotic substances such as polyethylene, polyurethane or nylon and are made to be as radio-opaque as possible. The wall thickness is reduced as far as possible to allow maximum lumen with the smallest outer diameter. However, the walls have to be thick enough to withstand the pressures required to inject contrast media and to provide torque control for manipulation.

Most catheters are introduced via the femoral artery and their length should be kept to the minimum required for the procedure. In practice 60–80-cm catheters are used for abdominal work and 100–120-cm catheters for the chest, neck, head and upper limbs. In adults most studies can be completed using 4-Fr or 5-Fr catheters and selection is dependent on the technical factors of flow rate requirement, catheter length, contrast medium viscosity and injection pump characteristics.

Clearly, the shape of catheter used for selective studies is very important and some radiologists still shape their own catheters for particular procedures. Some selections are shown in *Table 1* on pp. 81–83 but there is no substitute for experience.

Contrast media

A contrast medium for arteriography requires a high radiographic density, low viscosity, low toxicity and rapid excretion. The early contrast agents (e.g. thorium dioxide) were very toxic and were replaced by ionic iodinated compounds (iothalamate, diatrizoate and metrizoate) but these were viscous, caused a number of circulatory side effects, and were nephrotoxic. They have now been replaced by non-ionic iodinated compounds (iopamidol, iohexol and iopromide) which have a much lower osmolality (closer to that of plasma), virtually no cardiovascular side effects, and are thought to be less nephrotoxic. Patient acceptability is high. They still contain iodine and there is still a low risk of hypersensitivity reactions.

The radio-opacity of the compounds is related to the iodine concentration, which is indicated in milligrams per millilitre. For ordinary venous and arterial injections concentrations of 300–370 mg/ml are used, but where an arterial injection is being made in conjunction with digital subtraction radiography, 150–200 mg/ml is preferred.

The viscosity is lower in the lower concentrations and is also lowered by warming the contrast agent to body temperature. These factors are important in allowing hand injections, obviating the need for electrical pumps.

In general the total volume of non-ionic contrast used in an examination should not exceed 4–5 ml/kg of 300 mg/ml medium, i.e. 300–400 ml per patient. In some instances this guideline has been exceeded without difficulty in patients with normal renal function.

Drugs

Intravenous saline is required for flushing catheters and needles. Some operators add heparin to their flushing solution (1000–5000 units/l saline). Heparin may also be injected in higher concentrations during angioplasty procedures.

Sedatives such as diazepam (Diazemuls) may be given as a premedication or injected intravenously through butterfly cannulae during angiography for patient comfort. The author does not believe it is a necessary routine. Diazepam (Valium) can also be used as a premedicant.

Lignocaine (1–2%) is used in volumes of 5–10 ml for local anaesthesia at the puncture site. It can become toxic and larger volumes should be used with caution. Intravenous hyoscine butylbromide or glucagon may be used to reduce bowel movement in intravenous digital subtraction angiography of the abdomen. Blocking drugs for hypertensive crises and emergency medical support to treat cardiac arrests should be available.

In some parts of the world pharmacoangiography is used; the circulation being studied is altered before the injection of contrast medium but it is clinically beneficial in very few instances.

Injectors

While many selective injections can be made with a strong hand, a pressure injector is required when injecting large volumes of contrast into the heart, the pulmonary circulation, the aorta and its major branches.

A selection of commercial injectors which allow control of the volume, the flow rate and the pressure required is available. The injection can be linked with a trigger to radiographic exposure. Pressures of over 1000 p.s.i. can be tolerated by some catheters and these are needed for high injection rates through long narrow catheters. A means of warming the contrast medium to reduce its viscosity is important.

Radiographic equipment

A detailed description of radiographic apparatus is beyond the scope of this chapter but, in general, good results can only be obtained with good apparatus used to its maximum performance. The arteriographer needs to know what result is to be achieved and either have a thorough knowledge of radiographic equipment or trust in a first-class technician. It is very easy for the inexperienced to irradiate patients excessively and to waste quantities of film and contrast medium.

A good angiography room requires a high-output generator, high-quality fluoroscopy, a high-speed tube, fine focus, a suitable table, extensive movement facility and the means of recording rapid events with great detail. Most units are now mounted on a C arm or U arm to allow multiplanar imaging with minimal adjustment of patient position. For lumbar/lower limb arteriography a stepping tabletop movement is an advantage.

There are many ways of recording the procedure and the choice will depend very largely on the age of the equipment. Cine film, rapid-sequence cut film, multiformat small film, video, 105-mm rapid film and digital storage are all available and their advantages and disadvantages are hotly disputed. Where only cut film is available for a permanent record, a film changer capable of a rapid-sequence is required for most arteriography. Radiographic sequences need to be planned in advance of the injection and should be tailored to each procedure and to each patient. Digitalization of the fluoroscopic image with the ability to replay and to select which part of the examination is to form the permanent record has reduced the excessive use of rapid-sequence exposures. In the past, high-quality arteriography has only been available in a radiographic room but mobile C arm image intensifiers with high-quality digital subtraction images are now available for use in the operating theatre.

Radiation protection

This is a very important subject and refers not only to the protection of staff but to the protection of the patient from excessive exposure to ionizing radiation; it is governed by legislation in many countries. Local control of procedures involving ionizing radiation should be strict. Maintenance of equipment is important for the detection of radiation leakage and the maintenance of good performance. Suitable lead aprons and thyroid and eye protectors should be available and radiation protection authority well defined.

Preoperative

Preparation of patient

The patient should be assessed medically for the procedure, contraindications defined, risks explained and consent obtained. The site of puncture needs to be cleaned and shaved. It is wise to limit food intake for 2–4 h before arteriography but fluids should not be so restricted as to produce dehydration. If necessary, intravenous fluids should be provided in sick patients and intravenous access should be readily available if sedation is required.

Extra care should be taken when contemplating arteriography in patients with renal failure, hepatic failure, heart or respiratory failure, iodine hypersensitivity, sickle cell disease, diabetes or abnormal serum biochemistry. Patients with phaeochromocytomas may undergo a hypertensive crisis during arteriography and blocking drugs should be available. Arteriography should be carefully considered in patients with the Ehlers–Danlos syndrome and other connective tissue disorders including that caused by excess steroids. Where there is a previous history of iodine hypersensitivity the exact reaction should be ascertained and, where appropriate, steroid cover can be given and should be started 24 h before the arteriography.

The operator should be aware of the increased risks of infection from patients with hepatitis and human immunodeficiency virus infection, and appropriate safeguards should be taken for all staff.

Anaesthesia

The majority of arteriographic examinations are performed with the patient awake, using local anaesthesia at the puncture site. Oral or intravenous sedation may be used for patient comfort. Analgesia can be given, particularly to those patients suffering skeletal pain. General anaesthesia adds further risks to the procedure and should be reserved for the very young and for patients who cannot keep still. Pain or discomfort experienced during arteriography is an important warning sign and sedation should not interfere with a sensible rapport between the operator and the patient unless really necessary.

Techniques

Needle puncture

Intravenous

Intravenous digital angiography using a bolus technique may be performed from an intravenous cannula inserted into a good-sized vein at the elbow. Local anaesthesia is not usually required. A tourniquet is used to distend the vein and a 14-Fr or 16-Fr cannula/needle set is used to introduce a cannula into the vein for 1–2 cm. The cannula is fixed to the skin with tape and connected to an injector with flexible tubing capable of withstanding the pump pressure to be used – usually 150 p.s.i.

Arterial

Needle puncture of an artery should be performed at a site where the arterial pulse is easily palpable, the artery can be fixed in position, and the puncture site easily compressed following removal of the needle or catheter. Since the introduction of catheter procedures and digital subtraction angiography, direct puncture of the aorta, the carotid and the vertebral arteries is rarely warranted. Common sites for simple arterial puncture without catheterization are the common femoral and brachial arteries.

For femoral artery puncture the groin is shaved and cleaned. The femoral pulse should be examined and its strength assessed. Distal leg arterial pulsation and the state of the skin circulation of the feet should be noted. The skin is cleansed with antiseptic and the pulse identified high in the groin. Appropriate sterile gowns are applied. Local anaesthesia is infiltrated into the skin and around the artery. A small skin incision is made.

2a–c

A metal needle is held vertically between finger and thumb and inserted to rest on top of the artery when the pulse can be felt in the thumb. Experienced operators can attempt a single wall puncture but in most instances the needle is advanced through both walls of the artery. Support is given to the artery and soft tissues above the puncture site with the other hand while the hub of the needle is depressed gently in line with the artery over the upper thigh. The stylet is withdrawn and, using a gentle rotational movement, the needle is slowly withdrawn until a good pulsatile flow of bright red blood is obtained from the hub. If the flow is bright red but shows little pulsation the needle may need adjusting to lie centrally in the lumen. Non-pulsatile flow of bright red blood may occur distal to a stenosis, in which case it would be expected that a reduced pulse would have been noted before the procedure. The needle should be stabilized by the weight of saline-soaked swabs or be secured to the skin with tape and connected to a tap and flexible tubing. This should suffice for lower limb studies in most patients, but where the overlying soft tissue is deep the cannula needs to be advanced cranially in the artery, using an obturator or a short guidewire. Alternatively a polythene vessel dilator can be inserted over a guidewire. Free flow of blood should be checked with a syringe containing saline, which should be used to flush the needle regularly. A test injection of a few millilitres of contrast medium during fluoroscopy will confirm the correct position. Regular flushing with saline is required to prevent thrombus formation.

For a high brachial artery puncture the arm is abducted with the elbow extended. The radial pulse is noted. The brachial pulse is identified against the humeral shaft. The site is cleansed and draped and local anaesthesia is infiltrated. Pain or paraesthesia in the hand may be experienced if the adjacent nerves are irritated. A small skin incision is made and a 16-Fr or 18-Fr needle/cannula set is chosen. The brachial artery is stabilized with the index and middle fingers of one hand while a cannula needle is held in the fingers and thumb of the other. The artery is punctured obliquely through both walls in the line of the artery with the tip pointing centrally. The needle is slowly withdrawn until blood is obtained at the hub. The needle is held firm with one hand while the other gently advances the outer soft cannula into the arterial lumen. During this time flow from the hub will continue. The central metallic needle is withdrawn, and pulsatile blood should be seen from the hub of the cannula which is carefully connected to flexible tubing and lightly secured with tape. The cannula is flushed gently with saline, which should not cause pain. The patient may feel the cold saline pass to the hand. The intra-arterial position of the cannula is checked with a contrast injection under fluoroscopy. If a satisfactory intraluminal position of the tip is shown, the cannula can be further advanced into the artery for greater security and this is best performed

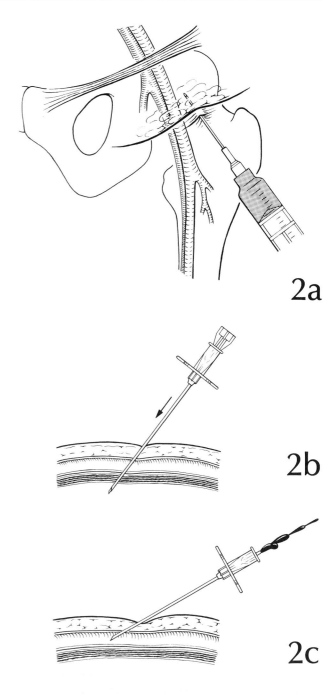

2a

2b

2c

while gently flushing with saline. The new position is checked as before and the cannula and connecting tube fixed with tape. The arm can now be moved to the patient's side and positioned for radiography.

For a low brachial artery puncture the same procedure is followed with the arm by the side and the hand supinated. Puncture is made into the brachial artery over the lower humerus.

The brachial artery is prone to spasm and a gentle and patient approach is required. The artery needs only light compression after the procedure and the radial pulse and the circulation to the fingers should always be checked.

Percutaneous arterial catheterization

The majority of catheter procedures are carried out through the common femoral artery with retrograde insertion of the catheter, but if this is impossible brachial and axillary routes may be used.

The preparation of the patient and the site of puncture is the same as described for arterial needle puncture except that it is often wise following skin incision in the groin to use a pair of fine pointed forceps to separate the soft tissues down towards the artery. This is particularly so where the tissues are fibrotic as a result of previous surgery, when there is an increased risk of damaging the tip of the catheter while introducing it. Before needle puncture, it should be ensured that the chosen guidewire and catheter are to hand and that the wire passes through the needle and catheter!

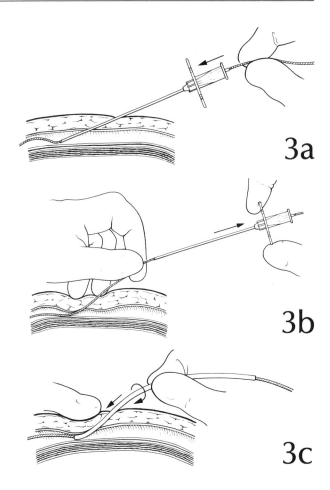

3a–c The needle is inserted through both arterial walls and withdrawn, as described in *Illustration 2b*, until a good pulsatile flow is obtained. While the hub of the needle is held close to the thigh the *soft* end of the wire is inserted through the cannula and passed into the iliac segment. This should occur with no resistance and only a gentle touch is required. If this is the case, the wire can be advanced into the lower aorta and its position checked by fluoroscopy. The needle is withdrawn over the wire and the wire held at the groin while gentle pressure is exerted over the artery. The wire is wiped with a saline-soaked swab and the catheter introduced over the wire. In general it is not necessary with 4-Fr and 5-Fr catheters to use dilators but if larger catheters are to be used serial dilatation over the wire is performed at this stage.

Before the catheter tip is inserted into the groin the caudal end of the wire should emerge from the catheter hub. If it does not, the wire should be withdrawn further until there is enough outside the patient to pass through the catheter. The catheter tip is then inserted into the femoral artery with a gentle rotational movement. The wire is slowly withdrawn as the catheter is advanced, and this can be monitored by fluoroscopy. The exchange of catheter over the wire is completed below the level of the renal arteries for aortography, but with some selective catheters the wire is maintained near the tip of the catheter until the correct position is obtained and the wire is then removed.

Flow through the catheter is checked and a tap is attached to the hub of the catheter. The catheter is flushed with saline and the tap is turned off while pressure is maintained on the syringe to prevent backflow of blood into the catheter tip.

Flushing of the catheter should be performed intermittently with a syringe. Pressure-bag continuous flushing is suitable for catheters with single end holes only.

If there is any resistance to the passage of the guidewire, fluoroscopy should be used to check its position. It may be necessary to change a straight wire for a J-tipped wire to pass through a tortuous iliac segment. If there is any doubt, the wire should be removed and the flow of blood from the needle tip reconfirmed. If resistance arises in the external iliac segment a retrograde injection of contrast medium under fluoroscopy should be made to check patency and possible stenoses. If the obstruction lies higher up it is possible to introduce a catheter over the wire in the external iliac artery and to inject contrast medium through the catheter while advancing it under fluoroscopic control. Usually, in this instance, it is wise to use a combination of a pigtail catheter and J wire. Alternatively, if the external iliac and common femoral segments are shown to be clear, a sheath should be introduced through which any combination of wire and catheter can be used, according to the circumstances prevailing.

Catheterization via arteriotomy

It is sometimes necessary to expose an artery surgically to introduce a catheter and this is often done in infants in preference to a percutaneous puncture of the brachial artery.

Protocols

Table 1 gives an indication of the standard protocols that can be used for arteriography. Much will depend on the type of radiographic equipment available, the expertise and experience of the operator and, above all, what is required of the examination.

Subtraction arteriography

This technique allows the subtraction of background data from images, providing a picture of the contrast distribution alone. For many years subtraction radiographs have been created from cut film by obtaining a negative film from an early mask radiograph without contrast and manually placing it over the radiograph of interest with contrast. A third radiograph is obtained by light exposure through the first two superimposed. This was time consuming and tedious but often valuable. Computer digitalization of data allows this process to be carried out instantaneously so that the result can be visualized during a contrast run. Furthermore, the mask may be changed easily and minor repositioning can be achieved electronically.

This system has significantly reduced the time and exposures required for arteriography and has greatly increased radiographic sensitivity so that similar images can be produced with a much lower concentration of iodine in the contrast medium. The technique has led to the development of intravenous digital subtraction angiography, avoiding the need for arterial puncture to study many of the major arteries. If arterial injection is preferred the concentration of the contrast medium can be reduced, allowing easier injections and reduced cost. Intra-arterial injections are still necessary to obtain fine detail and to study selected circulations.

The digital subtraction facility is now available on mobile image intensifiers and can be used in operating theatres. This opens new channels for intraoperative management of patients, allowing angioplasty or embolization to take place synchronously with surgery.

Aortography

The aorta can be readily visualized by intravenous digital subtraction angiography.

An intravenous cannula is placed into a vein at the elbow or, if needed, into the femoral vein. Contrast medium, 30–50 ml of 370 mg iodine/ml, is injected at 12–14 ml/s, followed immediately by 30 ml saline. This can be achieved from a single syringe using the 'layering' technique in which saline is first drawn into a syringe, followed by the required quantity of contrast drawn up with the syringe vertical and inverted. The contrast medium forms a layer below the saline. A flexible tube is used to connect the tube to a tap attached to the cannula. Injection of the total volume of contrast and saline bolus is made with the syringe maintained in this position. Care must be taken to ensure that the syringe and tubing are free of air. Alternatively, a multiple side-hole catheter can be introduced from an arm vein to lie in the superior vena cava and 30–50 ml of contrast medium injected at 15 ml/s.

Visualization of the aorta depends upon the bolus being maintained through the heart and pulmonary circulations. Time for this passage is allowed before imaging is started. Clearly the quality of the images obtained with this technique depends heavily on cardiac output. Poor output and dilated, poorly functioning heart chambers degrade the image. The thoracic aorta is visualized in right and left anterior oblique projections, and the abdominal aorta in frontal and occasionally lateral projections. Temporary bowel paralysis is usually required to avoid movement artefacts in the abdomen.

For intra-arterial studies a pigtail catheter is preferred for thoracic aortic injections. The catheter is placed in the ascending aorta well away from the aortic valve. High flow rates are required (20–24 ml/s) and the catheter chosen must be able to withstand the high pressures required (>1000 p.s.i.) without splitting. In the thoracic aorta 50–80 ml of high-concentration contrast medium are injected. If digital subtraction is being used in conjunction with an intra-arterial injection this volume is maintained but the contrast medium can be diluted to 150–200 mg iodine/ml, thereby reducing viscosity and the pressure required for high flows.

Table 1 Protocols for aortography and selective arteriography (normal sized adult)

Examination	Method			Contrast medium		
	Route	Needle or catheter	Imaging	Concentration (mg iodine/ml)	Volume (ml)	Rate (ml/s) (Pressure)
Thoracic aortography (AP, LAO, RAO)	Peripheral i.v. DSA	16-Fr PTFE cannula, antecubital fossa	5–10-s delay, 1/s	370	30–50 + 30 saline	12–14 (Low)
	SVC DSA	65-cm multiple side-hole 4–5-Fr catheter	5-s delay, 1/s	370	25–40	12–14 (Low)
	i.a. DSA	Pigtail 5-Fr 90-cm catheter	No delay, 3/s	300	60	20–25 (High)
	i.a. cut film	Pigtail 5-Fr 90-cm catheter	No delay, 3/s for 5 s	370	75–100	20–25 (High)
Abdominal aortography (AP, lateral)	i.v. DSA	16-Fr PTFE cannula	>8-s delay, 1/s	370	40–50 + 30 saline	12–14 (Low)
	SVC DSA	Multiple side-hole 4–5-Fr catheter	>8-s delay, 1/s	370	25–40	12–14 (Low)
	i.a.	Multiple side-hole 4–5-Fr catheter	No delay; arterial 2/s for 4 s; capillary 1/s for further 6 s; venous 1/2–3 s for further 12+ s	370	50–80	20–24 (High)
Lower limb angiography Aorta – ankle	i.v. DSA	16-Fr PTFE cannula, antecubital fossa	>8-s delay, 1/s	370	40–50 + 30 saline	12–14 (Low)
	SVC DSA	65-cm multiple side-hole 5-Fr catheter	>8-s delay, exposures 1/s at each level	370	25–50	12–14 (Low)
	i.a. DSA	Pigtail 4-Fr catheter	1–2/s at each level with overlap	150–200	50	15 (Medium)
	Aorta – ankle, stepping table, cut film	Pigtail 4-Fr or straight 4-Fr catheter below renals	1–2-s delay, 3 exposures 1/s at each level + 4 films at every other second at ankle	370	75–100	15 (Medium)
Femoral arteriography	Femoral i.a. ipsilateral retrograde	16-G needle 5-Fr dilator	DSA: 1–2/s at each level, delay as required for distal sites	150–200	20	Hand
			Cut film: moving table, 1/s in each position and delayed films at ankle	370	50	8 ml/s or hand
			Cut film: separate sites, 1–2/s	370	30	8 ml/s or hand (Strong)
	Contralateral catheter	Cobra 5-Fr, sidewinder 5-Fr catheters	DSA: 1–2/s at each level delay as required for distal sites	150–200	20	8 ml/s
			Cut film: moving table, 1/s in each position and delayed films at ankle	370	50	8 ml/s or hand
			Cut film: separate sites, 1–2/s	370	30	8 ml/s or hand (Strong)

Table 1 *Continued*

Examination	Method			Contrast medium		
	Route	*Needle or catheter*	*Imaging*	*Concentration (mg iodine/ml)*	*Volume (ml)*	*Rate (ml/s) (Pressure)*
Popliteal arteriography	Antegrade catheter	Multipurpose 5-Fr/4-Fr, cobra 5-Fr/4-Fr, Mani catheters	DSA: 2/s Cut film: 2/s for 3 s	150–200 300	10 10	Hand Hand
Selective abdominal angiography						
Coeliac axis (AP, lateral)	Femoral catheter	65-cm cobra 5-Fr, 90-cm sidewinder 5-Fr catheters	Cut film: 1–2/s for 4 s, 1/s for 6 s, 1/2–3 s for remainder (total 18–20 exposures); delayed exposures for portal vein	370	40–80	6–10 (Medium)
			DSA: 1/s for duration	300/150–200	40	10 (Medium)
Common hepatic	Femoral selective catheter	65-cm cobra 5-Fr catheter	As above	370	20–40	6–8 (Medium) or hand
Gastroduodenal	Femoral selective catheter	65-cm cobra 5-Fr catheter	As above	300	10–15	Hand
Splenic	Femoral selective catheter	65-cm cobra 5-Fr catheter	As above	370 for portal vein	50 60–100	6–8 6–8 (Medium)
Superior mesenteric	Femoral selective catheter	65-cm cobra 5-Fr, 90-cm sidewinder 5-Fr catheters	Cut film as above DSA: 1/s for duration	370 150–200	50–70 50	6–8 8
Inferior mesenteric	Femoral selective catheter	65-cm cobra 5-Fr, 90-cm sidewinder 5-Fr catheters	Cut film as above DSA	300 150–200	15–30 20	Hand Hand
Renal	Femoral selective catheter	65-cm femororenal 5-Fr catheter	Cut film as above DSA	370 150–200	6–15 6–15	4–6 or hand Hand
Upper limb						
Upper arm	Femoral catheter	90-cm sidewinder 5-Fr catheter	Cut film: 2/s for 4 s	300	10–15	4–8 or hand
Forearm	Femoral catheter	90-cm sidewinder 5-Fr catheter	Cut film: 2/s, 3–4/s for fistulae	300	10	4–6 or hand
	Brachial cannula	18–20-G PTFE cannula	DSA 3/s	150–300	10	Hand
Head and neck						
General	i.v. DSA	16-G PTFE cannula, antecubital fossa	1–2/s	370	30–50 + 30 saline	12–14
	i.a. DSA arch	Pigtail 5-Fr	1–2/s	300	60	20–25 (High)
	Femoral selective catheter	90-cm Mani, 90-cm side-winder 5-Fr	1–2/s	300	10–15	Hand
	i.a. arch, injection per femoral	Pigtail 5-Fr catheter	Cut film No delays, 3/s for 5 s	370	75–100	20–25 (High)

Table 1 *Continued*

Examination	Method			Contrast medium		
	Route	*Needle or catheter*	*Imaging*	*Concentration (mg iodine/ml)*	*Volume (ml)*	*Rate (ml/s) (Pressure)*
Selective						
Common carotid	Transfemoral catheter		2/s for 3 s	300	10–15	Hand
	Bifurcation	Mani or sidewinder 5-Fr, 90-cm	2/s for 3 s	300	10–15	Hand
	Cerebral	Mani or sidewinder 5-Fr, 90-cm	Cut film: 2/s for 2 s, 1/s for 6 s	300	10–15	Hand
Internal carotid	Cerebral	Mani or sidewinder 5-Fr, 90-cm	Cut film as above DSA: 2/s	300 150–200	8–10 8–10	Hand Hand
Vertebral	Cerebral	Mani or sidewinder 5-Fr, 90-cm	Cut film as above DSA: 2/s	300 150–200	4–8 4–8	Hand Hand

AP, anteroposterior; DSA, digital subtraction radiography; LAO, left anterior oblique; PTFE, polytetrafluoroethylene; RAO, right anterior oblique; SVC, superior vena cava

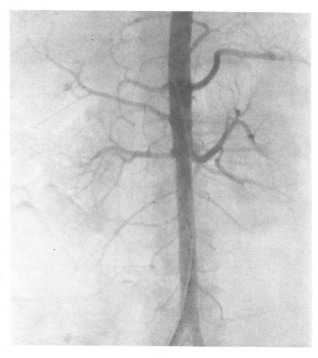

4 For the abdominal aorta either a straight flush or a pigtail catheter is suitable; it is placed over the 12th thoracic vertebral body and contrast medium, 50–60 ml of 370 mg iodine/ml, is injected at 20–22 ml/s. Imaging during the arterial phase only is often all that is required for 'plumbing' problems but for organ visualization imaging during the capillary and venous phases is also required. This may take over 20 s after injection and would carry a considerable radiation risk if the rapid rate of exposure required for arterial events were maintained throughout.

Lateral abdominal aortography is required when disease at the origins of the coeliac axis, superior mesenteric and inferior mesenteric arteries is suspected. Arterial phase imaging only is required.

A left axillary/brachial artery approach may be required when severe lower limb disease is present.

4

Selective arteriography

It is difficult to give comprehensive advice. Untutored, unsupervised and inexperienced selective arteriography can lead to major disasters. *Table 1* on pp. 81–83 gives outline details of the techniques used.

Carotid, vertebral and cerebral arteriography

5a–c Neurological sequelae may follow arteriography of the head and neck, whether by direct puncture (no longer advised) or by selective arteriography. Meticulous attention to detail is required here above all. Intravenous digital subtraction angiography or imaging from an aortic arch injection will often suffice to indicate atheromatous disease at the carotid bifurcation. Selective catheterization is required in many other instances and should only be undertaken by experts.

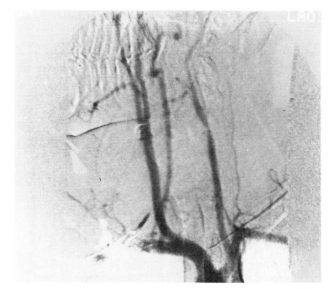

5a

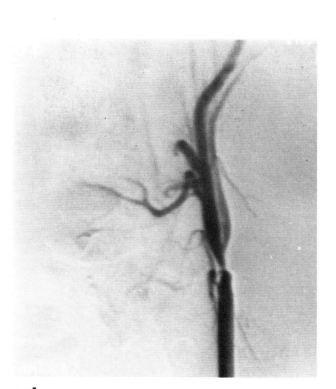

5b

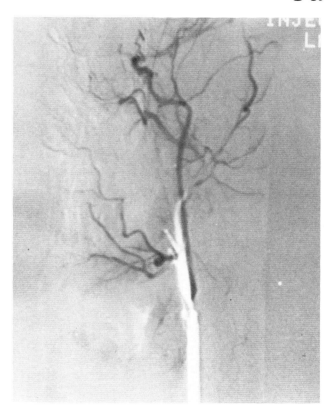

5c

Upper limb

6 Selective catheterization via a femoral puncture is the route preferred by many but it carries a risk of cerebral emboli from atheroma in the arch of the aorta or its major branches if these are traversed or inadvertently entered. An acceptable alternative for imaging of the forearm is a direct puncture of the brachial artery. A very rapid sequence of imaging may be required when investigating fistulae. Fine-focus detailed macroangiography is useful in examining the digital arteries.

Chest and neck

Selective studies of the thyroid, internal mammary and bronchial arteries can be performed for diagnostic and therapeutic (embolization) purposes. These studies may be difficult and should not be attempted by the inexperienced.

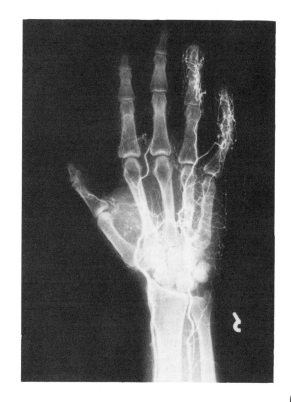

6

Abdomen

7a–d Selective studies of the abdominal organs are very common. It is wise to obtain an abdominal aortogram beforehand to identify the anatomy. There are many anatomical variations of arterial supply in the abdomen and the operator should be familiar with them to avoid excessive contrast injections and multiple radiation exposures. Cobra catheters will suffice for the majority and are easier to control and manipulate than the sidewinder type of catheter, which requires reformatting after introduction. However, the latter may be needed to get into the territory of the coeliac axis. Renal artery catheterization is relatively straightforward except when there is marked tortuosity or aneurysm formation of the abdominal aorta or iliac arteries.

Selective arterial studies of the adrenal glands have virtually been replaced by computed tomography and should not be undertaken lightly as there is a major risk of adrenal infarction.

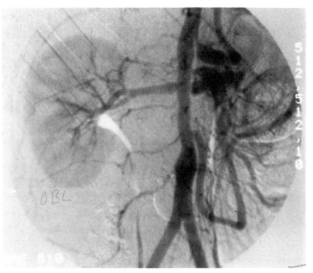

7a

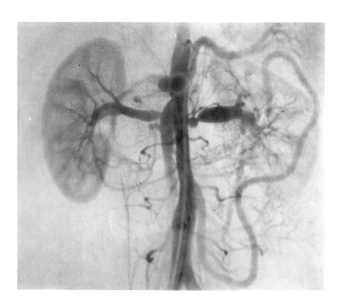

7b

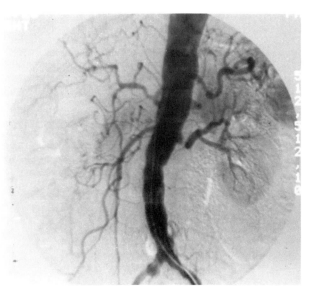

7c

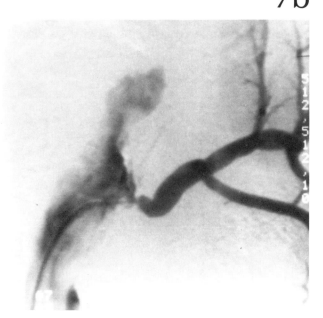

7d

8   Whenever selective catheterization of small arteries is performed great care must be taken to avoid thrombosis and embolization. The catheter may block the artery and, if continuous flushing is not used, thrombosis will ensue. Catheters should be withdrawn into a major artery as soon as possible. Thoraco-abdominal selective catheterization must always be carried out with a thorough knowledge of the variations of the arterial supply to the spinal cord. The main spinal artery of Adamkiewicz frequently arises at the thoraco-lumbar junction and damage to it must be avoided.

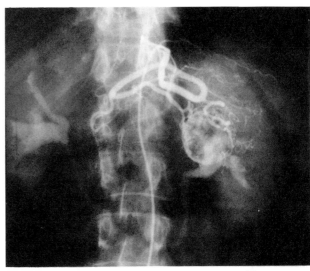

8

In general, selective catheterization is successfully performed by a combination of correct selection of catheter and gentle rotational and linear adjustment to the position of the catheter tip; on occasion, the judicious use of the guidewire to alter the shape and torque of the catheter is needed to gain access to the origin of an artery. Many of the newer thin-walled catheters are liable to kink at the groin during manipulation unless the guidewire is inserted through this segment. If catheter and guidewire are advanced together, with the tip of the guidewire proximal to the tip of the catheter, there is an increased risk of thrombus forming in the catheter tip and subsequently being flushed into the circulation. When flushing, blood should always be withdrawn into the syringe before saline is injected. If free flow is not obtained, the catheter is withdrawn into the aorta below the origin of the renal artery before a further injection is attempted. If in doubt, the catheter should be changed. In this situation, of course, the use of a sheath with a haemostatic valve at the groin avoids the need to pass a wire through the thrombosed segment of the catheter.

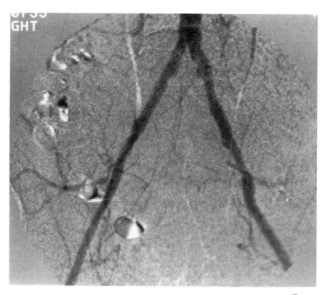

9a

Lower limb

9a–g Studies of the arterial supply to the lower limbs are very common and satisfactory images can be obtained by intravenous digital subtraction angiography in most patients, but only to the level of the popliteal trifurcation. Intestinal movement artefacts may be a significant problem over the aorta and the common iliac arteries. Many still prefer intra-arterial injections, whether or not digital subtraction is being used.

Alternatively, visualization of the lower aorta and the whole of both lower limbs can be achieved by a single aortic injection and a table top which moves in a stepwise fashion. This 'run' can be supplemented by further studies at single sites as necessary. The problem is to get the timing right for both limbs and to minimize the volume of contrast injected. Latterly this has become less of a problem with the use of non-ionic contrast media and digital subtraction. In most instances a multiple side-hole catheter is introduced into the lower abdominal aorta and the injection of 60–100 ml of high-concentration contrast medium at 15 ml/s is made. Three exposures at 1/s are made at each position of the table, allowing 1.5 s for movement between positions. More radiographs can be added at the ankle.

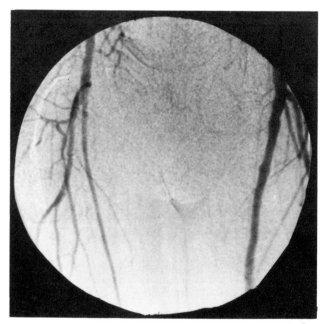

9b

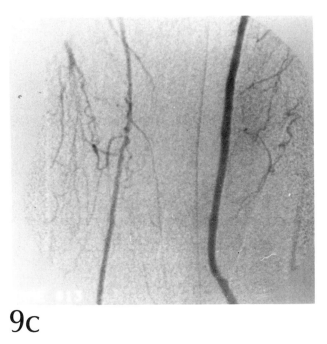

9c

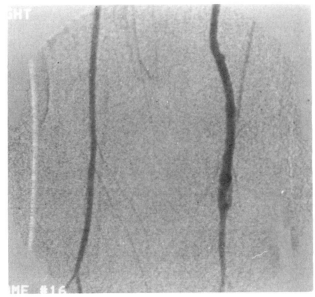

9d

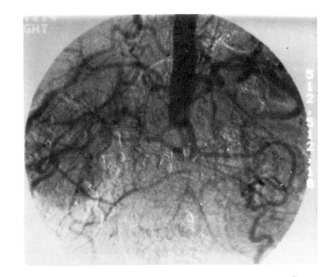

9e

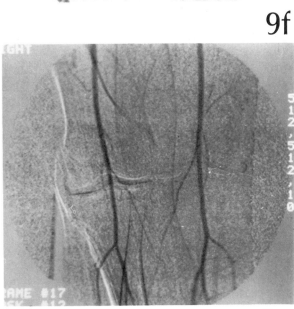

9f

9g

10a–d In many instances greater detail of distal arteries is required, necessitating unilateral injection into the common femoral artery. Ipsilateral needle puncture using a short cannula or dilator will often suffice. If there is no direct access, contralateral catheterization can be performed with a selective catheter which is manipulated over the aortic bifurcation and advanced antegradely down the affected limb. Similarly, catheters can be introduced via brachial or axillary puncture when necessary.

Direct antegrade catheterization of the common femoral artery can be performed for access to the superficial femoral and distal arteries for diagnostic arteriography, angioplasty and embolization. A high puncture of the common femoral artery is desirable to avoid entering the origin of the deep femoral artery which lies posterior to the main channel.

Contrast medium, 20–25 ml of 300–370 mg iodine/ml, is injected into the common femoral arteries and proportionately less more distally. Radiographic sequences other than 1/s are often necessary where stenosing disease causes significant delays in flow. Faster sequences are needed to study arteriovenous malformations.

Postoperative care

It is very important that haemostasis is obtained immediately after arterial procedures and this is achieved by exerting pressure on the puncture site for a minimum of 5 min. This time should be increased where there is a prolonged coagulation time and in the presence of hypertension. Excessive pressure is said to be a cause of distal thrombosis. The state of distal pulses and of the distal skin circulation at the end of the examination should be noted and brief details of the procedure, including the type and volume of contrast medium used, recorded. It is often useful, for future reference, to record which catheters were successfully used during the procedure.

It is possible to perform 4-Fr and 5-Fr single catheter arterial studies without the need for overnight hospitalization. The patient should rest for at least 4 h after arterial puncture and be accompanied for the next 24 h. Excessive movement of the leg should be discouraged but if good haemostasis has been obtained immediately after the procedure it is unlikely that haemorrhage will occur later. The patient is advised to apply light pressure to the puncture site when moving or coughing. Routine pulse and pressure records are not required after 4 h unless medically indicated.

Complications

General

Reactions to the contrast media used during arteriography occur in fewer than 3% of patients. Major reactions occur in fewer than 0.15% and fatalities in 0.005%. Hypersensitivity reactions are not dose related and therefore skin testing is not recommended. Toxic effects are dose related and are difficult to predict, but occur more frequently in dehydrated patients and those with renal and cardiac disease. Hypersensitivity reactions include bronchospasm and acute anaphylaxis. Toxic reactions include cardiac arrhythmias, cardiac arrest, pulmonary oedema and a feeling of peripheral warmth due to vasodilatation. Vasovagal attacks may occur during the procedure, particularly in nervous patients who are not adequately sedated. This can be a problem in elderly patients where diazepam can cause confusion.

In general most complications can be avoided, or at least the incidence reduced to a minimum, by meticulous attention to detail before, during and after arteriography.

Local

Embolization
Thrombotic embolization rarely occurs distal to an arterial puncture site unless there is local arterial disease present at the time of the examination. Distal small emboli may occur in the toes, reducing circulation and producing discoloration. Large emboli will block the popliteal artery or straddle the trifurcation. Surgical intervention or clot dissolution therapy needs to be rapid to be effective.

Thrombosis
Thrombosis of the femoral artery at the puncture site has not occurred in the author's experience but may occur from overzealous compression after the procedure.

Dissection
Intimal dissection at the puncture site may occur during introduction of a guidewire. The guidewire may be advanced some distance unless the operator is careful and sensitive to any resistance felt during the passage of the wire. If the wire and needle are withdrawn there are very rarely any significant sequelae. Repuncture is often successful but another site may be preferred.

Dissection also occurs during selective catheterization due to manipulation of the catheter or guidewire tip. The common hepatic artery seems particularly susceptible, possibly because of its shape.

Particular care should be taken where atheromatous plaques are present in the aorta or carotid arteries.

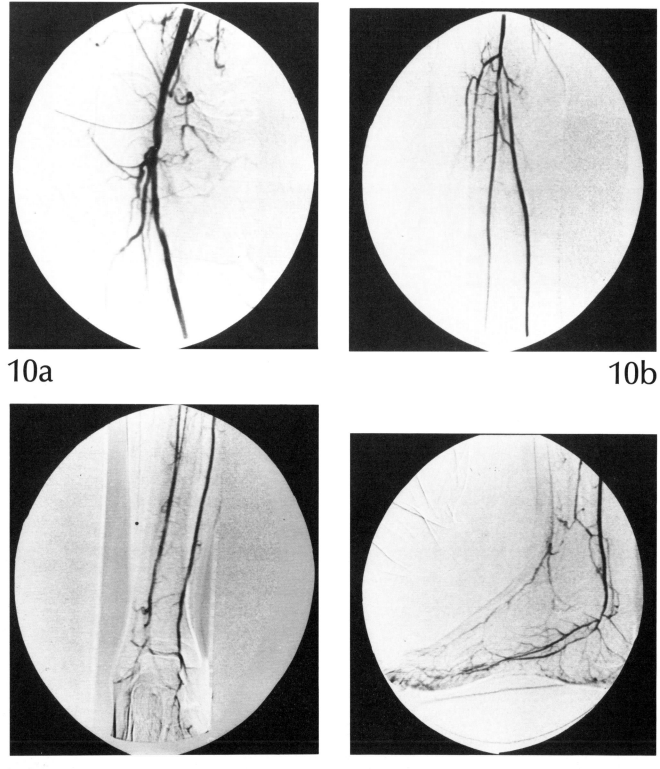

10a

10b

10c

10d

False aneurysm

A false aneurysm may be a late sequel at the puncture site, particularly if a subcutaneous clot is allowed to form or the patient is allowed to mobilize too quickly. Such aneurysms may be readily shown by colour flow ultrasonographic studies and careful compression over the neck of the aneurysm may be effective treatment. Otherwise surgical repair is necessary.

Arteriovenous fistula

A rare local complication in the groin is the formation of an arteriovenous fistula between the femoral artery and vein. Puncture of both structures, whether inadvertent or not, is necessary. Simultaneous ipsilateral catheterization of the femoral artery and vein should be avoided wherever possible.

Other imaging modalities

Whereas angiography may remain as a gold standard for arterial imaging, much can be achieved in selected situations by the other imaging modalities of ultrasonography, computed tomography and magnetic resonance. Ultrasonography and magnetic resonance imaging have the advantage of not subjecting the patient to exposure to ionizing radiation.

Ultrasonography

11a–c Simple ultrasonography is useful in the diagnosis and follow-up of aneurysms, the common sites for which are the abdominal aorta and the common femoral and popliteal arteries. The length and diameters (luminal and external) of the aneurysm are easily defined. In the aorta it can be difficult to define the relationship of an aneurysm to the origins of the renal arteries, and distended gas-filled loops of intestine degrade the quality of the examination. Duplex ultrasonographic scanning combines ultrasonography with Doppler analysis of blood flow and is very valuable at the carotid bifurcation. It may also be used to 'track' the femoral and popliteal arteries where stenoses and blocks may be analysed, but this is difficult and time consuming. Colour flow is an additional facility that has made flow analysis by Doppler much quicker and easier. Alterations in normal laminar flow due to stenoses are easily identified before spectral analysis. The technique is now also valuable in assessing organ flow, particularly in the liver, kidneys and their transplants.

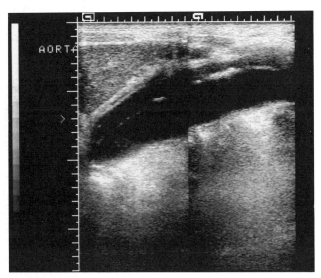

11a

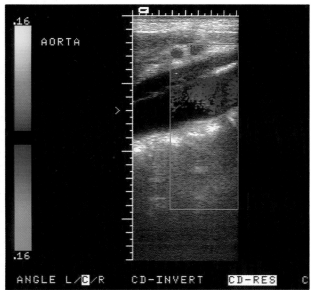

11b

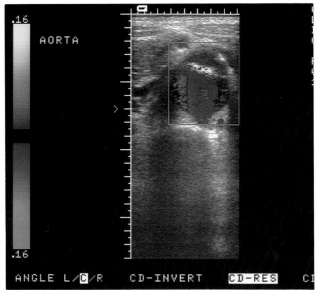

11c

Computed tomography

12a–e The aorta and major vessels can be visualized by computed tomography without contrast enhancement but excellent visualization of the lumen is obtained if dynamic scanning is performed during contrast infusion. Aortic rupture, dissection and aneurysm can be readily demonstrated in the thorax and abdomen. In the abdomen, details of luminal thrombus, wall calcification and periaortic fibrosis are shown much more clearly than by ultrasonography.

To avoid excessive radiation dose a combination of computed tomographic scanning and ultrasonography is recommended for the diagnosis and follow-up of abdominal aneurysms.

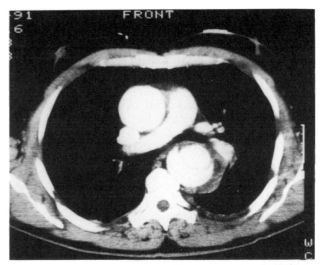

12a

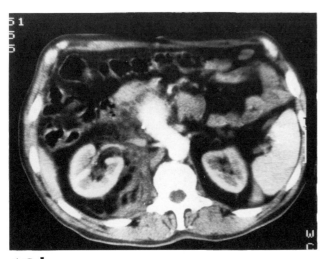

12b

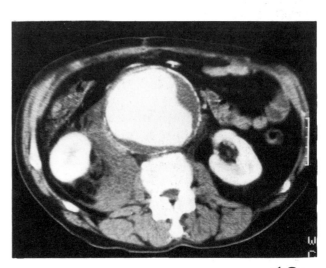

12c

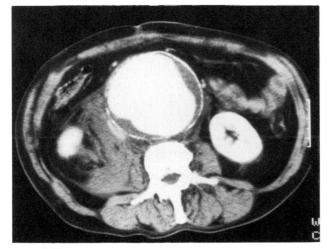

12d

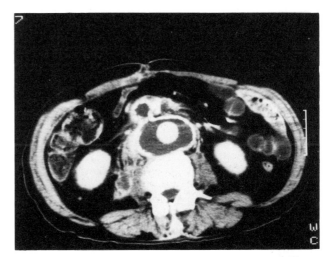

12e

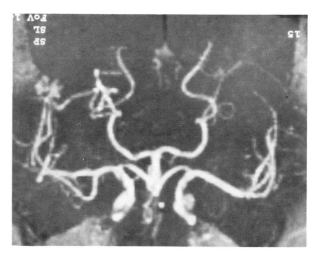

13a

Magnetic resonance imaging

13a–c This is a new technique which does not involve ionizing radiation and in which multiplanar cross-sectional images of the body are obtained. In most magnetic resonance image sequences moving blood is shown by a signal void but new sequences have been developed specifically to identify arteries. A new era of magnetic resonance angiography is emerging and the technique may become a major tool in the diagnosis of vascular diseases.

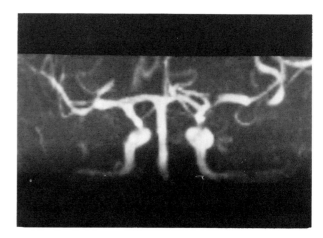

13b

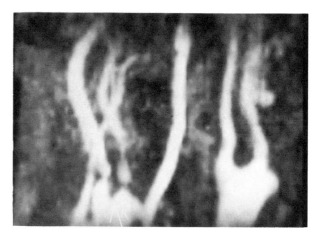

13c

Carotid body and cervical paragangliomas

J. W. Hallett Jr MD
Associate Professor, Section of Vascular Surgery, Mayo Clinic and Mayo Foundation, Rochester, Minnesota, USA

History

Carotid body or cervical paragangliomas are rare cases for most surgeons. In addition, these tumours have a reputation for being difficult to resect because of impressive vascularity, arterial adherence and local cranial nerve involvement. In fact, stroke and cranial nerve dysfunction remain sobering risks of surgical resection (*Table 1*). However, recent advances in preoperative evaluation and surgical technique have reduced perioperative complications to a reassuringly low level. The following surgical strategy and technique is based upon our long-term experience with over 150 carotid and cervical paragangliomas treated and followed at the Mayo Clinic over the past 50 years[1].

This chapter discusses three primary components of surgical management. First, which carotid body and cervical paragangliomas need resection? Second, what are the necessary preoperative tests before tumour resection? Third, what are the technical steps that maximize complete tumour resection but minimize neurovascular complications?

Table 1 Postoperative complications

	1935–1965	1966–1975	1976–1986
Tumours	70	46	37
Stroke	16(23)*	4 (9)	1(2.7)
Cranial nerve dysfunction	32(46)	14(30)	15(40)
Respiratory obstruction or tracheostomy	4 (6)	1 (2)	0
Mortality	4 (6)	1 (2)	0

*$P = 0.003$. Values in parentheses are percentages

Principles and justification

Indications

1 Regardless of age, nearly all patients with carotid body and cervical paragangliomas should undergo surgical removal of the tumour. This recommendation is not based upon the malignant potential since most of these tumours do not rapidly invade local structures or metastasize to distal sites. These tumours do, however, enlarge slowly but relentlessly to encase the carotid arteries and adjacent cranial nerves. They may be present for many years, even decades, before their growth causes symptoms. Eventually they cause local discomfort, cranial nerve deficits, dysphagia or death from metastases. Malignant invasion or metastasis is significantly more common in younger patients with familial, bilateral or multiple paragangliomas. Finally, neurovascular complications are much less common when tumours are resected at a smaller rather than a larger size. Stroke and cranial nerve deficits rise dramatically when tumours exceed a volume of 7 cm^3. Consequently, early resection is recommended.

In a few select situations, observation of a carotid body or cervical paraganglioma may be wiser than operation. Such an example would be an asymptomatic small tumour noted incidentally in a medically debilitated elderly patient with limited life expectancy. Observation is also appropriate in a patient with bilateral carotid body tumours when resection of one tumour has caused stroke or cranial nerve dysfunction on that side (vocal cord paralysis, swallowing dysfunction or unilateral tongue paresis). Finally, computed tomography (CT) and magnetic resonance image (MRI) scanning allow accurate monitoring of small paragangliomas that may arise high in the neck or near the skull

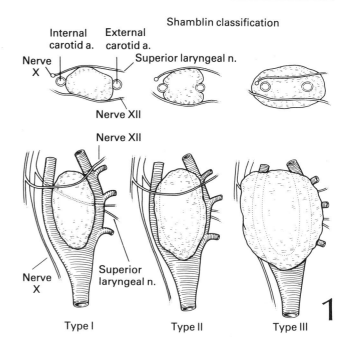

1

base where the risks of resection are heightened. Consultation with a neurosurgeon and a head and neck surgeon assists the general vascular surgeon in ascertaining the advisability of resecting such unusual glomus tumours.

Preoperative

Several important questions must be answered before operative intervention. What is the extent of the tumour? Are other cervical paragangliomas present? Is there any associated intrinsic carotid artery disease, especially associated atheromatous disease at the carotid bifurcation? Is there any preoperative cranial nerve dysfunction? Finally, is the tumour metabolically active, i.e. secreting catecholamines?

Tumour imaging

2 Several imaging methods can now diagnose and define the anatomy of a carotid body or cervical paraganglioma. The simplest method of ascertaining whether a neck mass is a carotid body tumour is colour flow duplex ultrasonography[2]. The tumour can be localized to the carotid bifurcation, and its vascularity can provide a rather impressive display of colour in the mass. Ultrasound can also be used to measure tumour size and search the carotid arteries for any sign of atheromatous stenosis. The limitation of colour-flow duplex ultrasonography is its inability to look low or high in the neck for other paragangliomas.

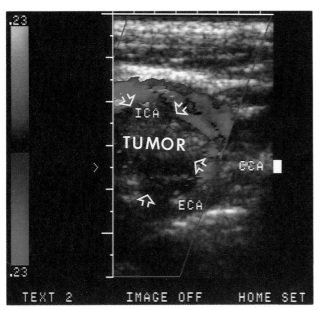

2

3a, b If multiple paragangliomas are suspected or if the identified tumour is extremely large, CT or MRI scanning is useful. These methods can clearly show the upper and lower limits of the neck region. They may also reveal tumour encasement of local structures or invasion into the skull. MRI and angiography are probably sufficient preoperative evaluation for many patients.

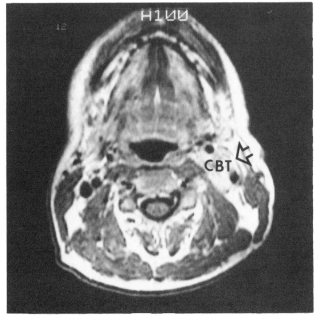

3a

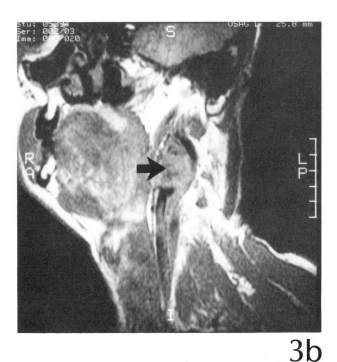

3b

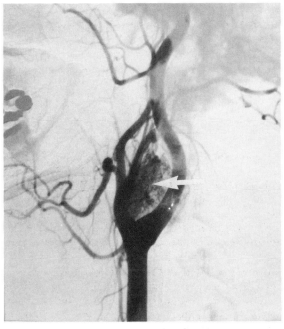

4

4 Finally, selective carotid arteriogaphy remains a useful adjunct in preoperative evaluation. Classically, the diagnostic method of choice has been arteriography since it demonstrates the characteristic hypervascularity of the tumour. An angiogram is also extremely sensitive in identifying additional cervical paragangliomas that are small and unsuspected. Of course, this remains an excellent method to delineate any atheromatous disease of the carotid bifurcation or internal carotid artery. For large tumours (Shamblin type III; *see Illustration 1*) the angiogram remains essential for preoperative tumour embolization that can decrease both troublesome vascularity and tumour size[3].

Cranial nerve involvement

Approximately 10% of patients with cervical paragangliomas present with a preoperative cranial nerve deficit. Consequently, careful assessment of these nerves is mandatory before operation. This examination should include indirect laryngoscopy to document vocal cord movement. When unilateral vocal cord paralysis is discovered and the hypervascular tumour appears adjacent to, but *not* in, the carotid bifurcation, a paraganglioma of the vagus nerve should be suspected.

Metabolic activity

Unlike other neural crest tumours, most carotid body and cervical paragangliomas do not secrete significant levels of catecholamines. Thus, routine urinary metanephrines or catecholamines are not necessary. In over 100 patients we have observed only three symptomatic patients with carotid body tumours and markedly elevated urinary catecholamines. They all had distinct symptoms, including headaches, palpitations, hypertension, photophobia, diaphoresis and dysrhythmias. All three patients had other paragangliomas. Consequently, preoperative catecholamine screening is indicated in patients who have symptoms suggestive of catecholamine excess, particularly those that have familial, bilateral or other associated paragangliomas.

Operative strategy

Our experience has been extensive enough to recommend ten key concepts that maximize complete tumour removal and minimize the risk of neurovascular morbidity.

Anaesthesia

General nasotracheal anaesthesia is recommended. A nasotracheal tube allows greater displacement of the floor of the mouth during retraction and dissection beneath the mandible. Although it is seldom necessary, subluxation of the mandible may improve exposure of large tumours that extend toward the base of the skull. Continuous electroencephalographic (EEG) monitoring is optional but does provide a sensitive method to detect hemispheric problems if internal carotid blood flow is interrupted for any reason (e.g. kinking by retraction, severe spasm with thrombosis or clamping during arterial repair). Elevation of the patient's head by 30–45° decreases jugular venous distension and may minimize cerebral oedema from any carotid clamping.

Operation

Internal carotid blood flow must be protected and maintained throughout the procedure. In the past, carotid artery ligation was utilized to control haemorrhage and allow complete tumour resection. Sacrifice of internal carotid blood flow resulted in a perioperative stroke rate that approached 25%. Such a high stroke rate is obviously no longer acceptable. None the less, some patients still require arterial repair or replacement. Consequently, a saphenous vein site should be prepared for possible arterial repair or replacement. Carotid shunts should also be ready.

Most patients (67%) require no arterial repair[1]. In about 10%, simple lateral suture repair of the carotid artery will be necessary. More complicated arterial reconstruction (patch, graft or end-to-end anastomosis) may be necessary in up to 25%. A carotid shunt is required in only 10%. The risk of neurovascular complications, however, is significantly higher in patients who require any type of arterial repair[1]. In fact, nearly all strokes occur in patients who have arterial repair or replacement during tumour excision. Advances in arterial management and repair have reduced the risk of stroke to approximately 2–3% for all cases[1] (*Table 1*).

Incision

5 The cervical incision must provide clear and adequate exposure for both vascular control and cranial nerve preservation. For small tumours (less than 3–4 cm in diameter), the best incision is along the anterior border of the sternocleidomastoid muscle, an approach that is relatively standard for carotid endarterectomy.

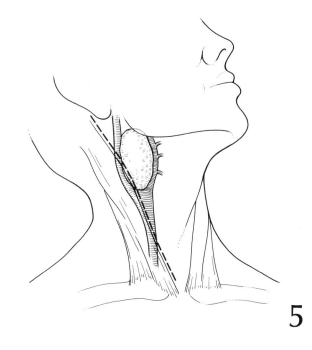

5

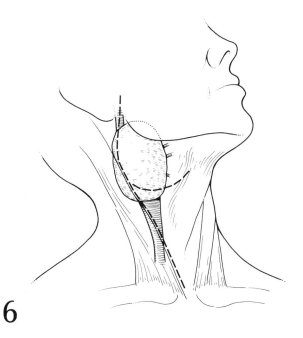

6

6 In contrast, larger tumours are more safely approached through a modified T radical neck incision.

Both these incisions generally result in good healing and satisfactory cosmetic appearance.

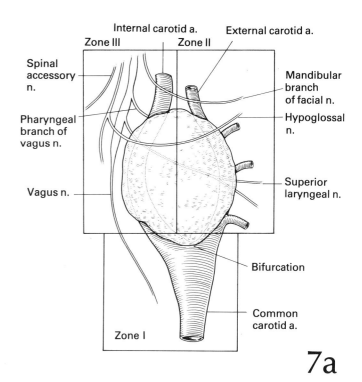

7a

Dissection

7a–c A systematic dissection around the tumour can minimize the risk of any cranial nerve injury. Dissection can be sequentially completed in three anatomical steps or zones (*Illustration 7a*). Zone I includes the common carotid artery, its bifurcation and adjacent vagus nerve. The initial step in the dissection is to identify the common carotid artery at the level of the omohyoid muscle and carefully dissect away from the adjacent vagal nerve (*Illustration 7a*). Near the carotid bifurcation, a myriad of small veins draining the tumour can be controlled with bipolar electrocautery. Zone II encompasses the external carotid artery territory and the overlying hypoglossal nerve, the underlying superior laryngeal nerve and the more superficial marginal mandibular branch of the facial nerve. Although these nerves may appear incorporated into the tumour, they can generally be separated from the surface and preserved (*Illustration 7c*). Zone III contains the internal carotid artery and the confluence of several cranial nerves: the proximal hypoglossal nerve, the upper vagus, the pharyngeal branch of the vagus, the spinal accessory nerve, and the glossopharyngeal nerve. Most serious cranial nerve injuries occur in this crowded zone. An experienced head and neck surgeon can be an invaluable assistant in safely resecting large tumours that extend high into zone III[4].

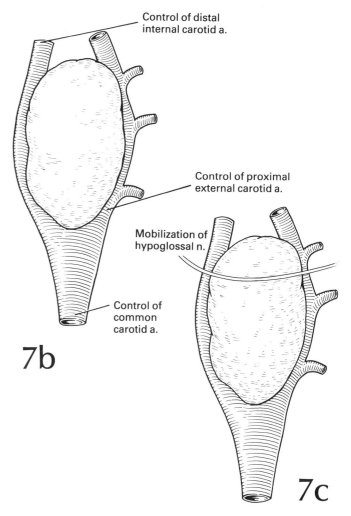

7b

7c

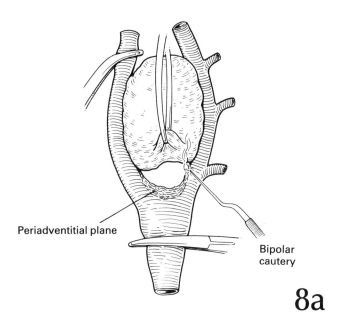

Periadventitial plane

Bipolar cautery

8a

Bipolar electrocautery

8a, b One of the most important instruments for safe tumour resection is bipolar electro-cautery (*Illustration 8a*). The usual standard electro-cautery allows for a zone of heat conduction around the cautery tip. Such heat can injure adjacent cranial nerves. On the other hand, the bipolar cautery only conducts energy between the tips of the bipolar forceps and allows nearly bloodless dissection along the tumour surface as the surgeon attempts to dissect it away from the adjacent arteries and nerves.

Periadventitial dissection

The tumour should be dissected in the periadventitial plane and not in the mistakenly recommended and treacherous subadventitial plane. Subadventitial dissection will either lead to intraoperative haemorrhage as one ventures into the arterial lumen or leave a weakened spot on the artery that is prone to disastrous carotid blowout.

Carotid clamping

Temporary carotid clamping after a small dose of heparin (2500 units) may be necessary for safe resection of tumours that are densely adherent to the carotid bifurcation. This area can be easier to dissect when the carotid bifurcation is not pulsating. This part of the tumour resection is often the most difficult point of dissection and an area where carotid injury is relatively common (*Illustration 8b*). Clamp time can be relatively short (5–10 min), and EEG changes seldom occur. Consequently, a shunt is usually not necessary. A small dose of heparin generally does not increase bleeding and is also useful when the internal carotid artery develops intense spasm. Such spasm is relatively common in younger patients and can be so intense that it causes local thrombosis or thromboembolism. A small dose of intra-arterial papaverine may also alleviate intense internal carotid spasm.

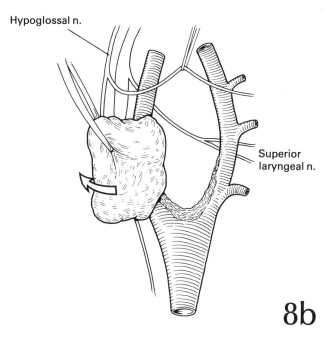

Hypoglossal n.

Superior laryngeal n.

8b

Ligation of external carotid artery

9a–d This may be necessary for complete and safe resection of some large tumours (*Illustration 9a*). Adequate superior tumour exposure may require identification of the facial nerve and its marginal mandibular branch, some parotid gland elevation, division of the digastric and stylohyoid muscles, and occasionally submandibular gland resection (*Illustration 9b*)[5]. Mandibular subluxation is an additional manoeuvre that may enhance high carotid exposure. In our experience, ligation of the external carotid artery may then be necessary in approximately one-third of patients with large tumours (greater than 5–6 cm in diameter; *Illustration 9c*). Such ligation decreases tumour vascularity and size, reduces bleeding and facilitates complete removal and dissection away from the internal carotid artery. The internal carotid artery in such cases is usually stretched and pushed laterally but not encased by the tumour (*Illustration 9d*). The internal carotid artery may be so tortuous after tumour resection that a segmental resection and reanastomosis of the artery may be necessary.

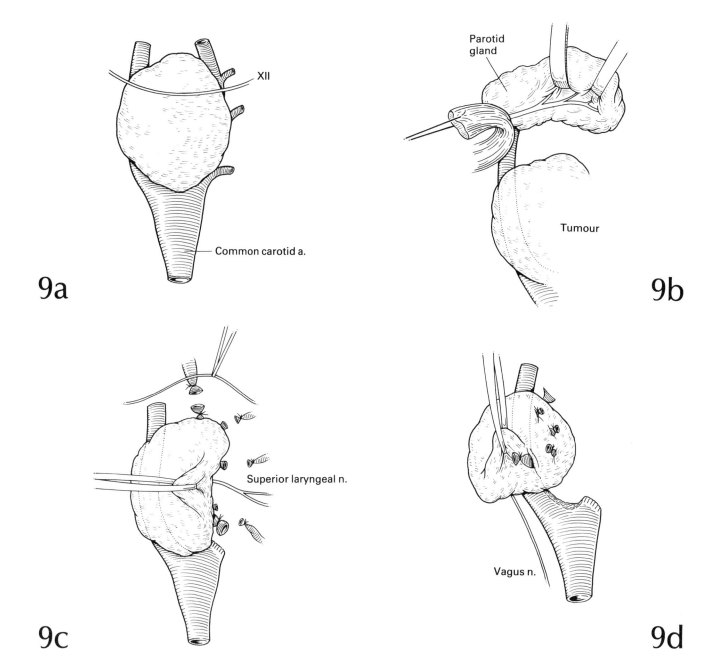

Closed suction drainage

A generous dead space is often left after resection of large tumours. Accumulation of blood or fluid in this dead space can cause some difficulty with the airway and also with swallowing. Consequently, we place a closed suction drain for 24–48 h.

Postoperative care

Patients should be monitored in an intensive care area for 6–12 h after operation. The major risks during this time are peripharyngeal haematoma and swelling that can compromise the airway. Rarely, unrecognized subadventitial injury to the carotid artery will result in catastrophic carotid blow-out that may not occur until several hours after leaving the operating room. If a sudden neurological deficit occurs, a bedside colour flow duplex carotid scan is recommended to ascertain patency of the carotid vessels and to detect any signs of intraluminal thrombus. Any arterial occlusion or technical defect should be corrected in the operating room. If no technical problems are identified, systemic anticoagulation should be considered as well as a CT or MRI scan to delineate any intracranial areas of embolism or infarct.

Outcome

Staging

Over 20 years ago, Shamblin and colleagues at the Mayo Clinic classified carotid body tumours according to the difficulty of surgical resection[6] (*see Illustration 1*). Type I tumours are well localized and easily resected. Type II tumours adhere to and partially surround the carotid vessels. Type III tumours surround the carotid arteries. This classification, however, did not necessarily correlate with malignant outcome. Since carotid body and cervical paragangliomas rarely metastasize to local lymph nodes, nodal involvement is inconsequential in most cases, even in those with large tumours. Distal metastases are also rare, but have been reported in bone, lung, liver, kidney, pancreas, thyroid and heart. Likewise, histological criteria for malignancy have been suggested, but both benign and malignant tumours may exhibit the same microscopic characteristics. Consequently, the only sure evidence of malignant behaviour is nodal or distal metastases. Preliminary DNA flow cytometry of carotid body tumours in our own recent experience (unpublished) suggests that most tumours have an abnormal non-diploid pattern that may portend more relentless growth. Such evidence substantiates our recommendation for both the early and complete resection of all carotid body tumours.

Results

Nearly all (95%) carotid body and cervical paragangliomas can be completely resected. Perioperative mortality rates are now low (2%), with no deaths in our past 15-year experience. Postoperative stroke is also unusual and affects approximately 2% of patients. These individuals are usually those with extremely large tumours or arterial repairs or replacement.

Cranial nerve dysfunction remains the primary risk of operation for these tumours. About 20% of patients still face a permanent cranial nerve deficit, usually related to tumours that originate in the vagus nerve which requires resection for cure. Temporary cranial nerve deficits are seen in another 20% of patients and usually involve the hypoglossal or marginal mandibular nerves.

The survival rate of patients after complete carotid body or cervical paraganglioma resection is encouraging (*Figure 1*). Essentially, the survival rate is equivalent to that of sex- and age-matched control subjects[7]. Metastatic disease has developed in only 2% of our patients in long-term follow up. Recurrence has been noted in approximately 6%. In our experience, all recurrent tumours have been observed in patients with multiple or familial cervical paragangliomas.

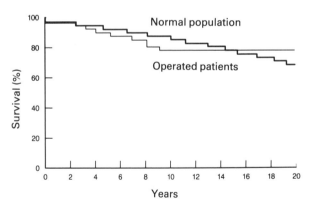

Figure 1   Survival rate after complete carotid body or cervical paraganglioma resection

References

1. Hallett JW, Nora JD, Hollier LH, Cherry KJ, Pairolero PC. Trends in neurovascular complications of surgical management for carotid body and cervical paragangliomas.: a fifty-year experience with 153 tumors. *J Vasc Surg* 1988; 7: 284–91.

2. Worsey MJ, Laborde AL, Bower T, Miller E, Kresowik TF, Sharp WJ. An evaluation of color duplex scanning in the primary diagnosis and management of carotid body tumours. *Ann Vasc Surg* 1992; 6: 90–4.

3. Smith RF, Shetty PC, Reddy DJ. Surgical treatment of carotid paragangliomas presenting unusual technical difficulties: the value of preoperative embolization. *J Vasc Surg* 1988; 7: 631–7.

4. Robinson JG, Shagets FW, Beckett WC, Spies JB. A multidisciplinary approach to reducing morbidity and operative blood loss during resection of carotid body tumor. *Surg Gynecol Obstet* 1989; 168: 166–70.

5. Meyer FB, Sundt TM, Pearson BW. Carotid body tumors: a subject review and suggested surgical approach. *J Neurosurg* 1986; 64: 377–85.

6. Shamblin WR, ReMine WH, Sheps SG, Harrison EG. Carotid body tumor (chemodectoma): clinicopathologic analysis of ninety cases. *Am J Surg* 1971; 122: 732–9.

7. Nora JD, Hallett JW, O'Brien PC, Naessens JM, Cherry KJ, Pairolero PC. Surgical resection of carotid body tumors: long-term survival, recurrence, and metastasis. *Mayo Clin Proc* 1988; 63: 348–52.

Vertebral artery reconstruction

Anthony M. Imparato MD
Professor of Surgery, New York University Medical Center, New York, USA

Thomas S. Riles MD
Professor of Surgery, New York University Medical
Center, New York, USA

History

1a, b Isolated vertebral arterial occlusions resulting in brain ischaemia are relatively uncommon when compared with the occurrence of combined carotid and vertebral lesions. Routine four-vessel angiographic studies performed in symptomatic patients for the Joint Study of Extracranial Arterial Occlusions demonstrated that lesions of vertebral origin were second in incidence only to those related to carotid bifurcation.

There has, however, been a reluctance on the part of vascular surgeons and neurologists to intervene aggressively in patients presenting with vertebrobasilar insufficiency syndromes. Surgeons have hesitated to perform angiographic studies in patients who are often extremely ill from brain stem ischaemia. The vertebrobasilar circulation may be difficult to outline angiographically without employing techniques specifically designed for its study. When vertebral arterial lesions are found, there is no universally applicable surgical operation which will correct all of the vertebral lesions. Furthermore, vertebrobasilar symptoms are frequently relieved by operations on the carotid system which are more attractive than vertebral operations since only 20% of total cerebral blood flow reaches the brain by way of the vertebrobasilar system. Nevertheless, the potentially great significance of the vertebral arteries in pathological states has been documented by Williams and by Hutchinson and Yates who, on the basis of postmortem studies, concluded that the incidence of severe cerebral infarction is higher with both carotid and vertebral involvement, suggesting that the term 'caroticovertebral' be applied to ischaemic brain syndromes as being more comprehensive.

Although relatively infrequently performed when compared with carotid operations, operations upon the vertebrobasilar system nevertheless constitute a significant and important approach to the relief of ischaemic cerebral symptoms, and perhaps preventing strokes and prolonging life.

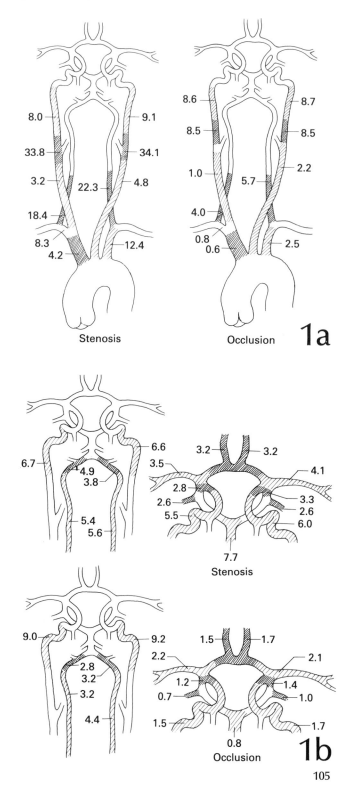

Stenosis   Occlusion   **1a**

Stenosis

Occlusion   **1b**

Principles and justification

Anatomy

Although the blood supply to the brain traditionally is described as being provided by an anterior (paired carotid arteries) and a posterior (vertebral arteries) circulation, the distinction between the two systems is artificial and arbitrary in view of the interdependence between the two systems by way of the normally occurring collateral pathways, as well as those persisting from embryonic life. This is further illustrated by the ability of the vertebrobasilar system to compensate for carotid vascular insufficiency, its flow increasing from physiological levels of 45 ml/min to levels which can compensate for deficiencies in the 750–800 ml total cerebral blood flow that can occur when severe carotid lesions exist. The vertebral arteries ordinarily originate from the subclavian vessels as their first branches, just proximal to and posterior to the thyrocervical trunks. A variation of this pattern of origin, necessary to properly evaluate nonvisualization of a vertebral artery, relates to the origin of the left vertebral artery from the arch of the aorta. The vertebral artery is divided into four segments: the origin, the intervertebral intraosseous segment, and the horizontal or distal atlantoaxial portions being extracranial, while the fourth segment is intracranial. The vascular surgeon is concerned with the relatively accessible extracranial portions, while the neuro-surgeons are concerned with the intracranial segments.

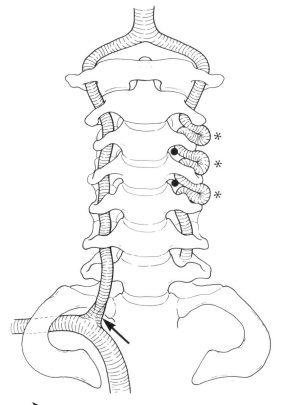

↖ Site of ostial stenosis/occlusion

● Sites of compression by osteophytes

✳ Sites of herniation out of vertebral canal

2

2 The first segment of the vertebral artery, origin-ating from the first part of the subclavian on its superior–posterior aspect, passes upward and backward between the anterior scalene muscle and the longus colli muscle. It enters the transverse foramen, usually on the sixth cervical vertebra, but occasionally on the fifth or the seventh. It is covered by the vertebral vein, usually just before its entrance into the transverse foramen, and is surrounded by a plexus of sympathetic nerves. The thoracic duct lies superficial to the artery on the left side. Frequently there is marked redundancy and curving of the first portion of the vertebral artery and, when this configuration is most marked, definite kinking of the vessel results. This portion of the vessel is the one most easily approached surgically. It is partially covered by the anterior scalene muscle, along whose anterior border courses the phrenic nerve. The thyrocervical trunk, recognizable from its branches (the first part of the vertebral having none), arises from the subclavian artery just anterior and distal to the vertebral origin, and must be differentiated from the vertebral artery which can easily be done if one remembers that it has branches. The internal mammary artery arises on the inferior border of the subclavian, while the costocervical trunk originates on the posterior aspect of the second

part of the subclavian artery. These facts are critical in attaining a dry field for a surgical approach to the origin through the subclavian artery.

The intraosseous or second segment ascends through the foramina of the transverse processes of the upper six cervical vertebrae. The course of the artery is relatively straight through the bony ligamentous canal. Occasion-ally there are significant redundancies of the vertebral artery which force it to protrude outside the bony canal through the ligamentous portions. Within the canal the artery is surrounded by a plexus of minute veins.

The third horizontal segment, also known as the distal atlantoaxial portion, emerges from the transverse foramen of the atlas and curves backward in a groove on the upper surface of the posterior arch of the atlas. It enters the vertebral canal as it angles forward to the free edge of the posterior atlanto-occipital membrane. The anterior ramus of the second cervical nerve lies behind the lower part of the vertebral artery in the C1–C2 interspace. A portion of the venous plexus encountered in the intraosseous portion of the vertebral artery may be encountered at this level. One or more small collateral branches may arise from the vertebral artery.

The fourth portion of the vertebral artery will not be described.

Pathology

3a–e, 4 Unlike the focal and almost un-varying disease encountered at the carotid bifurcation, the pathological conditions that affect the vertebral artery are more numerous. Most commonly, significant involvement occurs at the very origin of the vertebral from the subclavian artery where the atherosclerotic process, frequently rampant in the subclavian artery, impinges circumferentially upon the first 1–2 mm of the vertebral artery, producing marked stenosis. Except for the considerable redundancy of that portion of the vessel, the intima of the first part of the vertebral artery is otherwise uninvolved and is quite smooth and thin. The subclavian plaque may be quite extensive in an artery that can be friable and difficult to manage upon removal of plaque from its intimal surface. Where this involvement is of clinical significance there is usually an atrophic or rudimentary contralateral vertebral artery, or the pathological process may involve both vertebral origins which are very rarely ulcerated, unlike the situation when the carotid arteries are affected. Other lesions that result in impairment of flow through the vertebral system include compression of the intraosseous vertebral artery by osteophytes, atherosclerosis along the second and third portions of the vertebral artery and herniations of the vertebral artery from the intraosseous canal. Rarely there is thrombosis of the first part of the vertebral artery which may be patent in the intraosseous portion.

There is a wide variety of patterns of infarction of the brain in the distribution of the vertebrobasilar arterial system. Patients whose ischaemia progresses to the stage of infarction are very often beyond the stage where surgical intervention is helpful, but the areas of involvement may include the occipital lobes, the midbrain, the cerebellum and the medulla oblongata. In most instances in which surgical intervention is helpful, the patients have either very small infarcts due to infrequent and small emboli which may originate in the subclavian artery, or have symptoms in the anterior cerebral cortices unrelated to carotid occlusive disease. Primary haemorrhages in the distribution of the vertebrobasilar system are beyond the scope of the general vascular surgeon.

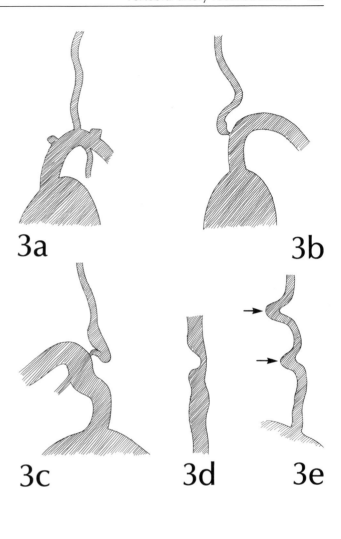

3a   3b

3c   3d   3e

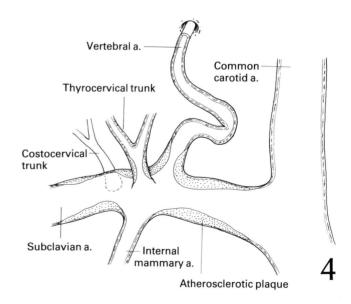

Vertebral a.

Common carotid a.

Thyrocervical trunk

Costocervical trunk

Subclavian a.

Internal mammary a.

Atherosclerotic plaque

4

Clinical syndromes

The clinical manifestations of interference with the arterial supply to the brain are ordinarily classified as either internal carotid artery territory ischaemia or vertebrobasilar territory ischaemia. Involvement of the vertebrobasilar system, although producing recognizable syndromes involving the brain stem and the cerebellar hemispheres and therefore relatively easily recognizable, may, however, occur as non-localizing symptoms, difficult to ascribe to the neural structures of the vertebrobasilar arterial system. Vertigo, ataxia, motor and sensory deficits which may be unilateral, bilateral or alternating, abnormalities of eye movement such as occur with dysfunction of cranial nerves III, IV and VI, Horner's syndrome, dysphagia associated with dysarthria, motor and sensory deficits of the face which may be unilateral, bilateral or alternating, are all strongly suggestive of posterior circulatory vascular insufficiency. On the other hand, severe or even mild dizziness, drop attacks without loss of consciousness, syncope of varying duration, headache and vomiting, are often ascribed to conditions other than that under discussion, yet may be associated with vertebral arterial lesions and be relieved by their correction. These are especially troublesome, either because their frequency means they are considered atypical of vertibrobasilar arterial insufficiency, or because they not infrequently occur in older individuals associated with other pathological conditions. Transient global amnesia, ascribed to a variety of conditions, may be a manifestation of vertebrobasilar insufficiency. If associated with other symptoms such as hemianopia, either unilateral or bilateral, then one might suspect that there are stenotic vertebral arteries. When it occurs in the absence of other symptoms, vertebrobasilar insufficiency as the source might be overlooked.

Preoperative

Symptoms

Who should be suspected of having significant vertebral arterial involvement sufficient to warrant angiographic studies and surgical intervention? In our series of over 3000 operations on the extracranial vessels for stroke prevention in which approximately 4% have been upon the extracranial vertebral arteries, the symptoms which led to diagnosis and operation can be classified as those which were (1) clearly cerebral hemispheric; (2) clearly brain stem; and (3) combined cerebral hemispheric and brain stem, with an appreciable number presenting with isolated seemingly non-focal symptoms. Dizziness, including vertigo, was the most common symptom, while focal cerebral symptoms, syncope, diplopia, drop attacks, headache, ataxia, confusion, generalized weakness, global amnesia, homonymous hemianopia, and aphasia accounted for the remainder. If more than one symptom complex is encountered with a non-focal symptom, the indication for aggressive investigation becomes stronger.

Physical examination and non-invasive studies

Physical examination may elicit the presence of carotid arterial occlusive disease with or without obvious involvement of the subclavian arteries manifested by blood pressure differentials in the upper extremities. Doppler scans of the neck and supraclavicular areas may reveal the presence of carotid occlusive involvement with impairment of flow antegrade in the vertebral arteries. The specific examination of the vertebral arteries non-invasively is difficult. Computed tomographic scans of the brain, positron emission tomographic (PET) scans and magnetic resonance imaging may each reveal areas of infarction of either the anterior or posterior parts of the brain or, with PET scanning, there may be focal areas of cerebral ischaemia of the posterior circulation. Ophthalmodynamometry, facial thermometry and transcranial Doppler studies are of limited value because the results are either not specific for vertebrobasilar arterial insufficiency or are difficult to interpret. The definitive study is radiographic.

Angiography

Patients suspected of having vertebrobasilar arterial insufficiency require visualization of the entire intra- and extracranial circulation to properly evaluate the mechanisms by which ischaemia is occurring, as well as to plan surgical procedures required for correction. Currently, the preferred technique is by catheter angiography of the aortic arch and its branches, with selective cannulation of the arch vessels to permit selective opacification of each of those arteries. Usually percutaneous puncture of the femoral artery is performed with retrograde passage of an appropriate catheter into the aortic arch. Contrast injection is made into each of the major vessels after cannulation of each of the origins of the arch vessels has been performed. In the visualization of the vertebral origins it is critical to realize that the areas of stenosis are at the very origin of the vessel, and these may be obscured by the overlying subclavian artery. Positioning the patient to project the vertebral origins is essential. The most common error involving failure to visualize markedly stenotic lesions of the vertebral origin can be avoided by appreciation of the fact that the normal vertebral origin angiographically is slightly flared, being widest at the origin from the subclavian artery. If the projection visualized reveals either parallel side walls of the first part of that vessel immediately beyond the subclavian or if there is tapering toward the subclavian artery, the true origin has not been visualized. In such instances retrograde brachial injections are performed through percutaneous punctures of those vessels.

A second area of importance involves visualization of the distal vertebral artery which occasionally terminates at the posterior inferior cerebellar artery, failing to join the basilar artery. Such a vessel is probably not operable, since a markedly stenotic vertebral artery would open into a very small anastomotic branch. The basilar artery must also be visualized because occasionally it is the site of advanced atherosclerotic narrowing, and this must be evaluated to determine the advisability of relieving vertebral arterial stenoses.

General evaluation

Cardiac

Except for the occasional younger patient who presents for surgery of the vertebral artery for non-degenerative conditions, most patients are in the age group and in a population in whom coronary artery disease is frequently encountered and may be severe. Cardiac evaluation studies include determinations of the left ventricular ejection fractions by radionuclide studies, thallium stress testing, prolonged monitoring for silent myocardial ischaemia and, ultimately, cardiac catheterization with angiographic study of the coronary arteries. In our experience cardiac catheterization is not primarily indicated unless one of the other tests indicates the presence of very advanced coronary artery disease. Left ventricular ejection fractions of 30% or lower, thallium stress testing that indicates transient deficits and silent myocardial ischaemia monitoring that indicates a high frequency and long duration of electrocardiographic abnormalities are indications to perform coronary angiography. When there is considerable involvement of the left main coronary artery or if unremitting angina pectoris is present, plans are made for performing the cerebral and myocardial revascularizations simultaneously. If not, then the cerebral revascularization is performed before any myocardial revascularization.

Renal

Evaluation of renal function is primarily by creatinine clearance studies. Creatinine clearance values greater than 15–20 ml/min, although markedly abnormal, are usually considered sufficient to perform relatively uncomplicated vertebral arterial operations unless it is necessary to repeat the injection of large quantities of radio-opaque iodinated compounds.

Other organ evaluations

Pulmonary function, coagulation parameters and evaluation of life expectancy in the presence of malignant neoplasms are as for other major surgical procedures. Patients whose life expectancy is estimated to be greater than 1 or 2 years are considered suitable candidates for surgical intervention on the vertebral arteries.

Anaesthesia

In general, operations performed on the first part of the vertebral artery are satisfactorily carried out under regional block anaesthesia. Those that require either opening the vertebral bony ligamentous canal or those on the third portion of the vertebral artery are better performed under general anaesthesia. The use of regional anaesthesia is recommended for its simplicity and for the ability to accurately monitor the cerebral status during the phase of clamping of the vertebral arteries. General anaesthesia is required for the more extensive operations where the bony canal may have to be unroofed or where the C1–C2 interspace needs to be exposed to permit distal bypass.

No shunts are used. In spite of the most extensive extracranial occlusive arterial involvement, vertebral artery clamping has been well tolerated.

Operations

SUBCLAVIAN VERTEBRAL ANGIOPLASTY

Subclavian vertebral angioplasty has been our preferred procedure to deal with ostial stenoses and their associated kinks. Avoidance of endarterectomy has obviated the need to deal with occasionally extremely friable subclavian arteries, does not require clamping the common carotid artery with the risk of producing cerebral ischaemia, and eliminates the risk of carotid antegrade embolization.

Incision

5 The incision is started one third of the way between the manubrium sterni and the mastoid process at the anterior border of the sternocleidomastoid muscle, and continued inferiorly and posteriorly parallel to the clavicle.

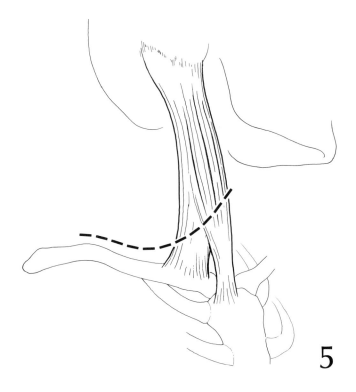

5

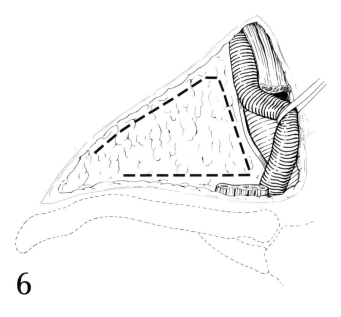

6

Division of muscle

6 The clavicular head of the sternocleidomastoid muscle is severed at its origin and permitted to retract, and the internal jugular vein is dissected free and retracted medially, avoiding the vagus nerve and the recurrent laryngeal nerve which lie between the vein and the common carotid artery. This exposes the scalene fat pad which is incised medially and by blunt dissection is freed from the underlying anterior scalene muscle on whose anterior surface rests the phrenic nerve covered by a thin fascial membrane.

The fat pad is developed so that it maintains only a lateral attachment.

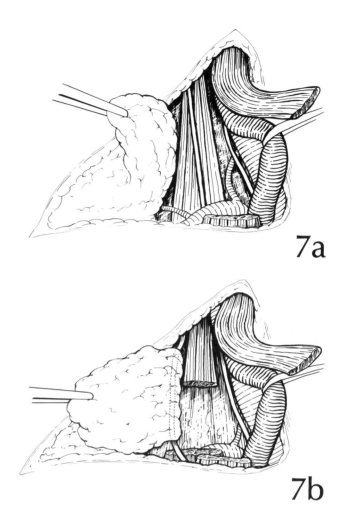

7a

Exposure of phrenic nerve

7a, b The phrenic nerve is dissected free to permit it to be retracted by the scalene fat pad, avoiding metal retractors or tapes to achieve its displacement from the operative field.

7b

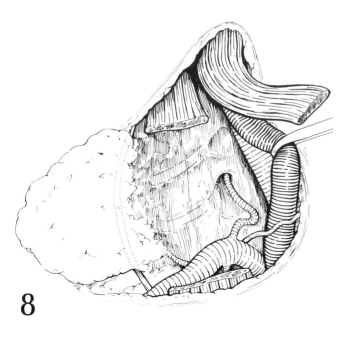

8

Exposure of vertebral artery

8 The anterior scalene muscle is divided inferiorly and permitted to retract upward. Branches of the thyrocervical trunk ordinarily cross anterior to the anterior scalene muscle and must be divided for access to the muscle.

The subclavian artery pulse is palpated medial to the anterior scalene muscle inferiorly and the four major branches dissected free. The vertebral artery is recognized from its location (first branch of the subclavian on the superior posterior aspect), absence of branches, tortuosity and finally entrance into the bony canal.

Arteriotomy

9 Arteriotomies in continuity of the vertebral and subclavian arteries are performed by excising an elliptical segment of the subclavian artery encompassing the origin of the thyrocervical trunk, continuing the opening upward on the anterior wall of the vertebral artery to beyond the kink. This ordinarily results in termination of the vertebral arteriotomy at least 1 cm short of its entrance into the transverse foramen of C6.

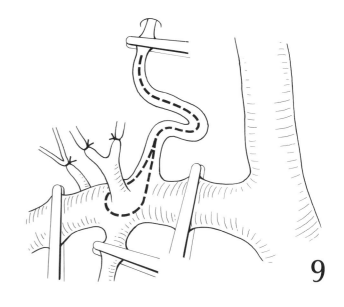

9

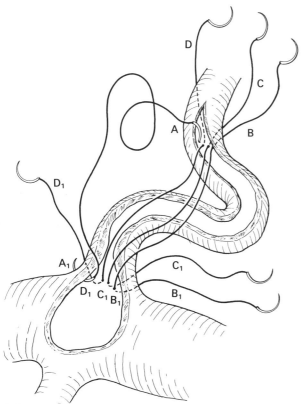

10

Scheme for closure

10 The resultant opening in the subclavian and vertebral arteries reveals the extent of the plaque, the normal intima of the vertebral artery beyond, and the placement of sutures to effect the plication which eliminates the kink. A goes to A_1, B to B_1, C to C_1 etc.

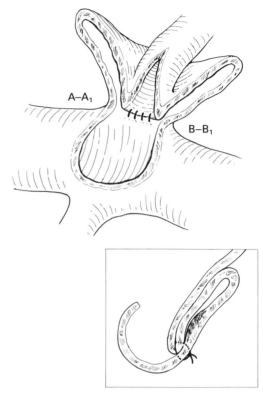

Plication

11 The plication is accomplished by ligating the sutures on the outside of the vessels, resulting in normal intima of the vertebral artery covering the ostial plaque and 'dog ears' from the redundant vertebral artery.

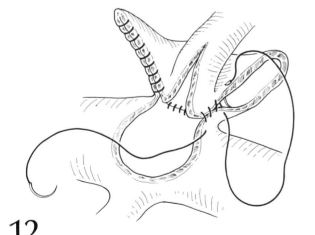

Correction of dog ears

12 The 'dog ears' are sutured to prevent bleeding, starting the closure at the subclavian–vertebral junction, continuing upward along the vertebral artery. A second row may be needed to secure haemostasis.

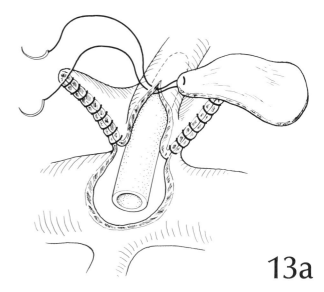

13a

Suture of vein patch

13a–c The segment of long saphenous vein excised from the groin is opened longitudinally and sutured as a vein roof patch closure of the subclavian vertebral arteriotomy, starting the closure at the distal angle of the vertebral arteriotomy, maintained widely open with a soft rubber catheter. The distal suture line is started with an everting horizontal mattress suture of 6/0 or 7/0 Dacron and continued downward as a continuous suture. The vein patch is sutured to the subclavian artery with 5/0 suture material.

Wound closure

Closure of the wound is achieved by releasing the phrenic nerve from its scalene fat pad retractor, repositioning the fat pad on top of the nerve and arteries, and suturing the manubrial head of the sternocleidomastoid muscle to its origin. The platysma and skin are closed in layers. Drainage with a 12-Fr red rubber catheter attached to suction is employed infrequently, and is removed in 24–48 h.

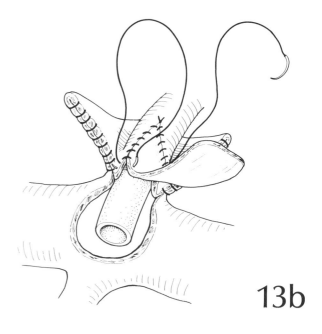

13b

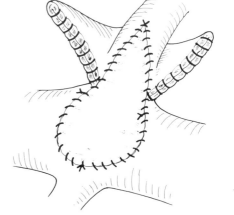

13c

VERTEBRAL TRANSPLANTATION OF THE CAROTID ARTERY

Incision

14 Incision for performing reimplantation of the vertebral artery into the common carotid artery is as for subclavian vertebral angioplasty. The clavicular head of the sternocleidomastoid muscle is divided, but the anterior scalene muscle is not. The internal jugular vein and vagus nerve are retracted laterally and the carotid artery medially.

The subclavian pulse is palpated medial to the medial border of the anterior scalene muscle after the scalene fat pad has been dissected from medially to laterally. The anterior scalene muscle is identified by palpation and resembles the sensation obtained by palpating the anterior aspect of the partially flexed proximal interphalangeal joint of the index finger.

The vertebral artery is dissected from its origin to its entrance with the transverse foramen of C6 and an estimate is made of the amount of redundancy and kinking which may be present. A 4-cm length of common carotid artery is cleared and controlled proximally and distally with tapes well below the carotid bifurcation to avoid the risk of embolization.

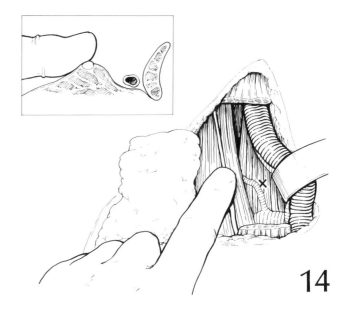

14

Anastomosis

15a–c Heparin, 3000 units, is given intravenously. The vertebral artery is clamped just below its entrance into the bony canal and divided just beyond its origin from the subclavian artery after having been doubly suture ligated. The transected end is swung medially to the carotid artery where a 3-cm segment is isolated between vascular clamps. A 4- or 5-mm aortic punch arteriotomy of the lateral wall of the common carotid artery can serve as the site of a terminolateral vertebral–carotid anastomosis using 6/0 or 7/0 non-absorbable suture, starting the anastomosis posteriorly with an everting mattress suture and continuing circumferentially with a continuous over and over everting suture.

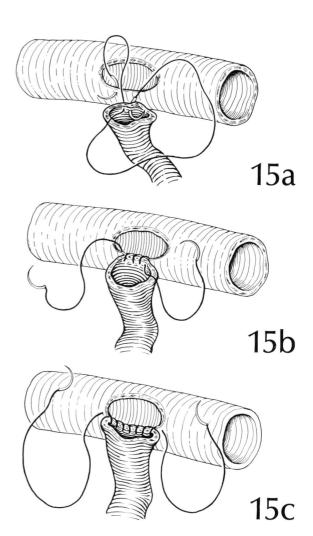

15a

15b

15c

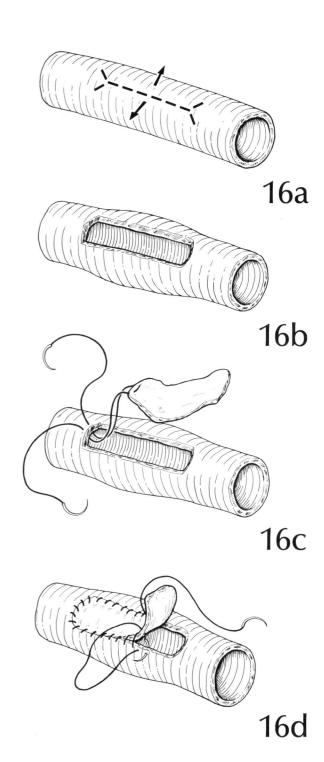

16a

16b

16c

16d

Use of Linton patch

16a–d To avoid producing ostial stenosis by suturing to an often thick walled common carotid artery it is our preference to interpose a 'Linton' venous roof patch on an arteriotomy of the common carotid artery.

17a–c The site for anastomosis of the terminal vertebral artery to the venous patch is then prepared as the direct vertebral–carotid anastomosis, either to a circular punch opening in the vein patch or through a 'trap door' opening.

The usual precautions for avoiding cerebral embolization are observed, flushing the carotid artery both antegrade and retrograde and the vertebral artery antegrade before making the final closure. The wound is closed in layers.

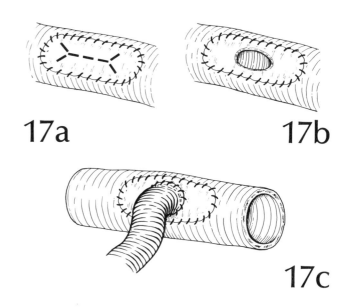

17a

17b

17c

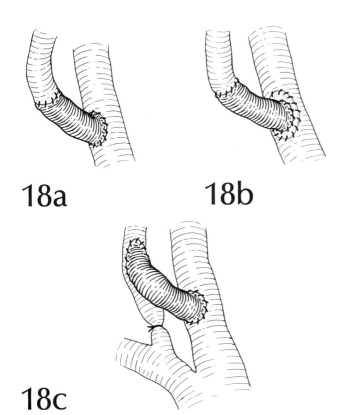

18a

18b

18c

Short vein graft

18a–c In the rare case in which the vertebral artery is too short to reach the carotid artery, reversed autologous saphenous vein can be used to achieve carotid–vertebral bypass.

OPERATION ON THE SECOND SEGMENT OF THE VERTEBRAL ARTERIES

Approach to the second segment of the vertebral arteries requires entering the bony canal formed by segments of the transverse processes of vertebrae C4–C6. The exposure is satisfactorily performed by the removal of the anterior portions of the bony and ligamentous canal. It is upon exposure of the vertebral artery that one encounters the extensive plexus of venules which surround the artery and make the dissection tedious. Nevertheless, this approach is feasible and can be used to bypass occlusions of the first portions of the artery, to relieve compressions from osteophytes, and to reduce multiple herniations of the vertebral artery between segments of the bony canal. It is not usually necessary to operate on this area for occlusive atherosclerosis.

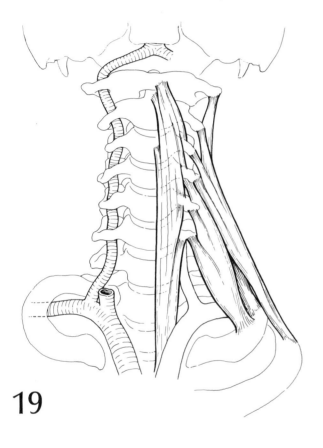

19

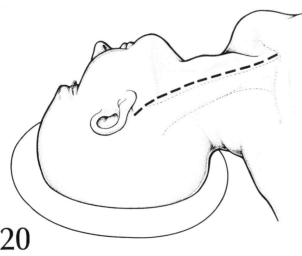

20

Anatomy

19 The anatomy relating to the surgical approach to the second part of the vertebral artery either for decompression or for carotid–vertebral bypass procedures relates to the tranverse processes of the vertebral bodies which form the bony canal and the complex longus colli muscle which has muscular fleshy attachments to the bodies and transverse processes of the cervical vertebral and tendinous attachments to the anterior scalene muscle.

Skin incision and exposure of vertebral artery

20 The skin incision extends from the mastoid process to the suprasternal notch anterior to the sternocleidomastoid muscle. The incision is deepened through the platysma and investing layer of deep cervical fascia, retracting the scalene fat pad laterally together with the sternocleidomastoid muscle, the clavicular insertion of which can be divided to improve exposure. The internal jugular vein, vagus nerve and carotid artery are freed and retracted medially, dividing the thyrocervical trunk branches if necessary.

The anterior tubercles of the transverse processes are palpated laterally and the vertebral bodies medially, and the depression between them identifies the roof segments of the transverse processes forming the transverse foramen. Overlying fascia is incised and, with a periosteal elevator, the attachments of the longus colli muscle are cleared from these depressions in the transverse processes C6–5–4–3.

The bony canal is unroofed with a small rongeur, carefully inserting it from below upwards at each level, staying against the posterior surface of the bone to avoid injury to the vertebral artery and to the numerous small veins which surround the vertebral artery. The vertebral artery is freed from the plexus of veins surrounding it, avoiding injury to the vertebral vein which lies posterolateral to the artery. This part of the dissection is tedious and results in annoying bleeding which must be patiently controlled with cautery, haemostatic agents and pressure.

Vertebral artery reconstruction

21 The vertebral artery can then be exposed over the number of segments necessary to either decompress the artery, or to achieve sufficient exposure to perform a bypass. The numerous veins are carefully clamped and cauterized. Venous bleeding occurs frequently, and is inevitable since the veins surround the artery.

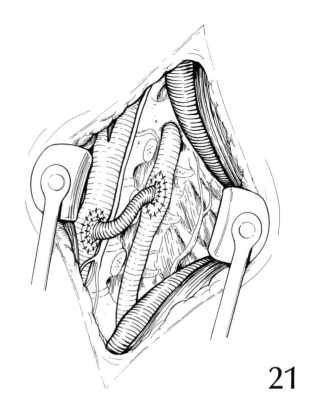

21

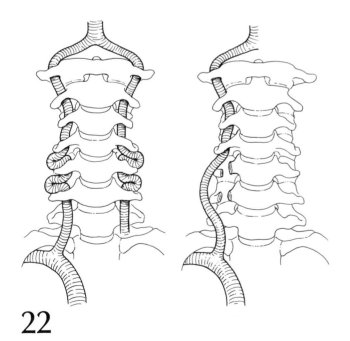

22

22 When decompression of the herniated artery is required, liberation over three segments is sufficient to convert multiple herniations into a relatively gentle curvature. On only one occasion has roof patch angioplasty been required. When osteophytes require to be resected they can be visualized. When a bypass procedure is needed the common carotid artery has been used as the origin of a long saphenous vein reversed autologous graft. In such instances a roof patch has been placed on the common carotid artery, and the smaller segment of long saphenous vein sutured to it. End-to-side anastomosis has been performed through trap door arteriotomies in the side of the vertebral artery.

Closure of the wounds is performed in layers. Heparin is not neutralized. Antiplatelet treatment is continued indefinitely.

RECONSTRUCTION OF THE DISTAL CERVICAL VERTEBRAL ARTERY

The direct surgical approach to the third segment of the vertebral artery, popularized by Kieffer and Bergeur, is a procedure that has been resorted to infrequently in our series, since most lesions requiring surgical intervention can be dealt with in the more easily approached proximal segments. It finds application most often for acute trauma and arteriovenous fistulae in which the vertebral artery can be ligated distally, but nevertheless has specific indications when the pathological process is of the mid and distal portions of the vertebral artery, when the segment between transverse processes C1–C2 offers the only segment for bypass procedures. Although the surgical approach has been known since Matas described it first in 1893, only recently has it achieved any popularity.

Position of patient

The operation is performed by placing the patient in the supine position, with the head turned away from the operated side, avoiding excessive extension and rotation.

Incision

23 The incision is made along the upper part of the anterior border of the sternocleidomastoid muscle, with an extension to the mastoid process. The external jugular vein is divided.

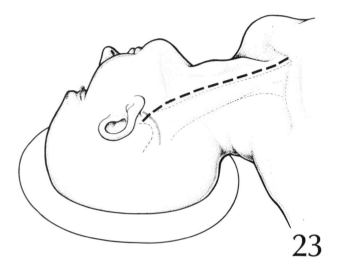

23

Exposure

24a–f The parotid gland is mobilized from the sternocleidomastoid muscle. The posterior part of the internal jugular vein is isolated to a level under the digastric muscle. The internal jugular vein and the sternocleidomastoid muscle are retracted apart, and the spinal accessory nerve identified approximately 3–4 cm below the mastoid process. The nerve needs to be mobilized to avoid trauma. The transverse process of C1 is palpated in the upper part of the incision, and the origins of the levator scapulae and the splenius cervicis muscles are exposed under the prevertebral fascia. The sympathetic fibres lie deep to this muscle plane and are retracted medially. The muscles described are divided along the lower border of the transverse process of C1. The vertebral artery then becomes accessible at the C1–C2 interspace where its pulsations can be felt. The anterior ramus of the second cervical nerve, which is behind the lower part of the vertebral artery, can usually be left in place. When it is on the anterior aspect of the artery it can be divided.

The superficial part of the vertebral artery comes into view. Its posterior aspect is dissected free to permit its control for the performance of an arteriotomy. If there are collateral branches arising from the vertebral artery they are preserved. The common carotid artery is isolated and a segment of reversed long saphenous vein is anastomosed to the side of the common carotid artery, and to the side of an arteriotomy performed in the arteriotomy of the vertebral artery. Occasionally an additional length of artery is required, whereupon the bony canal formed through the transverse process of C2 is rongeured away to expose an additional length of vertebral artery. This results in the need to deal with the plexus of veins surrounding the artery. End-to-side anastomosis appears to be preferable to end-to-end anastomosis which is technically more difficult to perform. If there is atherosclerotic disease of the carotid bifurcation it may sometimes be necessary to expose the subclavian artery for use as the starting point of an autologous saphenous vein graft.

The wounds are closed in layers. Antibiotics are continued for 3 days, and antiplatelet treatment indefinitely.

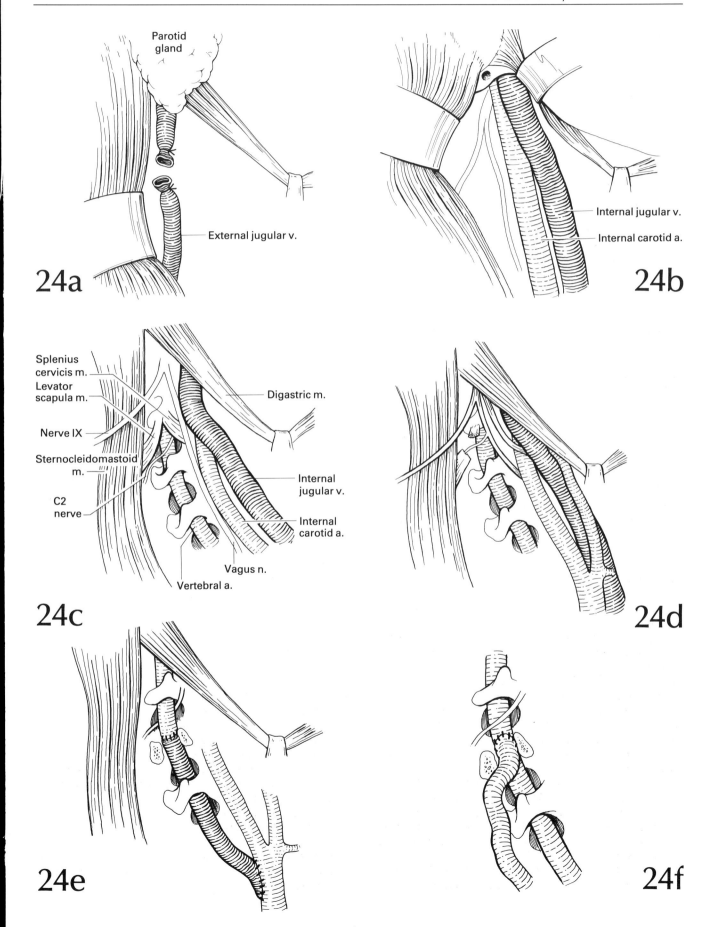

Parotid gland

External jugular v.

24a

Internal jugular v.

Internal carotid a.

24b

Splenius cervicis m.

Levator scapula m.

Nerve IX

Sternocleidomastoid m.

C2 nerve

Digastric m.

Internal jugular v.

Internal carotid a.

Vagus n.

Vertebral a.

24c

24d

24e

24f

BALLOON CATHETER TRANSLUMINAL DILATATION OF THE VERTEBRAL ARTERY

In 1978 Gruntzig performed dilatation of coronary artery stenosis with a flexible double-lumen balloon catheter, a technique that has become widely used for treatment of narrowed or occluded arteries in many parts of the body. Attempts have been made to establish the potential usefulness of this technique in the vertebrobasilar system. Stenoses that are beyond the usual operative fields, either at the junction of the vertebral artery to the basilar arteries or at the intracranial vertebral artery, have been successfully carried out by exposing the vertebral arteries at the level of the C1 and passing balloon catheters to the intracranial vertebral artery under fluoroscopic control.

Lesions at the origins of the vertebral arteries have also been dilated with balloon catheters. There are insufficient data at present to fully evaluate these procedures. The management of intracranial lesions in high-risk patients in whom it is inappropriate to carry out direct extracranial and intracranial bypass procedures would appear to be the area of recommended exploration.

Further reading

Berguer R. Distal vertebral artery bypass: technique, the occipital connection, and potential uses. *J Vasc Surg* 1985; 2: 621–6.

Edwards WH, Mulherin JL Jr. The surgical reconstruction of the proximal subclavian and vertebral arteries. *J Vasc Surg* 1985; 2: 634–42.

Giangola G, Imparato AM, Riles TS, Lamparello PJ. Vertebral artery angioplasty in patients younger than 55 years: long-term follow-up *Ann Vasc Surg* 1991; 5: 121–4.

Imparato AM. Vertebral arterial reconstruction: a nineteen year experience. *J Vasc Surg* 1985; 2: 626–34.

Reul GJ, Cooley DA, Olson SK *et al*. Long-term results of direct vertebral artery operations. *Surgery* 1984; 96: 854–62.

Carotid endarterectomy

Michael D. Colburn MD
Resident, Department of General Surgery, University of California at Los Angeles School of Medicine, Los Angeles, California, USA

Wesley S. Moore MD
Professor of Surgery, Chief, Section of Vascular Surgery, University of California at Los Angeles School of Medicine, Los Angeles, California, USA

History

Most cerebrovascular accidents (approximately 60%) are related to atheromatous disease of the extracranial carotid arteries[1]. The first carotid reconstruction was reported in 1954[2]. In 1988, the Rand Corporation published a report which reviewed the indications for carotid endarterectomy and concluded that the operation was being overused[3], and the role of carotid endarterectomy has been questioned. Recently, the efforts of a number of experts in the field have resulted in the initiation of several randomized prospective clinical trials designed to determine precisely the natural history and associated stroke risk of carotid artery atheromatous lesions[4-6]. The preliminary results of these trials are now available, and some 40 years after Eastcott's initial report describing operative repair of a carotid artery lesion, the proper role of carotid surgery is finally being clearly defined.

Pathology of carotid bifurcation occlusive disease

Atherosclerosis

Atherosclerosis is the most common pathological process affecting the cerebral circulation. The manifestations of atheromatous change in this area, however, can vary, and both occlusive and degenerative aneurysmal lesions are well known. Occlusive stenoses, however, are by far the most common. Clinically important histological characteristics include: the relative proportions of fatty, fibrous and calcified material; the presence of surface clot or ulceration; and the degree of intraplaque haemorrhage. Soft irregular fatty plaques which are not calcified represent high-risk lesions. On the other hand, smooth fibrous and calcified lesions are more stable and represent a lower embolic risk.

Fibromuscular dysplasia

The precise incidence of fibromuscular dysplasia is not known, but it is not common. Many different histological subtypes have been described, including intimal fibroplasia, medial fibroplasia, medial hyperplasia and perimedial dysplasia[7]. The most common subtype found in the extracranial carotid arteries is medial fibroplasia. Mural dilatations forming microaneurysms are common and form the basis of the classic 'string of beads' appearance observed angiographically. Intracranial aneurysms are commonly associated with carotid artery fibromuscular dysplasia and have been reported in approximately 30% of patients. In addition, a significant percentage of patients who present with a spontaneous carotid artery dissection are found to have evidence of fibromuscular dysplasia in the contralateral artery.

Intimal hyperplasia

Intimal hyperplasia is the abnormal sustained proliferation of cells and extracellular connective tissue matrix that occurs as the result of injury to the arterial wall. In the carotid bifurcation this injury typically occurs following an endarterectomy. Grossly, these lesions appear firm, pale and homogeneous. The involved area is smooth and uniformly located beneath the endothelium. Several mechanisms by which injury to the vascular endothelium may lead to activation of the medial smooth muscle cell have been suggested. Postulated theories include haemodynamic factors, alterations in lipid metabolism and complex interactions between the arterial wall and circulating factors such as platelets and components of the inflammatory system.

Radiation injury

Radiation therapy has become a common form of treatment for a variety of neoplasms, including those affecting the head and neck. Damage to the vascular wall alters its permeability to circulating lipids and impairs its ability to repair structural tissue. Over the course of the next few weeks endothelial regeneration and medial fibrosis begin to appear. Finally, within several months, the luminal surfaces become thickened and irregular. These changes are characterized by fatty infiltration, fibrosis and intimal regeneration. The medial fibrosis and intimal thickening are responsible for the eventual luminal narrowing seen following radiation injury.

Clinical patterns of cerebral ischaemia

Neurological events resulting from cerebrovascular pathology can conveniently be divided into three general categories based on the duration of symptoms. The first group of patients are those who experience a transient ischaemic attack (TIA), defined as an ischaemic event that lasts no longer than 24 h. Typically, the patient will report a focal neurological deficit, such as weakness in a limb or slurred speech. It is implied in this definition that neurological recovery is complete and no residual deficit is present. If the neurological deficit persists beyond 24 h, but completely resolves within 7 days, it is termed a resolving ischaemic neurological deficit (RIND). Lastly, if the ischaemic symptoms last longer than 7 days, the event is labelled a stroke. The clinical significance of a RIND is unclear, and it is considered by some to simply represent a stroke with rapid and full recovery. The term stroke implies irreversible brain tissue damage, even when clinically some patients appear to recover full function following a deficit which lasted longer than 7 days. It remains unclear whether a RIND represents permanent or reversible brain tissue damage.

Principles and justification

Indications

Atherosclerotic plaques

The role of carotid surgery in patients with asymptomatic carotid occlusive disease remains controversial. The case for endarterectomy in asymptomatic patients is based primarily on retrospective reviews studying patients with appropriate lesions who were followed but not operated on. To summarize the available data, the mean stroke rate/year in asymptomatic patients not treated by operations is about 5.0%, which could be expected to lead to a 5-year stroke rate of about 25%

(*Table 1*). In surgical patients, the mean operative mortality in patients with asymptomatic lesions is 1–2%, with a 30-day perioperative stroke rate of about 1.5%. The long-term stroke rate in operated patients is 1.3% in the first year and 0.5% each year thereafter (*Table 1*)[8]. This would predict a 5-year incidence of stroke of 4.8% (including perioperative strokes), which

represents an absolute reduction in the expected stroke risk of 20.2% in favour of surgically treated patients.

Unlike asymptomatic lesions, the indication for surgery in patients with symptomatic carotid lesions is no longer controversial. Three prospective randomized studies have now analysed the results of carotid surgery in patients with a symptomatic ipsilateral lesion (*Table 2*).

Fibromuscular dysplasia

The mechanism by which fibromuscular dysplasia of the extracranial carotid arteries causes symptoms is controversial. Platelet clots or cholesterol emboli may arise from the irregular luminal surface. Alternatively, decreased flow through a single critical stenosis, or through a number of non-critical stenoses aligned in series, may be the operative mechanism. It is likely that the true aetiology in any given patient varies, and combinations of these processes may also occur. Unfortunately, the natural history of fibromuscular dysplasia of the extracranial carotid artery in an otherwise asymptomatic patient is not known. Most authors agree, however, that currently asymptomatic lesions should be carefully followed and that surgical intervention should be reserved for those patients who later develop symptoms[1].

Recurrent carotid stenosis

The mean incidence of asymptomatic carotid restenoses ranges between 7% and 15%, and between 1% and 5% of developed restenoses are associated with recurrent

Table 1 Natural and modified history of atherosclerotic carotid bifurcation lesions

Symptoms at presentation	Stroke risk in first year (%)	Stroke risk yearly thereafter (%)	Stroke risk after 5 years (%)
Natural history			
Asymptomatic	5.0	5.0	25.0
Transient ischaemic attack	10.0	6.0	34.0
Completed stroke	9.0	9.0	45.0
Best medical therapy			
Asymptomatic	5.0	5.0	25.0
Transient ischaemic attack	8.5	5.0	28.5
Completed stroke	9.0	9.0	45.0
Surgical management			
Asymptomatic	1.3	0.5	3.3
Transient ischaemic attack	3.0	1.5	9.0
Completed stroke	7.0	2.2	15.8

Table 2 Prospective randomized trials comparing carotid endarterectomy with the best available medical treatment

Study	Number of patients	30-day operative mortality (%)	Percentage reaching endpoint (surgery group)	Percentage reaching endpoint (medical group)	Mean follow-up (months)
Asymptomatic*					
Veterans Administration Cooperative[4]	444	1.9			
Symptomatic					
Veterans Administration Cooperative[4]	189		7.7	19.4	11.9
>70% stenosis			7.9	25.6	
<70% stenosis			7.1	6.7	
North American Symptomatic Carotid Endarterectomy Trial[5]					
Stenosis (30–69%)*					
Stenosis (70–99%)	659	0.6	8.0	18.1	24
European Carotid Surgery Trial[6]					
Stenosis (0–30%)	374	1.4	11.8	6.2	36
Stenosis (30–69%)*					
Stenosis (70–99%)	778	0.9	12.3	21.9	36

*Results not yet available

symptoms[9, 10]. It has long been recognized that the natural history of recurrent carotid stenoses is not the same as that of the original lesion in a given patient. The risk of subsequent stroke or ischaemic events in these patients is clearly different from that of primary atherosclerotic lesions. This is probably related to the pathology of the recurrent lesion. Smooth, fibrous, intimal hyperplastic recurrent lesions, even of the same or greater degree of stenosis than the original atherosclerotic plaque, are well tolerated by most patients. This is probably due to the low risk of embolic events related to these lesions relative to the soft necrotic atherosclerotic plaques originally found in these patients.

Preoperative

Evaluation

Atherosclerosis is a systemic disease, and involvement in other vascular beds must be identified. The association between carotid and coronary involvement with atherosclerotic changes is well known and must be looked for. Any patient with a history of coronary artery disease, suggestive symptoms, or silent abnormalities on routine electrocardiography (ECG), should undergo a comprehensive cardiac assessment prior to any cerebrovascular reconstruction.

Traditionally, most surgeons have held to the belief that the complete evaluation of patients with cerebrovascular symptoms must include an accurate anatomical delineation of the aortic arch, carotid bifurcation and intracranial vasculature. Recently, however, the role of diagnostic arteriography has diminished and duplex scanning is emerging as an acceptable preoperative evaluation technique. The duplex scan is an accurate non-invasive imaging technique, and this, combined with increased knowledge of the natural history of these lesions, has caused the need for routine arteriography in all patients with cerebrovascular disease to be questioned. The arguments for carotid endarterectomy with or without preoperative arteriography have been outlined recently by Gelabert and Moore[11]. To summarize, there is no question that arteriography exposes patients to an increased risk which must be added to the operative morbidity when calculating the overall risk of surgical therapy; however, the need to image the entire cerebrovascular tree from the arch to the intracranial vessels is debatable. Clinically important proximal disease is uncommon and is usually apparent on physical examination. Furthermore, in the presence of a critical bifurcation lesion, identification of additional intracranial disease does not ordinarily alter the patient's management. Thus, the combination of a careful history and physical examination, combined with a reliable evaluation of the carotid bifurcation, should safely identify candidates for operative intervention.

Anaesthesia

Both local and general anaesthesia are accepted procedures for carotid surgery. Local techniques usually include a regional cervical block in combination with direct skin infiltration of anaesthetic agents. Initial sedation is normally achieved by gentle administration of parenteral diazepam or a related agent. Mental confusion, respiratory depression and hypoxia must be avoided. Regional cervical block is easily accomplished by infiltrating the cervical plexus with a mixture of 1% lignocaine hydrochloride and 0.5% bupivacaine hydrochloride. Rapid skin anaesthesia with a prolonged duration can also be obtained by this combination. Subcutaneous injections, as well as deep injections along the posterior border of the sternocleidomastoid muscle to anaesthetize the superficial nerves of the cervical plexus, complete the local block. Occasionally, additional injections within the carotid sheath may be required.

The advantages of local anaesthesia during carotid endarterectomy are related to avoidance of the cerebral and myocardial depressant effects of general anaesthesia. First, neurological assessment during carotid surgery is critical, and an awake patient is a very sensitive cerebral monitor. Secondly, neurological status in the immediate postoperative interval, a period during which patients who undergo general anaesthesia are not well monitored, is easily assessed. Finally, the improved tolerance of the elderly or cardiac-impaired patient to local anaesthesia allows a safer operation in these high-risk groups of patients.

Despite these advantages, most surgeons prefer general anaesthesia for patients undergoing carotid surgery. General anaesthesia provides the most controlled operative setting, including excellent airway control and less movement in the operative field. Physiological advantages include improved oxygenation, reduced cerebral metabolic demand and increased cerebral blood flow, particularly when halogenated anaesthetic agents are utilized.

Regardless of the method of anaesthesia, accurate blood pressure monitoring during carotid surgery is essential. Therefore, all patients should have a radial arterial catheter inserted prior to the induction of anaesthesia. This line can also be used to measure arterial blood gases and should be left in place to monitor blood pressure during the immediate postoperative period.

Operations

CAROTID ENDARTERECTOMY

Position of patient

The patient should be positioned supine on the operating table with the head rotated away from the operative side. The head of the table is raised 10–15° which reduces venous pressure and minimizes incisional blood loss. Depending on individual differences in body habitus, the neck can be extended by the placement of a small towel roll beneath the shoulders.

Incision

1 A longitudinal incision is made which follows the ventral border of the sternocleidomastoid muscle. The approximate position of the carotid bifurcation can often be determined from the preoperative diagnostic studies. Ideally, the incision should be centred longitudinally so that the bifurcation is below the midpoint. When necessary for additional exposure, this incision can be continued caudad to the sternal notch, and cephalad to the mastoid process[2].

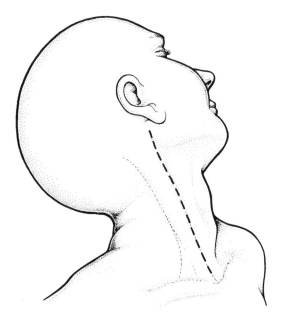

1

Dissection

2 The plane of dissection remains along the anterior border of the sternocleidomastoid until the belly of this muscle can be reflected off the carotid sheath. Often the posterior tail of the parotid gland is encountered at this level, and when this occurs further dissection is required. The gland should be mobilized and reflected anteriorly rather than divided, which can cause excessive bleeding and occasionally lead to a salivary fistula. Once the carotid sheath is visualized, it should be opened along the anterior border of the jugular vein, which can easily be identified through the sheath. The jugular vein is mobilized completely and any large branches identified. The common facial vein is a broad-based tributary, which commonly joins the jugular vein just above the carotid bifurcation. This vein provides a useful marker for the location of the carotid bifurcation and, once identified, it should be divided between ligatures. Particularly in high bifurcations, the hypoglossal nerve can also be located deep to the facial vein, and care must be taken to avoid inadvertent injury to this structure.

After dividing the facial vein, the jugular vein can be reflected laterally, providing exposure of the carotid vessels. The vagus nerve which is ordinarily posterior, can be located anywhere within the carotid sheath.

Therefore, in each case, its course must be identified and protected to avoid injury. The laryngeal nerve, which is usually recurrent, can arise directly off the vagus and cross anterior to the carotid artery at this level where it enters the vocal musculature. When not recognized, division of this nerve will lead to vocal paralysis. It should also be mentioned that, although this anomaly is more common on the left side, its presence has also been described on the right.

Once the sheath has been entered and all pertinent structures identified and protected, the common carotid artery is sufficiently mobilized proximally to allow complete delineation of the extent of disease, and to provide sufficient length in case a bypass shunt is required. The bifurcation, external and internal carotid arteries are then mobilized in a similar fashion. Reflex bradycardia can occur during manipulation of the carotid bulb due to stimulation of the carotid body. This can be prevented, or reversed when necessary, by local injection of an anaesthetic agent to block the nerves arising from the carotid body. The external and internal carotid arteries must be mobilized for a sufficient length to clearly identify the distal extent of the disease. The hypoglossal nerve must be carefully identified, particularly when mobilizing the internal carotid artery.

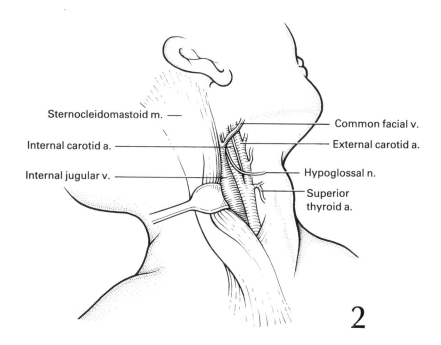

2

Carotid artery back-pressure measurement

3 Selective cerebral protection based on the measurement of distal internal carotid artery back-pressure was originally described by Moore *et al*. Using this method, the adequacy of the collateral blood flow to the ipsilateral hemisphere during proximal artery occlusion is determined by measurement of the back-pressure. A 22-Fr needle is bent 2 cm from the tip at an angle of 45° and connected to an arterial pressure transducer. The needle is inserted into the common carotid artery with the angulated tip lying longitudinally in the lumen and directed toward the bifurcation. First, an open carotid artery pressure is measured, and this should be compared with the radial artery line to ensure that the pressure transducer is functioning correctly. Then, with the external and proximal common carotid arteries temporarily occluded, the internal carotid artery back-pressure is recorded.

Although no precise consensus has been reached, most reviews define the range of 30–50 mmHg as the pressure below which cerebral protection is mandatory, If this is the case, the clamps on the external and proximal common carotid arteries are removed, and preparations are made for the use of an internal bypass shunt. Commonly cited objections to this method include the inaccuracy of extracranial pressures in the presence of an undiagnosed intracranial lesion and variations in the values obtained with different levels of anaesthesia, ventilation and other metabolic parameters.

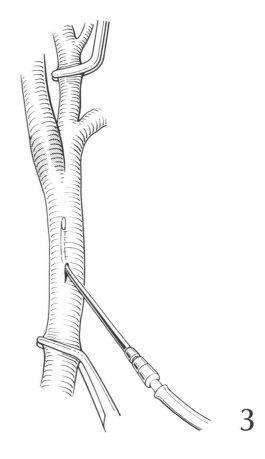

3

Insertion of shunt

4 When an internal carotid shunt is required, several principles should be appreciated. Most importantly, full exposure of all three major carotid vessels is mandatory. This allows for complete proximal common carotid control and full appreciation of the distal extent of disease in both the internal and external carotid arteries. With the internal and external carotid arteries controlled, the common carotid is occluded proximally with a soft clamp. The arteriotomy should extend comfortably beyond the distal extent of the luminal disease. The distal internal carotid is allowed to back-bleed, and an internal shunt with an appropriate diameter is gently inserted. The authors prefer to use the Javid shunt; however, other types are available. The shunt is flushed, clamped and subsequently inserted into the common carotid artery proximally. Snares (Rumel tourniquets) are used to secure the shunt at its insertion points, and the occluding clamp on the common carotid is removed. Thus in the final configuration, the shunt is in place with only a single occluding clamp in its mid portion. This clamp is removed slowly, watching carefully for air or debris which may be visible through the proximal portion of the shunt. Once the shunt is in place and cerebral protection accomplished, attention can be directed to the performance of a technically excellent operation.

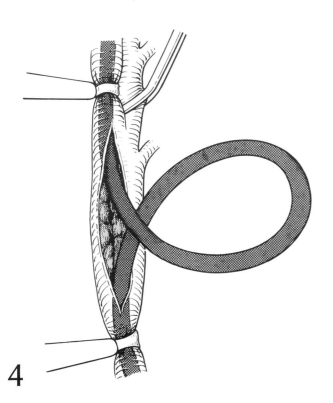

4

Clamping of carotid arteries

5 Performance of a technically perfect carotid endarterectomy requires appreciation of several time-honoured principles. Once adequate exposure is achieved and cerebral protection (if necessary) assured, the internal, external and finally common carotid arteries are clamped, in that order. The clamps should be placed in such a way that the bifurcation can be rotated exposing the lateral surface directly opposite the orifice of the external carotid artery.

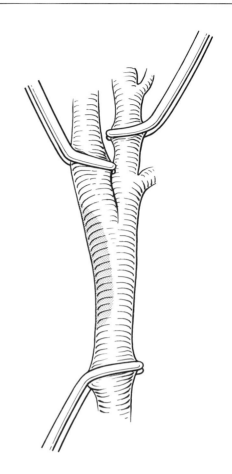

5

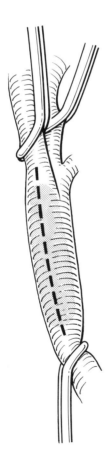

Arteriotomy

6 The arteriotomy is placed longitudinally along this surface. This minimizes the risk of damaging the bifurcation flow divider. Furthermore, by placing the arteriotomy here, there is less chance of narrowing the endarterectomized lumen during closure.

6

Endarterectomy

7a–c Once the arteriotomy is complete, a thorough inspection of the luminal surface is made, and any ulceration or mural thrombosis is noted. The precise depth of the endarterectomy plane is critical. Care should be taken to select the plane between the diseased intima and the circular fibres of the media. This allows complete removal of the atheromatous process without compromising the endpoint. More superficial planes risk incomplete removal of complex plaques, and deeper dissections inevitably lead to an abrupt step-up at the endpoint of the endarterectomy.

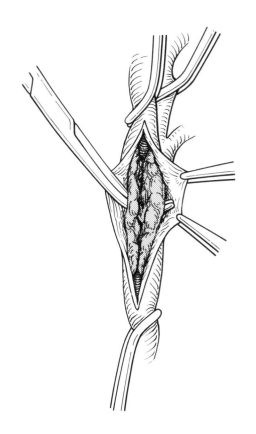

7a

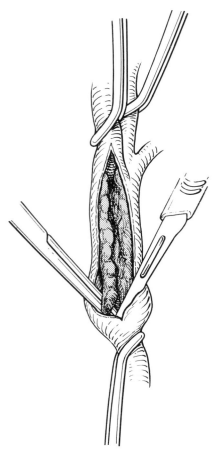

7b

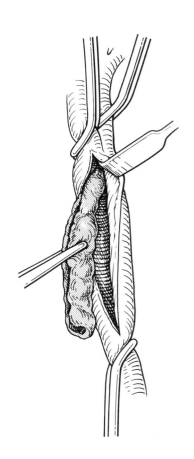

7c

Completion of endarterectomy

8 Once the endarterectomy is completed, including clearing of the external carotid artery and direct visualization of both the proximal and distal endpoints, the endarterectomy surface should be mechanically irrigated with liberal amounts of heparinized saline solution. This serves to remove small bits of atheromatous or medial debris and can help to identify occult intimal flaps. Any debris or small flaps that are identified should always be removed by gentle downward or lateral traction. Removing a fragment in the cephalad direction can lead to inadvertent extension of the dissection distally. It is of utmost importance to carefully examine the external carotid artery, as it is well known that technical failures in the orifice of this vessel can lead to serious postoperative complications.

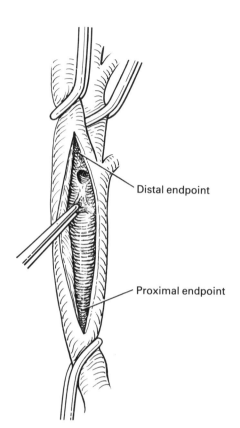

Distal endpoint

Proximal endpoint

8

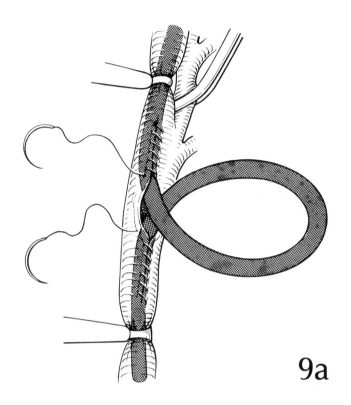

9a

Closure of endarterectomy

9a, b Closure of the endarterectomy site is critical, and the tendency to hurry this step of the procedure is perhaps the most common cause of postoperative complications. If an adequate evaluation of the collateral circulation has been made, and if appropriate cerebral protection (if necessary) has been instituted, there is absolutely no need to rush this portion of the procedure. Primary closure with 6/0 polypropylene suture is preferable and well tolerated. If a shunt has been placed, the arteriotomy is closed with the exception of an approximately 1-cm segment in the middle of the defect. The common carotid is again controlled, the shunt is clamped and removed, and the carotid vessels are again flushed, beginning distally as always. The arteriotomy closure is then completed, with the vessels temporarily occluded. Alternatively, a Satinsky partially occluding clamp can be used to maintain flow while the arteriotomy is repaired.

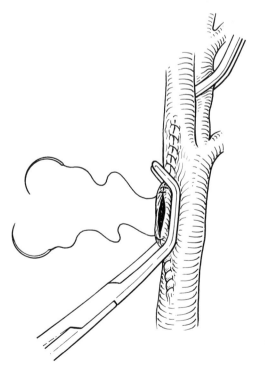

9b

PATCH ANGIOPLASTY

Patch angioplasty is appropriate for small vessels, particularly in women, and in reoperative cases. Prosthetic material is chosen in most situations (Dacron or expanded polytetrafluoroethylene (PTFE)), except in cases of recurrent carotid stenosis where autologous vein is preferable. An important principle when patching a bifurcation arteriotomy is not to attempt to construct the largest luminal diameter possible. Rather, the original size of the vessel should simply be approximated, and any unnatural luminal narrowing avoided. This prevents large patulous arteries which can become culs-de-sac for the later development of mural thrombi.

10a, b

Whichever method is chosen, the closure begins distally, and closely placed sutures incorporating small bites of artery are inserted until the carotid bulb and common carotid artery are reached. Proximally, a second suture is begun which proceeds distally. Before the suture line is completed, the internal, external and common carotid arteries are flushed. After the sutures are tied, the internal carotid artery is allowed to back-bleed and completely fill the carotid bulb. The proximal internal carotid artery is again gently occluded and flow is restored through the external system by removing the clamps on the external and common carotid arteries respectively. Finally, after several seconds the occluding clamp is removed from the internal carotid artery. When sutures are placed carefully and in an unhurried manner, suture line bleeding is seldom a problem. On occasion, pledgets of thrombin-soaked Gelfoam or fibrin glue may be necessary, particularly when prosthetic material is used.

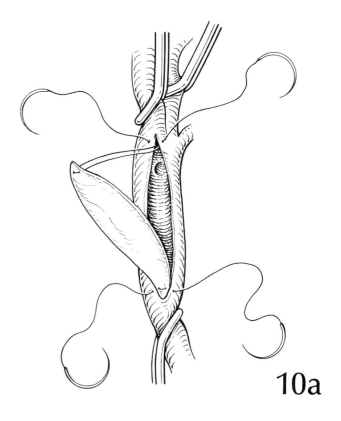

10a

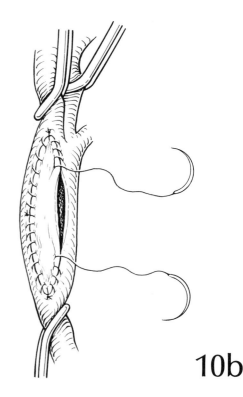

10b

EXTERNAL CAROTID ENDARTERECTOMY

Technique

Endarterectomy of lesions of the external carotid artery is indicated when flow reduction or ulceration in this vessel has been determined to be the cause of significant cerebrovascular symptoms. Most commonly this circumstance occurs following chronic occlusion of the internal carotid artery. In this setting, the external carotid artery can supply a significant portion of the intracranial circulation via well-developed collaterals. Therefore, embolization or the development of a flow-limiting lesion in the origin of the external cerebral circulation can cause significant symptoms in the distribution of the previously occluded internal carotid artery. This procedure is also very occasionally performed to repair a proximal lesion before an extracranial-to-intracranial bypass.

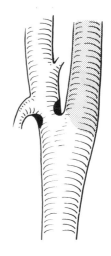

11 Dissection of the carotid bifurcation is carried out in a fashion similar to a standard carotid endarterectomy. After mobilizing the bifurcation and all its major branches, a moment should be taken to confirm that the internal carotid artery is totally occluded. Occasionally, this vessel will be found to be still patent, permitting a conventional carotid endarterectomy to be performed with restoration of antegrade flow through the internal cerebral circulation. If internal carotid occlusion is confirmed by direct inspection, the proximal carotid artery is clamped and the origin of the internal carotid artery is divided flush with the carotid bifurcation.

The arteriotomy through the orifice of the internal carotid artery is positioned on the posterior lateral aspect of the carotid bulb and continued distally onto the external carotid artery beyond the distal extent of the atherosclerotic lesion in that vessel. Under direct vision, an endarterectomy of the external carotid artery is performed. The plane of the dissection and the handling of the endpoints is managed in the same manner as a carotid bifurcation endarterectomy.

The arteriotomy is closed primarily. Great care should be taken to contour the repair to provide a smooth, tapered transition from the common carotid artery to the endarterectomized external carotid artery. Any residual luminal irregularities, such as a retained stump at the site of the divided internal carotid, may provide a cul-de-sac for the development of thrombotic or platelet aggregates, leading to emboli and recurrent cerebrovascular symptoms. If the external carotid artery is small, it may be necessary to close the arteriotomy with a patch. Either a prosthetic or autologous tissue patch may be used. Both vein and a segment of the chronically occluded internal carotid artery have been used successfully for this purpose.

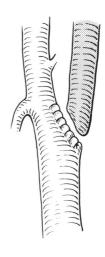

11

INTERNAL CAROTID ARTERY DILATATION

Technique

Early in the experience with the surgical management of fibromuscular dysplasia, most patients underwent resection of the diseased arterial segment and reconstruction by either primary anastomosis or construction of an autologous interposition graft. In 1968, Morris *et al.* described the technique of internal carotid artery dilatation, which has greatly simplified the surgical correction of these lesions.

This procedure is best performed while the patient is under general anaesthesia. The positioning, exposure and initial dissection of the carotid bifurcation are the same as for carotid endarterectomy. For this procedure, however, it is particularly important to mobilize the entire extracranial portion of the internal carotid artery. In this way, the dilatation can be carried out under direct visual and palpable control. Thorough mobilization of the carotid bifurcation will also aid in the cephalad passage of the carotid dilators by allowing caudal countertraction during the procedure.

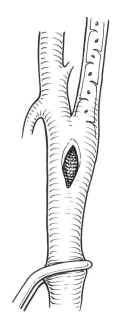

12   Once the arteries are all identified and mobilized, the patient is systematically heparinized and the common carotid artery is clamped proximally. A 1-cm longitudinal arteriotomy is made in the carotid bulb adjacent to the origin of the internal carotid artery. A 2-mm coronary dilator is then introduced into the orifice of the internal carotid artery proximally and carefully advanced. As mentioned, gentle caudal countertraction on the carotid bulb while advancing the dilator can be very helpful. The intraluminal position of the dilator should be assessed continually by a combination of visual inspection and external palpation. The dilator is passed to the base of the skull and then carefully removed. During the dilation, the surgeon will often feel the disruption of each intraluminal septum as the dilator is advanced.

Progressively larger diameter dilators of 0.5-mm increments up to a maximum of 4.0 mm are passed through the diseased arterial segment in a similar fashion. After each passage, the artery is allowed to back-bleed though the arteriotomy to remove any debris dislodged by the dilatation.

An alternative technique to progressive intraluminal dilatation is the use of intraoperative balloon angioplasty. One theoretical advantage of this method is avoidance of the potential arterial traction injury caused by the repetitive longitudinal motion of the intraluminal dilators. The results of this technique, however, though favourable, have not been shown to be superior to the standard dilatation procedure.

At the completion of the dilatation, the arteriotomy is closed and antegrade blood flow is restored. As always, completion arteriography is highly recommended to confirm an adequate technical result.

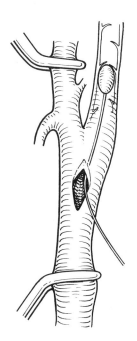

12

EXTENDED EXPOSURE TECHNIQUES

When a carotid artery bifurcates high in the neck, or when there is extensive distal disease involving the internal carotid artery, it may be necessary to obtain additional exposure in the superior aspect of the incision. Several techniques have been described to increase the length of internal carotid artery that can be approached. Surgeons performing carotid surgery should be familiar with these manoeuvres.

The simplest and most important technique is to extend the skin incision completely across the mastoid process behind the ear. This allows additional mobilization of the sternocleidomastoid muscle up to its tendinous insertion. The spinal accessory nerve enters the muscle at this level and must be preserved.

When additional exposure is necessary, the posterior belly of the digastric muscle can be detached from its insertion onto the mastoid process. The digastric muscle consists of two muscle bellies united by a rounded tendon. The posterior belly arises from the mastoid process and the anterior portion inserts on the mandibular symphysis. It is useful to appreciate the superficial anatomical position of the posterior digastric muscle when dissecting in this area. All important neurovascular structures lie deep to the digastric muscle at this level. Only the external jugular vein and branches of the facial and great auricular nerves pass superficial to the posterior belly of the digastric muscle. Below the muscle, particular care must be taken to avoid injury to the hypoglossal and spinal accessory nerves, as well as the facial branch of the external carotid artery. The stylohyoid muscle can also be divided. This muscle stretches between the styloid process and hyoid bone and its removal, along with the styloid process, can provide additional exposure of the distal internal carotid artery at the base of the skull.

When the disease extends very distally, it is possible to gain additional exposure by anteriorly subluxating the condylar process of the mandible. The displaced mandible can be secured in place with wires. This manoeuvre alters the geometry at the base of the skull by turning a triangular space into a rectangle and thereby enlarging the operative field.

Lastly, techniques by which the ramus of the mandible is divided have also been described. This is an involved procedure that greatly complicates the postoperative course, and the authors have never found this manoeuvre to be necessary.

RECURRENT STENOSIS

The incision and principles of exposure when approaching a recurrent carotid lesion are the same as described for a standard endarterectomy (page 127). The dissection is invariably more difficult due to scarring from the previous procedure, and extra care must be taken to avoid injury to the cranial nerves. The hypoglossal nerve is particularly vulnerable as it can be draped over the bifurcation by the scar tissue. Once completely dissected, the common, external and internal carotid vessels are clamped, and the bifurcation opened using a longitudinal arteriotomy.

The histological property of carotid bifurcation atherosclerotic lesions, which allows for the performance of a standard endarterectomy, is the ability to easily develop a plane of dissection between the plaque and the circular medial fibres of the arterial wall. Unfortunately, recurrent carotid lesions composed of hyperplastic intimal tissue do not share this property. These lesions are formed by intrinsic medial cells which migrate across the internal elastic lamina and replicate within the neointima. Thus, it is not possible to form a precise plane of dissection that allows the removal of the luminal narrowing disease without dangerously thinning the remaining arterial wall. The surgical approach to recurrent carotid lesions therefore, is patch angioplasty rather than endarterectomy. On the other hand, when the recurrent lesion is found to be composed of ordinary atheroma, a standard endarterectomy can be performed.

The choice of patch material includes prosthetic material and autologous vein. There is a theoretical argument that prosthetic material may contribute to the hyperplastic intimal process, but this has not been proved experimentally. In fact, it has been suggested that autologous vein, with its intact endothelium elaborating humoral growth factors, may be a greater stimulus to a continued hyperplastic reaction in the patched arterial segment. When vein is chosen, saphenous vein is most commonly used, as experience has shown that vein segments taken from the neck are ordinarily too thin and should be avoided. Regardless of the material chosen, the patch should always be constructed in such a way as to approximate the original size of the carotid bulb. Large patulous repairs may lead to the accumulation of laminar thrombus and result in distal embolism.

Occasionally, the recurrent disease is so advanced that patch angioplasty is not feasible. In these rare cases, reconstruction can be accomplished by the use of an interposition graft.

Wound closure

Closure of the incision following a carotid operation should be meticulous and adhere to all the basic principles of surgery. The wound should be irrigated generously with warm saline solution and perfect haemostasis confirmed. The platysma is reapproximated with a running suture, and the skin is closed with stainless steel staples. Some surgeons prefer to place a closed suction drain beneath the platysmal layer and bring it out through a separate stab wound. A sterile dressing is applied, and the patient is observed carefully while awakening from anaesthesia.

Postoperative care

Immediately after awakening from anaesthesia, a preliminary neurological assessment should be made. The patient is subsequently transferred to the recovery room followed by the intensive care unit for careful monitoring during the first 24 h following surgery. Particular attention should be made to assess systemic blood pressure and neurological function frequently during this period. In addition, careful wound observation is essential to detect the formation of a haematoma, which may compromise the reconstruction or threaten the airway. After 24 h, the intra-arterial line and the closed suction drain, if placed, can be removed, and the patient is returned to the general ward. Most patients undergoing carotid surgery are admitted to hospital the morning of surgery and are discharged home on the second or third day after operation. Before discharge, the skin staples are replaced with adhesive Steri-Strips and an appointment is made for the patient to return within 2–3 weeks for the first follow-up after the operation.

Complications

An uncomplicated carotid endarterectomy is a well-tolerated operation. Tissue trauma and operative blood loss are normally minimal, and patients are routinely discharged from hospital on the second or third day after surgery. For this reason, perioperative complications are particularly discouraging and must be avoided at all costs. Operative intervention, particularly in asymptomatic patients, will only continue to be justified by keeping operative morbidity and mortality to a minimum.

Technical errors

By definition, technical errors occurring during the operation are preventable by adherence to good surgical principles. One major cause of a technical complication is incomplete or inadequate removal of plaque from the endarterectomized segment. Distal intimal flaps are common if care is not taken to directly assess this endpoint. This complication can be minimized by extending the arteriotomy beyond the distal extent of the visible luminal disease. When a shunt has been inserted, this manoeuvre becomes critically important, otherwise it is not possible to adequately visualize the distal endpoint. Very occasionally, tacking sutures may be required to ensure a smooth transition to normal intima. Regardless of the visual appearance of the endarterectomized surface, a completion angiogram should always be obtained to document the absence of defects or narrowing following the arteriotomy closure.

Embolism occurring during or after carotid endarterectomy is probably the most common cause of postoperative neurological deficits. These events can occur while the carotid artery is being mobilized. Alternatively, embolism occurs during cross-clamping, following the insertion of the internal carotid artery shunt, or after restoration of flow. Placing the distal end of a shunt first allows back-bleeding and removal of any residual air or debris. Inserting the proximal portion while the shunt is clamped at its midsection, allows visualization of air or debris from the proximal common carotid artery while the shunt is slowly opened. Following completion of the endarterectomy, any residual plaque should be carefully removed. Irrigating the lumen with heparinized saline can be very helpful in identifying and completely removing small fragments. After closure of the arteriotomy, flow should first be restored into the external carotid system to capture any remaining intraluminal debris. Antegrade flow can then be safely re-established into the internal system by slowly removing the clamp on this vessel.

Cranial nerve injury

As described above, several peripheral nerves must be identified and protected during the exposure of the carotid bifurcation. Injury to these structures is another source of postoperative morbidity following carotid endarterectomy. In 1980, Hertzer reviewed the postoperative complications in a series of patients undergoing carotid endarterectomy and found a 16% incidence of cranial nerve injuries[12]. All cranial nerve injuries occurring during carotid surgery can be prevented by becoming familiar with the normal and possible abnormal anatomical neurovascular relationships and carefully protecting these structures during the procedure.

Hypertension/hypotension

Blood pressure changes, both during and immediately following carotid endarterectomy, are common and potentially serious if not treated appropriately. The aetiology of blood pressure fluctuations following carotid surgery is multifactorial. One proposed mechanism is damage to the baroreceptor mechanism located in the carotid sinus. Devascularization or interruption of the afferent nerves emerging from this structure potentially reduce the sensitivity of this receptor to changes in blood pressure. Conversely, endarterectomy of the carotid bifurcation may lead to overdistension of the thin-walled bulb and increased stimulation of the carotid sinus.

Intraoperative hypotension associated with bradycardia due to stimulation of the carotid body should respond promptly to the local injection of 0.5% lignocaine hydrochloride into the tissues adjacent to the carotid sinus. If this manoeuvre fails to restore normal haemodynamics, an immediate cardiac evaluation should be performed. Hypertension during or following carotid endarterectomy can usually be easily treated with intravenous sodium nitroprusside. The requirement for intravenous antihypertensive therapy seldom lasts beyond the first 24 h after operation, and patients with long-standing essential hypertension can be started on their oral medications following this interval.

References

1. Gelabert HA, Moore WS. Carotid endarterectomy: current status: *Curr Probl Surg* 1991; 28: 181–262.

2. Eastcott HHG, Pickering GW, Robb C. Reconstruction of internal carotid artery in a patient with intermittent attacks of hemiplegia. *Lancet* 1954; ii: 994–6.

3. Winslow CM, Solomon DH, Chassin MR, Kosecoff, J. Merrick NJ, Brook RH. The appropriateness of carotid endarterectomy. *N Engl J Med* 1988; 318: 721–7.

4. Towne JB, Weiss DG, Hobson RW. First phase report of cooperative Veterans Administration asymptomatic carotid stenosis study – operative morbidity and mortality. *J Vasc Surg* 1990; 11: 252–9.

5. North American Symptomatic Carotid Endarterectomy Trial Collaborators. Beneficial effect of carotid endarterectomy in symptomatic patients with high-grade carotid stenosis. *N Engl J Med* 1991; 325; 445–53.

6. European Carotid Surgery Trialists' Collaborative Group. MRC European Carotid Surgery Trial: interim results for symptomatic patients with severe (70–99%) or with mild (0–29%) carotid stenosis. *Lancet* 1991; 337: 1235–43.

7. Stanley JC, Gewertz BL, Bove EL, Sottiurai V, Fry WJ. Arterial fibrodysplasia: histopathologic character and current etiologic concepts. *Arch Surg* 1975; 110: 561–6.

8. Thompson JE. Carotid endarterectomy for asymptomatic carotid stenosis: an update. *J Vasc Surg* 1991; 13: 669–76.

9. Hertzer NR, Martinez BD, Benjamin SP, Beven EG. Recurrent stenosis after carotid endarterectomy. *Surg Gynecol Obstet* 1979; 149: 360–4.

10. Zierler RE, Bandyk DF, Thiele BL, Strandness DE. Carotid artery stenosis following endarterectomy. *Arch Surg* 1982; 117: 1408–15.

11. Gelabert HA, Moore WS. Carotid endarterectomy without angiography. *Surg Clin North Am* 1990; 70: 213–23.

12. Hertzer NR, Feldman BJ, Beven EG, Tucker HM. A prospective study of the incidence of injury to the cranial nerves during carotid endarterectomy. *Surg Gynecol Obstet* 1980; 151: 781–4.

Treatment of occlusion of branches of the aortic arch and subclavian arteries

Kenneth J. Cherry Jr MD
Consultant and Head, Division of Vascular Surgery, Department of Surgery and Associate Professor of Surgery, Mayo Medical School, Mayo Clinic, Rochester, Minnesota, USA

Innominate and aorto-carotid reconstructions

Principles and justification

Indications

The indications for arch reconstructions in the presence of appropriate lesions are anterior cerebral ischaemia, posterior circulation ischaemia, global ischaemia or upper extremity ischaemic symptoms. In the instance of innominate artery disease, there may be combinations of both neurological and upper extremity symptoms. Less commonly, asymptomatic but significant lesions of the innominate artery may be repaired in conjunction with coronary artery bypass or in preparation for planned major thoracic aortic, abdominal aortic or visceral artery reconstructions.

Atherosclerosis is the usual aetiology of these occlusive lesions; in the Western world, smaller numbers of patients will present with Takayasu's arteritis or giant cell (temporal) arteritis. The present-ing symptoms in those patients with atherosclerosis may be occlusive or atheroembolic in origin. The symptoms in patients suffering from one of the arteritides are occlusive by nature.

Contraindications

Contraindications to surgery include infections of the sternum, mediastinum or neck. Severe cardiac dysfunction may preclude direct repair of the great vessels, but combined coronary and great vessel reconstruction is more usual in these patients. Axillary–axillary grafts, subclavian–subclavian grafts, carotid–carotid grafts and contralateral carotid–subclavian reconstructions are alternatives in poor-risk patients and have been described. Their pretracheal or presternal locations and suspect long-term patency rates mitigate against them.

Preoperative

Evaluation

Patients presenting with cerebral or upper extremity lesions require full physical examination, with special attention to their neurological function, pulse status including auscultation, and upper extremities. Splinter haemorrhages or the small bluish discolorations typical of microemboli should be sought and noted if found. Allen's test or variants thereof may reveal digital artery occlusions. Blood pressure measurements should be obtained from both upper extremities. Chest radiographs, duplex scans of the extracranial cerebral vessels and evaluation of cardiac function if indicated should all be obtained. The patient should undergo evaluation in the vascular laboratory to provide documentation of the status of the upper extremities and as a baseline for postoperative evaluation. Aortography and views of the great vessels and their run-off beds are absolutely necessary to confirm the diagnosis, to localize and document the nature of the lesions and to plan operations.

Anaesthesia

These operations are performed with the patient under general anaesthesia. Barbiturate or hypothermic cerebral protection is rarely, if ever, necessary. Arterial lines should be used for monitoring the patient's blood pressure. Selection of cannulation sites, especially if the patient has multiple great vessel occlusive lesions, requires good communication between the surgeon and the anaesthetist. Central lines should not, as a rule, be placed from the patient's left side, as the left innominate vein is either mobilized extensively or divided primarily in many of these patients.

If available, electroencephalographic monitoring may be used to assess cerebral perfusion and activity. If, as in most cases, it is not available, stump pressure or some other form of assessing cerebral perfusion should be employed. Whichever method the surgeon finds most comfortable for carotid endarterectomies will work in this situation. Shunting is rarely necessary. Swan–Ganz monitoring is not usually required.

Operations

INNOMINATE ARTERY ENDARTERECTOMY

This operation is reserved for patients with atherosclerotic lesions of the innominate artery. There are two anatomical contraindications to performing innominate artery endarterectomy: (1) severe atherosclerotic or calcific disease of the aorta itself at the base of the innominate artery, precluding safe haemostatic clamping or the development of a safe endarterectomy plane proximally; and (2) inadequate distance between the origins of the innominate and left common carotid arteries, precluding clamping the former without impairing flow through the latter[1]. As an extreme example, a patient with a common brachiocephalic trunk would not be a candidate for endarterectomy.

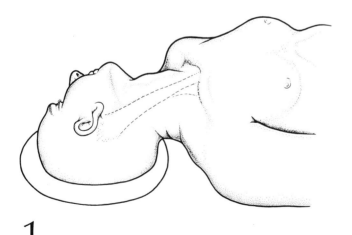

1

Position of patient

1 The patient is placed supine on the operating table with the head turned towards the left. The patient's back is elevated on towels placed longitudinally between the scapulae, and the head is supported in an extended position on towels or a foam ring. The neck, chest and upper abdomen are prepared and sterile drapes are applied. The inferior edges of the ear lobes are prepared and draped into the field as landmarks. The patient's arms are tucked to the side.

Incision

2 A full length sternotomy incision is made. The incision is extended into the right neck along the anterior border of the sternocleidomastoid muscle. The sternal attachments of this muscle may be taken down at this time and reattached at the conclusion of the operation.

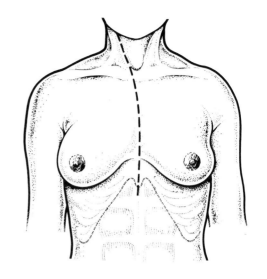

2

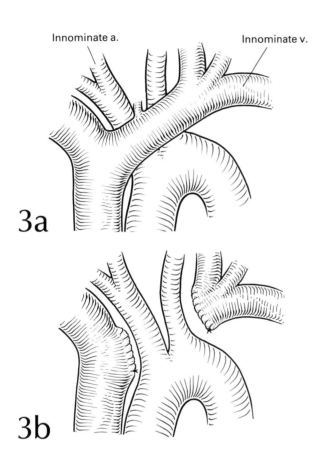

Innominate a.

Innominate v.

3a

3b

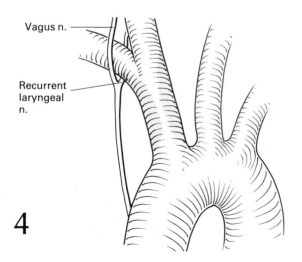

Vagus n.

Recurrent laryngeal n.

4

Exposure of innominate artery

3a, b The thymus and pericardial fat are mobilized as necessary. The left innominate (or brachiocephalic) vein may be mobilized by division and ligation of its tributaries. It is the author's preference to divide the vein primarily. Vascular clamps are placed across the vein as it courses anteriorly to the innominate artery and the vein is divided. The severed ends are oversewn with horizontal and over-and-over running 4/0 polypropylene sutures.

Dissection and exposure of carotid artery

4 The sternal retractor is opened gradually to avoid bony fractures and costochondral disruptions. Using sharp dissection, the ascending arch just proximal to the innominate artery, the origin of the innominate artery and the origin of the left common carotid artery are dissected free. The left common carotid artery needs only to be visualized and not dissected circumferentially. Visual and tactile inspection will reveal the state of the aorta at the base of the innominate artery and the distance between it and the left common carotid artery. If the aorta is healthy and the left common carotid artery sufficiently distant from the origin of the innominate artery, the dissection for innominate artery endarterectomy continues. The dissection is carried distally to the origins of the right common carotid artery and the right subclavian artery. The atherosclerotic process usually extends into the subclavian rather than the carotid artery. Intraoperative examination in conjunction with evaluation of the preoperative arteriogram allows precise determination of the extent of dissection needed. The vagus and recurrent laryngeal nerves must be identified and protected. Small vessel loops may be passed around them if desired. If more distal dissection along the course of the subclavian artery is necessary, the phrenic nerve must also be identified and protected.

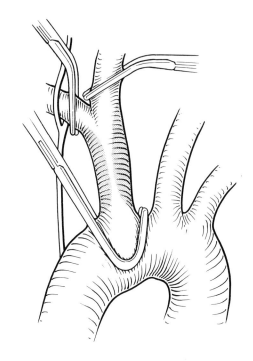

5

Aortic clamping

5 The patient is systemically heparinized. After the anticoagulant has had time to circulate, vascular clamps are first applied to the subclavian and carotid arteries. If the symptoms are atheroembolic in origin, clamping distally first is especially important. The origin of the innominate artery is clamped with a stout partial occlusion clamp that is narrow but deep, such as the Wylie J clamp (Pilling), to encompass the aorta as well as the origin of the innominate artery without impinging upon the origin of the left common carotid artery. It is the author's practice to wait a full minute at this point to ensure satisfactory flow through the left common carotid artery.

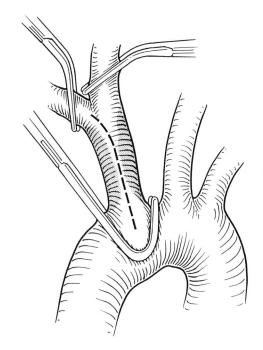

6

Arteriotomy

6 A vertical incision is made in the anterior innominate artery. Distally this incision extends at least 1 cm beyond the last grossly evident atherosclerotic plaque. If necessary, the incision is extended into the right subclavian artery, or more rarely the right common carotid artery. Proximally, the incision is carried down to the aorta.

Endarterectomy

7a–d If the proximal innominate artery is grossly free of disease, the endarterectomy plane is started just distal to the origin of the innominate artery. It is developed circumferentially at this point and the specimen divided. Using an arterial elevator, the diseased intima and the inner media are dissected free. The proper plane will have a yellow specimen side and a blue patient side. If the parent artery is purple rather than blue, the plane is too deep, and if the parent artery is a pale yellow rather than blue it is too shallow. Care is taken to do this on a broad front encompassing the entire arterial circumference rather

than to create salients of endarterectomized artery amid diseased artery. Such an approach allows more precise delineation and treatment of the distal end of the endarterectomy, which will usually end in a feathered tail of atherosclerotic plaque. Tacking sutures of 6/0 polypropylene are used distally if necessary. These are placed vertically using double-armed sutures placed from within the artery overlying the change of plane. The change of plane should be shallow, reflecting a well developed, feathered endpoint. It is incorrect simply to transect a thick plaque.

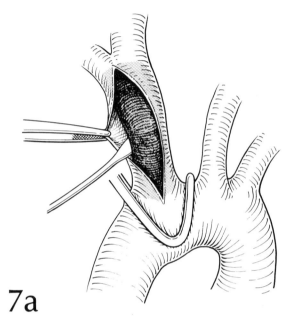

7a

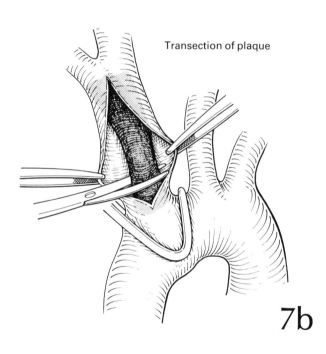

Transection of plaque

7b

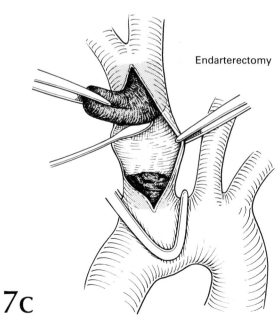

Endarterectomy

7c

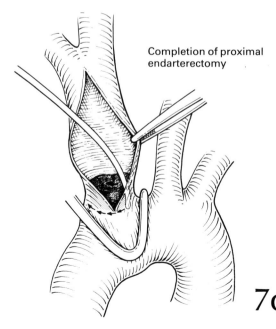

Completion of proximal endarterectomy

7d

Closure of arteriotomy

8 The artery is thoroughly irrigated with heparinized saline. Any floating attachments to the vessel wall are removed by pulling them perpendicular to the axis of the artery. It is well known that the innominate artery, like the subclavian artery, is a fragile structure. It is impossible to overemphasize the gentleness and precision with which the surgeon must work to achieve a satisfactory endarterectomy and closure of this vessel. If the artery is small, it may be patched with a woven Dacron graft using 5/0 or 6/0 polypropylene. In the author's experience most arteries may be closed primarily with these same fine polypropylene sutures. Suturing should begin from both ends of the arteriotomy. Just before completing the closure, careful partial opening of the proximal clamp is allowed, followed by back-bleeding, first from the subclavian artery and then the carotid artery. The lumen is flushed with heparinized saline again. The closure of the arteriotomy is completed and the subclavian clamp removed. There is ample retrograde flow from this vessel to determine suture line haemostasis. The proximal clamp is then removed. If there are bleeding sites requiring repair, the clamps are reapplied and appropriate repair is performed with very fine polypropylene sutures. Flow is restored first to the right subclavian artery and then to the right common carotid artery.

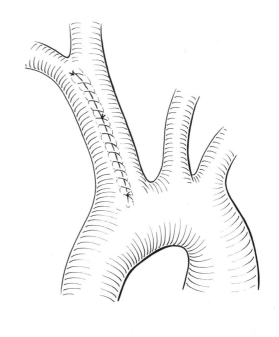

8

Wound closure

Protamine sulphate is not given unless satisfactory haemostasis cannot be achieved. A mediastinal drainage tube is placed and brought out through a separate inferior stab wound and secured to the skin with a heavy silk suture. If the pleural cavity has been entered, a chest tube is also placed. The sternum is closed with wire, the presternal fascia and subcutaneous tissue with polyglactin (Vicryl), and the skin with a running subcuticular suture of polyglactin. The patient should be awakened in the operating room to assess motor function of the extremities.

AORTOINNOMINATE ARTERY GRAFTING

Patients with arteritis, with failed previous arch reconstructions, those with atherosclerosis whose anatomy is not suitable for endarterectomy or, indeed, all patients with occlusive lesions of the innominate artery are candidates for aortoinnominate artery grafting. The indications for operation are the same as those for endarterectomy. Evaluation, anaesthesia and monitoring techniques, positioning and preparation of the patient are also identical.

Clamping of ascending aorta

9 Exposure of the mediastinal contents is initially the same as for innominate artery endarterectomy but the ascending aorta proximal to the innominate artery must be dissected free. The intrapericardial ascending aorta is most often soft and free of disease. A stout partial occlusion clamp is placed as far laterally as is possible. The author has found the Cooley curved multipurpose clamp (V. Mueller) to be especially well suited to this purpose. It is not necessary to heparinize the patient at this point. A vertical aortotomy is made, and the aortic wall separated with guy sutures of polypropylene.

Graft insertion

10 An 8-mm or 10-mm Dacron graft is chosen. Classically, woven Dacron grafts have been used in this position. More recently, the author has found collagen-coated knitted grafts to work well, and they are currently preferred at his institution for their handling and suturing characteristics. The graft is spatulated and fashioned to fit the aortotomy. Care must be taken to ensure that the aortotomy is not too long; equally important little, if any, aorta should be excised (unless needed for diagnosis) or the 'toe' of the graft will be flattened, rather than smoothly curved, when the aorta is opened. The anastomosis is performed using a running 3/0 or 4/0 permanent suture. Either polypropylene or Dacron is acceptable. When the anastomosis is completed, an arterial clamp is placed across the graft just distal to the anastomosis and the partial occlusion clamp is gently released to assess haemostasis. If more sutures are necessary the aortic clamp is resecured before repair. When haemostasis is achieved, the aortic clamp is removed. At this point, the patient is systemically heparinized. Control is obtained of the right subclavian and common carotid arteries, and then of the innominate artery. The innominate artery is divided just proximal to its bifurcation and prepared appropriately. The distal anastomosis is fashioned end-to-end with running 4/0 polypropylene or Dacron sutures. Just before completion of the anastomosis, appropriate antegrade and retrograde bleeding is allowed. The lumen is rinsed with heparinized saline

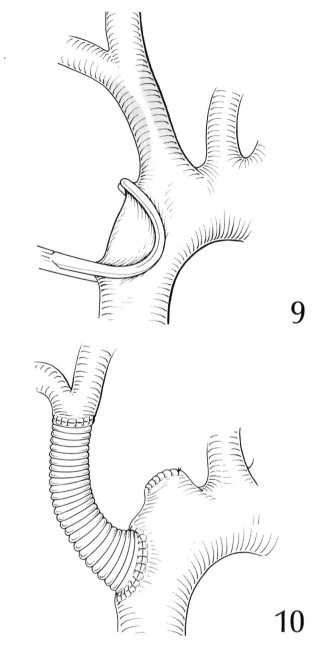

and the anastomosis completed. Flow is restored first to the subclavian artery and then to the carotid artery.

As much of the innominate artery as is possible is excised. The innominate stump is oversewn with horizontal and over-and-over permanent 3/0 or 4/0 sutures. Division of the left innominate vein and excision of the innominate artery allow maximum decompression of the mediastinum. These manoeuvres, plus lateral placement of the graft, help to prevent occlusion of the graft in the confined space of the anterior mediastinum when the sternum is reapproximated.

The conduct of the remainder of the operation is identical to that of endarterectomy.

AORTOCAROTID ARTERY GRAFTING AND AORTOSUBCLAVIAN ARTERY GRAFTING

With multiple arch lesions, or lesions extending well into the common carotid artery, as are often seen with Takayasu's arteritis, aortocarotid grafting rather than aortoinnominate grafting may be necessary. If both the innominate artery and the left common carotid artery are to be reconstructed, a Dacron graft may be sutured to the left lateral wall of the innominate graft as a side arm to the left common carotid artery. This is done in the upper mediastinum and is performed with a running or permanent suture. It is most practicable to perform this anastomosis before performing the distal innominate artery anastomosis. In order to ascertain the most advantageous location for this anastomosis, the sternal retractor may be relaxed to allow the grafts and the mediastinal contents to assume more nearly their permanent locations.

There are two schools of thought concerning the use of bifurcated grafts. Crawford and his colleagues at Baylor have favoured single limb grafts with side arms added as necessary[2, 3]. Practitioners at the Mayo Clinic have also been advocates of that method[4]. Surgeons at the Texas Heart Institute have found the use of bifurcated Dacron grafts preferable in their practice[5]. Both methods are probably equally effective. The author favours the use of single limb grafts because of their decreased bulk in the mediastinum and their angulation relative to the aorta.

If necessary, the carotid bifurcations are exposed through vertical incisions based on the anterior border of the sternocleidomastoid muscle. On the right, the sternal excision may simply be continued or a separate cervical incision made. On the left side, separate cervical incisions are most commonly performed. Tunnels along the native vessels are made, connecting the incisions. If the distal anastomoses are to the common carotid arteries, these are usually performed in an end-to-end manner using running 4/0 or 5/0 permanent sutures. Those to the carotid bifurcation are usually done in an end-to-side manner employing running 5/0 or 6/0 permanent sutures.

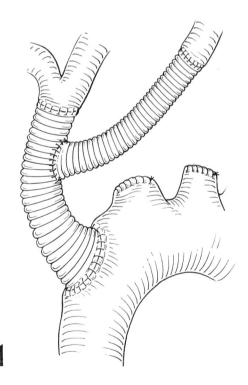

11

11 Side arms to the subclavian arteries may be added as necessary, although it is usually easier to reconstruct the left subclavian artery from a supraclavicular approach at the same or later operation. Again 4/0 or 5/0 running sutures are used for this purpose. It is best to reiterate at this point that care must be taken to avoid injuring the phrenic nerve, especially if bilateral subclavian artery reconstructions are necessary.

Postoperative care

Patients should be cared for as they would be following any thoracic procedure with haemodynamic and ventilatory monitoring. In addition, patients should be monitored as they are following carotid endarterectomy, with careful serial assessment of their neurological status. Pulse status of the right upper extremity should be monitored and the blood pressure determined. Deterioration of any of these parameters during the postoperative period requires appropriate medical response, whether surgical or not. Intravenous digital subtraction arteriography is usually obtained at the author's institution to document the status of the reconstruction. Patients are seen several times during the first year and annually thereafter.

Subclavian reconstructions

Principles and justification

Indications

Isolated proximal subclavian lesions are rarely symptomatic because of the rich collateral arterial pathways in the neck, upper chest and shoulder. Other synchronous lesions of the extracranial cerebral vessels are usually present in symptomatic patients. The notable exception is a proximal subclavian artery lesion which is the source of atheroemboli. Indications for reconstruction include claudication of the upper extremity, microemboli in the upper extremity from a subclavian lesion, or vertebrobasilar insufficiency. Subclavian or vertebral steal are terms often used to describe such vertebrobasilar symptoms in the presence of a subclavian lesion. The left subclavian artery is involved in 70% of the cases of subclavian artery occlusive disease.

Contraindications

Contraindications are few: current infection would be the most compelling. As an extra-anatomic reconstruction avoiding entry into a major body cavity, this operation is suited even for those patients with coronary disease.

Preoperative

Evaluation

Evaluation for these patients is the same as for patients with innominate artery occlusive disease.

Preparation of patient

If reconstructions to the distal axillary or brachial arteries are anticipated, the axillae and the upper extremities must be prepared and draped. One of the lower extremities should also be prepared and draped for harvesting of the long saphenous vein. Consideration should be given to first rib resection, performed from either a supraclavicular or transaxillary approach, to allow adequate space for the graft to pass through the thoracic outlet. These techniques are described in the chapter on pp. 470–474.

Shunting of the carotid arteries may be necessary. If the common carotid artery is still patent, the shunt may be placed in the standard manner in the native vessel. The patient's baseline flow is thereby maintained. If the parent vessel is not patent, the shunt may be placed and secured in a graft limb. After the suture line is started and a secure attachment assured, the shunt may be placed from the graft to the artery.

The conduct of the remainder of the operation is identical to those described previously. The cervical wounds are closed by reapproximation of the platysma with polyglactin and the skin with subcuticular polyglactin. Drains are not used in the cervical wounds. Again, these patients are awakened in the operating room to assess movement of all four limbs.

Anaesthesia and monitoring

General anaesthesia is used. An arterial line should be placed in the opposite extremity. Swan–Ganz catheters and central lines are rarely indicated. Electroencephalography, measurement of carotid stump pressure, or assessment of cerebral perfusion by whichever method works well for the surgeon, should be used. Shunting is necessary only rarely.

Operations

CAROTID–SUBCLAVIAN ARTERY BYPASS

Position of patient

The patient is placed supine with the back elevated on towels placed longitudinally between the scapulae. The head is extended, turned to face away from the lesion and supported on towels or on a foam ring. The neck and upper chest are prepared and the ear lobe partially exposed to provide a landmark.

Incision

12 Both the common carotid and subclavian arteries may be exposed through a single horizontal supraclavicular incision 7.5–9 cm in length placed 1–1.5 fingerbreadths above the clavicle. The medial border is placed over the clavicular portion of the sternocleidomastoid muscle. The incision is carried through the platysma. The lateral head of the sternocleidomastoid muscle is sharply divided. Any bleeding vessels are cauterized. The muscle may be reapproximated at the conclusion of the operation. The scalene fat pad is divided inferiorly between clamps and ligated. Some surgeons routinely seek out and ligate the thoracic duct. The author's preference is to ligate it if encountered. Its entry into the junction of the jugular and subclavian veins is usually caudad to the field and not seen. The anterior scalene muscle may easily be palpated at this stage.

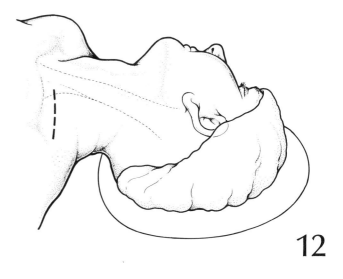

12

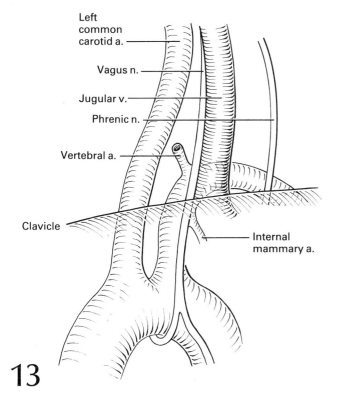

Left common carotid a.

Vagus n.

Jugular v.

Phrenic n.

Vertebral a.

Clavicle

Internal mammary a.

13

Exposure of phrenic nerve and subclavian artery and its branches

13 The brachial plexus and the phrenic nerve are identified and protected. The anterior scalene muscle is incised, and the dome of the subclavian artery identified just posterior to it. The dissection is extended both proximally and distally to allow comfortable placement of clamps and a generous anastomosis. Branches of the subclavian artery may be divided between clamps and ligated to facilitate this mobilization. If at all possible, the internal mammary artery should be preserved in case coronary grafting becomes necessary later. The vertebral artery is usually quite proximal to this dissection and left undisturbed. If the presenting symptom is one of atheroembolization or if the subclavian artery is not immediately preocclusive, the artery must be dissected free proximal to the vertebral artery to allow for ligation at that level.

Graft anastomosis

14 Medial retraction allows exposure of the common carotid artery. The jugular vein and the vagus nerve are identified and protected. A tunnel is created posterior to the jugular vein and the sternocleidomastoid muscle. A knitted Dacron graft, usually 7–8 mm in diameter, is clotted and the patient heparinized. The carotid artery is clamped. The arteriotomy is made in the lateral wall. Care is taken that the incision is not too long lest the anastomosis be narrowed, as the graft is not spatulated but brought off at a right angle. If shunting is necessary, the intraluminal shunt is placed at this stage. The anastomosis is performed with a running 4/0 or 5/0 polypropylene or Dacron permanent suture. Appropriate antegrade and retrograde flushing is allowed before completion of the anastomosis. When completed, a clamp is placed on the graft and flow is restored to the carotid artery.

The graft is brought through the tunnel posterior to the jugular vein and the sternocleidomastoid muscle, taking care not to injure the thoracic duct by traction. Depending on the patient's anatomy, the graft may be placed posterior or anterior to the phrenic nerve. The latter position is probably preferable. The position of the nerve in relation to the graft should be specified in the surgical notes in case reoperation becomes necessary. Control of the subclavian artery is obtained and a vertical arteriotomy made in its superior aspect. The graft is spatulated and sutured end-to-side with a running 4/0 or 5/0 polypropylene suture. Braided suture material should be avoided when repairing the delicate subclavian artery. Again, appropriate antegrade and retrograde bleeding is allowed. If atheroembolization is the aetiology or if the subclavian lesion is not immediately preocclusive, a ligature is placed proximal to the origin of the vertebral artery. Retrograde flow through the subclavian artery into the vertebral artery and antegrade flow into the extremity are thus ensured.

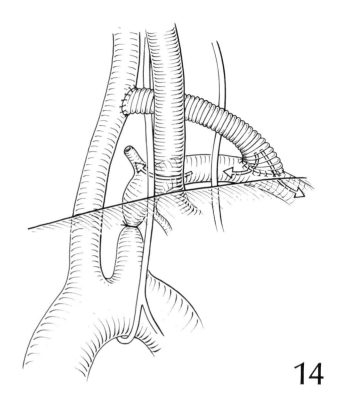

14

SUBCLAVIAN–CAROTID ARTERY BYPASS

Isolated lesions of the proximal common carotid artery, usually the left common carotid artery, in the presence of a healthy, patent, ipsilateral subclavian artery are best treated by subclavian–carotid artery bypass graft. The operation is essentially the same as that of carotid–subclavian artery bypass, obviously with reversed inflow and outflow tracts. The subclavian anastomosis is performed first in this instance. The distal anastomosis is often at the level of the carotid bifurcation.

TRANSPOSITION OF THE SUBCLAVIAN ARTERY

The indications for subclavian artery transposition into the common carotid artery are the same as those for carotid–subclavian artery bypass grafting. This alterna-tive for the correction of proximal left subclavian artery lesions is appealing because prosthetic material is not used and there is only one anastomosis[6]. More extensive dissection proximal to the vertebral and internal mammary arteries down into the thorax is necessary. The same incision as for carotid–subclavian artery bypass is used, and the carotid artery is exposed in the same manner. The proximal dissection is aided by the use of long, narrow retractors such as short Wylie renal vein retractors which allow focused retraction in a relatively deep space. When the dissection is complete, the patient is given sodium heparin. The tunnel created is the same as in the operations described above, i.e. behind the jugular vein and the sternocleidomastoid muscle.

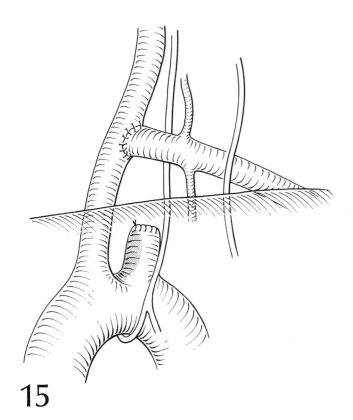

15

15 The proximal subclavian artery, the vertebral and internal mammary arteries and the distal subclavian artery are clamped. The subclavian artery is divided as far proximal to the vertebral artery as practicable. The stump is oversewn with horizontal and over-and-over 4/0 or 5/0 polypropylene sutures. The cut open end is then transposed and brought behind the jugular vein and the sternocleidomastoid muscle. Control of the carotid artery is obtained. The arteri-otomy is made laterally and slightly posteriorly. Again, this anastomosis is made at a right angle. The arteriotomy should not be too long lest the anastomosis be narrowed. The anastomosis is sutured with running 4/0 or 5/0 polypropylene. The same manoeuvres of antegrade and retrograde bleeding are performed.

The remainder of the conduct of the operation is the same as for the previously described procedures.

Postoperative care

Patients should be cared for as they are following any reconstructive operation for the arteries with careful monitoring of the pulse status. In addition, the neurological status of the patient should be assessed on a frequent serial basis. As for the innominate artery reconstructions, deterioration of any of the parameters requires appropriate medical response. Again, before discharge intravenous digital subtraction arteriography is obtained to assess the baseline status of the reconstruction.

References

1. Carlson RE, Ehrenfeld, EK, Stoeny RJ, Wylie EJ. Innominate artery endarterectomy. A 16-year experience. *Arch Surg* 1977; 112: 1389–93.

2. Crawford ES, DeBakey ME, Morris GC Jr, Howell JF. Surgical treatment of occlusion of the innominate, common carotid, and subclavian arteries: a 10-year experience. *Surgery* 1969; 65: 17–31.

3. Crawford ES, Stowe CL, Powers RW Jr. Occlusion of the innominate, common carotid, and subclavian arteries: long-term results of surgical treatment. *Surgery* 1983; 94: 781–91.

4. Cherry KJ Jr, McCullough JL, Hallett JW Jr, Pairolero PC, Gloviczki P. Technical principles of direct innominate artery revascularization: a comparison of endarterectomy and bypass grafts. *J Vasc Surg* 1989; 9: 718–24.

5. Ruel GJ, Jacobs MJHM, Gregoric ID, Calderon M, Duncan JM, Ott DA *et al*. Innominate artery occlusive disease: surgical approach and long-term results. *J Vasc Surg* 1991; 14: 405–12.

6. Sandman W, Kniemeyer HW, Jaeschock R, Hennerici M, Aulich A. The role of subclavian–carotid transposition in surgery for supraaortic occlusive disease. *J Vasc Surg* 1987; 5: 53–8.

Takayasu's arteritis: indications for surgery and appropriate procedures

Yoshio Mishima MD
Professor, IInd Department of Surgery, Tokyo Medical and Dental University, Yushima, Bunkyoku, Tokyo, Japan

Surgical intervention should preferably avoid active inflammatory episodes and the best guide is the erythrocyte sedimentation rate (ESR). Stenoses developing during acute inflammatory attacks, however, may require urgent surgical treatment, in which case it is advisable to attempt to maintain the ESR below 40 mm/h with anti-inflammatory steroid therapy.

Principles and justification

Extracranial vessels

The indications are similar to those in atheromatous carotid disease, ranging from critical stenoses of the internal carotid artery or arch vessels associated with appropriate symptoms, to stenosis in the brain with visual disturbance, transient ischaemic episodes, syncope and evidence of retinal emboli, plus the presence of small retinal aneurysms. Advanced cases, with arteriovenous retinal fistulae, are a contraindication to surgery. Surgery may be considered for asymptomatic critical carotid stenoses when other surgery, such as for aortic stenoses due to vasculitis, must be undertaken. These carotid reconstructions should precede the definitive and more major procedure.

The best technique of reconstruction avoids direct endarterectomy of the inflamed and stenosed segment, and should consist of resection with end-to-end replacement with autogenous vein, or aortocarotid or subclavian–carotid bypass.

It is usually satisfactory to reconstruct flow in only one side even if both sides are involved, and simultaneous bilateral reconstruction is not advisable.

Atypical coarctation of the aorta

Surgery is indicated when the systolic blood pressure is higher than 180 mmHg at rest, or when it rises higher than 200 mmHg after gentle exercise, and is particularly indicated when medical treatment fails to control hypertension. Patients who respond well to medical treatment should not be treated surgically unless the stenosis becomes worse. The procedure of choice is bypass of the stenosed area with an aortoaortic Dacron graft.

Renal artery reconstruction

The indications for surgery are systolic hypertension above 180 mmHg or diastolic hypertension above 110 mmHg. A renin ratio of more than 1.5 between involved and uninvolved renal vein samples, or a renal vein/peripheral vein renin coefficient of 0.24 or higher are also indications for surgery.

The procedure of choice is transluminal angioplasty, though its success rate is only 50%. Failure is an indication for aortorenal bypass, with either autogenous vein or a synthetic graft. Nephrectomy may be required in patients with severe renal atrophy and poor or negligible renal function on that side.

Aortic incompetence

Surgery is indicated when regurgitation is more than 3° on Seller's classification and the left ventricular ejection fraction is also more than 0.4. The procedure of choice is aortic valve replacement, which may include replacement of the aneurysmal ascending aorta by Bentall's technique.

Subclavian artery

Subclavian and innominate reconstruction is indicated in patients with symptomatic cranial steal syndrome (either left subclavian steal or, on the right side, carotid plus vertebral steal to the subclavian artery) when this is associated with persistent troublesome symptoms. Bilateral simultaneous procedures are occasionally indicated. The technique of choice is carotid–subclavian bypass; in diffuse disease involving most of the arch vessels, branched bypass from the ascending aorta to both subclavian arteries or subclavian and carotid arteries may be required.

Coronary artery surgery

The only indications for coronary artery bypass surgery in Takayasu's disease correspond to those in atheroma. The techniques of choice are percutaneous angioplasty, which may have a lower success rate than in atheromatous disease or, should this fail or be contraindicated, aortocoronary bypass.

Aneurysms

Saccular aneurysms must be treated by urgent surgery as they have a very high risk of rupture. The indications for surgery in fusiform aneurysms are comparable with those in atheromatous disease, i.e. symptoms or definite evidence of increase in size. The treatment involves resection and replacement with a synthetic graft.

Extracranial intracranial bypass

K. G. Burnand MS, FRCS
Professor of Vascular Surgery, St Thomas' Hospital, London, UK

Principles and justification

This operation was devised by Yasargil and Donaghy in 1967[1] to provide an additional blood supply to an ischaemic cerebral hemisphere. Its advent appeared to provide surgeons with the ability to revascularize the brain in patients with carotid occlusions which until then were untreatable. Other indications for extracranial intracranial bypass are for high intracranial carotid stenoses, or where a stenosis is present in the main stem of the middle cerebral artery[2]. A rare indication is to provide an alternative blood supply to a portion of brain where the primary arterial supply has to be sacrificed as part of therapy, for example, a patient having an arteriovenous malformation removed from the brain.

Many of these operations were performed in the 1980s for patients with few symptoms who simply had a carotid occlusion, on the grounds that this type of patient would benefit from an improved blood supply to an underperfused brain[3]. Studies of cerebral blood flow were seldom, if ever, performed to confirm this hypothesis. A large multicentre study was organized by Barnett in North America to examine the clinical value of extracranial intracranial bypass in preventing stroke and extending life[4]; 1377 patients were admitted to the study, but a further 1695 were operated on outside the trial on the grounds that surgical treatment was considered 'essential' and it would have been unethical to include these patients in the 'medical' arm of the study[5]. Patients were followed for a mean of 55.8 months, and at this point there was no difference in the morbidity or mortality rates of the operated group compared with the medically treated group, who mostly received aspirin. Strokes occurred with equal frequency in both groups, and the mortality rates were almost identical. Only 30%, however, were having or had had transient ischaemic attacks at the time of entry to the study, the majority having had a minor stroke. No measurements were made of cerebral perfusion. Despite its many flaws, this study appeared to signal the end of extracranial intracranial bypass.

Smaller studies, however, have subsequently shown that a subgroup of patients with reduced cerebral reserve who have intractable symptoms of cerebral hypoperfusion (repeated disabling transient ischaemic attacks; ten or more per day) causing episodes of unconsciousness can benefit considerably from extracranial intracranial bypass[6].

Preoperative

Selection of patients and investigation

Cerebral hypoperfusion is the probable cause of transient ischaemic attacks that occur on a frequent daily basis and are brought on by effort or exercise. Cerebral autoregulation may be severely embarrassed when both carotid arteries are occluded, and under these circumstances an increased demand for peripheral blood flow may temporarily reduce cerebral perfusion. There may also be a reduction in perfusion to a single cerebral hemisphere when the circle of Willis is incomplete. The cerebral reserve may be measured by positron emission tomography[7], xenon clearance following carbon dioxide stress and transcerebral Doppler velocity measurements of the middle cerebral artery, also in response to a carbon dioxide stress[8].

Patients with appropriate symptoms being considered for extracranial intracranial bypass must have evidence of an occluded carotid artery related to the hemisphere from which the symptoms are arising. They must also have 'hypoperfusion' confirmed by one of the investigations listed above. Carotid occlusion can be determined by duplex ultrasonography, but should be confirmed by arteriography (intravenous digital subtraction arteriography or arch aortography). Computed tomography or magnetic resonance imaging of the brain should exclude other conditions such as a meningioma or a chronic subdural haematoma, which may give rise to similar symptoms. A neurological opinion is also essential. These tests should identify the small number of individuals who have severe disabling 'hypoperfusional' cortical symptoms with critically reduced cerebral reserve. These patients, who cannot be helped in any other way, benefit considerably from the improved local cortical flow produced by an extracranial intracranial bypass[6].

Preparation of patient

Patients must be assessed for their fitness for operation. This includes taking a careful history, which should elicit any symptoms of atheromatous disease at other sites such as the coronary, splanchnic or limb arteries. A careful enquiry must also be made into their past or present history to exclude associated disease. A full examination should detect abnormalities in the heart, lungs and peripheral circulation as well as determining any permanent neurological damage. A full blood count, chest radiography and electrocardiography are essential preoperative investigations in all patients. The anaesthetist should see the patient before the operation and confirm fitness for general anaesthesia.

Anaesthesia

After induction of anaesthesia the patient is paralysed, intubated and then ventilated. The endotracheal tube is attached to a long connecting tube to ensure that the head and neck are free from all impedimenta. A cannula is inserted into a peripheral vein, and an intravenous infusion of crystalloid is commenced. A single dose of broad-spectrum antibiotic is given intravenously (amoxycillin with potassium clavulanate (Augmentin), a cephalosporin, or amoxycillin alone).

Operation

Position of patient

The head is shaved with electric clippers, and the patient is placed in the full lateral position with the head supported on a padded ring.

1   The course of the superficial temporal artery is determined before the operation using a portable Doppler ultrasonographic probe and indelibly marked on the skin surface. The skin is then prepared with chlorhexidine or povidone–iodine, and the head is draped to expose the appropriate side of the scalp from the ear to the vertex.

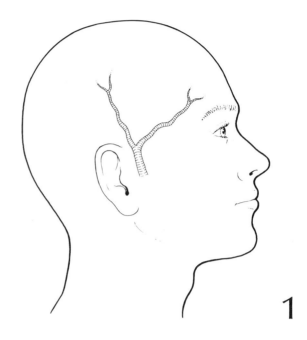

1

Incision

An incision is made over the trunk of the superficial temporal artery, either just above or just in front of the ear. The incision should only divide the skin, because the artery often lies just beneath the deep layers of the dermis. The edges of the wound can be retracted with skin hooks until a suitable length of incision is available to insert a self-retaining retractor. Small iris scissors are used to bluntly part the skin edges. The superficial temporal artery lies on the temporal fascia, and its position can be confirmed by palpation. The surgeon may wish to wear magnifying loupes during this part of the dissection, but those with good natural vision will not require this aid. The superficial temporal fascia is divided and the artery freed from the surrounding muscle.

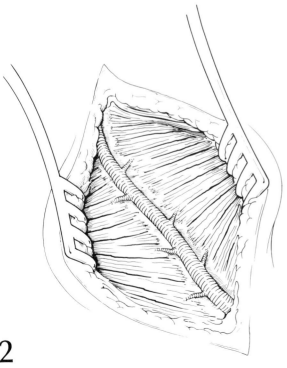

2

2   The skin incision is extended as the artery is dissected upwards. The vessel should be left within its fascial sheath in order to avoid damage. Branches should therefore be divided and sealed by diathermy well away from the main trunk. Side branches can be safely coagulated with bipolar diathermy. There are few branches coming off the front or the back of the vessel, most arising from either side, and once these side branches have been divided a pedicle can be raised containing the vessel. Either the posterior or anterior division of the main artery is followed depending on which branch appears to be the dominant vessel as judged by Doppler mapping and arteriography. The selected vessel is followed for a suitable distance towards the vertex of the skull.

3 A cortical branch of the middle cerebral artery must now be prepared to receive the bypass. The alternative approaches are a simple burr hole (which may be enlarged) or to turn a skull flap. The former is much simpler. The burr hole should be centred about 5 cm above the external auditory meatus or about 1–2 cm above the apex of the pinna. It can usually be made through the same incision that has been used to mobilize the superficial temporal artery.

The temporal fascia is divided in the line of the skin incision, and the fibres of the temporalis muscle are split in the same direction using diathermy. The cranium is exposed by separating the temporalis muscle off the bone with a periosteal elevator. A self-retaining retractor is then inserted to expose an appropriate area of skull. A perforator is applied to the brace and a hole is bored into the skull through the exposed cranium. It is again centred approximately 5 cm above the external auditory meatus. Firm downward pressure on the brace cuts out a cone of bone through the skull. As the tip of the perforator passes through the inner table of the skull

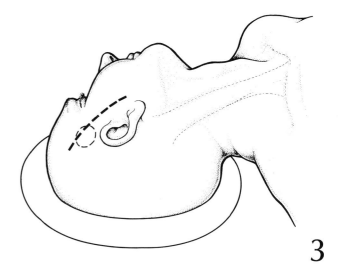

3

into the extradural space, the brace is felt to 'rock' slightly. When the bone chips are removed, a Mc-Donald's dissector can be carefully inserted between the bone and the dura mater. A burr is then used to widen the defect in the skull. The burr hole may then be enlarged still further using bone-nibbling forceps.

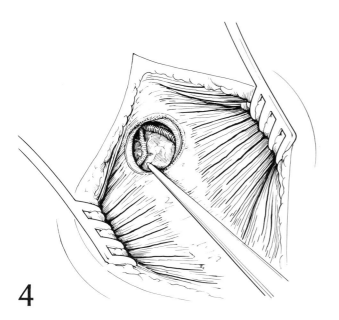

4

4 Once a reasonable area of dura has been exposed, a hook is inserted into the dural membrane which is incised with a scalpel. This initial incision is extended with scissors into a cruciate shape. The four points of the dura can then be retracted and sutured to provide easy access to the brain. At this point a cortical artery can often be seen with the naked eye crossing the surface of the brain. The artery appears bright red and is easily distinguished from cortical veins, which are dark blue in colour. The burr hole may be extended if an artery is not seen. Alternatively, gentle dissection of the pia mater using blunt forceps may demonstrate a vessel, particularly if the operating microscope is used to view the surface of the brain. The burr hole must be enlarged if the artery lies to one side of the field or if it is not easily visible.

5 Once an artery is clearly seen, the operating microscope is moved into position and focused on the surface of the brain. Both the surgeon and the assistant should be comfortably seated on either side of the microscope, which is adjusted using an automatic focus and zooming pedal until the surface vessels are clearly visible. The pia mater is gently teased off the artery using blunt dissection with watchmaker's forceps and microdissecting scissors. Between 1 and 2 cm of vessel should be freed from the surface of the brain. Small side branches can be cauterized with a bipolar diathermy before being carefully divided. Again, care is taken to apply the diathermy well away from the main vessel.

The distal end of the superficial temporal artery is then prepared. A small bulldog clamp is applied proximally, and the artery is divided distally and ligated. The end of the vessel is dissected out of the surrounding tissues in the pedicle, so that a 'clean' portion is available for the anastomosis. The bulldog clamp is released to ensure that there is a good blood flow from the end of the artery.

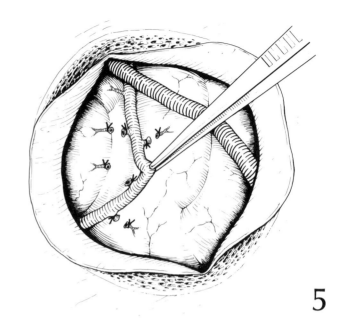

5

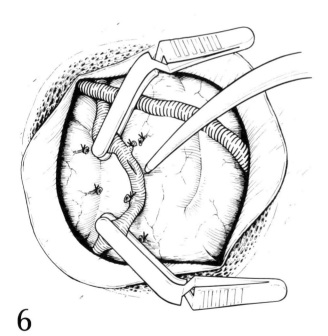

6

6 Microvascular bulldog clamps are applied to either end of the prepared segment of cortical vessel, using a special spring applicator to apply and release them. A longitudinal incision is then made into the cortical vessel with a diamond knife and extended with microscissors for 2–3 mm (an appropriate length to match the cross-sectional diameter of the transected superficial temporal artery).

The cut end of the superficial temporal artery is then brought into close apposition with the cortical vessels. Both of the lumens are flushed with heparinized saline, and it is extremely useful to have a device that both flushes and sucks away any blood clots. This is primed with heparinized saline.

7 A suture is inserted into the apex of the free end of the superficial temporal artery, from outside to inside and this is then brought through the arteriotomy in the cortical vessel from in to out.

This first suture is tied and another suture is put into the heel of the anastomosis before being tied. All knots are tied using needle holders by a microsurgical technique, which must be learnt and practised regularly. A third suture is then placed halfway between the first two on one side and held out. This ensures that both walls of the vessel are not inadvertently picked up during subsequent suturing. Long ends are left on all the sutures, and these can be used as retractors.

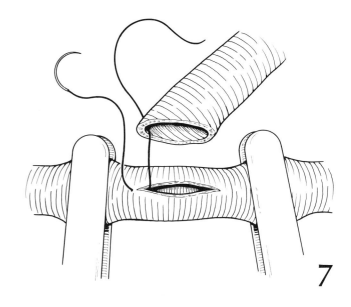

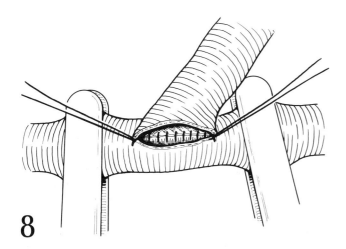

8 An assistant then holds the long ends of the middle and apical sutures, and it is a simple matter to insert two or three sutures on either side of the middle suture to complete the back layer.

The superficial temporal artery is then turned forwards and a middle suture is placed in the centre of the far side. This is gently pulled up and other sutures are inserted in the same way. Other techniques that have been used include placing each individual suture next to the initial suture all the way round or placing the two original sutures 160° rather than 180° apart. Each surgeon has his or her own preference.

9   When the anastomosis has been completed the clamps are removed from the cortical vessel and the presence of any suture line bleeding is observed. If large quantities of blood escape additional sutures must be inserted to close the gap.

Eventually the suture line should be dry, and the dura may be loosely closed around the superficial temporal artery with 2/0 catgut. The bone chippings removed at the time of making the initial burr hole are placed around the vessels and the skin is closed with interrupted 4/0 nylon sutures. A thin gauze dressing is placed over the suture line and fixed with plastic spray.

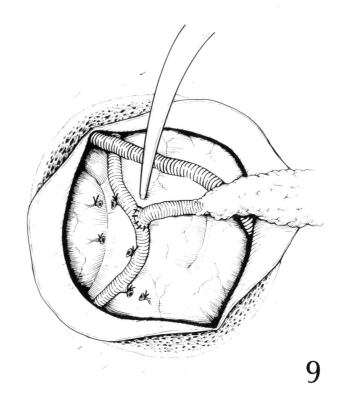

9

Postoperative care

The patient should be awake as the last suture is placed and the neurological state can be rapidly assessed. Intravenous fluids are given for 24 h, and patients can start on oral fluids in the recovery room. Neurological observations should be made every 30 min to 1 h for the first 24 h, and anticonvulsants should be given for 6 weeks. Sutures can be removed on the seventh day, and the patient may leave hospital before this if the recovery is uncomplicated. The major complication of the operation is stroke, usually associated with occlusion of the bypass. Haemorrhage may also require reoperation. Infection and epilepsy are rare. By carefully selecting appropriate patients, good results are obtained.

References

1. Yasargil MG. Experimental small vessel surgery in the dog including patching and grafting of cerebral vessels and the formation of functional extra-intracranial shunts. In: Donaghy RMP, Yasargil MG, eds. *Microvascular Surgery*. St Louis: CV Mosby, 1967.

2. Andrews BT, Chater NL, Weinstein PR. Extracranial-intracranial arterial bypass for middle cerebral artery stenosis and occlusion: operative results in 65 cases. *J Neurosurg* 1985; 62: 831–8.

3. Sundt TM, Whisnant JP, Fode NC, Piepgras DG, Houser OW. Results, complications and follow-up of 415 bypass operations for occlusive disease of the carotid system. *Mayo Clin Proc* 1985; 60: 230–40.

4. The EC/IC Bypass Study Group. Failure of extracranial-intracranial bypass to reduce the risk of ischemic stroke. *N Engl J Med* 1985; 313: 1191–200.

5. Sundt TM. Was the international randomized trial of extracranial-intracranial arterial bypass representative of the population at risk? *N Engl J Med* 1987; 316: 814–16.

6. Bishop CCR, Burnand KG, Brown M, Ross-Russell RW, Browse NL. Reduced response of cerebral blood flow to hypercapnia: restoration by extracranial-intracranial bypass. *Br J Surg* 1987; 74: 802–4.

7. Gibbs JM, Wise RJS, Leenders KL, Jones T. Evaluation of cerebral perfusion reserve in patients with carotid-artery occlusion. *Lancet* 1984; i: 182–6.

8. Bishop CCR, Powell S, Insall M, Rutt D, Browse NL. Effect of internal carotid artery occlusion on middle cerebral artery blood flow at rest and in response to hypercapnia. *Lancet* 1986; i: 710–12.

Surgical technique for aortic dissection

P. Michael McFadden MD
Cardiovascular and Thoracic Surgeon, Department of Surgery, Ochsner Clinic, New Orleans, Louisiana, USA

John L. Ochsner MD
Chairman Emeritus, Department of Surgery, Chief, Division of Thoracic and Cardiovascular Surgery, Ochsner Clinic, New Orleans, Louisiana, USA

History

Aortic dissection is the most common catastrophe involving the aorta. It occurs in approximately one in every 300–500 patients and is more frequent than rupture of an abdominal aortic aneurysm. Two important contributing factors in the development of aortic dissection are hypertension and disease of the aortic media; an abnormality of the aortic media is present in almost all cases. Lesions of the aorta which predispose to dissection have been classified as elastic tissue defects, muscular lesions or combined lesions of the media. Marfan's syndrome is a classic example of an elastic tissue defect. Approximately 71% of patients with cardiovascular manifestations of this syndrome have aortic dissection. Elastic lesions are the most common finding in patients presenting with aortic dissection under the age of 40 years, while muscular lesions predominate in patients over 40. Medial degeneration is occasionally caused by a combination of elastic and muscular lesions. Conditions such as rheumatoid arthritis, scleroderma, giant cell arteritis, granulomatous arteritis and ankylosing spondylitis are associated with combined medial degeneration. Degeneration of the aorta with ageing and atherosclerosis predisposes to dissection. Hypertension has been identified in approximately 70% of patients with aortic dissection. Dissection occurs with increased frequency in conditions in which hypertension is common, such as pregnancy, congenital bicuspid aortic valve and coarctation of the aorta. Iatrogenic causes secondary to aortic cannulation, catheterization procedures or intra-aortic balloon placement are seen with increasing frequency as the number of invasive procedures performed on the cardiovascular system rises.

The condition is characterized by the development of a haematoma which dissects longitudinally for variable distances within the aortic wall. The source of the haematoma is most often a transverse intimal tear. The majority of aortic dissections begin subintimally and progress to involve the middle to outer third of the aortic media. A dissection may occur at any point along the course of the aorta and progress circumferentially, proximally or distally. This condition has the potential to affect any organ system. The dissection may remain patent as a false channel, terminate in thrombosis, re-enter the true lumen by fenestration, or rupture into the pericardial, pleural or peritoneal cavities. Complications that result from aortic dissection are often life threatening; early diagnosis and treatment are therefore essential. Associated complications such as myocardial infarction, cardiac tamponade, aortic valvular insufficiency, stroke, paralysis and visceral or extremity ischaemia may initially obscure the diagnosis and delay definitive treatment. A thorough history and physical examination as well as a high index of suspicion best serves the patient and leads to early diagnosis. Untreated, 21% of patients will die within the first 24 h, 60% within 2 weeks, and 90% within 3 months.

Classification

1 Multiple classifications and subclassifications of thoracic aortic dissection have been proposed. The majority are found to be detailed, cumbersome and unnecessary. The classification which has been used most commonly in the past is that proposed by DeBakey. The classification proposed by the Stanford University group we find to be simple and the most useful. This classification is based solely upon the presence or absence of involvement of the ascending aorta, regardless of the site of origin of the intimal tear. Dissections involving the proximal ascending aorta are classified as Stanford type A, and dissections distal to and not involving the ascending aorta are classified as Stanford type B. This classification not only relates to prognosis but assists in therapeutic decision making.

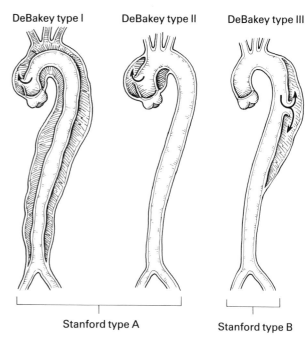

DeBakey type I   DeBakey type II   DeBakey type III

Stanford type A   Stanford type B

1

Principles and justification

The general management of all patients with aortic dissection, whether acute or chronic, begins with medical therapy. The plan is to alter the pathophysiology of dissection and prevent secondary complications. It is our recommendation that operative intervention is indicated in virtually all patients with acute type A (ascending) aortic dissections and in the majority of acute type B (descending) thoracic dissections. In addition, most chronic type A dissections will ultimately require surgical therapy. The majority of patients with chronic type B descending dissections can be managed medically. In all patients who do not undergo initial surgical management close surveillance is indicated in order to detect late sequelae of dissection that may require surgical intervention. Contraindications for surgical therapy can be relative or absolute. Relative contraindications include age and the degree of physiological abnormality of vital organs. An absolute contraindication to operation is a concomitant life limiting condition, the course of which is similar to the natural history of aortic dissection.

Management of the patient with aortic dissection is a coordinated effort involving the emergency physician, medical specialist, radiologist, cardiovascular surgeon and cardiac anaesthesiologist. The patient will require invasive monitoring for continued assessment and management of both haemodynamic and laboratory parameters while the evaluation is in progress. Provided the patient is not hypotensive, drugs such as sodium nitroprusside, trimetaphan camsylate or intravenous propranolol are administered intravenously to lower the mean arterial blood pressure and to decrease the shear forces and dp/dt on the aortic wall. The target mean arterial blood pressure should be in the range of 50–80 mmHg. Beta-antagonists have been most useful in attaining the desired pharmacological effect. Nitroprusside is effective in rapidly lowering the blood pressure but has been shown to increase dp/dt in some instances. Pharmacological management is tempered should myocardial ischaemia, oliguria, or mental confusion occur. Delay in evaluation, diagnosis and initiation of treatment must be avoided.

The preferred diagnostic examination to confirm the presence, location and extent of aortic dissection remains the contrast aortogram. This examination can be performed easily and is relatively undemanding for the patient. Medical attention to the patient need not be impeded during the conduct of this procedure. Magnetic resonance imaging is an extremely sensitive non-invasive procedure which may, when combined with cine imaging techniques, provide not only the diagnosis but information as to blood flow characteristics within the false lumen. Its application, however, is limited due to the time required to perform the procedure and the technical difficulties encountered in physically managing these critically ill patients during the examination. The efficacy of transthoracic echocardiography has also been demonstrated in this condition and may provide a rapid method of establishing a diagnosis at the bedside. Transoesophageal echocardiography has been particularly useful in determining dissections involving the descending aorta. The sensitivity of these modalities is limited and a negative examination does not rule out aortic dissection.

Operation

TYPE A DISSECTIONS AND DISSECTIONS OF THE TRANSVERSE AORTIC ARCH

The authors believe that deep hypothermic circulatory arrest and replacement of both the ascending aorta and transverse arch to a point distal to the left subclavian artery is the preferred approach to the repair of type A and transverse aortic arch dissections. This approach addresses the immediate possibility of retrograde dissection resulting in aortic valvular incompetency or death, as well as the late sequelae of vascular compromise of the brachiocephalic circulation or pseudoaneurysm formation. Surgical management is the same as for repair of transverse arch aneurysms.

Incision

2 A median sternotomy incision is used, with extension into either the right or left neck to provide adequate distal exposure of the innominate vessels. The incision is carried along the anterior border of the sternocleidomastoid muscle. The sternal and clavicular attachments of the sternocleidomastoid muscle and the strap muscles may be divided. The innominate vein may also be divided but this is rarely necessary and may result in swelling of the left upper extremity postoperatively.

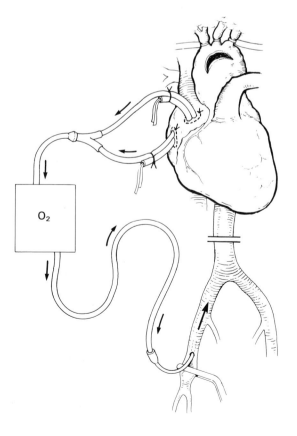

2

Cardiopulmonary bypass

3 Standard cardiopulmonary bypass techniques are employed. This involves femoral arterial cannulation and cannulation of the superior and inferior vena cavae or right atrium. Cardiopulmonary bypass is initiated and the patient is cooled systemically to a nasopharyngeal temperature of 18°C. Simultaneously, the heart is cooled topically with 4°C iced saline or slush. A primary concern in these patients is preservation of neurological function during the phase of circulatory arrest. The patient's head is packed in ice while deep core cooling is accomplished. Phenobarbitone is often added to the anaesthetic regimen, as it has been demonstrated to provide a degree of cerebral protection. Once cooling has been achieved, the usual perfusion flow rates of 25–50 ml/kg per min are reduced to less than 500 ml/min or more commonly discontinued altogether.

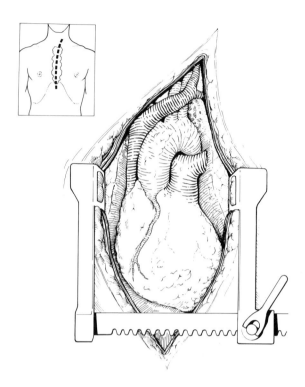

3

Aortotomy

4 The aorta is opened and inspected. A false lumen is often encountered initially, which may be circumferential or partial. The wall of the true lumen is opened and the coronary ostia are identified. The myocardium is protected by administration of 500–1000 ml of 4°C hyperkalaemic cardioplegia solution instilled by handheld cannulae or by a retrograde perfusion catheter placed in the coronary sinus. Topical hypothermia with ice slush or continuous iced saline irrigation affords additional myocardial protection throughout the period of circulatory arrest. The goal is to maintain the myocardial temperature in the range of 4–17°C.

Transection of aorta

5a, b The aorta is transected proximally and distally. Clamping of the aorta or innominate vessels is usually not required during circulatory arrest. The intimal tear is sought and, if present, is included in the resected aortic segment. The tear is commonly located anteriorly and to the right in type A dissections. However, the intimal tear in type A dissections need not be located in the ascending aorta. A cuff of transverse aortic wall containing the innominate vessels is preserved.

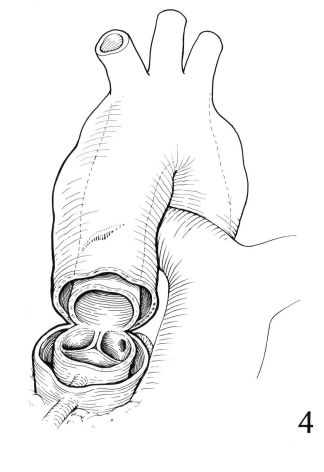

4

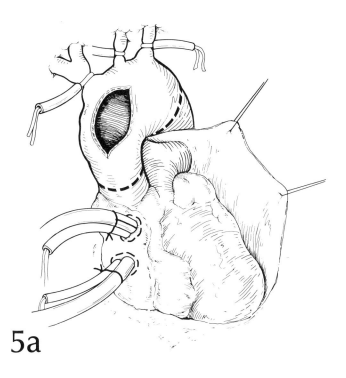

5a

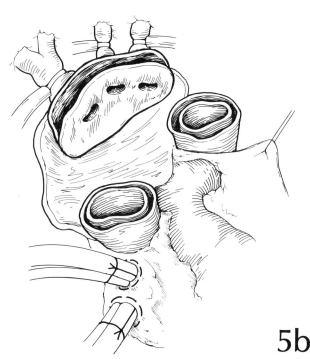

5b

Evaluation of the aortic valve

6 Aortic valvular regurgitation may be associated with type A dissections. Inspection of the aortic valve and coronary arteries is performed to rule out involvement of these structures. A thorough evaluation of the aortic valvular apparatus and coronary arteries at this stage of the operation allows for planning and choice of conduit for the repair. When the aortic valve apparatus is irreparably damaged, replacement is required. More commonly, regurgitation results from prolapse of the aortic leaflets due to loss of commissural support. Salvage of the native valve is preferable to replacement, and this is feasible in the majority of type A dissections. Even when the dissection involves the right or non-coronary cusps, resuspension of the valve to the graft is possible with polytetrafluoroethylene (PTFE; Teflon) felt pledgets, preserving native valve tissue and function. Valvular replacement rather than reconstruction is recommended in type A dissections resulting from Marfan's syndrome or aortoannular ectasia due to the primary underlying pathology in these patients. A decision to repair or replace the aortic valve is based on the anatomical findings. A tube graft or valved conduit is then chosen. Reconstruction of the proximal aorta and valvular apparatus is reserved until after the distal aorta and arch repairs are completed and cardiopulmonary bypass is reinstituted. This technique minimizes duration of cerebral ischaemia.

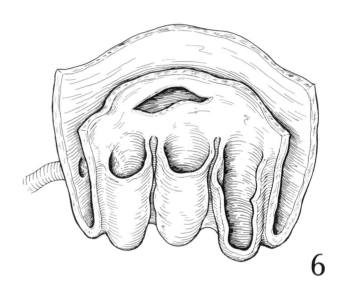

6

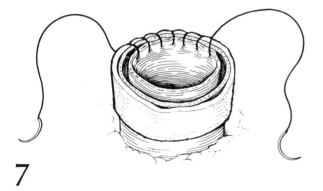

7

Distal aortic repair

7 The distal aorta is reconstructed using a 'sandwich' technique. PTFE felt strips are placed on both the adventitial and intimal surfaces to buttress the dissected aortic wall. Felt may also be placed between the dissected layers when necessary. The false lumen is obliterated with a continuous 4/0 polypropylene suture. A Dacron interposition graft is then tailored to approximate the size of the distal aorta. This may require an oblique transection in order to fashion the graft to approximate the diameter of the distal aorta. Recent experience in Europe with the use of vascular glue in the management of aortic dissection has been shown to be effective.

Distal aortic anastomosis

8a, b The distal anastomosis is performed first. The anastomosis is performed with a long (140 cm) 3/0 polypropylene suture. A very low porosity woven Dacron graft is recommended (Ochsner–Woven 50 porosity). These grafts are haemostatic and do not require preclotting. They allow for proper selection of graft size while the patient is anticoagulated and on cardiopulmonary bypass. However, we prefer to make the graft completely non-porous by autoclaving the graft after soaking it in heparinized blood or albumin. The posterior suture line is begun by taking a narrow horizontal mattress suture from the outside to the inside of the graft and carrying the needle from the intima to the adventitia of the aorta through the PTFE felt buttresses. The anastomosis is begun at the mid-portion of the posterior wall of the aorta and is carried bilaterally in a running fashion. Meticulous attention to technique in the presence of friable aortic tissue is necessary to prevent haemorrhagic complications. An aortic cross-clamp or balloon occluder may be utilized if necessary to control backbleeding from the distal aorta. This is unnecessary in the majority of cases.

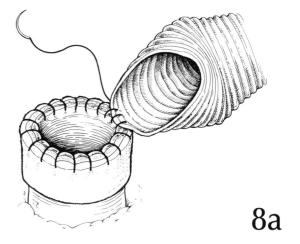

8a

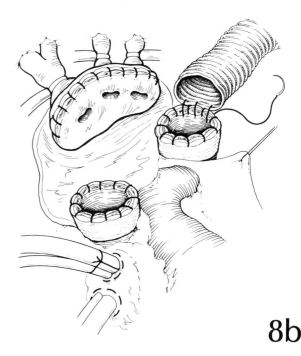

8b

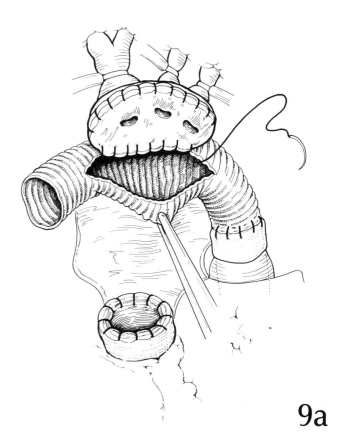

9a

Proximal arch implantation

9a, b Following completion of the distal anastomosis the cuff of aorta including the innominate vessels is prepared with PTFE felt buttresses in a manner similar to the distal aorta. A window of appropriate size is created in the superior aspect of the graft. The aortic cuff is then sutured to the window in the superior aspect of the Dacron graft using a long (140 cm) 3/0 polypropylene suture.

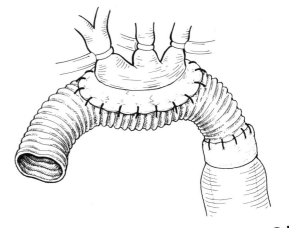

9b

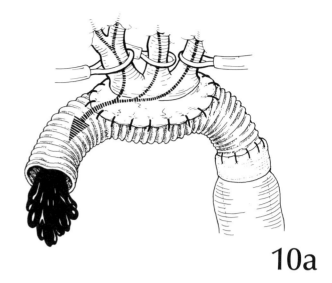

10a

10a–c Before performing the proximal anastomosis the innominate vessels are flushed through the proximal limb of the graft to remove retained air and debris. These vessels are then temporarily controlled with clamps to prevent cerebral embolism as cardiopulmonary bypass is slowly reinstituted to allow retrograde filling of the aorta. The distal aorta is flushed through the graft. The graft is then cross-clamped just proximal to the origin of the innominate artery and the clamps on the innominate vessels are released. This technique allows retrograde perfusion to the innominate vessels while the proximal aortic anastomosis is completed. Rewarming to 37°C is begun once cerebral reperfusion is reinstituted using standard cardiopulmonary bypass techniques. Rewarming is performed at a rate not exceeding 1°C every 3 min. Blood temperature is not allowed to exceed the core temperature by more than 6°C in order to preserve the integrity of cellular membranes.

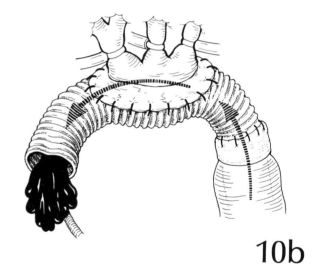

10b

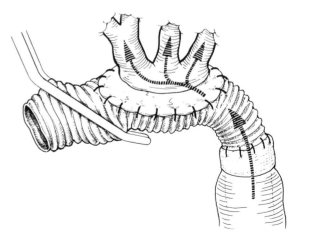

10c

Fenestration technique

11 In chronic dissection, the outer wall of the aorta becomes fibrotic, secondary to the dense inflammatory process and healing of the adventitia. The false lumen is often larger than the true lumen and major branches of the aorta may be fed by the false channel. Obliteration of the false lumen in the chronic stage may not be possible or advisable because of the disparity in diameters of the true and false lumen and the potential for ischaemia in branches that may now be fed by the false lumen. Fenestration or resection of a portion of the false septum is often preferable.

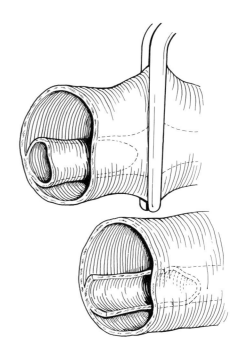

11

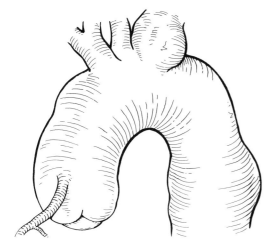

12a

Repair of pseudoaneurysm

12a, b Pseudoaneurysm formation may necessitate resection and interposition grafts to one or more of the innominate branches.

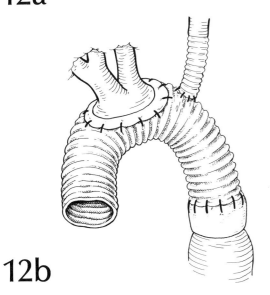

12b

Stabilization of aortic valve at proximal anastomosis

13a, b Reconstruction of the proximal aortic root is designed to accomplish both stabilization of the aortic valve apparatus and prevention of recurrent proximal dissection. To accomplish this a 'sandwich' technique is commonly employed. The adventitial surface of the aorta is buttressed with a PTFE felt strip while a second felt strip is placed on the intimal surface. An additional felt strip may be placed between the walls of the true and false lumen. The layers are then approximated circumferentially with a running 4/0 polypropylene suture, thereby obliterating the false lumen. Care must be taken not to compromise the coronary ostia or arteries, and tailoring of the PTFE strip to accomplish this is often necessary. Preservation of the aortic valve is accomplished with this technique.

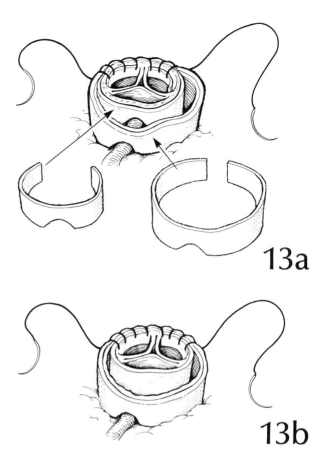

13a

13b

14a, b The proximal aortic anastomosis is performed while the patient is re-warming.

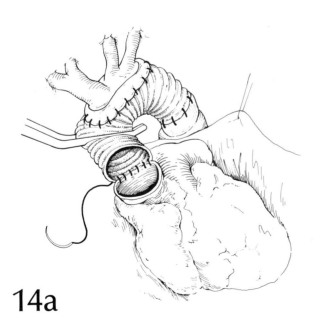

14a

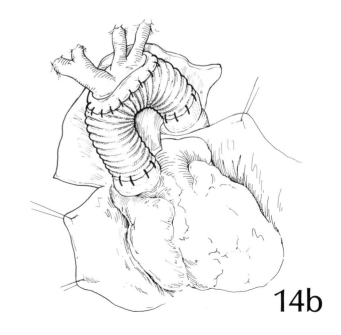

14b

Aortic valve replacement

15a, b In patients with type A dissection in whom valvular repair is not possible, replacement of the aortic valve is necessary. When the integrity of the supra-annular aorta is good the proximal aorta may be scalloped to preserve the coronary ostia. Prosthetic aortic valve replacement is performed. This is accomplished with a 3/0 mattress non-absorbable suture. Either a mechanical or bioprosthetic valve may be employed. The possibility of bioprosthetic valve failure and reoperation must be taken into consideration when selecting a tissue valve. The Dacron graft is sutured in a supracoronary position. Replacement of a failed valve can be accomplished through an incision in the Dacron graft and would not necessarily require replacement of the graft.

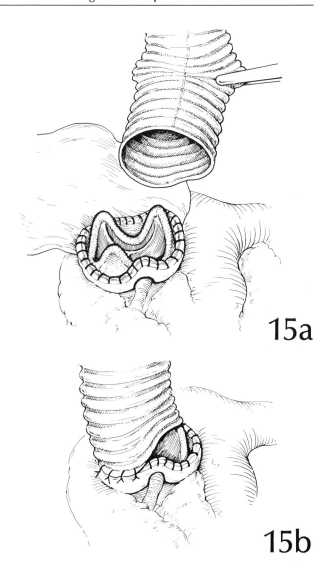

15a

15b

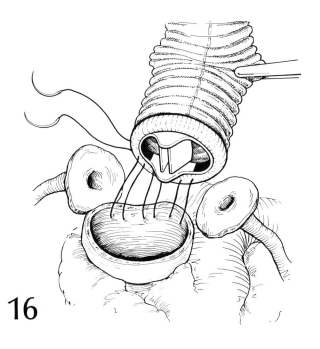

16

16 In the presence of insufficient supra-annular tissue, or involvement of the coronary arteries, a valved conduit must be utilized. Reoperation for a failed composite valved conduit would require replacement of both the valve and the conduit. A mechanical valved conduit is therefore recommended in this situation as it is more durable and less likely to require reoperation. A separate valved conduit is usually required. After the proximal anastomosis and valve implantation are completed the valved conduit can be tailored and sutured to the distal Dacron graft in an end-to-end fashion.

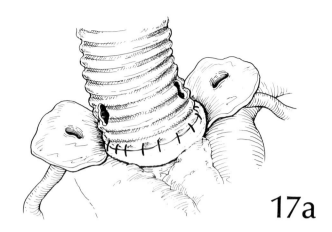

17a

Reimplantation of coronary arteries

17a–c Reimplantation of the coronary arteries is required in the presence of a composite valved conduit. This may be accomplished by the method described by Bentall in which a portion of the aortic wall is left attached to the coronary arteries. Direct reimplantation of the coronaries to the graft is performed with a 'button' of aorta around the coronary ostia. Aneurysmal formation of the residual aortic tissue has been decribed, so a small PTFE felt 'washer' may be tailored to externally buttress the anastomosis of the aortic 'button' to the composite graft. When it appears that too much tension will be present on the coronary graft anastomosis the authors employ Cabrol's modification and insert a tubular graft (8-mm Gore-tex) end-to-end to both coronary buttons and side-to-side to the aortic graft.

Once graft placement has been completed, the heart is resuscitated in the usual fashion. Heparin anticoagulation is reversed with protamine administration. Judicious use of intravenous procoagulants and topical thrombogenic agents is recommended as bleeding from the interstices of the graft is frequently encountered. Postoperative coagulopathy is always a problem following deep hypothermic arrest and is magnified in the presence of aortic dissection. Procoagulants and component therapy including fresh frozen plasma, platelets, cryoprecipitate, packed red cells and, occasionally, factor IX are necessary in the majority of cases. Frequent reassessment of the coagulation status is mandatory until adequate haemostasis has been achieved. This assessment is performed by utilization of the activated clotting times (ACT), prothrombin time (PT), partial thromboplastin time (PTT), platelet count and thrombelastogram (TEG).

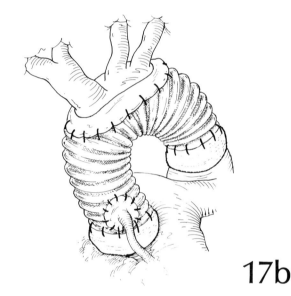

17b

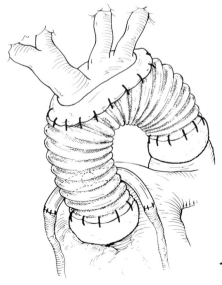

17c

Limited repair for type A dissection

18a–d Traditional repair of type A aortic dissection is mentioned for completeness. Standard cardiopulmonary bypass techniques with moderate systemic hypothermia and myocardial preservation are employed. In this repair the ascending aorta is clamped proximal to the innominate artery. Replacement of the ascending aorta is performed in the manner described under type A and arch dissections (page 165). The proximal anastomosis is performed first with this technique. The aortic valve is repaired or replaced as indicated and concomitant coronary revascularization procedures may be performed if necessary.

This technique allows for continuous cerebral perfusion. The authors reserve this technique for patients with very limited type A dissections involving the proximal or mid ascending aorta with no involvement of the transverse arch. However, the authors feel strongly that the majority of patients will have a better repair and long-term result with ascending and arch aortic replacement under deep hypothermia and circulatory arrest.

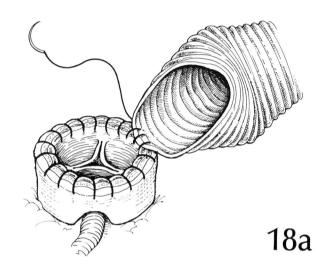

18a

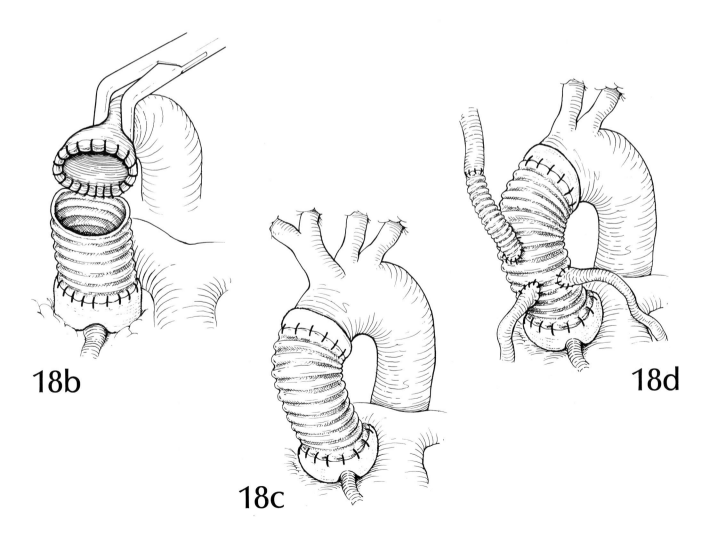

18b

18c

18d

TYPE B AORTIC DISSECTION

Prevention of death and morbid sequelae are the objectives in the management of patients with type B aortic dissection. This includes aortic rupture, aneurysm formation and extension of the dissection which can result in paraplegia or vital organ ischaemia. The principles of surgical therapy are to perform replacement of the most involved portion of the descending aorta and to restore vital organ and extremity perfusion.

Incision

19a, b Exposure of the descending thoracic aorta is accomplished through a standard left posterolateral thoracotomy.

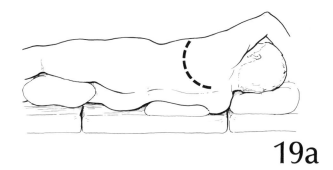

19a

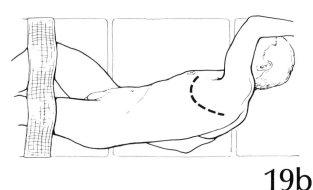

19b

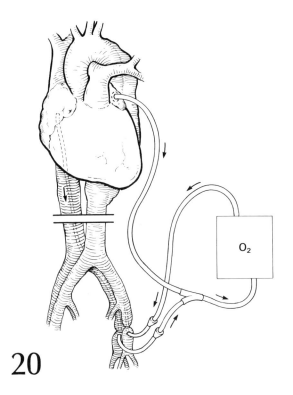

20

20 Circulatory support in all cases is achieved with partial femorofemoral cardiopulmonary bypass or left atriofemoral bypass via right superior pulmonary vein cannulation.

The incidence of renal insufficiency and spinal cord injury has been lessened with the use of partial cardiopulmonary bypass in aortic dissection. This technique gives the best chance of renal and spinal cord preservation. Systemic heparin anticoagulation required for this type of circulatory support has not been a problem. Exposure of one or both groins when positioning the patient allows access for femoral arterial and venous cannulation. A long fenestrated venous cannula is advanced to the level of the right atrium. It is rarely necessary to supplement the venous return with a separate superior vena cava or pulmonary artery cannula, since only partial cardiopulmonary bypass is required. Surgical exposure of the descending thoracic aorta should be limited to the immediate area of dissection and greatest involvement. Extensive dissection may interrupt spinal cord collateral vessels and predispose to paraplegia. Postoperative haemorrhage, a potential complication due to the friable periaortic tissue and anticoagulation, is also minimized with a limited surgical exposure.

Aortic clamping

Once partial cardiopulmonary bypass is initiated the aorta may be clamped either proximal or distal to the left subclavian artery, whichever affords best exposure for the proximal repair. When a clamp is placed proximal to the left subclavian artery, which is usual, a separate clamp must be applied to the left subclavian artery. The distal aortic clamp is then placed at the appropriate level for distal repair. Injury to the left recurrent laryngeal nerve is avoided. Application of the aortic clamp in acute dissection may itself result in intimal injury and must be performed carefully. The use of clamps fitted with rubber padded inserts may minimize this potential problem.

Aortotomy

21 The aorta is divided proximally and distally. An attempt is made to preserve as many intercostal branches as possible in order to minimize the risk of spinal cord ischaemia. Small intercostal vessels are oversewn with figure-of-eight 2/0 non-absorbable sutures. Reimplantation of large intercostal vessels, as is practised in descending aneurysm repairs, is rarely indicated in dissections. The posterior aortic wall remnant is left *in situ* to avoid the complications outlined previously.

Obliteration of dissection

22a, b In acute type B dissections, obliteration of the proximal and distal false lumen is accomplished with a 'sandwich' technique. Intimal and adventitial PTFE felt strips are placed to buttress the wall and all layers are oversewn with a running 4/0 polypropylene suture.

The patient incurs a greater risk of paraplegia in type B dissection than with a descending thoracic aneurysm. This difference has been attributed to non-perfusion of the spinal cord during isolation and clamping procedures. Atherosclerotic thoracic aneurysms often demonstrate progressive thrombotic occlusion of the intercostal vessels without neurological impairment. This implies development of an adequate collateral which is rarely present in aortic dissection.

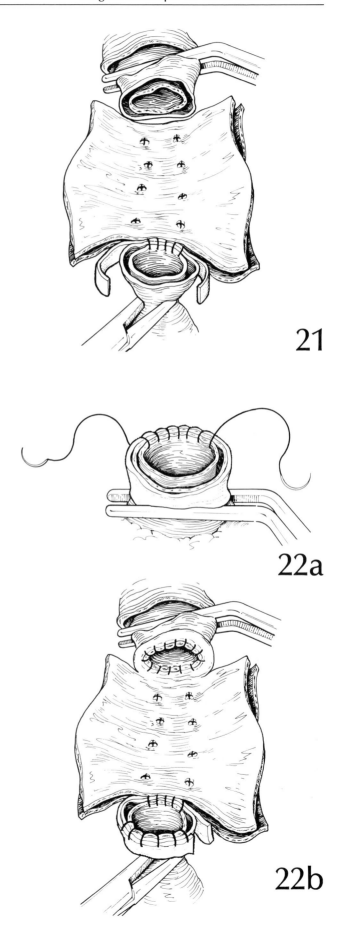

21

22a

22b

Graft replacement

23a–f The graft of choice is a preclotted very low porosity Dacron graft (Ochsner–Intravascular 50 porosity). The proximal anastomosis is performed first (*Illustrations 23a and 23b*) A long running (140 cm) 3/0 polypropylene suture is placed in a horizontal mattress fashion in the graft and then sewn to the aorta as described in the technique for type A dissection repair.

Disparity in graft to aorta size can be corrected by tailoring the distal graft. Before completion of the distal aortic anastomosis, the graft is vented in a retrograde manner by removing the distal aortic clamp (*Illustration 23c*). This procedure allows for evacuation of air and particulate debris within the graft. The distal clamp is reapplied and the aorta is flushed antegrade. The distal anastomosis is then completed (*Illustration 23d*). Before re-establishing circulation through the graft the suture lines are examined for bleeding by removing the distal aortic clamp. If necessary, reinforcement of the suture line is accomplished at this time with 3/0 felt pledgeted horizontal mattress sutures while the aortic pressure is low. The proximal clamp is then removed. In most instances the wall of the *in situ* residual aorta will require a running haemostatic suture to minimize perioperative haemorrhage (*Illustrations 23e* and *23f*).

Postoperative haemostasis is accomplished as outlined in the section on type A dissections.

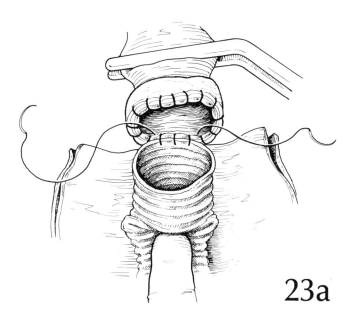

23a

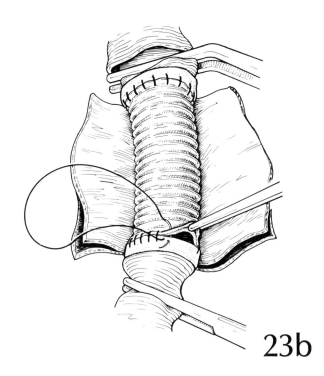

23b

Outcome

Operative mortality rates following repair of aortic dissections are approximately 15% even at institutions where there is wide experience in the management of this condition. Postoperative cerebrovascular deficits range from 7% to 10%. Postoperative follow-up and evaluation on a routine basis must be continued, since these patients are at risk indefinitely for redissection, aneurysm formation and vascular compromise. The use of computed axial tomography and cine magnetic resonance imaging in this condition has been of great assistance in non-invasive postoperative evaluation. In most institutions postoperative angiography has been reserved for situations which need clarification after non-invasive techniques have been inconclusive.

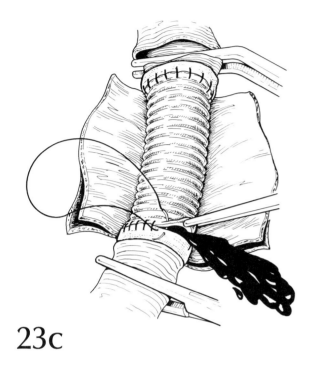

23c

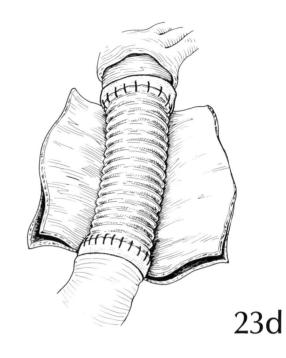

23d

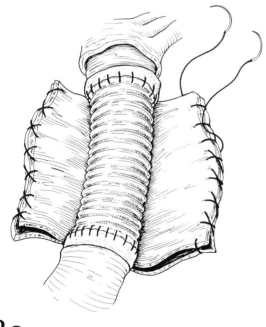

23e

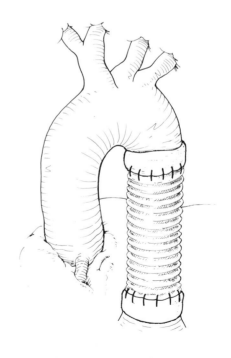

23f

Descending and suprarenal aortic aneurysms

Samuel R. Money MD
Department of Surgery, Ochsner Clinic, New Orleans, Louisiana, USA

Larry H. Hollier MD, FACS
Department of Surgery, Ochsner Clinic, New Orleans, Louisiana, USA

Principles and justification

Descending thoracic, thoracoabdominal, and suprarenal aortic aneurysms present a challenge to the vascular surgeon. Despite many advances in recent years, the mortality and morbidity rates of surgical intervention are high when compared with other vascular procedures. Non-operative treatment of patients with thoracoabdominal aortic aneurysms or descending aortic aneurysms has a poor prognosis with about one-quarter of patients surviving for more than 2 years, while the operative mortality rate for repair of thoracoabdominal and descending aortic aneurysms varies from 3% to 20% depending on the extent of the aneurysm[1,2]. It is therefore clear that operative repair offers a better chance of long-term survival for the patient. We believe an aggressive approach should be taken towards repair of these aneurysms, especially in mild to moderate risk patients.

Preoperative

Most patients with thoracic and thoracoabdominal aneurysms are asymptomatic, although some patients complain of chronic or intermittent back pain. Patients may report a worsening or a new onset of back pain before rupture which may be due to intramural dissection, rapid expansion of the aneurysm, or even a contained perforation. Chest radiography provides the first suggestion of aneurysm in many patients but is often misinterpreted as aortic tortuosity. Palpation of an abdominal aneurysm that extends to the costal margin may also be suggestive of a suprarenal or thoracoabdominal aneurysm. Magnetic resonance imaging (MRI) or computed tomography (CT) should be carried out to determine the extent of the aneurysm, location of the intramural thrombus, and potential relationships to the visceral vessels. Patients frequently require a biplane angiogram to evaluate disease in the visceral vessels.

Patients with aortic aneurysms are generally elderly and have several coexisting diseases. The most common risk factors are coronary artery disease, chronic pulmonary disease and renal dysfunction. In order to reduce operative risk, full evaluation should be carried out for these and any other problems suggested by the history and physical examination.

Minimum preoperative evaluation includes chest radiography, measurement of serum electrolytes, complete blood count, platelet count, coagulation profile and arterial blood gas measurement. We routinely include a duplex evaluation of the carotid arteries. If no significant cardiac symptoms are present the patient will usually undergo a stress electrocardiogram or dipyridamole thallium scan as a screening test. If either of these tests is positive, or if the patient has a significant history suggestive of coronary artery disease, the patient will undergo coronary angiography before operative intervention. The presence of significant coronary artery disease as demonstrated on cardiac catheterization will be treated before aortic replacement. The diagnosis of significant carotid artery disease on duplex scanning (>70%) will lead to cerebral angiography and, if confirmed, carotid endarterectomy before aortic surgery. Patients are requested to refrain from smoking for 2 weeks before the planned operation. They are admitted to the hospital 24–48 h before surgery for bowel preparation, pulmonary toilet, and intravenous antibiotics.

Anaesthesia

The participation of a skilled anaesthesiologist is critical to the operative management of these patients[3, 4]. If the procedure involves entering the chest cavity, a double-lumen endotracheal tube is inserted using bronchoscopic control. This will facilitate complete collapse of the left lung, thus providing better exposure of the descending aorta. Multiple monitoring lines are placed, including a pulmonary artery line, radial arterial line, and two large bore intravenous lines for infusion of fluids via a rapid infusion device. In patients with impaired cardiac function, transoesophageal two-dimensional echocardiography is utilized during the procedure. A lumbar intrathecal catheter is placed to drain cerebrospinal fluid (CSF) both during and after the operation, keeping the CSF pressures below 10 mmHg. Steroids, thiopentone and mannitol are administered before aortic cross-clamping to protect a potentially ischaemic spinal cord. In addition, a Foley catheter with a thermistor attachment is placed in the bladder. The operating room is cooled and the patient is passively cooled to 32–34°C; cooling the patient will reduce the metabolic demand of the spinal cord, thereby affording additional protection of the cord against ischaemic injury.

Operation

1 Aneurysms that involve the abdominal aorta and extend to above the renal arteries are suprarenal aortic aneurysms. Aneurysms that occur between the left subclavian artery and the diaphragm are classified as descending aneurysms. True thoracoabdominal aortic aneurysms involve both the thoracic as well as the abdominal aorta and are classified into four groups based on the extent of aortic involvement. Type I thoracoabdominal aortic aneurysms involve the aorta distal to the left subclavian artery and extend down to the visceral vessels. Type II aneurysms involve most of the descending and abdominal aorta. Type III aneurysms involve less than one-half of the descending thoracic aorta and the abdominal aorta. Type IV aneurysmal involvement is all intra-abdominal; however, to gain proximal control the lower thoracic aorta must be clamped.

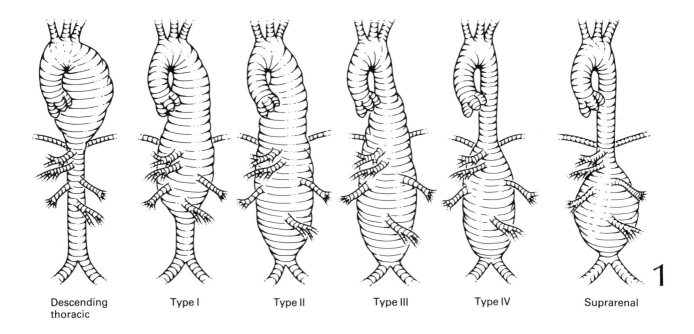

| Descending thoracic | Type I | Type II | Type III | Type IV | Suprarenal |

1

Incision

2 Descending aortic aneurysms are usually amenable to resection through a standard fourth or fifth interspace lateral thoracotomy. Sometimes, separate incisions at the fourth and seventh interspaces are required. Thoracoabdominal aortic aneurysms are approached with the patient in the right lateral decubitus position on an air controlled 'bean bag', with the hips being permitted to fall into a semisupine position. The incisions for thoracoabdominal aortic replacement vary according to the type of aneurysm. The incision for types I and II is made through the fifth interspace and is connected to an upper midline or paramedian abdominal incision. Types III and IV aneurysms are usually approached through the eighth interspace and the incision is continued obliquely across the left side of the abdomen. The incision and approach for a suprarenal aneurysm is by a standard extraperitoneal approach below the diaphragm. The dissection progresses in an extraperitoneal fashion.

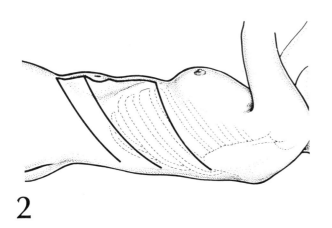

2

Dissection

3 The dissection is continued through the diaphragm with the diaphragm cut in a circumferential fashion. To facilitate later closure of the diaphragm, alternating coloured sutures are used along the diaphragmatic incision so that they can be matched by colour at closure. The crus of the diaphragm is divided and the entire aneurysm is examined and proximal and distal control established.

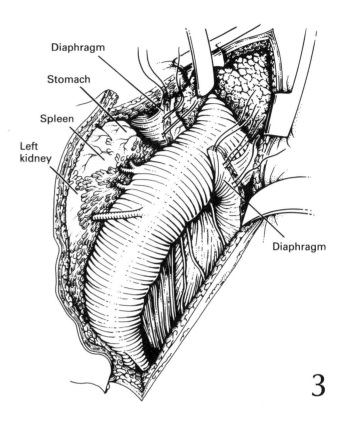

3

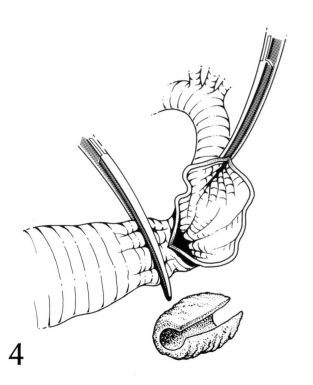

4

Aortic clamping

4 Systemic heparinization is not used; however, 1000 units of heparin are given intra-arterially through the aorta. The distal aortic clamp is placed first, then the proximal clamp is placed and the occluded segment of aorta is opened vertically. If a segment of narrowing is noted along the aorta between two large segments of aneurysm an intermediate clamp may be placed, and therefore the proximal portion of aorta can be opened first. The laminated thrombus is removed from the opened aneurysmal sac.

Intercostal reimplantation

5 A tightly woven graft of appropriate size is selected. The proximal anastomosis is performed with 0 polypropylene (Prolene) on a V-7 needle. In order to incorporate intercostal arteries near the anastomosis, the graft is frequently bevelled posteriorly; the anastomosis is then performed obliquely to include intercostals with a posterior tongue of aortic tissue. We attempt to revascularize as many pairs of intercostals as is technically feasible. This may require multiple cuffs to be reimplanted on the graft, or even a separate smaller graft from the aortic graft to revascularize intercostals. The clamp is sequentially moved distally in order to restore the critical spinal cord blood flow as soon as possible.

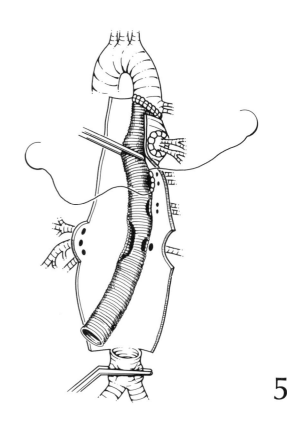

5

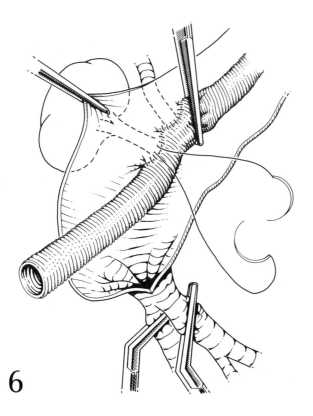

6

Visceral vessel reimplantation

6 The visceral vessels can be reimplanted into the graft after excising an island of graft wall of appropriate size to match the cuff of aorta containing the visceral vessels. When possible, the coeliac, superior mesenteric, and renal arteries are included in the aortic graft as a single cuff. Alternatively, two cuffs are utilized, usually including the left renal artery as a separate anastomosis. In type I aneurysms the visceral vessels can frequently be incorporated as an anterior tongue of the distal anastomosis in a fashion similar to the way in which the intercostals are incorporated as a posterior tongue of the proximal anastomosis. Following reimplantation of the visceral vessels, care must be taken to release the clamp slowly to minimize sudden hypotension. Hypotension can be minimized by volume loading with blood and crystalloid before declamping and by the rapid transfusion of blood with a rapid infusion system. Administration of bicarbonate, fresh frozen plasma, and platelets is also required. The visceral anastomoses are then closely inspected to ensure patency and to check for excessive bleeding.

Distal anastomosis

7 The distal anastomosis can then be performed as either a single distal aortic anastomosis or as a bilateral iliac reconstruction (adding a bifurcation graft), depending on the extent of disease.

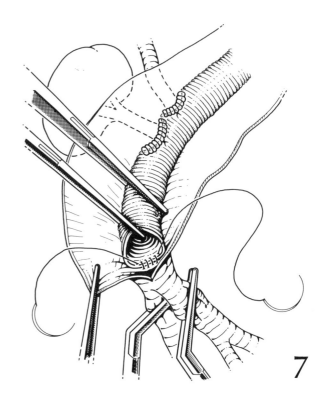

7

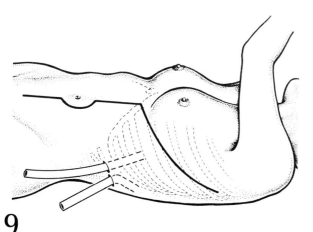

8

PTFE membrane

9

Closure of aneurysm sac

8 When all the anastomoses are complete, the sac of the aneurysm is tightly closed over the graft with a running polypropylene suture. In some patients there may be insufficient aortic wall remaining to close the aneurysm sac over the graft. In these instances we use a thin-walled polytetrafluoroethylene (PTFE) membrane to completely cover the graft to provide tamponade of any further bleeding. This is particularly helpful when fibrinolysis or other coagulopathy exists and bleeding occurs from needle holes or through the interstices of the graft.

Wound closure

9 The diaphragm is repaired with interrupted mattress sutures of non-absorbable material. High and low lying posterior chest tubes are placed and brought out through stab wounds in the midaxillary line inferior to the incision. The wound is closed with interrupted sutures of non-absorbable material.

Postoperative care

After surgery the patient remains intubated, with no attempts being made to wean from the respirator for the first 24 h. Maintenance fluid is given at an initial rate of 125 ml/h, reduced in a stepwise fashion to 60 ml/h by the third postoperative day. Urine replacement is started immediately after operation and is stopped after the first 12–24 h. By the third postoperative day mobilization of fluid will occur and frusemide may be used to reduce pulmonary congestion. During the first 24–48 h the patient is given low-dose dopamine (2.5 mg/kg) to aid in renal and visceral perfusion. The chest tubes are ordinarily removed on postoperative day 2–5. The intrathecal catheter is left in place for 24–72 h and the CSF pressure is kept below 10 mmHg.

Outcome

We recently reported our first 150 consecutive cases of thoracoabdominal aortic aneurysm replacement[3]. Over 96% of patients survived long enough to determine the status of postoperative neurological function and the overall 30-day mortality rate was 10%. Cardiac problems and coagulopathy were the leading causes of early mortality; late mortality was most often caused by multiorgan system failure. The most common cause of morbidity was pulmonary insufficiency, occurring in over 20%. Previous reports from other institutions have indicated a high rate of neurological injury following thoracoabdominal aortic aneurysm repair, with para-plegia reported to be as high as 30% in some studies[5]. In our series[3] only 4% of the patients developed lower extremity neurological deficits. The authors believe this is due to our routine attempts to completely reimplant intercostal arteries as well as to the use of the multiple adjunctive measures which we have described above.

In summary, repair of descending thoracic, thoracoabdominal or suprarenal aneurysms is a high-risk procedure. Proper preoperative evaluation of the patient, coupled with appropriate perioperative care and expeditious surgical technique, can reduce these risks to acceptable levels.

References

1. Hollier LH, Symmonds JB, Pairolero PC, Cherry KJ, Hallett JW, Gloviczki P. Thoracoabdominal aortic aneurysm repair: analysis of postoperative morbidity. *Arch Surg* 1988; 123: 871–5.

2. Crawford ES, Crawford JL, Safi HJ, Coselli JS, Hess KR, Brooks B et al. Thoracoabdominal aortic aneurysms, preoperative and intraoperative factors determining immediate and long-term results of operations in 605 patients. *J Vasc Surg* 1986; 3: 389–404.

3. Hollier LH, Money SR, Naslund TC et al. The risk of spinal cord dysfunction in 150 consecutive patients undergoing thoracoabdominal aortic replacement. *Am J Surg* 1992; 164: 210–14.

4. Hollier LH, Marino RJ. Thoracoabdominal aortic aneurysms. In: Moore WS, ed. *Vascular Surgery: A Comprehensive Review*. 3rd ed. Philadelphia: WB Saunders, 1991: 295–303.

5. Crawford ES, Svensson LG, Hess KR, Shenaq SS, Coselli JS, Safi HJ et al. A prospective randomized study of cerebrospinal fluid drainage to prevent paraplegia after high-risk surgery on the thoracoabdominal aorta. *J Vasc Surg* 1991; 13: 36–46.

Thoracic aorta to femoral artery bypass

James S. T. Yao MD, PhD
Magerstadt Professor of Surgery, Division of Vascular Surgery, Department of Surgery, Northwestern
University Medical School, Chicago, Illinois, USA

Walter J. McCarthy MD
Assistant Professor of Surgery, Division of Vascular Surgery, Department of Surgery, Northwestern University
Medical School, Chicago, Illinois, USA

History

Arterial bypass from the descending thoracic aorta to the femoral artery provides successful perfusion to the lower extremity when a transabdominal approach to the abdominal aorta is undesirable. The first reported operation was performed in 1956 by Stevenson et al.[1]. Several years later, in 1961, Blaisdell et al. used this type of bypass around an infected abdominal aortic prosthesis[2]. Since then, fewer than 160 cases have been reported in the world literature[3-5]. In patients with good surgical risk this procedure provides an alternative inflow source for femoral artery reconstruction with a long-term patency rate superior to the traditional axillofemoral bypass.

Principles and justification

Indications

The indications for operation can be divided into three categories:

1. Failed grafts: reconstruction after two previously failed aortobifemoral bypasses.
2. Conversion of existing or recently failed axillary popliteal or axillary femoral bypasses originally placed for septic abdominal aortic conditions, e.g. infected aortic grafts or aortoduodenal fistulae.
3. Hostile abdomen: this category includes patients who had complex or multiple major abdominal procedures or intra-abdominal infection, and those who have received radiation therapy.

Preoperative

Assessment

Arteriographic detail of the femoral outflow is often best provided by either transaxillary retrograde arteriography or, in the face of aortofemoral graft occlusion, direct puncture of the axillary femoral or popliteal grafts if these are patent. Arteriographic visualization of the descending thoracic aorta is not absolutely necessary, and this area can be studied using infusion computed tomographic scanning.

Preoperative selection should be that used for standard thoracotomy; without pulmonary resection, the operation is less stressful than usual. Evaluation usually includes a preoperative pulmonary function test, cardiac assessment and arterial blood gas measurement. If indicated, a Swan–Ganz catheter is placed for intraoperative and postoperative monitoring.

Anaesthesia

Anaesthetic management is similar to that used for a routine thoracotomy. In addition, a double-lumen endotracheal tube allows collapsing of the left lung and simplifies exposure of the supradiaphragmatic aorta. The double-lumen tube is useful but not essential.

Operation

Position of patient

1 The patient is positioned on the operating table with the pelvis flat and the left side of the thorax elevated 30° from horizontal. Position is maintained with sandbag elevation of the left side of the chest. The left arm is elevated and attached to the ether screen or held in an arm holder. The prepared surgical field extends from the left axilla to the lower thighs, bilaterally.

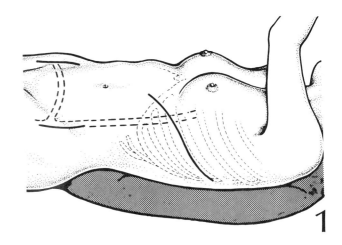

Incision

The thoracoabdominal incision is placed in the 7th interspace, crosses the costal cartilages and runs obliquely on the abdominal wall, ending just beyond the costal cartilage.

Exposure of thoracic aorta

Transection of the left rectus abdominis muscle is followed by entry into the retroperitoneum beneath the internal oblique fascia. Opening the peritoneum is avoided. The diaphragm is incised directly beneath the cut costal cartilage radially toward the aorta. The diaphragmatic incision is made with the electrocautery and is limited to the very periphery of the diaphragm. The inferior pulmonary ligament is incised to expose the aorta above the diaphragm. Circumferential control of the aorta is gained with sharp and blunt dissection, and a Silastic sling is placed. A nasogastric tube should be placed to aid in the identification of the oesophagus.

Exposure of femoral artery

The groin incisions are performed after the aorta is controlled. If a functioning axillary–femorofemoral graft is in place, this may only entail isolating the existing femorofemoral graft.

Retroperitoneal tunnelling

2 The left groin incision is extended with transection of the inguinal ligament to gain entry to the retroperitoneum. Blunt dissection by the surgeon's right and left index fingers completes the retroperitoneal tunnel along the anterior axillary line. Even with an obese patient this tunnel is short enough to allow easy approximation of the surgeon's right and left index fingers. The tunnel is anterior to the spleen and left kidney, and this approach avoids major retroperitoneal veins.

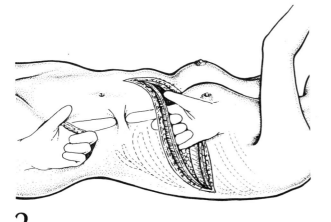

Femoral tunnelling

If a femorofemoral tunnel is required, it is usually placed in the subcutaneous position.

Aortic anastomosis

3 After an adequate dose of heparin has been administered, the thoracic aorta is clamped with a partial occlusion clamp. If the aorta is large and the patient is hypertensive, intraoperative control of the blood pressure with a sodium nitroprusside drip must be obtained. A 10-mm or 12-mm polytetrafluoroethylene prosthesis is anastomosed to the aorta in an end-to-side manner with 4/0 or 5/0 polypropylene sutures.

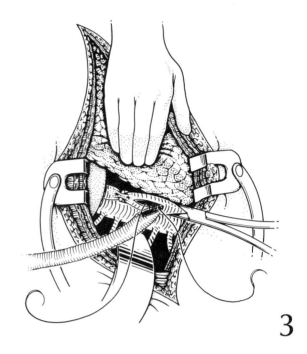

3

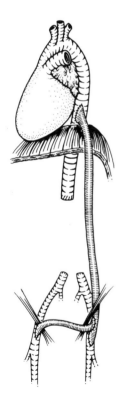

4

Femoral anastomoses

4 The graft is brought over the diaphragm and through the retroperitoneal tunnel, and the distal anastomoses are completed in an end-to-side manner.

Wound closure

Any existing axillary grafts are transected and oversewn at the groin level and allowed to thrombose. The diaphragm is closed around the graft with non-absorbable sutures. The chest is drained with two chest tubes, which are removed early after the operation. Closure of the thoracoabdominal incision is often aided by excising a portion of the costal cartilage.

Postoperative care

Complications

Most complications are related to blunt dissection during the tunnelling manoeuvre. These include rupture of the spleen, bladder injury and bleeding from the iliac vein.

Outcome

Since the initial report[6], descending thoracic aorta to left femoral bypass with femorofemoral bypass has been employed in 21 patients over a 10-year period. This surgical experience has recently been reported[7]. These bypasses were placed to convert an axillopopliteal or an axillofemoral graft to a more permanent inflow source in 12 patients, after multiple failed attempts (at least two) at intra-abdominal aortic repair in five patients, and to avoid exploring the abdomen after extensive retroperitoneal dissection or radiation in four patients. In this series there was no perioperative mortality. Perioperative myocardial infarction, stroke, or renal failure requiring haemodialysis was also not encountered. With the follow-up of 1–120 months (mean, 44 months) the 4-year patency was 100%. A single graft failed at 49 months, but was reopened by thrombectomy and femorofemoral bypass. Thus, the extended patency was 82% but the secondary patency remains 100% throughout. Since their thoracic operations, patients have required five femoropopliteal, three femorotibial, two deep femoral and two femorofemoral operations.

Descending thoracic aorta to femoral grafting is a safe, extremely durable arterial bypass. It is an excellent reconstruction for survivors of aortic graft infection, those with repeatedly failed aortic grafts, and for patients for whom re-entering the abdominal cavity would be hazardous.

Acknowledgements

Supported in part by the Alyce F. Salerno Foundation.

References

1. Stevenson JK, Sauvage LR, Harkins HN. A bypass homograft from thoracic aorta to femoral arteries for occlusive vascular disease: case report. *Am Surg* 1961; 27: 632–7.

2. Blaisdell FW, DeMattei GA, Gauder PJ. Extraperitoneal thoracic aorta to femoral bypass graft as replacement for an infected aortic bifurcation prosthesis. *Am J Surg* 1961; 102: 583–5.

3. Criado E, Johnson G Jnr, Burnham SJ, Buehrer J, Keagy BA. Descending thoracic aorta-to-iliofemoral artery bypass as an alternative to aortoiliac reconstruction. *J Vasc Surg* 1992; 15: 550–7.

4. Branchereau A, Magnan P-E, Moracchini P, Espinoza H, Mathieu JP. Use of descending thoracic aorta for lower limb revascularisation. *Eur J Vasc Surg* 1992; 6: 255–62.

5. Bowes DE, Youkey JR, Pharr WP, Goldstein AM, Benoit CH. Long-term follow-up of descending thoracic aorto-iliac/femoral bypass. *J Cardiovasc Surg* 1990; 31: 430–7.

6. McCarthy WJ, Rubin JR, Flinn WR, Williams LR, Bergan JJ, Yao JST. Descending thoracic aorta-to-femoral artery bypass. *Arch Surg* 1986; 121: 681–8.

7. McCarthy WJ, Mesh CL, McMillan WD, Flinn WR, Pearce WH, Yao JST. Descending thoracic aorta-to-femoral artery bypass: ten years' experience with a durable procedure. *J Vasc Surg* 1993; 17: 336–48.

Aortoiliac reconstruction: thromboendarterectomy and bypass grafting

John J. Ricotta MD
Professor of Surgery and Director, Division of Vascular Surgery, State University of New York at Buffalo, Buffalo, New York, USA

James A. DeWeese MD
Professor of Surgery and Chief Emeritus of Cardiothoracic and Vascular Surgery, University of Rochester Medical Center, Rochester, New York, USA

History

Aortoiliac reconstruction began with thromboendarterectomy of the aortoiliac and femoral segments. Open endarterectomy was developed first by Dos Santos, followed by the semiclosed technique and, finally, eversion endarterectomy, still used by some. Concerns about the technical challenge of thromboendarterectomy and the better long-term patency of aortofemoral bypass have caused many surgeons to abandon this procedure. In recent years, attention has turned to extending the bypass more proximally to adequately address disease in the perirenal and visceral aorta, most commonly through an extended retroperitoneal approach. At the same time there has been a resurgence of interest in iliofemoral bypass for patients with unilateral iliac occlusion. Stenotic iliac lesions are now often treated by percutaneous balloon angioplasty, sometimes accompanied by distal cross-femoral reconstruction. An axillobifemoral bypass is occasionally used. Thus, there are now many alternatives in aortoiliac reconstruction, and the approach is currently tailored to each clinical situation[1,2].

Principles and justification

Reconstruction of the aortoiliac segment is usually justified in patients with symptomatic arterial insufficiency of one or both lower extremities. The relatively low morbidity and mortality rates associated with aortofemoral bypass (2–5%) and excellent long-term patency rates (about 90%) justify this approach in patients with symptoms of claudication who are otherwise fit for surgery[3]. Patients with claudication who are at increased risk for aortofemoral bypass can often be treated by lower risk procedures, e.g. iliofemoral bypass, cross-femoral bypass, axillobifemoral bypass, or percutaneous angioplasty with or without cross-femoral bypass. If there is an indication from the physical assessment that one of these approaches is possible, then angiography is appropriate to evaluate higher risk patients with claudication for such intervention.

Impending tissue loss with severe aortoiliac disease is a firm indication for arterial reconstruction. Because amputation is often the alternative in these patients, a higher degree of operative risk is acceptable. As in patients with claudication, however, the treatment selected must be matched to the patient's arterial anatomy and clinical condition.

As a general guideline, patients with diffuse aortoiliac involvement are best treated by aortofemoral bypass. Unilateral iliofemoral reconstruction is reserved by the authors for those patients with significant disease restricted to a single iliac system and a relatively normal aortic bifurcation. Percutaneous angioplasty has been helpful in patients with discrete (usually less than 5 cm) stenosis or occlusions of the iliac vessels. While some clinicians advocate angioplasty in lesions up to 10 cm in length, iliofemoral bypass is preferable if possible in these cases. In poor-risk patients with bilateral iliac disease, i.e. occlusion with contralateral discrete stenosis, the authors have not hesitated to employ unilateral angioplasty with cross-femoral bypass. In these cases, a Palmaz stent is currently employed in conjunction with angioplasty to protect the downstream reconstruction.

Preoperative

Assessment

In addition to a thorough history and physical examination non-invasive vascular evaluation is important. This should include segmental limb pressures and Doppler waveform recording from the common femoral arteries. Duplex ultrasonography may be helpful in some patients to identify discrete iliac lesions amenable to angioplasty, but it cannot currently replace biplane angiography[4]. Angiography should include antero-posterior views of the entire abdominal aorta including the visceral vessels. Lateral aortic views are important when perirenal disease is suggested on the anteroposterior aortogram or when a meandering mesenteric artery is identified. Lateral aortography is the only way to identify posterior aortic plaque and to visualize the orifices of the coeliac and superior mesenteric arteries. If stenoses of the iliac arteries are suggested, oblique films may be necessary to delineate the extent of disease further. Finally, when questions still remain as to the significance of aortoiliac disease, pullback pressure measurements may be necessary, often with the use of a vasodilator such as papaverine. A pressure gradient of more than 10 mmHg following injection of a vasodilator is diagnostic of a haemodynamically significant lesion. Distal films should include tibial run-off.

From the foregoing it is obvious that transfemoral aortography is preferred whenever possible. This provides the best information on distal run-off and permits pressure measurement. In some cases of severe iliac disease or aortic occlusion, transfemoral aortography is not possible. Transaxillary or translumbar aortography is an acceptable alternative. Use of small catheters and the digital subtraction technique has reduced complications from the transaxillary approach. Lateral aortography is often needed in these cases and may be cumbersome if a translumbar approach is used. Intravenous digital subtraction techniques are seldom detailed enough to provide information not available after a thorough physical examination and non-invasive study.

General evaluation focuses on the heart, lungs and abdominal viscera. A history of angina, exertional dyspnoea, postprandial abdominal pain, or hypertension is sought. Laboratory evaluation includes chest radiography, electrocardiography, clotting profile and serum creatinine concentrations. A history of untreated angina, unstable angina, or unexplained cardiographic abnormalities requires further evaluation, currently by stress nuclear cardiography or 24-h electrocardiographic monitoring. Patients with ischaemic myocardium at risk may require coronary angiography, particularly before elective surgery for claudication. Significant dyspnoea or abnormal chest radiographic findings should prompt preoperative pulmonary function tests. Patients with hypertension and abnormal or borderline serum creatinine concentrations should have a creatinine clearance performed before surgery, particularly if angiography suggests renovascular disease.

Patient preparation

Patients should be admitted on the evening before surgery for hydration. Intravenous hydration is particularly important if angiography is performed on the day before operation. Intensive preoperative monitoring (including peripheral arterial and pulmonary artery catheters) is indicated in patients with visceral vessel involvement as well as in those at increased cardiac risk. Optimal preoperative control of intravascular volume, cardiac performance and vascular resistance is essential in these patients to reduce perioperative morbidity.

Prophylactic antibiotics are administered within 1 h before skin incision and continued until all invasive monitoring is removed. General anaesthesia is preferred for these procedures. Supplemental epidural anaesthesia may be useful in some patients, and this can be continued for 24–48 h after surgery in selected cases.

Operations

Aortoiliac endarterectomy is still indicated in some patients whose disease is limited to the distal aorta and common iliac arteries. Although it may be technically more challenging than bypass procedures, it avoids the use of a prosthetic material. The more extensive dissection of the aortic bifurcation required with this procedure may increase the frequency of ejaculatory dysfunction in men and is used sparingly in men for this reason. Cases of aortic hypoplasia are best treated by aortofemoral bypass. Endarterectomy is occasionally useful when re-establishing flow in a contaminated field or treating a graft infection. Thromboendarterectomy can be performed through a standard retroperitoneal or transabdominal approach.

STANDARD RETROPERITONEAL APPROACH

Position of patient and incision

1 For the standard retroperitoneal approach, the patient is positioned with the left side elevated to 30–45°. This is readily achieved by a rolled towel or bean bag. Reverse flexion of the table (jack-knife position) is helpful for additional exposure. The incision is begun just below the umbilicus just medial to the lateral border of the rectus muscle and extends laterally to the tip of the 12th rib.

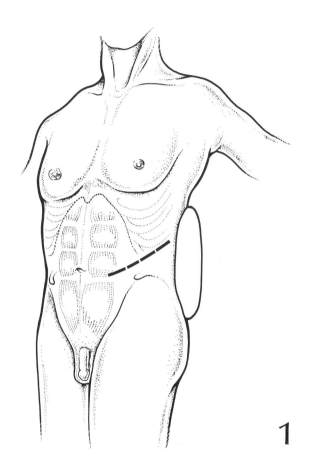

1

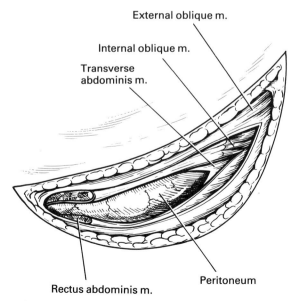

External oblique m.

Internal oblique m.

Transverse abdominis m.

Rectus abdominis m.

Peritoneum

2

2 The anterior rectus sheath is incised and the rectus muscle is retracted (or occasionally transected) for adequate medial exposure. The medial portion of the incision is the most usual point at which the peritoneal cavity is entered, and care should be taken to avoid this. If the peritoneum is incised, it is immediately closed with a running absorbable suture (3/0 or 4/0). The external oblique, internal oblique and transverse abdominis muscles are transected along the line of the skin incision.

Exposure of the aorta and iliac vessels

3 The retroperitoneal space is entered laterally and the peritoneum and its contents are swept medially using a gauze laparotomy pad. Mobilization proceeds above the retroperitoneal fat and psoas muscle and the genitofemoral nerve. In this approach, dissection is anterior to the left kidney. The inferior mesenteric artery is identified and divided for additional exposure. From this point on the operation is identical to the transperitoneal approach. At the conclusion of the endarterectomy the rectus sheath, transverse abdominis and oblique muscles are closed individually with 0 or 2/0 absorbable sutures.

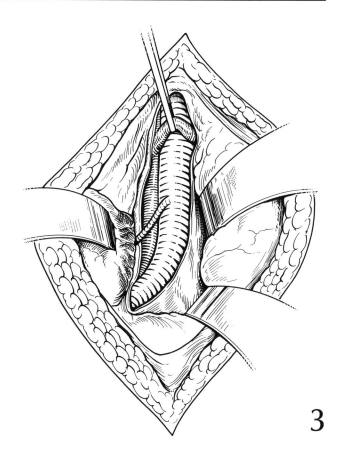

3

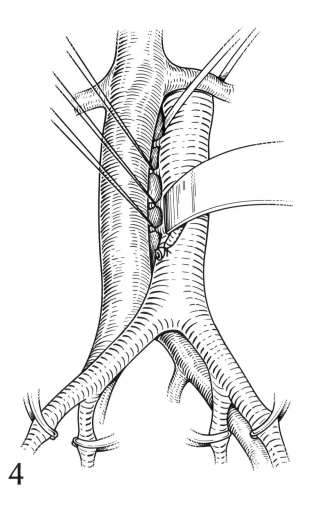

4

Mobilization of the aorta and iliac vessels

4 Completion of the thromboendarterectomy requires extensive mobilization of the aorta and iliac arteries including their tributaries. Mobilization should extend 2–3 cm proximal and distal to the known area of disease and may include the distal abdominal aorta, common external and internal iliac arteries, middle sacral and lumbar arteries. The smaller arteries can be controlled by Pott's ties or small bulldog clamps.

Arterial incision

5   Incisions are made to encompass the proximal and distal aspects of the proposed thromboendarterectomy. This can be accomplished by using two incisions: one placed to the right of the inferior mesenteric artery and extending down the right common iliac vessel and a separate longitudinal incision on the left common iliac artery. This technique minimizes disruption of the preaortic autonomic plexus, which is located to the left side of the aortic bifurcation.

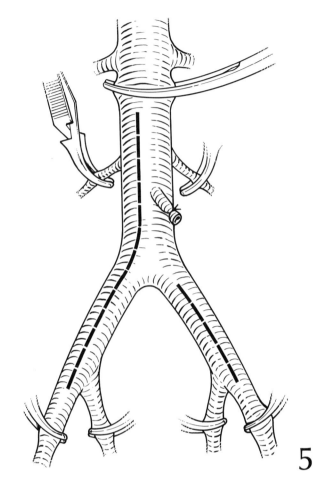

5

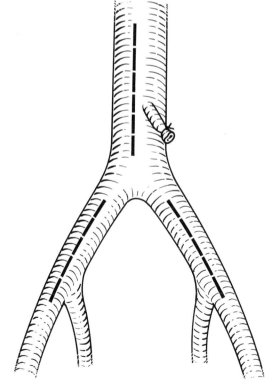

6

6   Alternatively, three incisions can be made, separating the aortic and right iliac arteriotomies. In either event the iliac arteriotomies must extend distally past the end of the endarterectomy (usually at the iliac bifurcation).

Endarterectomy

7 The plane of cleavage is identified just deep to the intima. This plane is developed using a clamp or endarterectomy spatula. The dissection is carried circumferentially throughout the diseased segment. The inner core is divided proximally and distally with scissors and the plaque is removed. Endarterectomy may be facilitated by dividing the plaque proximally early in the procedure to aid in developing the cleavage plane. The endarterectomy is completed in a semiclosed fashion using an intraluminal dissector between the incisions. The endarterectomy is ended where the plaque becomes attenuated, most often at the common iliac bifurcation. The intima is cut flush at this point with Pott's scissors to avoid loose flaps.

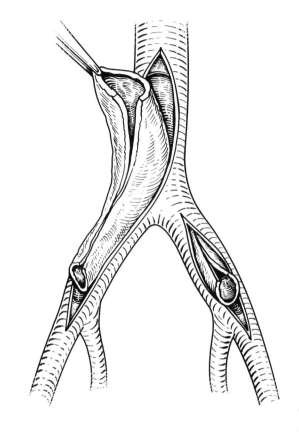

7

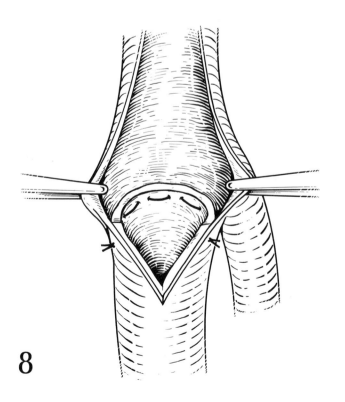

8

Securing the intima

8 Following transection of the intima, it is inspected closely and the area irrigated with heparinized saline solution. If the intima is loose at its distal cut margin, it should be anchored to the vessel with a series of interrupted mattress sutures tied outside the vessel. After inspection of the distal operative site, the entire endarterectomy is flushed with heparinized saline to remove any loose debris and thrombus.

Closure of arteriotomies

9 The arteriotomies are closed with running 4/0 or 5/0 monofilament sutures. Before completion of the closure, clamps are momentarily released first distally and then proximally to flush out residual debris or thrombus.

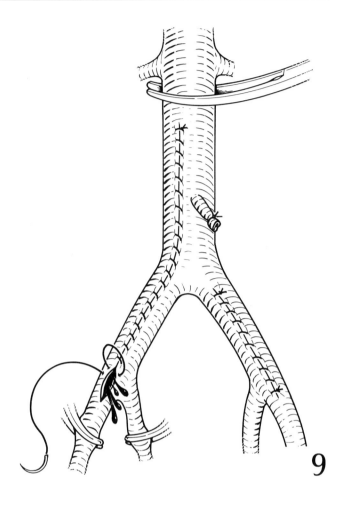

9

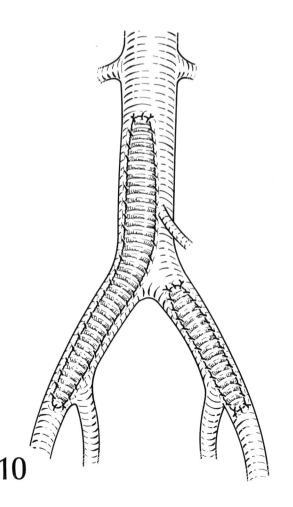

10

10 If necessary, the arteriotomies may be closed with a patch of Dacron or polytetrafluorethylene (PTFE). This is particularly helpful when the aorta is small. The ends of the patch are rounded or squared off to widen the distal ends of the arteriotomy. After release of the clamps, bleeding is controlled by packs with light pressure. Liquid thrombin or microcrystalline collagen may occasionally be required. Significant suture line leaks are repaired with interrupted 6/0 sutures.

Alternative methods of endarterectomy

11 Eversion endarterectomy and semiclosed endarterectomy have been used as alternatives to the method described here. Eversion endarterectomy involves complete mobilization and transection of the vessel involved, which is then turned back on itself.

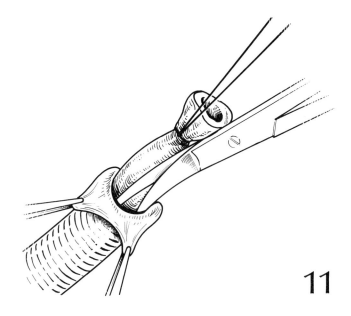

11

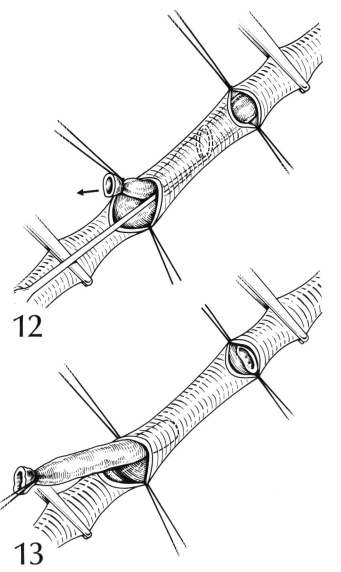

12

12, 13 The semiclosed technique usually involves multiple transverse arteriotomies and the use of a looped endarterectomy stripper. These techniques are difficult for long segments unless the operator is very familiar with them. They offer no advantages over the approach described above.

13

TRANSPERITONEAL AORTOILIAC AND AORTOFEMORAL BYPASS GRAFT

This remains the most common procedure performed for aortoiliac occlusive disease. A variety of prosthetic materials is used. Currently, the authors' preference is collagen-impregnated Dacron or PTFE because of the impermeable nature of the material. If standard knitted or woven Dacron is used, it must be preclotted before implantation. Using this approach, the proximal anastomosis is infrarenal; while the distal anastomosis can be to the common iliac, external iliac, or femoral arteries, the authors believe that common femoral anastomosis is indicated in the overwhelming majority of operations performed for occlusive disease and is associated with better long-term patency.

Incision

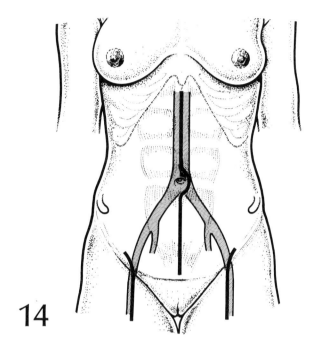

14 The preferred incision is a long midline one extending from the xiphoid process to the pubic symphysis, although a left paramedian or even a transverse incision is employed by some surgeons. When the graft is to be carried to the femoral arteries, these are exposed by longitudinal incisions beginning above the level of the inguinal ligament and extending down over the femoral arteries low enough to expose the common femoral bifurcation. Additional proximal exposure of the distal external iliac artery can be gained by curving the incision laterally parallel to the inguinal ligament. The ligament can be retracted superiorly and the artery exposed, often without transecting the ligament.

Exposure of the abdominal aorta

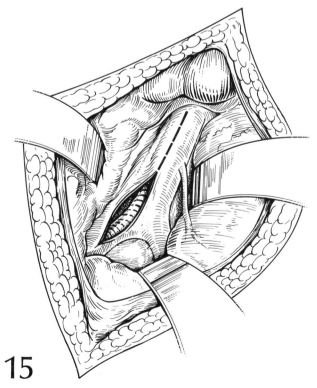

15 The retroperitoneum is entered by incising the retroperitoneal attachments of the duodenum and mobilizing the ligament of Treitz. This incision is begun as close to the duodenum as possible and continued down the right side of the aorta. A flap of posterior peritoneum is developed based to the left of the aorta. This flap is used after completion of the bypass to separate the graft from the visceral organs. The lymphatic vessels overlying the aorta are divided between ligatures or clips. Dissection proceeds proximally until the renal vein is identified. Failure to encounter this structure must alert the operator to the possibility of a retroaortic renal vein. During dissection the inferior mesenteric vein is mobilized and retracted. Although the inferior mesenteric vein may be ligated if necessary, this has not occurred in operations for occlusive disease in the authors' experience.

Infrarenal aortic dissection begins just below the renal vein and continues for 2–3 cm distally. The importance of placing the proximal (aortic) anastomosis high on the infrarenal aorta cannot be overemphasized. This area is most often free of disease and most amenable to precise anastomosis. One or more pairs of lumbar arteries may be sacrificed to obtain adequate mobilization of the aorta. The aorta is encircled using finger dissection if possible, although a curved vascular clamp may be required. During these manoeuvres care must be taken to avoid damage to the vena cava or lumbar veins.

Mobilization of the renal vein

16, 17 In especially high lesions, additional exposure can be gained by mobilizing or dividing the renal vein. The authors prefer mobilization to division and ligature. Mobilization may require division of the gonadal vein to allow the renal vein to be retracted superiorly. If the renal vein must be divided this should be done close to its junction with the vena cava and the ends oversewn with a double layer of 5/0 monofilament suture. When dividing the renal vein it is important to preserve both the gonadal and adrenal veins to provide venous outflow for the left kidney. Whenever possible the decision to transect the renal vein should be made before the gonadal vein is sacrificed during mobilization of that structure.

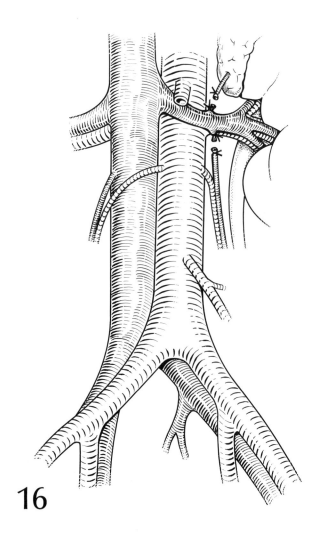

16

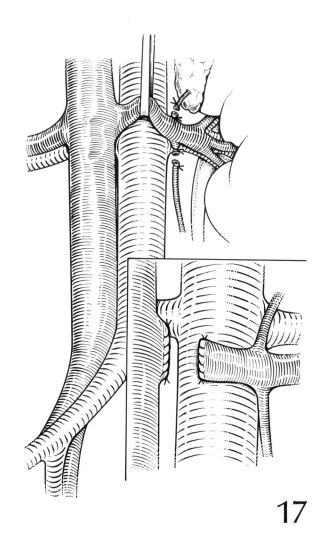

17

Clotting the graft

This step is always necessary when a non-coated knitted Dacron graft is used, although it is not as important when the less porous woven grafts are employed. Preclotting serves two purposes: to seal the graft effectively against leakage and to provide a smooth fibrin lining at the blood–graft interface. When newer impervious prosthetics are used, this step is not required.

18, 19 Before systemic heparinization, fresh blood, 100 ml, is withdrawn from the aorta or vena cava and placed in a basin. An appropriately sized graft is selected for use. The graft should be isodiametric or slightly smaller than the artery for aortic reconstruction. In the authors' experience the graft selected is more often too large than too small for the vessels. One end of the graft is clamped, and fresh blood is forced through the graft using a catheter-tipped or bulb syringe. This procedure is continued until leakage through the prosthesis is minimal. The prosthesis is then flushed with heparinized saline to remove any loose debris.

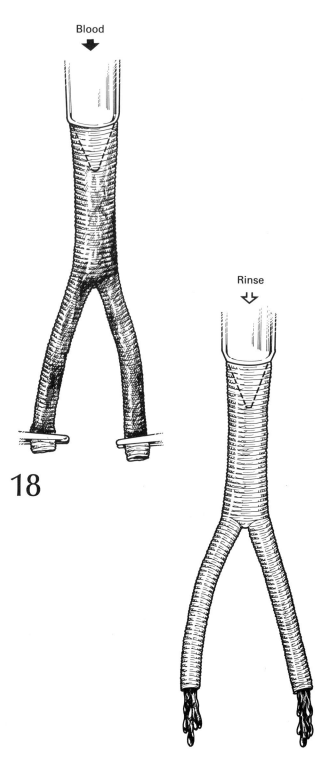

Making the tunnel

20 Following removal of blood for clotting, the retroperitoneal tunnel is made using blunt dissection. Tunnelling is accomplished using finger dissection from the abdominal and femoral incisions. The tunnel begins in the abdomen behind the ureter and directly over the iliac artery. Failure to remain behind the ureter can result in postoperative ureteric obstruction. In the groin, the plane is found immediately over the femoral artery. Tunnelling is completed bluntly and a long vascular clamp is guided through the tunnel from below upwards. Dacron tape is left in the tunnel.

The patient is anticoagulated with intravenous heparin, 100–150 units/kg. The arteries are clamped distally first to avoid embolism, and the prosthesis is inserted. At this point the inside of the prosthesis is inspected, and any loose fibrin or clot is removed using forceps or flushing techniques. After completion of the proximal anastomosis, the graft will be filled with blood to test for leakage and then flushed with blood to remove debris before performing the distal anastomosis.

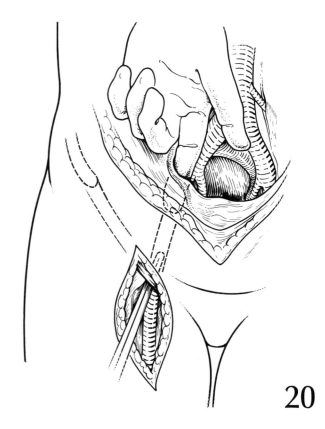

20

End-to-end proximal anastomosis

The proximal anastomosis may be end-to-end or end-to-side. The former is preferable because of less turbulent flow and more accurate suture placement. End-to-end anastomoses have a particular advantage when there is extensive juxtarenal aortic disease, as they permit inspection of the proximal aorta, limited thromboendarterectomy, and accurate placement of sutures in the proximal anastomotic line. Every effort is made to locate the proximal anastomosis high on the infrarenal aorta.

21 The aorta is clamped proximal and distal to the area proposed for anastomosis, and the aorta is transected. The distal end of the aorta is oversewn with a double layer of 3/0 or 4/0 polypropylene (Prolene).

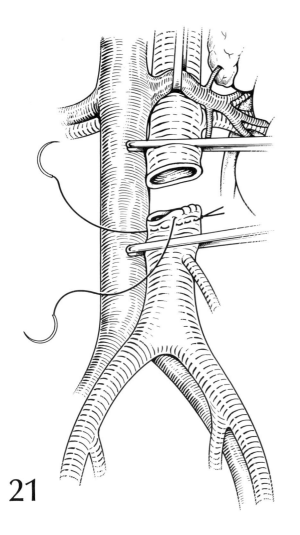

21

22 A preclotted graft of appropriate size is then anastomosed to the cut end of the aorta using a running 3/0 or 4/0 polypropylene suture. The anastomosis is begun on the posterior wall of the aorta. This suture may be tied or a running parachute technique may be used. The two ends of the suture are then continued posteriorly and anteriorly to complete the suture line. Whenever possible, the sutures proceed from intima to adventitia on the aorta.

Alternative techniques include placing two equidistant sutures to bisect the anastomosis or using interrupted mattress sutures for the posterior wall or the entire circumference of the anastomosis. While these methods have their advocates, the authors have not found them to be particularly advantageous in the usual aortic reconstruction. It is most important that the aortic sutures are placed in relatively good aorta with a single motion whenever possible. Excessive torque on the artery can result in needle hole bleeding or even disruption of the proximal suture line.

End-to-side proximal anastomosis

End-to-side grafts are indicated in specific circumstances where it is important to preserve prograde flow to the pelvis through the hypogastric vessels[5]. This is most common when there are bilateral external iliac occlusions with less disease in the aorta and common iliac vessels. If inferior mesenteric flow is to be preserved, proximal end-to-side anastomosis may be used, although an end-to-end anastomosis with reimplantation of the inferior mesenteric artery may be preferable. End-to-side anastomosis is also preferred in patients with a small aorta. It may be used in patients where the aortic segment to be used is soft and disease-free. The exposure of the aorta is identical to that already described.

23 A side-biting partial occlusion clamp may be used; however, two aortic occlusion clamps are preferred because this allows better exposure of the arteriotomy. The upper clamp is applied in the standard fashion above the level of anastomosis. The lower clamp is applied from below in the axis of the aorta to occlude the lumbar vessels as well as the distal aorta. End-to-side anastomosis does not require mobilization of the posterior aortic wall. An elliptical incision is cut in the graft and the suture is begun at the distal aorta and the 'heel' of the graft as a mattress suture, which is tied and then carried up each side. One suture is carried around the apex of the graft so that this critical area can be completed under direct vision. Suturing should always proceed from inside to outside on the artery to avoid raising a flap of intima. When the anastomosis is complete, it is tested as described below.

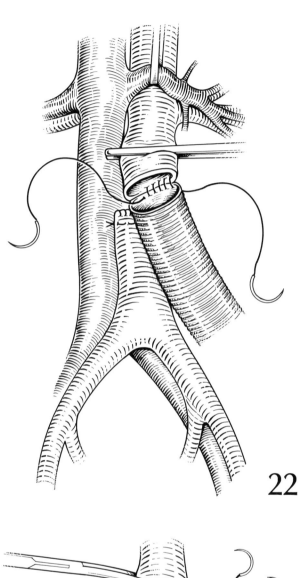

22

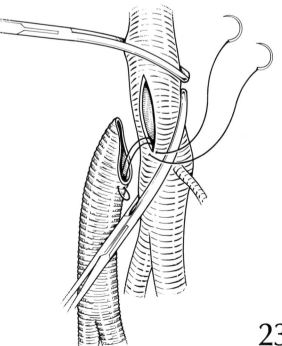

23

Testing the proximal suture line

24 The limbs of the aortic graft are clamped and the aortic clamp briefly removed to allow the graft to fill with blood. The graft is reclamped close to the suture line and the aortic clamp again released to test anastomotic integrity. Bleeding from needle holes is usually controlled with pressure. Any large leaks, however, are best repaired with interrupted sutures at this point. Once the suture line is secure, the proximal aorta is reclamped.

Prolonged clamping of the graft should be avoided unless the character of the aorta precludes reclamping the vessel safely. A cuff of graft may be placed over the limbs of the bifurcation graft and brought proximally to cover the anastomosis. This is particularly helpful when the aortic cuff is friable and has been used routinely by some surgeons with the hope of decreasing aortoenteric fistulae.

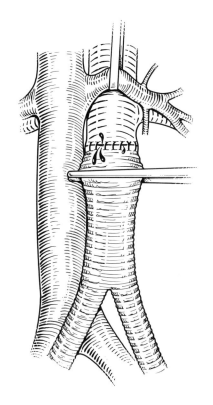

24

End-to-side distal anastomosis

The distal anastomosis may be performed to the common iliac, external iliac or common femoral artery. While there are some advantages to avoiding an anastomosis in the groin (lower incidence of wound problems and avoiding an area of flexion), the long-term patency of aortofemoral grafts may be superior to that of aortoiliac grafts when performed for occlusive disease. For this reason the distal anastomosis is usually carried to the common femoral artery. As progressive disease is frequent in the superficial and common femoral arteries, it is important to site the femoral anastomosis low on the common femoral artery over the orifice of the deep femoral artery. A long vascular clamp is pulled through the tunnel with the umbilical tape previously placed. Each limb of the graft is grasped and pulled down into the groin, care being taken not to twist it.

25 The distal end of the graft is carefully bevelled for the distal anastomosis. The graft should be cut in an S shape with heavy scissors. The distal end should be tailored to accommodate the distal arteriotomy. The distal anastomosis can then be performed.

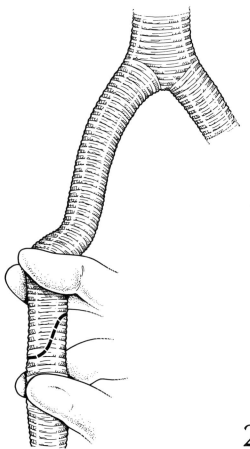

25

26 The technique of distal anastomosis is the same in the iliac and femoral arteries. A segment of artery is isolated between clamps and a longitudinal arteriotomy made. In the femoral artery the origins of the superficial and deep femoral arteries are dissected free, and these arteries are clamped. As stated above, the incision should extend down to the common femoral bifurcation so that the orifice of the deep femoral artery is visualized. If the superficial femoral artery is occluded or there is disease at the orifice of the deep femoral artery, the arteriotomy can be extended down the deep femoral artery, and the distal anastomosis can be extended as a tongue over the deep femoral artery as a deep femoral reconstruction. The anastomosis is begun by placing double-ended 5/0 or 6/0 polypropylene sutures at each corner of the graft. These are carried from the inside to the outside of the artery.

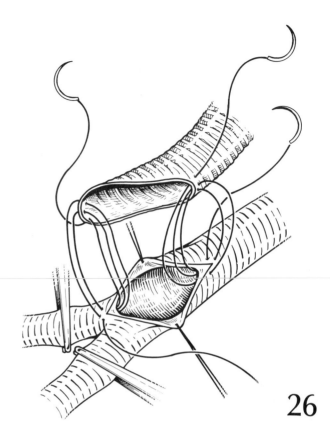

26

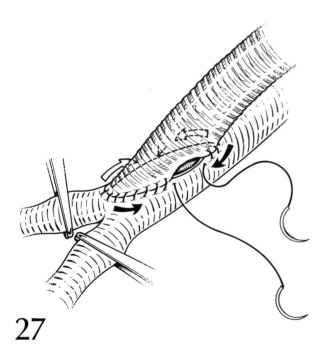

27

27 With the graft suspended, three or four sutures are placed at each corner under direct vision. The sutures are then drawn taut, the graft brought down to the artery, and the anastomosis completed by running sutures placed towards the middle of the suture line from each apex. This technique permits optimal visualization of the corner stitches, which is important to avoid compromising both inflow and outflow.

In an alternative technique, a mattress suture is placed at the 'heel' of the graft and then run around the top of the graft under direct vision. Following completion of one anastomosis the distal clamp is removed, allowing retrograde flow to flush out clot and debris through the opposite limb of the graft. This contralateral limb is then clamped near the bifurcation, and the proximal clamp is slowly released to prevent a drop in systolic blood pressure of more than 20 mmHg. The same procedure is carried out after completion of the second anastomosis.

Reimplantation of inferior mesenteric artery

In most patients the inferior mesenteric artery can be sacrificed with impunity, but in a small number the collateral circulation is inadequate. A large meandering artery seen on preoperative arteriography may help to identify these patients. Larger arteries (5 mm diameter or more), particularly those without back-bleeding, are more likely to require reimplantation.

28 If reimplantation is necessary, a button of aortic wall with the inferior mesenteric artery at its centre is excised and sewn onto the side of the graft. At operation the inferior mesenteric artery may be tested by temporary occlusion. During this time the colour of the intestine is observed and Doppler flow can be studied in the inferior mesenteric artery and along the antimesenteric border of the intestine.

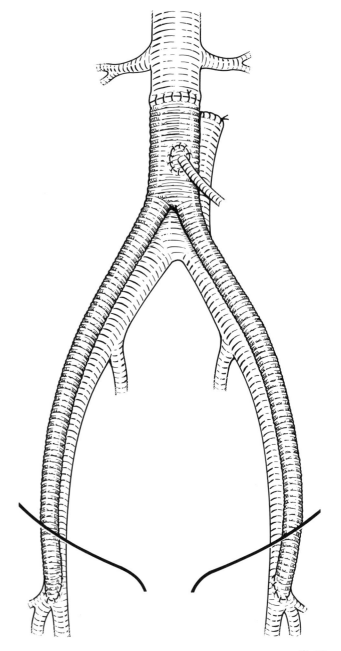

28

Closure of retroperitoneum

29 Following insertion of the graft, the retroperitoneum is closed. The purpose is to prevent contact of the intestine, particularly the duodenum, with the aortic prosthesis. The retroperitoneal incision is approximated with a running absorbable suture. A double-layer closure has been suggested to separate the aorta more effectively from the abdominal viscera. Every attempt is made to leave the mobilized duodenum free rather than to reattach it to its retroperitoneal position. If necessary, an omental pedicle may be placed between the aorta and the intestine to provide further coverage.

The groin wounds are closed meticulously in layers. At least two subcutaneous layers are employed. Haemostasis and avoidance of lymphatic leaks are of utmost importance in prevention of wound complications. Subcuticular closure of the skin avoids transcutaneous sutures in the groin.

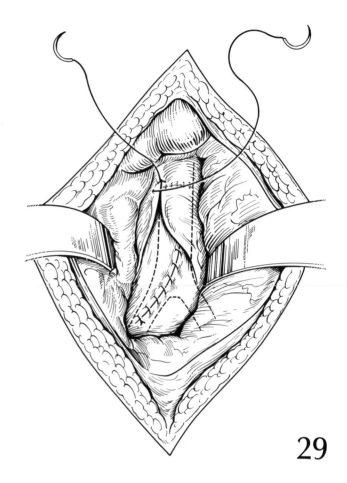

29

TREATMENT OF JUXTARENAL AORTIC OCCLUSIONS

Following aortic occlusion, thrombus may extend to the level of the renal vessels. In these instances the atherosclerotic plaque ends below the renal arteries, but the perirenal artery is occluded by organized thrombus. A standard aortofemoral bypass can be accomplished using minor modifications of the techniques just described. The goal of these modifications is to establish a segment of infrarenal aorta suitable for anastomosis.

30 Exposure is identical to that described for transperitoneal aortic procedures. In this case, however, the renal vein is mobilized and both renal arteries, as well as the suprarenal aorta, are exposed. After heparinization, the renal arteries are controlled by bulldog clamps or soft loops, and the aorta is transected 3–4 cm below the renal vein. The occluded proximal aortic segment is then transposed anterior to the left renal vein to facilitate exposure and a thrombectomy is begun. The dissection plane is between the organized plug of thrombus and the intima. This proceeds circumferentially until the thrombus is extruded from the aorta by the combined forces of dissection and prograde aortic flow. It should be noted that the aorta is *not* clamped during this portion of the dissection, but rather controlled by the operator's fingers or an open clamp.

When prograde flow is established, the aorta is occluded by digital pressure followed by application of a vascular clamp. The thrombectomized portion of the aorta is inspected and flushed to remove debris and the aortic clamp is reapplied below the renal vessels. The aorta is then repositioned behind the renal vein and a standard end-to-end bypass is performed as previously described.

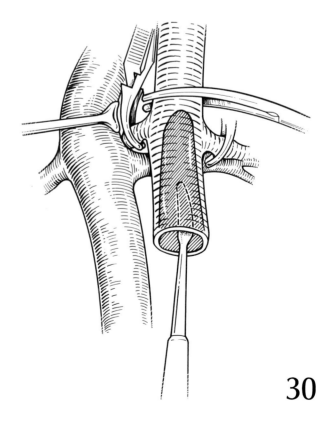

30

SUPRACOELIAC CONTROL OF AORTA

Not uncommonly, the aorta is significantly diseased at the level of the renal vessels or in the portion involving the origins of the mesenteric arteries. This is often not appreciated on standard anteroposterior angiography. While infrarenal aortofemoral bypass is often performed in these cases, clamping a diseased infrarenal aorta may result in embolism, bleeding from the proximal suture line, or late false aneurysm. If significant perirenal disease exists, it is better to clamp the aorta above the renal vessels. When this is done the proximal anastomosis can often be placed just distal to the origins of the renal arteries, avoiding visceral revascularization. The authors prefer to obtain aortic control above the coeliac axis at the level of the diaphragm. This can be done either transperitoneally or by an extended retroperitoneal exposure.

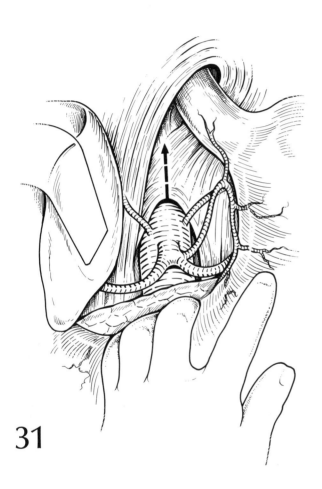

31

Transperitoneal exposure of supracoeliac aorta

31 The supracoeliac aorta is approached through the gastrohepatic ligament[6]. The triangular ligament is incised and the left lobe of the liver is mobilized and retracted to the right. The aorta is located by palpation, and the muscular fibres of the aortic hiatus are divided by ligature or cautery. It is not necessary to isolate the oesophagus at this point, as the aorta is easily distinguished from this structure. After the crural fibres are dissected away from the aorta, the vessel can be encircled by finger dissection. A tape is not placed around the aorta; when the clamp is to be applied, the vessel is encircled by the thumb and index finger of the left hand, lifted off the spinal column and occluded with a straight vascular clamp.

Treatment of perirenal aortic disease

32 With the aorta clamped above the coeliac artery, the aorta is transected below the renal vessels. In most instances an anastomosis can be performed at the level of the renal vessels without further manipulation. If necessary, an endarterectomy of this segment can be performed, although the plane is somewhat more superficial than is usually taken in peripheral vessels. Back-bleeding encountered from the mesenteric vessels is usually modest and can be controlled by pressure, or the field can be kept clear with suction. Use of autotransfusion is suggested in these cases. After the aorta is deemed satisfactory, anastomosis is performed.

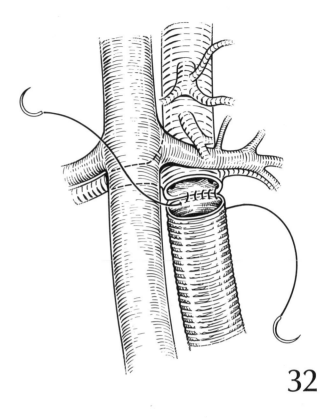

32

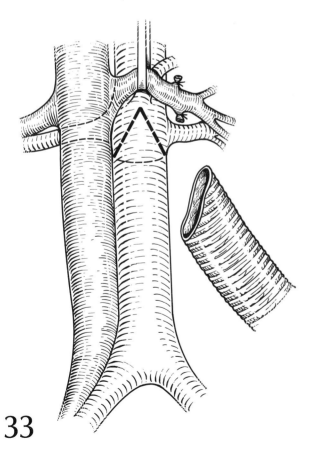

33 Very occasionally, endarterectomy must be continued just above the orifices of the renal vessels. If this can be anticipated the retroperitoneal approach is preferred. Additional exposure, however, can be gained by incising the anterior aspect of the aorta to just below the superior mesenteric artery. After endarterectomy, the proximal portion of the graft is bevelled to facilitate closure of this defect.

33

EXTENDED RETROPERITONEAL APPROACH TO THE AORTA

When the aorta at the origins of the mesenteric and renal vessels is involved in the atherosclerotic process, the extended retroperitoneal approach is preferred[7]. In this exposure, the supracoeliac aorta is approached on its posterolateral aspect and the viscera are reflected anteriorly. By dividing the diaphragm at the aortic hiatus, the aorta can be exposed to the level of the 10th thoracic vertebra. A thoracoabdominal incision is avoided, along with its attendant morbidity. The major drawback of this approach is limited access to the visceral and right renal vessels. Therefore, it should only be used when disease is confined to the origin of these arteries and can be treated by endarterectomy.

Patient position and incision

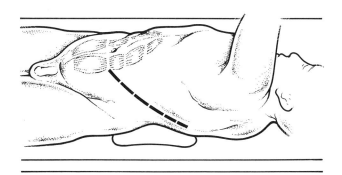

34 The patient is placed in a modified left thoracotomy position with shoulders almost perpendicular to the operating table but hips rotated as much as possible parallel to the plane of the table. A bean bag is used to stabilize this position. Exposure is facilitated by placing the table in a jack-knife position. The operating surgeon is positioned at the patient's back.

The incision begins 3–5 cm below the umbilicus at the lateral border of the rectus muscle and extends laterally between the 10th and 11th or 11th and 12th ribs, depending on the level of aortic control desired. The authors initially carried this incision to the border of the paraspinous muscles, but in recent years have shortened its posterior extent considerably. This appears to have decreased the incidence of intercostal neuralgia and 'pseudohernia' from denervation of the lateral abdominal musculature. It is important to try to spare the intercostal bundles as much as possible. When the superior incision is used, the chest is commonly entered at the lateral border of the incision. This is of no great consequence and the fibres of the diaphragm are reapproximated over a temporary tube at the conclusion of the operation while the lungs are expanded.

34

35 The oblique and transverse abdominis muscles are divided in the line of the skin incision, and the retroperitoneal space is entered. Mobilization begins laterally and extends medially as described for the standard retroperitoneal approach. In this case, however, dissection is carried behind the left kidney, which is displaced anteriorly with the other viscera. In the unusual circumstance of a retroaortic renal vein, the kidney is left posteriorly.

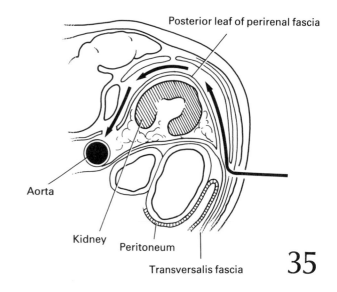

Dissection of the aorta

36 A large lumbar vein is usually encountered, which helps identify the origin of the left renal artery. Dissection of the aorta begins along the vertebral column and continues posteriorly. The most important landmark is the left renal artery, which should be identified early. The aortic dissection should proceed posterior to this vessel. Lymphatic and lumbar vessels are ligated in continuity as necessary with 3/0 silk ligatures. Dissection is carried through the diaphragm, diaphragmatic crura and, if necessary, to the lower thoracic aorta. This allows the aorta to be clamped in a disease-free area. No attempt should be made to dissect the aorta circumferentially from this approach, as this could result in troublesome venous bleeding. The vessel is mobilized enough to allow placement of a larger vascular clamp above the level of disease and below the renal arteries.

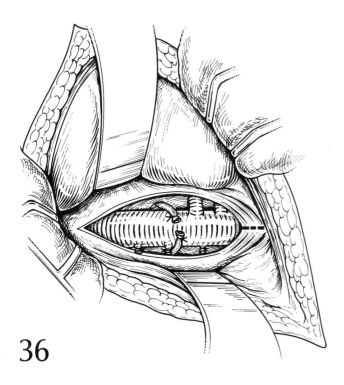

Endarterectomy of suprarenal abdominal aorta

37a, b The aorta is incised posterior to the left renal artery. An endarterectomy plane is established at this point. This plane is more superficial than would be taken in the femoral or carotid systems. Back-bleeding from the renal and superior mesenteric and coeliac arteries is controlled with Fogarty balloon catheters. If necessary, endarterectomy of one or more of the renal and visceral arteries may be carried out at this point. After the aortic segment has been end-arterectomized, the repair proceeds in one of two ways.

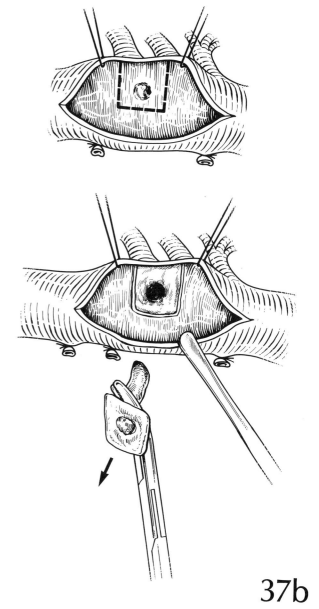

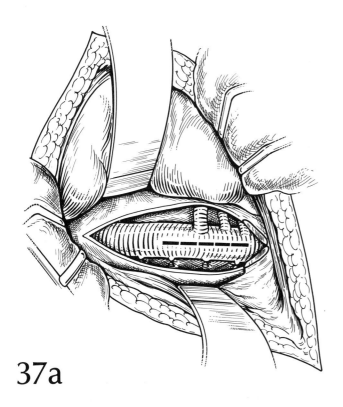

37a

37b

38 If the distal aorta is normal, the arteriotomy may be closed with 4/0 or 5/0 monofilament after the distal intima has been secured to avoid dissection. This approach is only applicable in a small minority of patients.

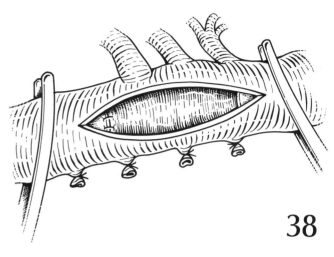

38

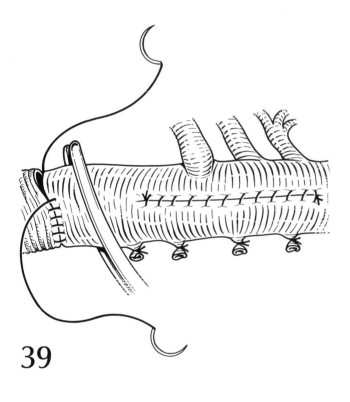

39

Endarterectomy with aortofemoral bypass

39 When there is extensive aortoiliac disease, this procedure may be combined with standard aortofemoral bypass. The endarterectomy is extended into the proximal cuff of the infrarenal aorta (without extending the arteriotomy), which is then transected 2–3 cm below the renal arteries. The aortotomy is closed with a running 5/0 polypropylene suture, and the transected endarterectomized aorta is reclamped below the renal arteries. Following this, a standard end-to-end aortofemoral graft is placed. Once again, however, 4/0 or 5/0 polypropylene on a fine needle is used for the proximal suture line. Fine sutures and use of felt pledgets to buttress the aortic closure diminish bleeding problems.

40 Alternatively, the aortic anastomosis can be made directly to the visceral aorta by bevelling the graft. Although this extends the suprarenal clamp time minimally, it avoids two suture lines and in recent years has become the authors' preferred approach. The aorta is usually clamped above the renal arteries for no more than 30–45 min, and this is tolerated without ill effects in most patients.

Wound closure

Following completion of the reconstruction, the wound is closed in layers. If the pleura has been entered, it is closed around a 20-Fr red rubber catheter which is then removed. The muscle layers are then closed individually using running 0 or 1 absorbable sutures. Scarpa's fascia is closed with a 3/0 running suture, and the skin is approximated in the usual fashion.

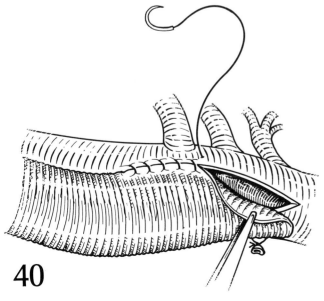

40

ILIOFEMORAL BYPASS

This procedure is reserved for patients with significant disease limited to one iliac artery. Ideally, a portion of common iliac artery should be available for the proximal anastomosis. This procedure can still be performed, however, if the origin of the involved iliac vessel is occluded, provided that the aortic bifurcation is free of disease. The authors prefer this procedure to cross-femoral bypass in appropriate cases, because it avoids operation on an asymptomatic limb and involves a single groin incision. Long-term patency of this type of reconstruction is comparable with or superior to that reported with cross-femoral bypass.

Exposure of iliac artery

41 The involved iliac artery is exposed retroperitoneally as previously described on page 38. On the right side the vena cava does not interfere with exposure.

When the origin of the common iliac vessel is patent, the artery is clamped at this point after heparinization. If the ipsilateral hypogastric artery is perfused in a prograde fashion, an end-to-side anastomosis to the common iliac artery is performed as previously described.

If the common iliac artery is occluded, the iliac artery is transected and an end-to-end anastomosis is constructed. This is done with a 4/0 monofilament suture using an 8-mm or 10-mm prosthesis. Tunnelling and distal anastomosis are as described on page 202.

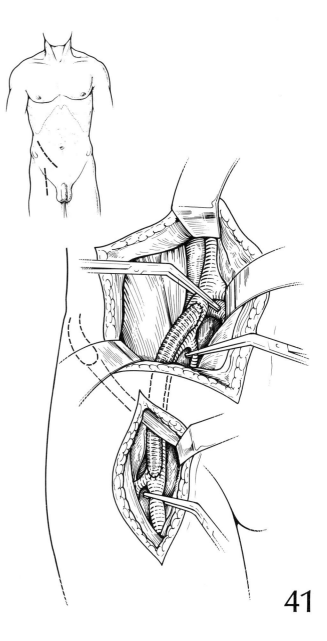

41

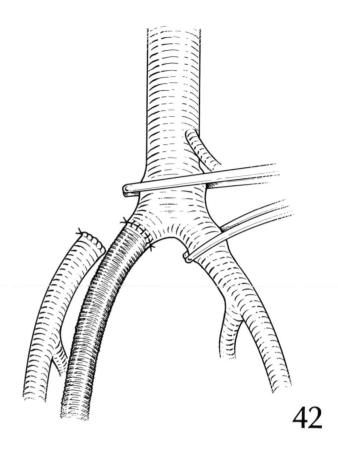

42 If the common iliac artery is completely occluded but the aortic bifurcation is not severely diseased, control is obtained by clamping the distal aorta and contralateral iliac vessel. In these cases, the common iliac artery is transected and its origin thrombectomized. An end-to-end anastomosis can be performed to the disobliterated proximal common iliac vessel. Tunnelling and distal anastomosis are performed and wounds closed.

42

Postoperative care

Patients who undergo aortic reconstruction are monitored for 24–48 h in an intensive care unit. The authors routinely use indwelling urinary catheters, radial arterial lines and measurements of central venous pressure. In patients with cardiac dysfunction, pulmonary artery catheters are employed, and this is routine in patients in whom supracoeliac manipulation has been performed.

Complications

Major postoperative problems are hypovolaemia, bleeding and distal ischaemia. These are best anticipated by aggressive monitoring and treated early. The authors routinely reverse anticoagulation with protamine sulphate and assume that continued blood loss is due to a technical error. While this is a rare event, prompt re-exploration is required. Alteration in distal perfusion can be diagnosed by physical examination and confirmed by Doppler blood pressure measurement. When it occurs, prompt re-exploration is required, which can usually be performed transfemorally. Operative angiography may be required to identify the cause of

graft failure. Prophylactic fasciotomy may be required if the ischaemic interval exceeds 4–6 h. Patients with evidence of atheroembolism and intact pulses are treated expectantly.

Colonic ischaemia may occur, often heralded by bloody diarrhoea, and is best documented by flexible sigmoidoscopy[8]. Ischaemia limited to the mucosa may be treated non-operatively with nasogastric suction, intravenous antibiotics and repeated endoscopic evaluation. Transmural ischaemia requires prompt resection and colonic diversion.

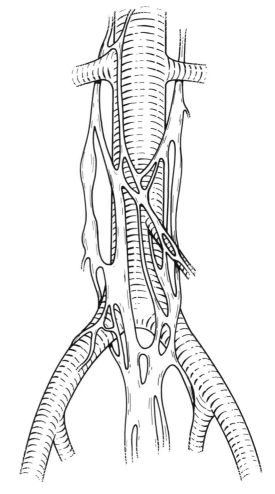

43 Impotence, or more commonly retrograde ejaculation, can occur as a result of disruption of the parasympathetic nerves around the aortic bifurcation. This can be prevented by careful dissection in this area.

Pelvic ischaemia can occur after revascularization of the infrarenal aorta and can be associated with ischaemia of the distal spinal cord. It is often due to pelvic devascularization caused by a proximal end-to-end aortic anastomosis in the face of bilateral external iliac occlusions, which prevent retrograde perfusion of the hypogastric arteries and distal aorta. This can be prevented by attention to the preoperative arteriogram and use of an end-to-side aortic anastomosis in these cases. If an end-to-side anastomosis is technically difficult, some attempt to revascularize at least one hypogastric artery is warranted.

43

References

1. Davies AH, Ramarkha P, Collin J, Morris PJ. Recent changes in the treatment of aortoiliac occlusive disease by the Oxford Regional Vascular Service. *Br J Surg* 1990; 77: 1129–31.

2. Brewster DC. Clinical and anatomical considerations for surgery in aortoiliac disease and results of surgical treatment. *Circulation* 1991; 83(Suppl): 142–52.

3. Szilagyi DE, Elliott JP Jr, Smith RF, Reddy DJ, McPharlin M. A thirty year survey of the reconstructive treatment of aortoiliac occlusive disease. *J Vasc Surg* 1986; 3: 421–36.

4. Langsfeld M, Nepute J, Hershey FB, Thorpe L, Auer AI, Binnington HB *et al.* The use of deep duplex scanning to predict hemodynamically significant aortoiliac stenoses. *J Vasc Surg* 1988; 7: 395–99.

5. Picone AJ, Green RM, Ricotta JJ, May AG, DeWeese JA. Spinal cord ischemia following operations on the abdominal aorta. *J Vasc Surg* 1986; 3: 94–103.

6. Green RM, Ricotta JJ, Ouriel K, DeWeese JA. Results of supraceliac aortic clamping in the difficult elective resection of infrarenal abdominal aortic aneurysm. *J Vasc Surg* 1989; 9: 124–34.

7. Shepard AD, Tollefson DF, Reddy DJ, Evans JR, Elliott JP, Smith RF *et al.* Left flank retroperitoneal exposure: a technical aid to complex aortic reconstruction. *J Vasc Surg* 1991; 14: 283–91.

8. Zelenock GB, Strodel WE, Knol JA, Messina LM, Wakefield TW, Lindenauer SM *et al.* A prospective study of clinically and endoscopically documented colonic ischemia in 100 patients undergoing aortic reconstructive surgery with aggressive colonic and direct pelvic revascularization, compared with historic controls. *Surgery* 1989; 106: 771–80.

Femorofemoral and axillofemoral bypass techniques

F. Quigley MS, FRACS
Staff Specialist, Vascular Surgery, Royal Adelaide Hospital, Adelaide, South Australia

I. Faris MD, FRACS
Chairman, Department of Surgery, University of Adelaide, and Head of Unit, Vascular Surgery, Royal Adelaide Hospital, Adelaide, South Australia

Femorofemoral bypass

History

Femorofemoral subcutaneous grafts were popularized by Vetto in 1962 as an alternative to aortoiliac reconstruction in high-risk patients with unilateral iliac disease and patients with occlusion of one limb of an aortobifemoral graft. The use of the opposite limb as a donor artery had previously been described by McCaughan and Kahn in 1960 but these authors used the external iliac system as the donor artery and tunnelled the graft extraperitoneally above the bladder.

Principles and justification

The main reason for using a femorofemoral bypass rather than an aortobifemoral bypass is the lower morbidity and mortality rates associated with the lesser procedure. Initial concern that this would lead to a high failure rate due to progression of disease in the donor iliac system has been shown to be unnecessary, as excellent long-term patency figures have been reported. In patients with unilateral iliac disease alternative surgical procedures include iliofemoral bypass, iliac endarterectomy, and unilateral aortofemoral bypass or unilateral axillofemoral bypass. Endovascular procedures may also be used to treat stenoses or short occlusions. Critics of femorofemoral bypass have been concerned with the potential for a 'steal' phenomenon to occur on the donor side. The excellent patency of aortobifemoral bypass is partly offset by significant morbidity rates. This includes the cardiac risks of aortic clamping, the pulmonary risks of major abdominal surgery, and compromised sexual function. Femorofemoral grafting can also be used to treat unilateral occlusion of an aortobifemoral graft.

Preoperative

Assessment

The assessment of the severity of iliac stenosis may be difficult. Preoperative arteriography may be carried out via the donor artery. Uniplanar radiographs may underestimate the severity of the disease in the common iliac arteries because the disease is most severe along the posterior wall of the artery and, in addition, it is hard to predict the haemodynamic effect of changes seen on the arteriogram. When there is concern that the donor iliac artery may be diseased, the aortofemoral pressure gradient can be assessed at the same time as arteriography is performed. If pullback pressures cannot be done at the time of angiography a direct puncture of the femoral artery can be made for comparison of femoral and brachial pressures. If the femoral/brachial index is less than 0.85 or decreases by more than 0.15 after hyperaemia induced by intra-arterial papaverine (30 mg) or 5 min of tourniquet ischaemia to the thigh, the donor iliac system is probably inadequate.

Alternatively, a 50% or greater stenosis on arteriography in the donor limb can be taken as a contraindication for the procedure unless the iliac stenosis can be treated by a balloon angioplasty. Assessment of the iliac arteries using duplex ultrasonography is being investigated, but has not yet reached the stage of widespread clinical use.

Anaesthesia

The operation may be performed under light general, spinal or epidural anaesthesia. Occasionally the procedure may be done under local anaesthesia but the tunnelling of the graft across the pubic symphysis is painful and requires some form of sedation.

Operation

All patients receive perioperative antibiotics (cephalothin 1 g intravenously 6-hourly for 24 h) and heparin, 5000 units, at the time of surgery. The operating table should be suitable for obtaining a radiograph of the inguinal area without shifting the patient.

The operation is performed with the patient in the supine position. The abdomen below the umbilicus and both legs to the ankles are prepared by applying povidone-iodine and sealing the feet in transparent bowel bags. This allows assessment of circulation of both legs throughout the operation. The pubic area is excluded by suturing a drape in place.

Incision

The femoral bifurcation is exposed with a longitudinal incision extending distally from the mid inguinal point. If there is no pulse the femoral artery may be felt as a cord in the femoral triangle and the incision placed over it. If there has been a previous exposure of the femoral arteries, the former incision should be used.

1   The proximal limit of the exposure is the inguinal ligament. There are no major structures superficial to the common femoral artery except that a tributary of the external iliac vein may cross the artery at the level of the inguinal ligament. Damage to this vein may be difficult to control. Tapes are passed around the common femoral and superficial femoral arteries before the deep femoral artery is dissected. Traction on the tapes will allow the origin of the deep femoral artery from the posteromedial aspect of the common femoral artery to be dissected. A tape can be placed around this vessel. Smaller branches are preserved and controlled with a double loop.

When the common femoral artery is occluded or the origin of the deep femoral artery is stenosed on the recipient side an adequate length of deep femoral artery is exposed. It is better to anticipate the need for this dissection because it is more difficult, and damage to the veins more likely, if the dissection is undertaken after the clamps have been applied and the arteries opened. The major structure encountered is the deep femoral vein, which emerges deep to the superficial femoral artery and crosses superficial to the deep femoral artery on its way to join the femoral vein. The upper edge of the vein is usually within 1 cm of the origin of the deep femoral artery and the vein may be 1 cm wide. It must be dissected carefully before it is divided. If the vein is large it is safer to divide it between vascular clamps and oversew the ends with a 5/0 polypropylene (Prolene) suture. Division of the vein displays the proximal segment of the artery down to its first major branch. It is desirable to dissect and tape both the branch and the continuing trunk of the artery.

The first section of the deep femoral artery is the preferred site for anastomosis but more distal segments may be used if necessary. An indication of the severity of

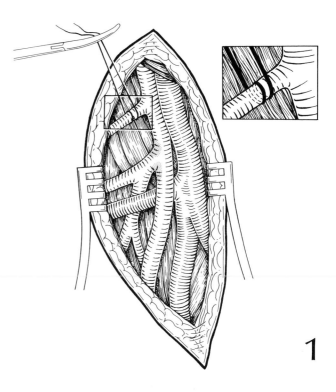

1

the atheroma in the artery can be gained from passing a pair of scissors or curved clamp behind the artery and palpating the thickness of the wall against the clamp or scissors.

Graft

Polytetrafluoroethylene (PTFE) or Dacron (woven or knitted) 8 mm or 10 mm diameter are the grafts of choice. Reversed saphenous vein is probably best preserved for femoropopliteal bypass which may be required later. Vein may be used when the recipient groin is infected. There is probably no advantage in using externally supported grafts in this situation.

Anastomoses

After administration of heparin, 5000 units intravenously, and the application of clamps, arteriotomy is performed.

2 The usual configuration is described as a C where the toe of the anastomosis is downstream so that blood flow reverses direction from the donor femoral artery up the graft.

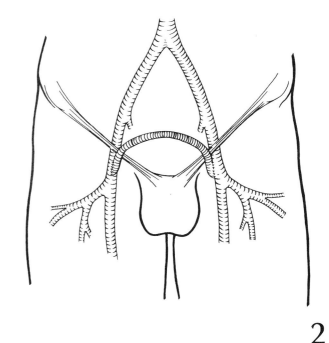

2

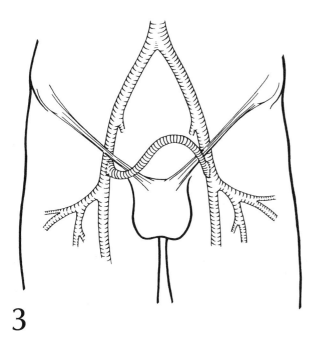

3

3 The alternative S-shaped configuration with the toe of the donor anastomosis placed proximally in the external iliac artery is more difficult to carry out and has no significant haemodynamic advantage.

When the crossover graft is being used to overcome unilateral occlusion of an aortobifemoral graft the C-shaped configuration can be associated with kinking near the anastomosis to the donor graft limb and, in this situation, an anastomosis either with the crossover graft at a right angle to the established graft or an S configuration is advised.

The anastomosis on the donor side is performed first, after opening the recipient artery to confirm that the bypass can proceed. The graft is bevelled to allow an oblique angle and the anastomosis is sutured with 5/0 polypropylene. Suturing should begin at the proximal end of the anastomosis because the acute angle between graft and artery makes access difficult later in the procedure. Before completion of the anastomosis the clamps are momentarily released to flush any clot that has formed. The graft is then clamped close to the anastomosis and flow restored to the donor limb. Major leaks are repaired and minor leaks through suture holes in the prosthesis are packed with a gauze swab, with or without absorbable haemostatic material.

4 The anastomosis on the recipient side is most easily made to the common femoral artery in an end-to-side manner with the toe of the anastomosis placed distally and the heel of the anastomosis a few millimetres from the proximal end of the arteriotomy on the medial side in exactly the same way that the donor anastomosis is sutured.

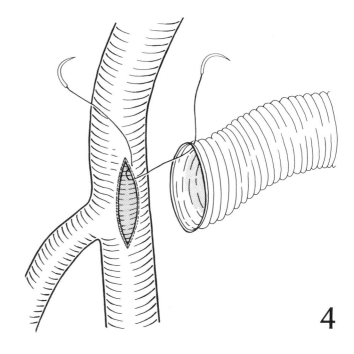

4

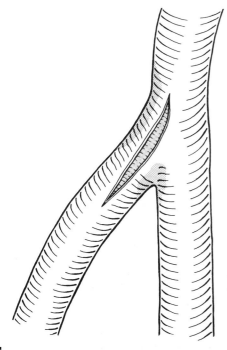

5

5 As with aortobifemoral bypass, it is important to ensure flow into the deep femoral artery and this may be achieved by extending the arteriotomy in the common femoral artery across the origin of the deep femoral artery using the apex of the graft as a patch across any stenosis that is present. The use of the graft as a patch rather than performing an endarterectomy of deep and common femoral arteries provides adequate blood flow into the deep femoral artery and decreases the likelihood of false aneurysm formation. Extensive disease in the proximal portion of the deep femoral artery may be overcome by an endarterectomy.

6 A useful alternative, when it is known on the preoperative arteriogram that the common and superficial femoral arteries are occluded, is to make an arteriotomy in a distal, disease-free segment of the deep femoral artery and to anastomose the graft to the artery with a Miller cuff. In such cases when it is known that the middle third rather than the proximal segment of the deep femoral artery is to be exposed, the artery can be approached directly by dissecting in the same plane as the superficial femoral artery about 10 cm from its origin. The dissection may be made either medial or lateral to the superficial femoral artery which has few branches at this point and is easily pushed to one side. The Miller cuff is formed by making a longitudinal arteriotomy in the usual way. A strip of long saphenous vein is then harvested and opened longitudinally. One edge of the strip of vein is then sutured the whole length of the arteriotomy with the cuff completed by suturing the two ends of the vein strip together.

Completion angiography is performed when the recipient anastomosis includes a profundaplasty or is directly into the deep femoral artery. Angiography is performed by injecting 10–20 ml of contrast medium (sodium and meglumine ioxaglate (Hexabrix) or iopamidol) directly into the graft via a 21-gauge butterfly needle after the clamps have been removed, taking a single exposure as the last few millilitres of contrast medium are being injected. If the PTFE graft is used it will be necessary to suture the puncture in the graft, usually with a single 5/0 polypropylene suture.

Tunnelling graft

The graft is placed subcutaneously anterior to the external oblique muscle and rectus sheath and runs a curved course above the pubic symphysis. A bimanual technique is used to form a tunnel. The ends of the tunnel are formed by sharp dissection beginning over the inguinal ligament above and medial to the femoral artery. The spermatic cord, which is inferomedial to this dissection, should be avoided. A finger is inserted from each side as far medially as possible and an empty pair of sponge-holding forceps or a pair of scissors are used to break across the midline raphe to complete the tunnel. The graft is then carefully pulled through the tunnel. If the graft is not to be placed in the tunnel immediately, a tape can be placed in the tunnel and this facilitates the subsequent placement of the graft.

The exact sequence of the procedure may differ if there are two surgeons to perform the anastomoses. It is quicker if surgeons operate synchronously on each side.

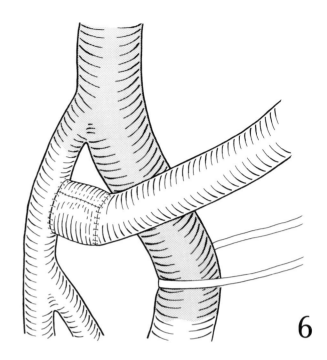

6

With two surgeons the graft is placed in the tunnel before the anastomoses begin. The surgeon on the donor side begins suturing the anastomosis and, when the proximal end of the anastomosis is secure, the surgeon on the recipient side trims the graft to the appropriate length and begins suturing. It is important that the graft should not be too tight. The anastomosis on the medial aspect of the donor side is sutured from within the lumen because with the graft placed in its tunnel it is no longer possible to move the graft sufficiently to suture from the outside on this aspect of the anastomosis.

With one surgeon the anastomosis on the donor side is performed first and then the graft placed in its tunnel. To ensure that no kinking is present the graft is flushed before commencing the recipient anastomosis. The graft is again flushed just before completing the recipient anastomosis to ensure no clot has formed in the graft while the anastomosis has been performed. The same precaution against clot formation in the recipient artery is also made by momentarily releasing clamps on recipient vessels before completion of the anastomosis. Closed suction may be placed in each wound at completion of the operation.

An inguinal hernia may hinder the formation of the tunnel which passes above the external inguinal ring. It is not difficult to repair the hernia through the same incision, if necessary by extending the incision proximally a short distance in the normal fashion and then proceeding with the operation as before.

Haemodynamic considerations

There must be a sufficient pressure gradient between the sides to maintain flow in the graft. There have been reports of early graft failure due to abolition of pressure differential between donor and recipient arteries when an endarterectomy of the recipient artery (distal external iliac or common femoral) which restored inflow was carried out at the same time. Where disease is limited to the common femoral or distal external iliac artery it is preferable to carry out an ipsilateral endarterectomy rather than perform a femorofemoral bypass.

Stealing blood from the donor limb, which may result in worsening of ischaemia in the donor limb, may occur if there is stenosis of the donor iliac arteries associated with severe donor limb outflow disease in the presence of a normal recipient limb outflow bed. A normal iliac inflow system has sufficient capacity to supply both limbs. If there is stenosis in the inflow system the lower vascular resistance in a normal recipient limb may result in diversion of blood flow from the donor limb. Symptomatic steal is rare in reported series of femorofemoral bypasses despite objective evidence of it occurring in up to 45% of cases[1].

The more common form of haemodynamic failure is where the graft remains patent but does not relieve symptoms, usually due to inadequate inflow. Angioplasty of the affected iliac segment or the addition of an aortofemoral or axillofemoral component may rectify the problem.

Postoperative care

Drains can be removed the morning after the operation. The procedure is well tolerated by patients who may be sitting out of bed the next day and walking the day after. The patient is usually ready for discharge 5–7 days following operation. There is a small but significant mortality rate resulting from the associated cardiopulmonary disease.

Outcome

Late graft failure is usually due to progression of disease in the outflow tract rather than donor iliac disease, but is not as common as was initially expected when the procedure was first described. Plecha[2] reported a 5-year primary patency rate of 72%. Patency is best for grafts placed when the runoff is good (patent superficial femoral and deep femoral arteries) and worst when the runoff is poor or performed after one limb of an aortobifemoral graft has occluded.

The donor artery side may also be affected by the same complications common to any vascular bypass of infection, haemorrhage, occlusion or false aneurysm formation. The occurrence of such a complication in the 'good' leg is a disaster but is no more frequent in femorofemoral bypass than aortofemoral bypass.

Axillofemoral bypass

History

First introduced by Blaisdell in 1961, the operation was initially used as an alternative to direct aortic reconstruction in patients who were of high operative risk because of either cardiac disease or aortic sepsis. The first patient to have the procedure by Blaisdell was originally planned to have aortic reconstruction but suffered a myocardial ischaemic event on induction and so had the lesser procedure of axillofemoral bypass. Louw reported the use of this technique at the same time as Blaisdell as an alternative to aortofemoral bypass for patients with severe occlusive disease of the aortoiliac segment.

Principles and justification

Bypass of the aorta is achieved with a lower morbidity rate than with direct methods because no major body cavity is entered and the haemodynamic stress associated with aortic crossclamping is avoided. Indications include infected aortic prosthesis, aortoenteric fistula, mycotic aortic aneurysms, a 'hostile' abdomen due to multiple previous intra-abdominal operations, abdominal radiation, morbid obesity, and where there is thought to be a high risk associated with aortic surgery in a patient with severe cardiac, renal or respiratory disease.

Preoperative

The use of an axillary artery as a donor vessel in the presence of subclavian or innominate disease may result in diversion of blood flow from the distal part of the donor limb (upper limb steal). Bilateral brachial artery pressure measurements and auscultation for supraclavicular bruits are usually sufficient to detect donor vessel disease but angiography or duplex scanning may be necessary.

Anaesthesia

General anaesthesia is the preferred method although local anaesthesia can be used in very frail patients. The donor arm is placed at right angles, taking care to avoid hyperabduction which may result in injury of the brachial plexus.

Operation

Draping

The anterior aspect of the shoulder, the lateral chest wall and axilla, and the side of the abdomen on the donor side as well as the whole of the abdomen below the umbilicus and both legs to the ankle are prepared with povidone-iodine and draped. Because of the large operative field that needs to be prepared the drapes may best be held in place with either staples or povidone-iodine impregnated 'Ioband' adhesive drape.

Incision and exposure of arteries

7 An oblique incision is made about 2–3 cm below the middle third of the clavicle, the lateral extent being the medial border of the deltoid muscle. This incision is deepened through subcutaneous tissue and fascia overlying pectoralis major. The cephalic vein, which should be preserved, may be encountered at the lateral end of the wound. The transversely running fibres of the pectoralis major muscle are split in the direction of the incision and a self-retaining retractor placed. The clavipectoral fascia is incised and the upper border of the pectoralis minor muscle displayed. Exposure of the contents of the axilla is much easier if this muscle is divided. Division is performed as close as possible to its attachment to the coracoid process of the scapula.

The axillary artery is palpated deep in the axilla. As the dissection proceeds, the first major structure encountered is the axillary vein which lies anteroinferior to the artery. The vein is dissected from the artery, dividing tributaries of the vein as necessary. Care needs to be taken in dissecting the artery to preserve the thoracoacromial and subscapular branches. The brachial plexus lies above and behind the artery at this point and is at risk from direct trauma and retraction.

A suitable length of the artery is isolated and encircled with tapes. The donor site is usually the first or second part of the axillary artery and, to simplify the anastomosis and the position of the graft, it is recommended that the pectoralis minor muscle be divided. Alternatively, the muscle can be retracted laterally while the anastomosis is completed. The preferred site of the anastomosis is to as proximal a part of the axillary artery as possible. At this level there is very little motion of the artery or graft with movement of the arm and this may decrease the risk of false aneurysm formation due to dislodging of the artery from a graft tethered by fibrous tissue.

The femoral vessels are exposed in the usual way as described above.

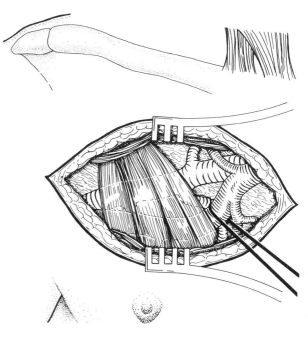

7

Choice of graft

Similar patency rates have been obtained using either Dacron or PTFE grafts, 8 or 10 mm in diameter. Several studies suggest an advantage with the use of externally supported grafts[3].

Axillary anastomosis

8 The axillary artery is lifted forward by the encircling tapes and after administration of heparin clamps are applied. The arteriotomy in the axillary artery should be placed in a longitudinal direction on the anteroinferior rather than anterior aspect of the artery to avoid a kink or acute curve as the graft goes behind the lateral border of pectoralis major. The graft is bevelled to give an oblique anastomosis that avoids a T-shaped configuration and allows the graft to run laterally to the axilla without kinking or the need to penetrate the pectoralis major muscle. The wall of the axillary artery is much thinner than the wall of a diseased common femoral artery so that sutures must be placed and held gently lest they cut out of the wall. When the anastomosis is completed the circulation is restored to the arm by placing a clamp on the graft just beyond the anastomosis before placing the graft in the tunnel. This allows the graft to be moved about for access to the posterior aspect of the suture line if any bleeding is present.

Tunnelling graft

With the pectoralis minor muscle divided the graft is tunnelled behind the lateral border of pectoralis major and then subcutaneously down the chest in the mid-axillary line. The lower part of the graft swings forward medial to the anterior superior iliac spine to the groin. Ideally this tunnel is made without the need for a counter incision between axilla and groin. The mid-axillary line is recommended rather than a course further anteriorly to avoid kinking whenever the patient bends over.

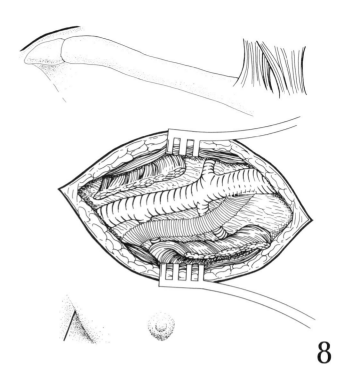

8

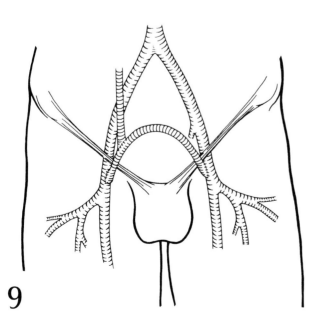

9

Femoral anastomosis

There is good evidence that the patency of axillo-bifemoral grafts is superior to that of axillounifemoral grafts. The explanation is probably the greater flow through the axillofemoral component when the outflow is to both lower limbs. The anastomosis between axillary limb and crossover should be as close as possible to the femoral artery.

Various configurations are possible.

9 The axillary graft may be anastomosed to a standard femorofemoral graft in an end-to-side fashion on the ipsilateral side. This is the preferred configuration if there are two surgeons operating. One surgeon performs the axillary anastomosis while the second surgeon performs the anastomosis between femoral artery and crossover prosthesis on the ipsilateral side. The second surgeon then goes to the opposite side of the operating table and performs a similar anastomosis between crossover graft and femoral artery. The first surgeon tunnels the graft and anastomoses its distal end to the side of the crossover graft. In this way each surgeon performs two anastomoses and this shortens the procedure considerably.

10 Alternatively, the axillary portion may be anastomosed to the ipsilateral femoral artery and the graft to the other femoral artery taken off the axillary graft in a side-to-end fashion above the femoral anastomosis.

The graft-to-graft anastomosis should be made close to the femoral artery anastomosis because the portion of the axillofemoral limb that lies distal to the side arm anastomosis will have only about half the flow in the proximal portion and appears to have a higher thrombosis rate.

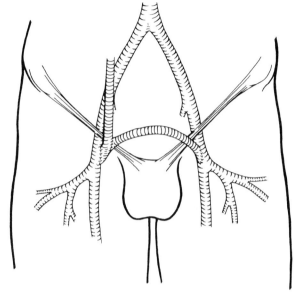

10

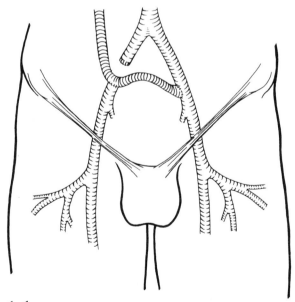

11

11 As a third option, the femoral artery on the ipsilateral side may be divided and the proximal stump oversewn. The axillary graft is then anastomosed to the distal femoral artery side-to-end and the part of the axillary graft distal to this anastomosis is tunnelled to the opposite groin and anastomosed to the femoral artery in an end-to-side fashion. This configuration is only possible where there is no significant common femoral or deep femoral origin disease on the ipsilateral side.

Outcome

Most reports indicate a much poorer patency rate for axillofemoral grafts than with aortofemoral bypass; however, a recent report[3] suggested improved patency using externally supported PTFE with a patency of 85% at 4 years. External compression due to body positioning during sleep has been implicated as a cause of thrombosis of axillofemoral grafts and this may be an explanation for the reported improvement in patency using externally supported grafts.

Patency rates are best for grafts carried out for non-occlusive disease (e.g. infected aortic prosthesis) followed by cases in which the run-off is good (patent superficial femoral artery) and worst when the runoff is poor.

False aneurysm at the axillary anastomosis may occur due to infection or technical reasons. Sullivan *et al.*[4] reported two cases of mechanical disruption of the axillary anastomosis when the patients fully abducted the affected arm. When the axillary anastomosis is made too far laterally the graft anastomosis will be under tension when the arm is in full abduction.

A periprosthetic fluid collection may occur due to the accumulation of lymph around the graft. Treatment is by aspiration, rerouting of the graft or drainage of the collection by a pedicle of omentum placed in the cavity around the graft.

Apart from a higher rate of thrombosis than aortobifemoral grafts, the operation has a long-term complication rate of around 2% made up of false aneurysm formation, embolization to the brachial artery and axillary artery thrombosis[5].

References

1. Harris JP, Flinn WR, Rudo NR, Bergan JJ, Yao JST. Assessment of donor limb hemodynamics in femorofemoral bypass for claudication. *Surgery* 1981; 90: 764–73.

2. Plecha FR, Plecha FM. Femorofemoral bypass grafts: ten year experience. *J Vasc Surg* 1984; 1: 555–61.

3. Harris EJ, Taylor LM, McConnell DB, Moneta GL, Yeager RA, Porter JM. Clinical results of axillobifemoral bypass using externally supported polytetrafluoroethylene. *J Vasc Surg* 1990; 12: 416–21.

4. Sullivan LP, Davidson PG, D'Anna JA, Sithian N. Disruption of the proximal anastomosis of axillobifemoral grafts: two case reports. *J Vasc Surg* 1989; 10: 190–2.

5. Bunt TJ, Moore W. Optimal proximal anastomosis/tunnel for axillofemoral grafts. *J Vasc Surg* 1986; 3: 673–6.

Abdominal aortic aneurysm resection

Averil O. Mansfield ChM, FRCS
Consultant Vascular Surgeon, St Mary's Hospital, London, UK

Principles and justification

The decision to operate on an abdominal aortic aneurysm is made on consideration of two factors: the size of the aneurysm and the fitness of the patient. If an aneurysm ruptures, the community mortality rate is in the region of 90%. If the patient reaches hospital and has an operation, the mortality rate is around 50%. If, however, the operation is elective and the aneurysm is intact, the operative mortality rate should be under 5%.

It is generally accepted that the risk of rupture becomes significant when the transverse diameter of the aneurysm reaches about 5 cm, hence a patient with an aneurysm of this size or greater should be offered an operation unless general fitness for major surgery precludes this.

Preoperative

General assessment

Ischaemic heart disease is a commonly associated problem and is the most common cause of postoperative mortality. The author prefers patients to have an exercise test and, if this reveals a problem, guidance about further tests is sought from the cardiologist. When necessary the operation is delayed in order to improve the patient's fitness; an aortocoronary bypass may be performed if indicated.

Renal function is routinely assessed and if the creatinine is elevated further investigation of the cause is undertaken with the assistance, where necessary, of the nephrologist. This may involve renal scans, arteriography and sometimes biopsy.

Pulmonary function tests are performed when indicated and, when necessary, treatment including drugs and physiotherapy is given.

Specific investigations

Clinical examination will be comprehensive but particular attention must be paid to other common sites of aneurysm, e.g. the popliteal arteries. Occlusive disease in the legs is sometimes associated, in which case ankle pressure indices should be recorded. The abdomen should be auscultated in order to detect bruits and particularly to detect an aortocaval fistula by the mechanical murmur which is sometimes audible. Rectal examination will be routine but may occasionally demonstrate a pelvic aneurysm.

Ultrasonography is a useful screening test and in some centres is the only specific preoperative test carried out routinely. It is operator dependent and a skilled ultrasonographer not only can measure the aneurysm but can demonstrate the renal arteries and their relationship to the aneurysm.

Computed tomography is the author's preferred routine preoperative investigation and will demonstrate the size, relationships, characteristics and extent of the aneurysm as well as other intra-abdominal problems. Particularly useful features to note are: the wall thickness (if greatly thickened anteriorly it will give warning of an inflammatory aneurysm); the course of the ureters; the site of the left renal vein (whether anterior or posterior to the neck of the aneurysm); the origin of the visceral arteries and their relationship to the sac; and the presence of iliac aneurysms.

Magnetic resonance imaging may in time replace other investigations as, in addition to providing transverse sections, it supplies some information equivalent to that of arteriography, while avoiding irradiation and administration of contrast media.

The specific indications for arteriography in the author's work-up are involvement of the visceral arteries and intermittent claudication.

Prophylactic antibiotics, usually flucloxacillin or a cephalosporin, are administered.

Anaesthesia

The operation is performed under general anaesthesia. The patient is monitored by means of an arterial line, a central venous line and, in the author's unit, a Swan–Ganz catheter.

An epidural catheter is inserted at the end of the operation for the delivery of epidural opiates for pain control. A bladder catheter is essential for the close monitoring of urinary output.

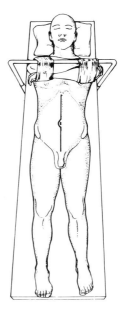

1a

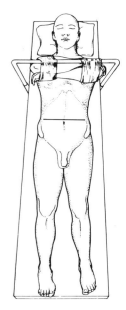

1b

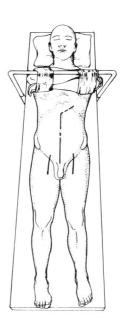

1c

Operation

Incision

1a–c Normally the incision is made in the midline from the xiphisternum to the pubic symphysis (*Illustration 1a*).

Occasionally, when preoperative investigations indicate that a straight graft is definitely all that will be needed and there have been no previous abdominal operations, a transverse incision sited just above the umbilicus can be used (*Illustration 1b*).

If there is doubt about the upper limits of the aneurysm provision should be made to extend the incision across the costal margin if necessary (*Illustration 1c*).

Occasionally the external iliac arteries are aneurysmal and in this case the graft will have to be taken down to the groins. These should always be prepared but will seldom be incised.

Laparotomy

The peritoneal cavity is carefully examined for any additional pathology. In the author's experience the most common additional findings are gallstones, diverticular disease and colonic cancer.

Throughout the laparotomy care must be taken to avoid manipulation of the aneurysm because of the danger of macroemboli and microemboli, the latter being commonly referred to as 'trash'. Individual decisions will need to be taken if additional unexpected problems are revealed but no procedure that might spill organisms can be carried out at the same operation as the insertion of a prosthesis into the aorta.

Exposure of the aorta

The author stands on the patient's right but other surgeons find it easier to stand on the left.

2 The whole of the small bowel has to be mobilized to the right of the abdomen. The base of the mesentery runs across the posterior abdominal wall and overlies the aorta. This process of moving the gut to the right may be visualized as turning the pages of a book with the spine of the book being the base of the mesentery. This must be done completely in order to avoid danger to the vessels in the small bowel mesentery.

When adhesions are encountered these must be dealt with very carefully as invasion of the gut lumen will result in the need to abandon the operation in an unruptured case.

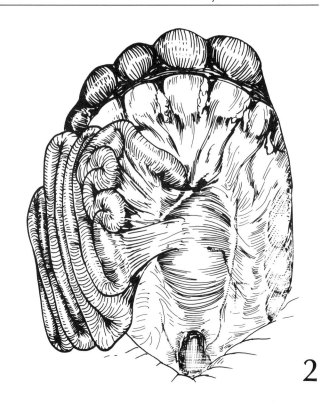

2

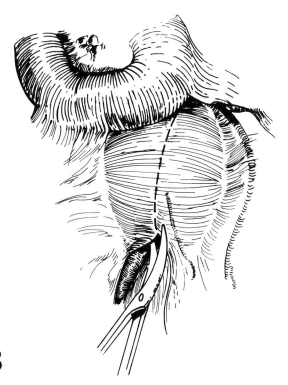

3

3 The posterior peritoneum is divided along the line of divide between the small bowel mesentery to the right and the large bowel mesentery to the left, avoiding the blood supply of both. Division is continued upwards to the duodenojejunal junction, easily identified by the inferior mesenteric vein. Great care is needed to avoid damage to the serosa of the duodenum.

4 The most important landmark in the exposure of the aorta is the left renal vein. This normally crosses the aorta at or above the neck of the aneurysm. Occasionally it runs behind the aorta and may have been identified there by computed tomography. Failure to recognize a retroaortic renal vein can result in severe haemorrhage.

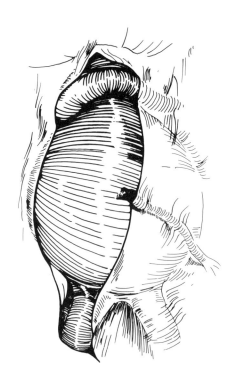

4

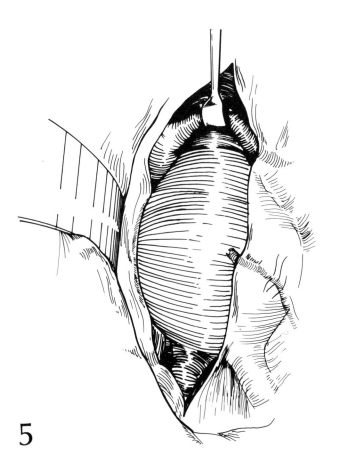

5

5 The lower edge of the left renal vein and its junction with the inferior vena cava is displayed. It can be gently freed from the underlying aorta so that it can be displaced upwards if necessary before clamping. Tributaries should be left intact at this stage because it is occasionally necessary to divide the left renal vein and the tributaries are then important collaterals.

Preparation of the neck of the aneurysm

The area of the aorta where normal aorta suddenly expands to become aneurysmal is first identified. If possible 1 cm of normal aorta is needed in order to place the clamp. The dissection is entirely limited to the sides of the normal aorta. The dissection never needs to extend to the posterior surface of the aorta, and to trespass there with finger, instrument or sling is to invite disaster from bleeding lumbar arteries or veins.

During the preparation of the sides of the aorta the aim is to clear an area big enough to place the clamp and to be able to reach the lumbar spine on either side. The renal arteries are nearby and may even be arising in whole or in part from the neck of the aneurysm, and the possibility of a lower pole renal artery arising here or even from the aneurysmal segment should be recognized. The renal arteries must be carefully preserved.

Once it is clear that the clamp can be placed when required, the other end of the aorta is approached.

Tilting the table towards the surgeon, if standing on the patient's right, is a considerable advantage.

Exposure of the iliac arteries

The lower end of the aorta is uncovered, care being taken to avoid the inferior mesenteric artery which arises from the anterior surface of the aorta towards its left side.

6 At this stage the gut may be wrapped in a towel and placed in a gut bag. Some surgeons are able to cope with the gut packed into the right iliac fossa but the author prefers to wrap it and lift it outside the abdomen.

It is difficult to identify the nerves which run over the aortic bifurcation but in males this area should be avoided for fear of subsequent abnormal sexual function. Male patients should be warned of the possibility during preoperative counselling.

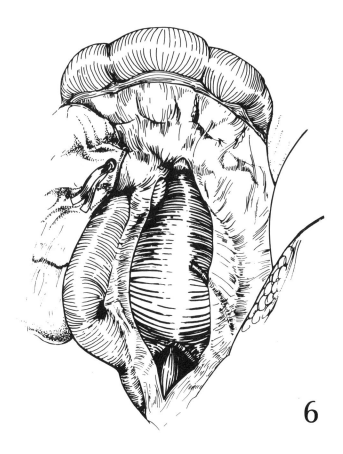

6

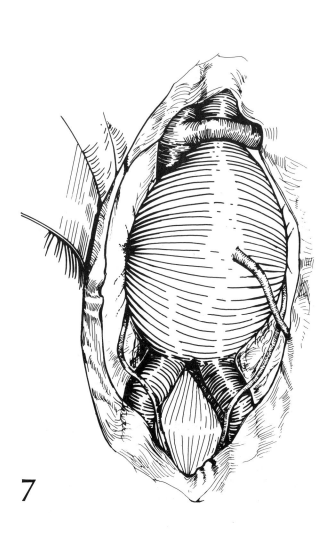

7

Right iliac artery

7 The ureter is the only structure of importance lying anterior to the iliac artery apart from the gut. The ureter obviously should not be damaged but perhaps less obviously nor should its blood supply. Hence it should be identified but not moved and the dissection should take place on each side of it. This is particularly important when it is stretched out over a large iliac aneurysm and there is a great temptation to mobilize it off the aneurysm. The ureter must, however, be left undisturbed in the certain knowledge that when the aneurysm is deflated by the operation the ureter will no longer be stretched and its blood supply will be intact.

Left iliac artery

8 This is more difficult as the sigmoid colon and its mesentery is a barrier to extensive dissection from above. The iliac artery can easily be clamped above the sigmoid colon but, if it is aneurysmal and the whole artery needs to be explored, it is easier to divide the peritoneal reflection lateral to the sigmoid colon and reflect the sigmoid colon towards the aorta. This enables the whole of the left iliac artery and the ureter to be displayed.

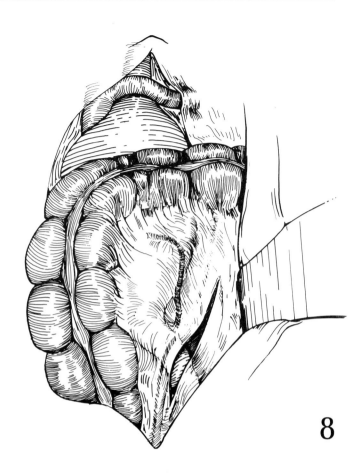

8

Site of distal clamping

This site will depend on the presence and extent of iliac aneurysms and will be beyond them. If the common iliac artery is aneurysmal but there are no aneurysms beyond the bifurcation, then both internal and external iliac arteries need to be displayed. Care must be taken to avoid dissection around these arteries because of the risk of bleeding from the closely applied vein. Venous injury in the depths of the pelvis from the internal iliac vein can cause haemorrhage which is difficult to control. It is better to accept the possibility that both the vein and the artery may be clamped than to risk tearing the vein by separating the two.

An alternative to iliac clamping is intraluminal balloon tamponade introduced from the aorta.

Iliac aneurysms

When these are present the first essential is to exclude them from the circulation so that they do not pose a future threat. The second aim is to leave one internal iliac artery in circulation. It this is impossible because of bilateral internal iliac aneurysms then the deep femoral arteries assume great importance and must be preserved. Consideration will also need to be given to the reanastomosis of the inferior mesenteric artery.

Insertion of the graft

If a woven graft is used there is no need to preclot the graft before heparin is given. If a knitted graft is preferred then preclotting is very important and in these cases a graft would be selected and 20 ml of blood from the aorta placed in the graft at this stage. If the patient has a coagulopathy then a sealed graft which is impervious to blood may be employed. Grafts can be sealed with gelatin, collagen or albumin.

When everything is prepared for clamping the anaesthetist gives heparin intravenously. The author uses a standard but rather unscientific dose of 5000 units.

9 After allowing time for circulation the iliac arteries are clamped with Dardik clamps.

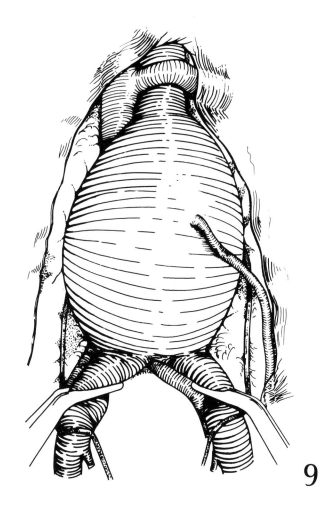

9

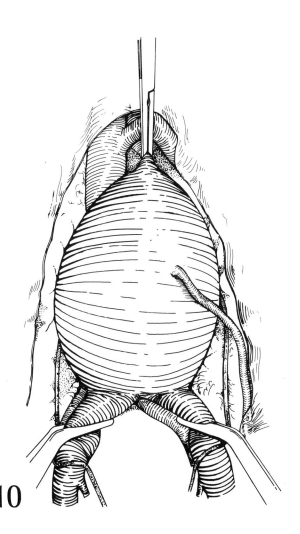

10

10 A clamp is placed on the aorta in the normal segment just above the neck. A Glover's coarctation clamp may be used and placed from front to back and not from side to side. It should be closed only as tightly as is necessary to stop the aortic pulsation below it. It can be steadied by the use of a tape or sling.

11 The aorta is opened towards its right side in order to avoid the origin of the inferior mesenteric artery. The incision passes upwards to the midline at the neck and the edge of the neck is transected with scissors in its anterior half. A Dardik clamp is placed across the free edge of the aortic wall to control the inferior mesenteric artery.

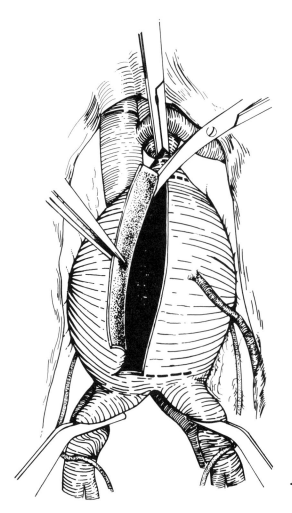

11

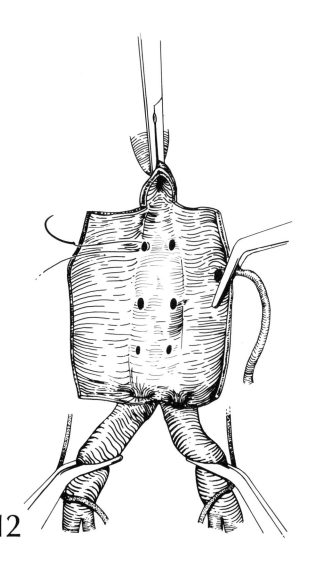

12

12 The incision is extended down to the bifurcation. The thrombus is scooped out and a specimen sent for culture. There may be quite profuse haemorrhage at this time from the lumbar arteries. These need to be oversewn but if they are surrounded by atheroma it may be more efficient to remove some of this in order to be able to place an accurate and effective suture. A silk suture may be used. All bleeding from lumbar arteries must be completely controlled because they will not be in continuity with the circulation hereafter and bleeding can be an avoidable cause for a return to theatre.

If a graft has not yet been prepared, one is now selected to match as far as possible the size of the arteries.

Straight graft

13 The proximal anastomosis is between the neck of the aneurysm and the edge of the Dacron graft. Using 3/0 polypropylene (Prolene) the suture line is begun in the middle of the back. Each bite goes through the artery and graft separately and the bites are about 1 mm apart. The depth from the edge should vary so as not to produce a neat and fragile row of perforations, but each bite needs to be at least 1 mm and often 2 or 3 mm deep. Any tendency to slip onto the aneurysmal section must be resisted as this will result in a future weakness of the wall.

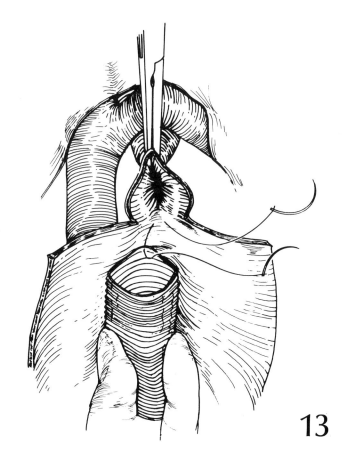

13

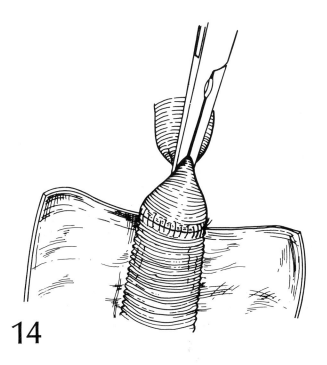

14

14 The knot should be placed towards the left lateral wall so that it is away from the duodenum.

15a–e When the proximal anastomosis is complete it can be tested by clamping the graft and releasing the aortic clamp. The advantage of this test is that any leak at the back becomes impossible to get to once the lower anastomosis is completed. The clamp may be left on the graft until the completion of the second anastomosis.

The graft is stretched and cut to fit. It should not be left so long that it bulges forwards when flow is restored, nor should it be so tight that there is tension. The distal anastomosis on the aortic bifurcation is similar to the proximal anastomosis and can be started either in the middle of the back or at a lateral corner. The bites need to be substantial, as at the proximal anastomosis, but one should bear in mind the fact that the left common iliac vein may be a close posterior relation.

The parachute technique may be used for both anastomoses when polypropylene or similar suture material is being used. In this method a number of sutures are placed before being tightened, giving the benefit of clear vision in a difficult corner.

Before completion of the distal anastomosis all the components are allowed briefly to flush back to remove thrombus or debris and air. It is usual to allow flow into only one iliac artery initially and to remove the second iliac clamp when the anaesthetist is ready. Back-bleeding from the inferior mesenteric artery is checked and, if satisfactory, the artery is oversewn from within. This avoids damage to its first branch which might be responsible for the continuity of the vascular supply to the colon from the superior mesenteric artery.

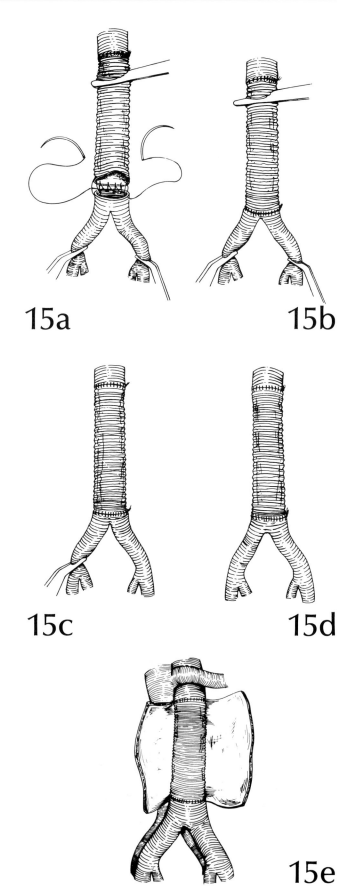

15a

15b

15c

15d

15e

16 The sac is closed around the graft thus avoiding direct contact between graft and gut.

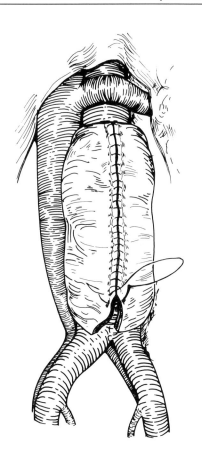

16

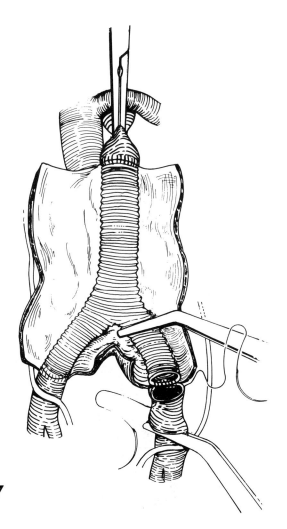

17

Bifurcation graft

The trunk of the bifurcation graft is cut short but should be long enough to enable a branch to be joined onto it should the need arise.

The top anastomosis is identical to that of the straight graft.

17 Each distal anastomosis is placed at the most proximal point consistent with excluding all the aneurysms. Ideally, if there are no aneurysms beyond the iliac bifurcation, the anastomosis is onto the conjoined orifices of the external and internal iliac arteries. The graft then lies inside the opened iliac aneurysm or is tunnelled through it and always lies behind the ureter.

18 If the internal iliac artery is not aneurysmal but the bifurcation is diseased it is sometimes possible to join the proximal external iliac artery to the proximal internal iliac artery and then to join the graft end-to-side onto the external iliac artery, thus preserving internal iliac flow.

If the internal iliac artery is aneurysmal then it must be ligated or oversewn and the distal anastomosis is end-to-end to the external iliac artery.

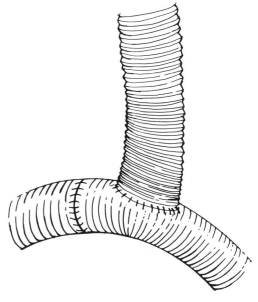

18

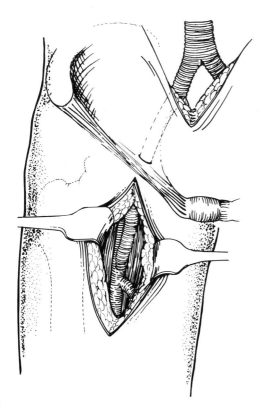

19

19 Very occasionally even this level proves to be unsatisfactory and the distal anastomosis is in the groin onto the common femoral artery.

In aneurysmal disease it is important to avoid longer grafts than necessary so that the intervening structures are still supplied with blood. Dacron, unlike arteries, does not have branches.

Aortocaval fistula

20, 21 Operative management, especially if the condition is unexpected, may prove difficult because of profuse haemorrhage. The communication between aorta and inferior vena cava should be closed with a running 3/0 polypropylene suture from within the aorta.

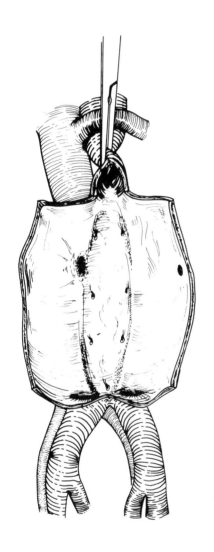

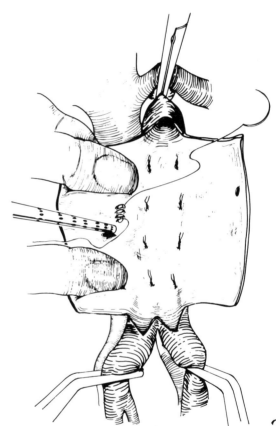

20

21

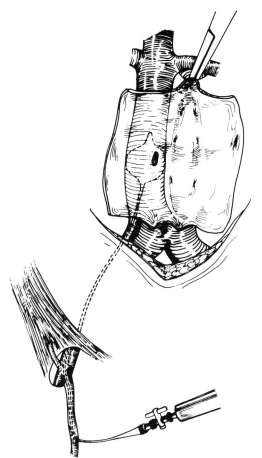

22 Digital pressure as in *Illustration 21* is usually enough to control the venous bleeding but when in difficulty a useful technique is to use balloon tamponade, either introduced directly through the fistula or remotely inserted. The latter is a most useful adjunct to the control of venous bleeding and a caval occlusion catheter is passed up from the saphenous vein while packs control the bleeding. When correctly positioned they are inflated and the bleeding is usually easily controlled. Sometimes there is more than one fistulous opening.

22

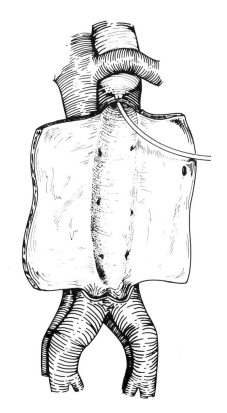

Variation when aneurysm is ruptured

The patient is not paralysed until the drapes are in place and the operation can begin. Heparin is omitted in most cases.

The proximal clamp is placed first.

23 Occasionally a balloon catheter is used for proximal control on a temporary basis.

Very rarely the aorta is controlled by a clamp at the hiatus. Although regarded by some as a useful emergency measure the author has not found it to be required in the great majority of operations. It is not as easy as it sounds, it results in considerable haemodynamic disturbance, and because it is above the renal arteries it probably increases the risk of renal failure.

When the graft is inserted some time should be spent looking for vessels such as lumbar arteries which may not have bled when the patient was hypotensive initially but which can cause postoperative problems with bleeding.

23

Postoperative care

All patients require close postoperative monitoring, ideally in an intensive care unit. The latter is essential in the emergency case. It is unusual in the author's unit for a patient to be ventilated after surgery for an unruptured infrarenal aneurysm but it would be routine to ventilate the patient for a period after an emergency operation.

Urinary output is closely monitored and appropriate support such as renal dopamine given as necessary.

Clotting parameters need to be measured and when necessary corrected. After emergency operations it is often necessary to give platelets and fresh frozen plasma.

Cardiac and respiratory monitoring and treatment are given as required and as the patient warms up every effort is made to maintain a stable blood pressure and cardiac function.

Adequate pain control is essential and is usually satisfactorily taken care of by epidural opiates. The method of choice will depend on local preference but reliable relief from pain must be provided.

Antibiotics are continued until the lines are removed. Heparin is used for prophylaxis against thromboembolism unless there is a contraindication.

Complications

Early problems are usually technical and most often concerned with bleeding. Occasionally patients will have to return to theatre for this problem but every effort must be made at the original operation to avoid this.

Renal dysfunction is one of the more frequent problems, especially in cases of rupture, and occasionally patients will require dialysis.

Prolonged ventilation, usually following massive transfusion, can be a problem and some patients may eventually need a tracheostomy.

Myocardial infarctions may occur after the repair of an aneurysm, hence the desire to improve cardiac function before operation when this is possible.

'Trash' embolization should be prevented as far as possible by avoiding manipulation of the aneurysm, by using heparin, by clamping distally before proximally, and by flushing the vessels before flow is restored. If, in spite of this, problems occur embolectomy will sometimes help, but when this is not appropriate an infusion of prostacyclin may be given.

Infection is a major concern and graft infections are usually later problems which can be life threatening and generally require the removal of the graft.

False aneurysms can sometimes occur at the anastomoses and again these are usually late complications.

Aortoenteric fistula, when it occurs, is usually a very late complication and when a patient with an aortic graft presents with gastrointestinal haemorrhage it should be the major component of the differential diagnosis.

Outcome

The majority of patients can expect to have a normal life span after repair of the aneurysm.

Future work on abdominal aneurysm resection should address the following key issues: (1) what size of aneurysm requires operation; (2) should patients be screened for abdominal aortic aneurysm; (3) which graft should be used; (4) is there a familial genetic disposition; and (5) will endoluminal methods become the treatment of choice?

Transfemoral intraluminal graft implantation for abdominal aortic aneurysms

Juan C. Parodi MD
Chief, Department of Vascular Surgery, Instituto Cardiovascular de Buenos Aires, Buenos Aires, Argentina and Adjunct Associate Professor of Surgery, Bowman Gray School of Medicine, Wake Forest University, Winston-Salem, North Carolina, USA

History

Since Dubost first introduced surgical grafting technique in 1952[1], refinement of graft material and techniques has made the operative approach using prosthetic grafts to repair aneurysms a very safe procedure. Even so, in some patients with multiple and severe co-morbidities the risks are prohibitive for surgical intervention. Alternative treatment for these patients includes the exclusion technique followed by extra-anatomical bypass[2]. Others have combined this approach with catheter occlusion techniques[3]. Unfortunately, these alternative techniques have neither eliminated the risk of rupture nor decreased the incidence of death in these patients[4, 5].

The rapid development of endovascular technology has prompted the development of a transluminal graft technique in the treatment of patients with an abdominal aortic aneurysm who are poor surgical risks. Preliminary animal and clinical experience has been promising[6, 7]. It is expected that, with further refinement, this technology will emerge as an alternative technique for treating patients with an abdominal aortic aneurysm.

Principles and justification

Indications

At present the indication for this procedure is strictly confined to those patients with prohibitive surgical risks, such that standard surgical intervention is deemed undesirable. As experience grows and there is more extended follow-up demonstrating the safety and patency of these grafts, the indication may be extended to patients who are considered for elective replacement of an abdominal aortic aneurysm.

Certain anatomical conditions should be present to make the procedure technically feasible. These are: (1) a proximal and distal neck (or cuff) of more than 2 cm; (2) a suitable iliac axis and at least one patent iliac artery. The iliac artery should be more than 7 mm in diameter with a straight or nearly straight axis.

Preoperative

Assessment

In addition to routine studies to evaluate patients for aortic surgery, all patients require infusion computed tomographic (CT) scanning and complete arteriography. The CT scan cut should be at 5-mm intervals for precise diameter determination. Three-dimensional reconstruction, particularly with the new spiral CT scanning technique, will help to assess the actual diameter and length of both the neck and distal aorta. Arteriography will help to locate precisely the neck of the aneurysm and its proximity to orifices of the renal artery and the actual length of the aorta measured from the renal arteries to the aortic bifurcation. The status of the visceral artery, the presence of a meandering mesenteric artery or dual renal artery, and the patency of the inferior mesenteric artery are also best assessed by arteriography. Arteriography also gives vital information about the status of the iliac artery and its patency.

Instrumentation

The device consists of a graft–stent combination. The current approach is based on the concept that stents may be used in place of sutures to secure the proximal and distal ends of a fabric graft along the length of the aneurysm. Experimental studies have shown that stents could replace surgical sutures and could act as a friction seal to fix the ends of a graft to the vessel wall. These friction seals were developed by creating a transluminal graft–stent combination, by suturing a modified Palmaz balloon expandable stent to the partially overlapping ends of a tubular, knitted Dacron graft. This was done so that stent expansion would press the graft against the aortic wall, creating a watertight seal.

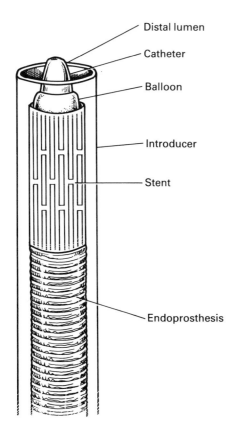

Distal lumen

Catheter

Balloon

Introducer

Stent

Endoprosthesis

1

1 The assembly kit contains one balloon expandable stent, 5.5 mm in diameter and 3.5 cm in length. These are stainless steel, modified Palmaz stents. A specially made, thin-walled, crimped knitted Dacron graft (Barone Industries, Buenos Aires, Argentina) is sutured to the stent, overlapping half of the length of the stent.

Patient preparation

The procedure should be performed in an operating room equipped with fluoroscopic equipment. A mobile C-arm image intensifier providing real-time digital subtraction with instantaneous replay of each digital exposure and roadmapping is ideal. The patient should be prepared and draped as for aortic surgery. The anaesthesia team should be alerted about the possibility of immediate surgical intervention.

Operation

Incision

2 Under local or regional anaesthesia, the common femoral artery is exposed through a standard groin incision. In general, the common femoral artery is chosen on the side of the iliac artery with a straighter course and with fewer atherosclerotic changes.

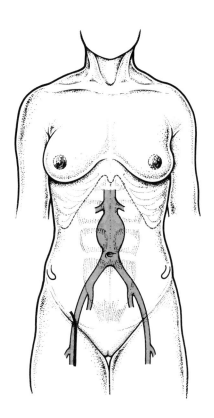

2

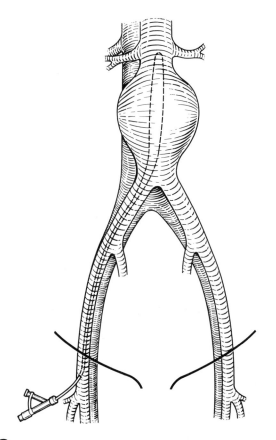

3

3 After heparin, 5000 units, has been given intravenously, an 18-gauge Cournand needle is inserted cephalad into the common femoral artery. A soft-tip (0.38 inch) guidewire is advanced through the needle into the distal thoracic aorta, and a 5-Fr pigtail catheter is introduced over the guidewire. Once the catheter is positioned in the visceral segment of the abdominal aorta, the guidewire is removed and peroperative arteriography is performed. The pigtail catheter has radio-opaque calibrations at 20-mm intervals. In order to obtain measurements from the arteriogram, a radio-opaque rule is placed behind the patient parallel to the axis of the aorta.

After the intraoperative measurements have been compared with those determined preoperatively, the appropriate size of endoluminal device is selected. The graft overlaps the proximal stent by one-half and is attached to it using braided, synthetic suture material.

4 After the stent has been mounted over the balloon, the graft is folded and the entire assembly is introduced into an 18-Fr polytetrafluoroethylene sheath through a transverse arteriotomy.

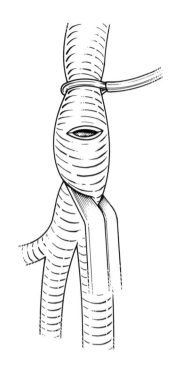

4

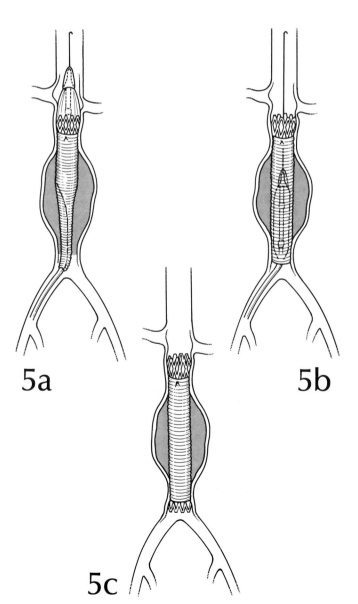

5a

5b

5c

5a–c A guidewire is reintroduced, the pigtail catheter is removed, and the wire is replaced with a super-stiff wire. The sheath containing the device is advanced over the wire to the level of the proximal neck of the aneurysm. The sheath is then removed, leaving the graft, stent and balloon in the aortic lumen. At this time, attention is paid to lowering blood pressure. The author prefers to keep mean blood pressure below 80 mmHg by intravenous infusion of glyceryl trinitrate. As soon as blood pressure is stable at this value, the proximal balloon is inflated for less than 1 min to whatever volume is necessary to attain the proper diameter for that particular patient. In order to apply a perfectly cylindrical shape to the stent, the balloon can sometimes be inflated again at both ends of the stent. In some instances, the shape of the stent may be adapted to an irregular aneurysm neck by repeated inflations under low pressure along the entire length of the stent.

After the proximal stent has been deployed, the balloon is inflated along the shaft of the graft to distend it under low pressure. Provided all previous measurements were correct, the distal radio-opaque calibrations on the graft should be level with the aortic bifurcation. A second stent is then applied to the distal end to establish a seal preventing reflux around the graft.

A completion aortogram is then obtained by introducing an arteriographic catheter over the guidewire. Arteriography confirms the success of the procedure and patency of the renal arteries. After removal of the guidewire and overlying catheter, the arteriotomy is closed with 6/0 polypropylene suture. Great care is taken to ensure complete haemostasis.

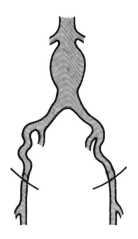

6 When both iliac arteries are very tortuous, a 'pull-down manoeuvre' can be used, which consists of dissection of the common femoral artery circumferentially. By ligating some of the small branches, the external artery is then dissected bluntly. This manoeuvre allows the external iliac artery to be free of the surrounding tissue, and a gentle pull towards the feet would allow a straighter course of the artery for instrumentation.

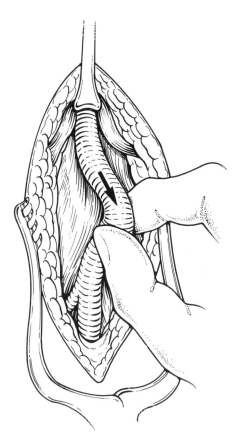

6

7a, b If the above manoeuvre is not sufficient to allow passage of the device to the aorta, the alternative approach would be a separate incision above the tortuous area. A transverse incision similar to kidney transplantation is used to expose the common iliac artery. A Dacron graft is then anastomosed in an end-to-side manner and brought to the groin for instrumentation.

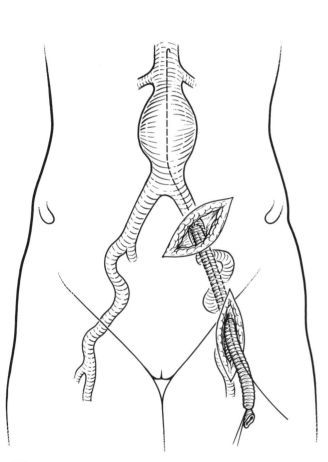

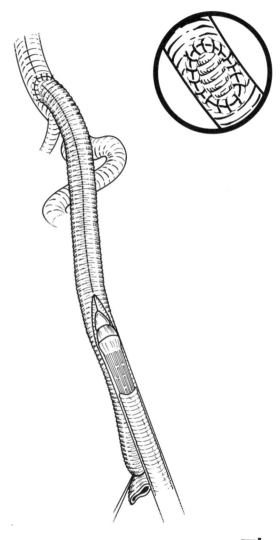

7a

7b

Postoperative care

Postoperative care is similar to that for any aortic surgery. Ankle pressure is measured to confirm patency of the graft. Evidence of microembolization must be sought. Special attention must be paid to urine output because proximity of the device to the renal artery may cause a problem. When the patient is ambulatory, a colour duplex scan and an infusion CT scan are obtained to confirm proper placement of the graft. If necessary, arteriography can give further information. Because the procedure is new, patients must be closely monitored during the first year after the operation with repeated colour duplex scanning.

References

1. Dubost C, Allary M, Oeconomos N. Resection of an aneurysm of the abdominal aorta: reestablishment of continuity by preserved human arterial graft with results after 5 months. *Arch Surg* 1952; 64: 405–8.

2. Blaisdell FW, Hall AD, Thomas AN. Ligation treatment of an abdominal aortic aneurysm. *Am J Surg* 1965; 109: 560–5.

3. Berguer R, Schneider J, Wilner HI. Induced thrombosis of inoperable abdominal aortic aneurysm. *Surgery* 1978; 84: 425–9.

4. Schanzer H, Papa MC, Miller CM. Rupture of surgically thrombosed abdominal aortic aneurysm. *J Vasc Surg* 1985; 2: 278–80.

5. Kwann JHM, Dahl RK. Fatal rupture after successful surgical thrombosis of an abdominal aortic aneurysm. *Surgery* 1984; 95: 235–7.

6. Parodi JC, Palmaz JC, Barone HD. Transfemoral intraluminal graft implantation for abdominal aortic aneurysms. *Ann Vasc Surg* 1991; 5: 491–9.

7. Laborde JC, Parodi JC, Clem MF *et al.* Intraluminal bypass of abdominal aortic aneurysm: feasibility study. *Radiology* 1992; 184: 185–90.

Retroperitoneal approach to aortic aneurysms

Robert P. Leather MD
Albany Medical College, Vascular Surgery Section A61, Albany, New York, USA

Benjamin B. Chang MD
Albany Medical College, Vascular Surgery Section A61, Albany, New York, USA

R. Clement Darling III MD
Albany Medical College, Vascular Surgery Section A61, Albany, New York, USA

Dhiraj M. Shah MD
Albany Medical College, Vascular Surgery Section A61, Albany, New York, USA

History

Many surgeons prefer the retroperitoneal approach to repair of aortic aneurysms only in 'high-risk' patients but the authors apply this approach to *all* patients in an effort to minimize operative trauma and shorten hospital stay. The approach used at this centre is usually the 'extended' retroperitoneal approach first reported by Williams *et al.*[1] because this posterolateral exposure of the aorta affords the widest and most flexible exposure. Use of a more anterior retroperitoneal exposure (as originally reported by Rob[2] and more recently advocated by others) limits aortic exposure and in many instances is more technically difficult to perform. However, it is very similar anatomically to that gained by transperitoneal techniques and many surgeons feel more comfortable with the anterior approach, rather than the relatively unfamiliar posterolateral approach.

The retroperitoneal approach actually consists of a family of exposures and incisions to the abdominal aorta and its branches. Although transperitoneal approaches to the aorta have traditionally been employed, an increased appreciation of the virtues of the retroperitoneal approach has evolved over the past several years. There is continued debate as to the physiological merits of the two classes of approach: in many cases a retroperitoneal approach is clearly superior, if only for simplifying the technical conduct of the operation. Thus it benefits the vascular surgeon to be familiar with and experienced in these alternative exposures.

In this chapter current techniques of aortic surgery employing the retroperitoneal approach in several clinical settings are presented, including ruptured and elective abdominal aortic aneurysms, suprarenal aneurysms, associated renal and visceral artery disease and infected aortic grafts.

Principles and justification

Indications

Left peritoneal approach

The potential advantages of the retroperitoneal approach are both technical (operative) and physiological (intraoperative and postoperative). Properly employed, the retroperitoneal approach may be used in most aortic surgery, often with better and more flexible exposure than is gained transperitoneally, even in patients with ruptured aneurysms, suprarenal aneurysms and infected aortic grafts.

The physiological advantages of the retroperitoneal approach may translate into a shorter and smoother postoperative course for the patients, thereby minimizing hospital stay. A marked decrease in blood loss with the combination of the retroperitoneal approach and aneurysm exclusion (described below) often avoids transfusion.

Although the retroperitoneal approach is appropriate to almost all operations on the subdiaphragmatic aorta and its branches, this approach is especially useful in cases involving aneurysms with a 'high' or suprarenal neck, concomitant disease of the visceral aorta and its branches, repeat operations, inflammatory aneurysms, an associated horseshoe kidney, and pulmonary insufficiency. Aortic surgery in obese patients, patients with intra-abdominal adhesions and/or inflammatory processes (diverticulitis or cholecystitis) is greatly facilitated using this exposure.

Right retroperitoneal approach

An alternative to the left-sided retroperitoneal approach is the exposure of the infrarenal aorta through a right retroperitoneal approach. This approach is analogous to the anterolateral approach reported by Rob. Specific indications for this approach, rather than the left retroperitoneal approach, fall into two general categories: (1) the right-sided approach may be used to gain better access to structures on the right side such as the renal or common iliac arteries or where tortuosity of the aorta makes an exposure from the right technically advantageous; (2) it may be used to avoid scarring or inflammation in the left retroperitoneal space from previous operations or infections.

Ruptured aneurysm

The treatment of ruptured aneurysms through a left retroperitoneal approach was developed at the authors'

institution as a direct result of experience during elective cases. Initially used in cases in which there was contraindication to a midline approach (such as dense adhesions), the retroperitoneal approach has become the preferred method of management in such cases.

Aortic graft infections

The treatment of infected aortic grafts usually involves the removal of the infected graft, suture closure and tissue coverage of the aortic stump and axillobifemoral bypass. Treatment in this manner carries a relatively high morbidity and mortality rate, partly because of rupture of the aortic stump and the morbidity of occlusion of the axillofemoral bypass.

In an effort to circumvent these problems, the extended left retroperitoneal approach may be utilized in these cases.

Preoperative

Preparation

All patients undergo arteriography before surgery. Patients with aneurysmal disease also undergo computed tomography. The need for either has been questioned, but intraoperative assessment of major arterial lesions is difficult from the retroperitoneal approach unless vessels are specifically exposed. In addition, arteriography may be performed with minimum morbidity and mortality in the modern setting. Having this information available before the start of surgery allows the surgeon to plan the operative approach and reconstruction carefully.

A heating blanket and suction bean bag (Olympic Vac-Pac) are placed on the operating table and covered with a blanket. The Vac-Pac should extend from the top of the patient's shoulders to just below the buttocks.

The patient is then positioned on the table and lines are inserted. Central venous catheters and Swan–Ganz catheters are best inserted into the right internal jugular vein: catheters inserted in either subclavian vein may occlude after the patient is positioned.

Anaesthesia

General endotracheal anaesthesia is used.

Operations

LEFT RETROPERITONEAL APPROACH

Position of patient

1   The patient's torso is lifted, carried towards the left and then rotated so that the left shoulder is elevated 30–60° from the horizontal. The pelvis is minimally rotated, allowing for easier access to the groins. The bean bag is then positioned around the left chest and evacuated in order to hold the patient in position. The left arm is supported by folded blankets or a cross-arm sling. The left thigh is elevated 30–45 cm by folded blankets or a second bean bag; this relaxes the ipsilateral iliopsoas muscle and permits easier access to the distal aorta and iliac arteries. Finally, the table is extended 10–30° to open the space between the ribs and iliac crest. While this is being performed, intravenous prophylactic antibiotics and mannitol (25 g intravenous bolus and 5 g/h intravenous drip) are administered.

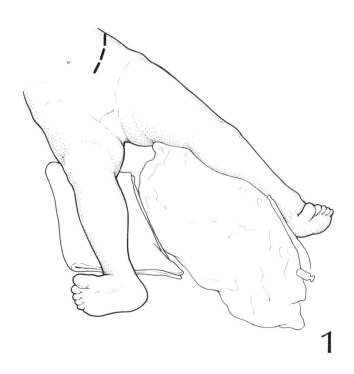

1

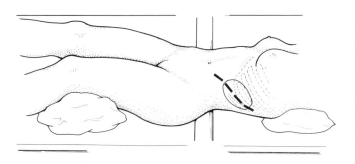

2

Incision

2   The skin is incised along the 10th or 11th intercostal space. The 10th interspace is used when access to the perirenal or visceral aorta is thought necessary. The incision is usually extended posteriorly to the mid axillary line, but may be carried to the posterior axillary line if more cephalad exposure is desired. The incision is lengthened anteriorly to the edge of the ipsilateral rectus abdominis muscle. The three lateral muscles of the lateral abdominal wall are divided. The transversus abdominis is divided laterally at first, allowing the surgeon to separate the peritoneum from the muscle, and then incised medially. The intercostal muscles are divided along the top of the 10th rib. The pleura can be identified and preserved or, if opened, closed at the end of the case after suction evacuation of the pleural space over a catheter, without deleterious effects.

Exposure

3 Once the incision is complete, the peritoneum and
   left kidney are swept together anteriorly and
medially, exposing the psoas and periaortic tissue. A
self-retaining retractor is invaluable in maintaining
exposure.

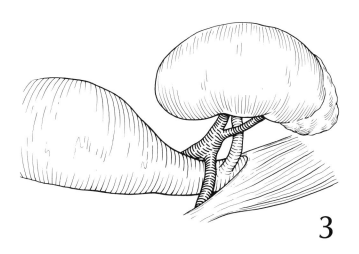

3

Dissection

4 If the aorta is patent, the outflow vessels (usually
   iliac arteries) are controlled initially in order to
minimize distal embolization from the aorta caused by
manipulation and dissection. The femoral vessels are
exposed through standard vertical groin incisions. The
right external iliac artery is exposed through a
counter-incision made just above the inguinal ligament.
The left iliac arteries are accessible through the primary
incision. The right common iliac artery is accessible but
not usually readily exposed through this type of
retroperitoneal approach. After the outflow vessels are
isolated, the patient is given intravenous heparin, 30–35
units/kg, and the arteries clamped.

At this stage the immediate infrarenal aorta is isolated.
The surrounding periaortic lymphoareolar tissue and
nerve plexus invariably obscure this area. The end of the
left crus of the diaphragm usually marks the level of the
left renal artery, which is often palpable under the
periaortic tissue. Dissection of this tissue should begin
immediately below these landmarks. The lumbar branch
of the left renal vein tranverses the aorta perpendicularly and immediately caudad to the renal artery. This
should be secured carefully before division. The
remaining tissue may be divided with impunity,
although not without annoying bleeding, thereby
revealing the neck of the aneurysm. If suprarenal or
supracoeliac control of the aorta is required, the left
crus of the diaphragm should be divided parallel to the
aorta, revealing the entire visceral aorta and its
branches.

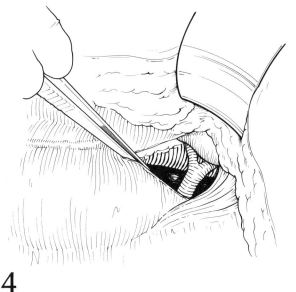

4

Exposure of aorta

5   The left lateral side of the aorta is exposed,
    followed by the anterior and then the posterior
aorta; lumbar arteries are ligated and divided as
necessary.

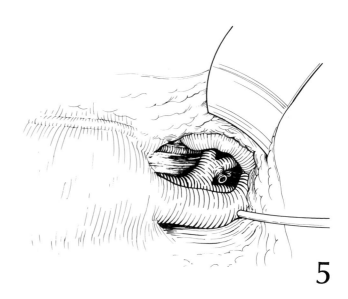

5

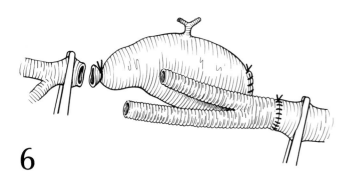

6

Aortic clamping

6   The aorta may now be cross-clamped and the
    aneurysm opened for conventional endoaneurys-
morrhaphy. Control of intraluminal bleeding and
anastomosis may be undertaken in the usual manner.
However, in an effort to further simplify the operative
procedure and minimize blood loss, the authors
routinely use a procedure termed 'aneurysm exclusion
and bypass'. This procedure is conceptually similar to an
aortobifemoral bypass performed for occlusive stenotic
disease of the aortoiliac arteries, with the addition of
ligation of the iliac arteries.

Transection of aorta

7 Aneurysm exclusion requires a second clamp to be placed across the aorta 2–3 cm distal to the first clamp, often across the aneurysmal aorta. The aorta is then transected between the two clamps flush with the distal clamp. The vena cava is usually separated from the aorta at this point but it may be damaged if the aorta is carelessly transected. The division should always be performed under direct vision up to the end.

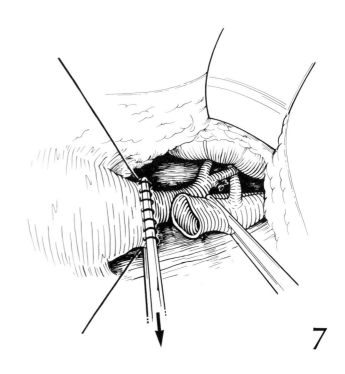

Closure of aortic stump

8 The distal clamp is then undersewn or oversewn with two layers of continuous 3/0 polypropylene sutures. The clamp is removed and the suture ends drawn up and tied. The oversewn aorta is then retracted distally. It should be noted that the retroaortic veins are especially well visualized and preserved from the posterolateral exposure; thus patients with a retroaortic left renal vein are preferentially treated by the extended left retroperitoneal approach.

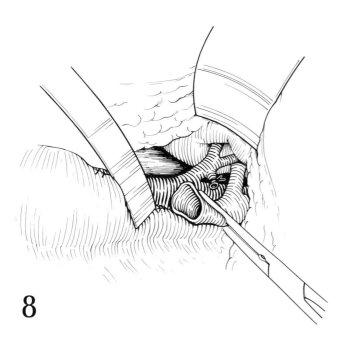

Proximal anastomosis

9 The proximal anastomosis is then performed. Although some surgeons may feel uncomfortable with a completely transected aorta, it is easier to ensure good suture placement in this situation as the entry and exit of all bites can be seen easily. The anastomosis is performed with a 60-cm 3/0 polypropylene suture using a 'parachute' technique. The initial bites are taken at the most distant portion of the aorta and are carried anteriorly a short distance before the posterior suture is used to complete the bulk of the anastomosis. Care should be taken when tightening the suture not to tear the aorta by overzealous tensioning. Usually one-third to two-thirds of the anastomosis is completed before drawing the graft to the aorta. The anastomosis is tested by occluding the graft and slightly opening the proximal clamp. Any defects are repaired at this stage.

When a tube graft is used in an 'exclusion', the distal aorta is then transected between two clamps and the proximal clamp oversewn. The vena cava is closely applied to the aorta and may be easily injured by the incautious operator. The distal anastomosis is then completed using the similar technique and suture.

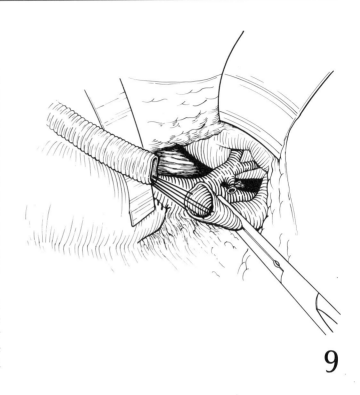

9

Insertion of bifurcation graft

10 If a bifurcated graft is used the left common iliac artery is either interrupted without division by two layers of 3/0 polypropylene continuous mattress sutures or divided and the proximal end oversewn. Ligation in continuity is to be avoided because occlusion may be incomplete. The graft is then anastomosed to the iliac or femoral arteries as necessary. The right graft limb is usually tunnelled retroperitoneally along the right iliac vessel to the right external iliac or femoral artery; the space of Retzius anterior to the bladder may also be used. The tunnelling of the right graft limb must be performed carefully, under direct vision or with gentle finger dissection; penetration of the peritoneal cavity with perforation of viscera may result if the operator blindly forces a blunt instrument along the proposed course of the graft limb. The proximal artery is again interrupted or oversewn, thereby completing the exclusion of the aneurysm. The distal anastomoses are completed with 5/0 or 6/0 continuous polypropylene sutures.

Once the anastomoses are complete the clamps are removed sequentially, usually perfusing one leg at a time to minimize haemodynamic disturbance. Distal perfusion is assessed by Doppler ultrasonographic examination, inspection of the extremities, and use of on-table volume plethysmography.

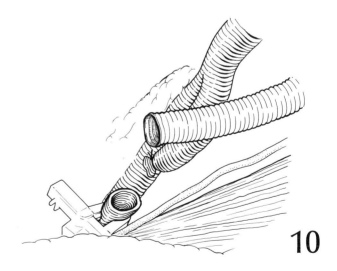

10

Wound closure

The incision is closed in layers with continuous 0 polypropylene sutures. Closure is facilitated by flexing the table, thereby bringing the flat muscles of the flank into apposition.

RIGHT RETROPERITONEAL APPROACH

Position of patient

The exposure of the aorta from the right side requires the same preparation of the table. After intubation, the patient's right side is elevated 30–45° from the horizontal. The table is extended as with the contralateral approach.

Incision

The incision is usually made from the anterior axillary line in the 10th or 11th intercostal space going anteriorly to the ipsilateral rectus fascia. This fascia is usually partially divided.

Exposure

11 After the retroperitoneal space has been entered, the plane between the peritoneum and Gerota's fascia should be identified and opened. The right kidney and ureter are left in place while the peritoneum is mobilized to the left. This exposes the aorta from an anterolateral aspect. The overlying lymphatic tissue is divided, thereby exposing the neck of the aneurysm. The left renal vein may be mobilized and retracted cephalad or divided if necessary. The vena cava may be gently retracted laterally. Small retroperitoneal venous branches to the vena cava are suture ligated before division to prevent later avulsion. The remainder of the operation may be completed as desired by exclusion or endoaneurysmorrhaphy techniques.

The aorta may be exposed only to the base of the superior mesenteric artery with this approach. Recovery is identical to that seen with the left retroperitoneal approach.

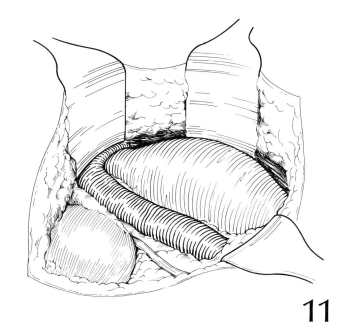

11

CONCOMITANT RENAL AND VISCERAL ARTERY RECONSTRUCTION

One of the great advantages of the left posterolateral retroperitoneal approach is the ability to perform simultaneous reconstruction of the renal and visceral arteries.

Incision

The incision is made in the 10th interspace. After the peritoneum is retracted, the left crus of the diaphragm is divided parallel to the aorta, but the left hemidiaphragm may be left intact, exposing the visceral portion of the abdominal aorta. The coeliac, superior mesenteric and the right renal arteries may then easily be exposed. Access to the right renal artery from the left side may be performed transluminally or extraluminally after division of the infrarenal aorta.

Renal artery bypass

12 If renal artery reconstruction is undertaken during the placement of an aortic graft, the easiest option is to sew short sidearms of 6-mm polytetrafluoroethylene (PTFE) to the body of the aortic graft before aortic cross-clamping. The sidearms are then anastomosed (end-to-end or end-to-side) to the renal arteries after flow is established to the lower extremities once the aortic anastomosis is completed. Alternatively, the renal artery may be reimplanted directly into the body of the graft.

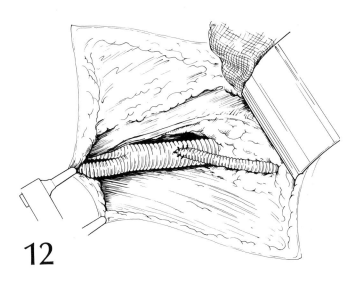

12

Transaortic endarterectomy

13a, b The other major option for revascularization of the renal and visceral arteries is transaortic endarterectomy. After division of the crus the supracoeliac aorta is clamped. The renal and/or visceral arteries are isolated and controlled and the aorta is then incised. The type of incision used varies with the extent and type of endarterectomy undertaken: usually an aortotomy is made vertically along the posterolateral side of the vessel but an alternative approach is to make a U-shaped 'trap-door' aortotomy around the arteries to be endarterectomized. The reader is referred to the work of the San Francisco group for a full understanding of the important technical features of this operation[3].

Completion of the endarterectomy is the most problematic aspect of this procedure. The arteries may be mobilized and everted into the aortic lumen, allowing direct visualization of the end point. The aortotomy is closed with 5/0 or 6/0 polypropylene. If an aortic graft is to be used the endarterectomized infrarenal aorta may be clamped and the supracoeliac clamp removed to restore flow to the renal and visceral vessels. After the involved arteries are reperfused, the end point should be checked preferably with intraoperative duplex ultrasonography.

If the end point is not satisfactory or if the occlusive disease extends down the length of the visceral arteries, the left kidney is placed posteriorly. Further dissection of the visceral arteries may be performed, exposing the coeliac artery and its primary branches as well as the proximal 8–12 cm of the superior mesenteric artery. Bypass to these arteries may be performed from the aorta or the aortic prosthesis.

Currently, unilateral renal artery stenosis is managed via a retroperitoneal approach on the affected side. With bilateral renal disease the left retroperitoneal approach is used as long as the right-sided lesion is in the proximal half of the artery.

Isolated visceral artery disease may be treated with endarterectomy or bypass. Although the aorta is commonly used for an inflow source other visceral, renal and iliac arteries may also be utilized.

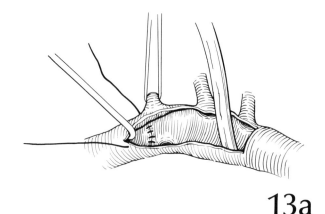

13a

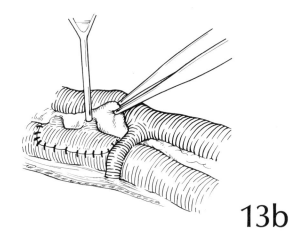

13b

RUPTURED ANEURYSMS

Position of patient

The patient is intubated and positioned as with elective cases.

Incision

The incision is made from the posterior axillary line in the 10th intercostal space.

Once this is completed, the supracoeliac aorta is bluntly approached by elevating the peritoneum from the diaphragm while keeping the left kidney in place. By not entering the infrarenal retroperitoneal space, the haematoma is not decompressed. The supracoeliac aorta is easily palpated through the overlying crus and may be compressed by the operator's fingers. The crus is divided transversely to expose the aorta, which may be then clamped as necessary.

After the proximal clamp has been placed, the lower retroperitoneal space is entered. The neck of the aneurysm may be isolated and clamped in the usual fashion, after which the proximal clamp is removed. The aneurysm is opened and the iliac arteries controlled, and the graft placed intraluminally in the usual fashion.

Treatment of ruptured aneurysms via a retroperitoneal incision is best attempted only after gaining experience with this approach in elective settings. Control of the aorta can be gained within 5 minutes in all cases.

AORTIC GRAFT INFECTIONS

After the diagnosis is made, the patient is anaesthetized and positioned in the normal fashion.

A retroperitoneal incision is made in the 10th intercostal space.

The perirenal aorta is exposed. This dissection is sometimes facilitated by exposure of the suprarenal aorta away from previous scarring. Once the proper plane of dissection has been identified, further dissection caudad into the area of the proximal anastomosis may be accomplished more safely. The proximal clamp is placed just below or above the renal arteries as necessary. A second clamp is placed slightly below the first, the aorta divided, and the distal end oversewn with continuous polypropylene. This manoeuvre should isolate the contaminated area from the operative field. A PTFE aortic bifurcation graft is anastomosed to the proximal aorta; this may require anastomosis to the suprarenal aorta with subsequent revascularization of both renal arteries. It is very important to perform the proximal anastomosis to uninfected aorta. Immediate Gram stains of the area are obtained as well as cultures.

Tunnelling of graft limbs

Tunnelling the graft limbs requires some ingenuity. For the left graft limb, the inguinal ligament is typically crossed laterally by entering the fascial sheath under the sartorius muscle.

The right graft limb is tunnelled anatomically if the original prosthesis is a tube graft but if the infected graft is a bifurcated graft, the new right graft limb is tunnelled anteriorly in the space of Retzius just along the cephalad border of the pubic ramus and anterior to the bladder. The groin is entered medially.

Anastomosis

The distal anastomoses are performed distally into the superficial or deep femoral arteries. If the deep femoral arteries are used, the distal incisions are made along the lateral border of the sartorius muscle starting just distal to the level of the common femoral artery. The dissection elevates the sartorius muscle medially, thereby exposing the deep femoral artery in a clean tissue plane with fascial separation from an infected femoral artery. The new graft is perfused, the incisions closed and then covered with adhesive plastic drape.

Removal of graft

The patient is then repositioned into a supine posture, the abdomen and groins prepared and draped, and a midline incision made. The infected graft is isolated and the proximal anastomosis reduced. The short piece of aorta that remains is debrided. The distal anastomoses are exposed and detached and the infected graft is removed.

The groins are debrided and branches of femoral artery controlled. The bed of the aortic graft is debrided and omentum is sewn down to this area. The incisions are then closed.

This method obviates the need for extra-anatomic bypass and avoids a contaminated aortic closure. It also allows for an in-line aortic graft without the contamination seen with *in situ* replacement of the infected graft.

Postoperative care

Care of the patient differs little in principle from the care of any major aortic reconstruction. The patients are typically extubated the next morning, as a high-dose narcotic anaesthetic technique is usually employed. Nasogastric tubes are used infrequently and removed at the time of extubation.

An effort is made to minimize cardiac work for the first few postoperative days. Filling pressures are optimized to maintain cardiac output, usually with crystalloid. Transfusions are given to maintain adequate oxygen delivery, usually maintaining a haematocrit in the range 25–30%. Most elective patients do not require transfusions.

One of the most important measures is the maintenance of body temperature, as shivering markedly increases oxygen consumption and hypothermia begets acidosis and peripheral vasoconstriction, leading to increased demand upon a depressed myocardium. All solutions and the inspired air are heated. Warming lights, heaters, or blankets should be used liberally.

After extubation, the patients are discharged to the ward. Ambulation and feeding begin 24–36 h after completion of the surgery. Patients are discharged home 5–9 days after surgery.

Complications

Complications related to the retroperitoneal approach include incisional hernia. The incision may often produce a bulge in the area of the operation that is noticeable to the patient. Intercostal neuralgia is occasionally seen and usually responds to serial nerve blockade. Three patients required operative resection of the 12th intercostal nerve under local anaesthesia for pain relief.

More onerous complications include organ rupture caused by overzealous retraction, usually in very thin patients.

Outcome

The retroperitoneal approach has become the authors' preferred method of exposure of the infradiaphragmatic aorta and its branches. Over a 6-year period, 569 elective abdominal aortic aneurysms were repaired using this approach, with 559 survivors (98%). In addition, 133 aortic grafts for occlusive disease were performed, with 128 survivors (96%). One ureter required repair after injury during reoperation. There was also one blunt injury to the bladder due to blind tunnelling in the space of Retzius.

The retroperitoneal approach provides the surgeon with the ability to expose the entire subdiaphragmatic aorta and its branches. This flexibility, one of the principal advantages of this approach, serves to simplify the operative conduct of these cases. Therefore, knowledge of the uses of this approach can only benefit the surgeon and should prove to be the impetus to become familiar with this technique.

Ruptured aneurysms

Patient survival over the last 5 years has been 86%.

Aortic graft infections

The method described has been used in nine patients over a 5-year period without residual or recurrent sepsis or bypass occlusion.

References

1. Williams GM, Ricotta J, Zinner M, Burdick J. The extended retroperitoneal approach for treatment of extensive atherosclerosis of the aorta and renal vessels. *Surgery* 1980; 88: 846–55.

2. Rob C. Extraperitoneal approach to the abdominal aorta. *Surgery* 1963; 53: 87–9.

3. Stoney RJ, Reilly LM, Ehrenfeld WK. Chronic mesenteric ischemia and surgery for chronic visceral ischemia. In: Wilson SE, Veith FJ, Hobson RW III, Williams RA, eds. *Vascular Surgery. Principles and Practice*. New York: McGraw-Hill, 1987; 672–84.

Further reading

Chang BB, Paty PSK, Shah DM, Leather RP, Kaufman JL. The right retroperitoneal approach for abdominal aortic surgery. *Am J Surg* 1989; 158: 156–8.

Chang BB, Shah DM, Paty PSK, Kaufman JL, Leather RP. Can the retroperitoneal approach be used for ruptured abdominal aortic aneurysms? *J Vasc Surg* 1990; 11: 326–30.

Leather RP, Darling RC III, Chang BB, Shah DM. Retroperitoneal in-line aortic bypass for treatment of infected infrarenal aortic grafts. *Surg Gynecol Obstet* 1992; 175: 491–4.

Leather RP, Shah DM, Kaufman JL, Fitzgerald KM, Chang BB, Feustel PJ. Comparative analysis of retroperitoneal and transperitoneal aortic replacement for aneurysm. *Surg Gynecol Obstet* 1989; 168: 387–93.

Renal artery reconstruction

R. H. Dean MD
Director, Division of Surgical Sciences, Professor and Chairman, Department of General Surgery, Bowman Gray School of Medicine, Winston-Salem, North Carolina, USA

K. J. Hansen MD
Assistant Professor, Department of General Surgery, Bowman Gray School of Medicine, Winston-Salem, North Carolina, USA

A variety of operative techniques has been used to correct renal artery stenoses in the past 20 years. These techniques include aortorenal bypass using saphenous vein, autogenous hypogastric artery or synthetic material, endarterectomy, renal artery reimplantation, and extra-anatomical procedures such as splenorenal anastomosis and hepatorenal bypass. Whereas thromboendarterectomy and renal artery reimplantation are only suitable for proximal or orificial lesions, aortorenal bypass can be employed for either atherosclerotic disease or fibromuscular dysplasia of the renal artery.

Although each of these techniques has its proponents, the most important point to be made is that no single method is applicable to all situations and that any one of these techniques may be the superior method of renal revascularization in a given patient. Generally speaking, the indications for operation and use of these respective procedures are for the treatment of hypertension and/or renal insufficiency caused by renal ischaemia. Detailed descriptions of the preparations for evaluation and conduct of studies used to identify candidates for operation are outlined elsewhere in detail[1-3].

Preparation

Several measures should be considered routine in the preparation for operation and in perioperative management. Since approximately one-third of patients will have a contracted blood volume from diuretic therapy or the disease itself, preoperative overnight intravenous hydration is important. Similarly, operations should be delayed after diagnostic studies such as arteriography until it is proven that any adverse consequence of such studies has stabilized or resolved.

We routinely use pulmonary artery catheters and an indwelling radial artery catheter to monitor fluid balance, blood pressure and myocardial performance closely during the operation. Similarly, these monitoring methods are continued for the first 48 h after operation.

Operation

Certain measures are applicable in almost all renal arterial operations. Mannitol, 12.5 mg, is administered intravenously at least 10 min before renal crossclamping and heparin, 100–200 units/kg, is given intravenously. Occasionally, protamine is required for reversal of the heparin at the end of the reconstruction. Finally, accurate monitoring of blood loss and fluid replacement during the operation is mandatory, because episodes of hypotension are especially detrimental to renal function under these circumstances.

EXPOSURE OF RENAL ARTERY

Adequate exposure is the most difficult but important aspect of renal artery surgery.

Skin incision

1 A midline incision from the xiphoid to the pubic symphysis provides excellent access to either renal artery. This incision is carried to the side of the xiphoid process to gain an additional 3–4 cm of proximal exposure.

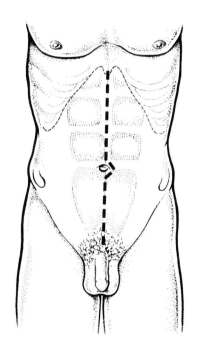

1

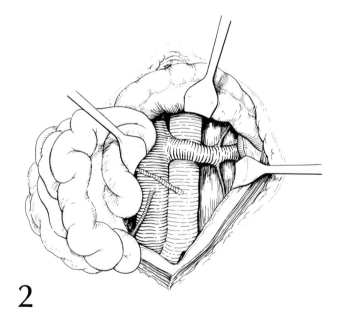

2

Exposure of left renal artery

2 To expose the left renal artery, the posterior peritoneum overlying the aorta is incised longitudinally and the duodenum is reflected to the patient's right. By extending the posterior peritoneal incision to the left along the inferior border of the pancreas, an avascular plane behind the pancreas can be entered. This allows excellent exposure of the entire renal hilum on the left and is of special significance when distal lesions are to be managed. The renal artery lies behind the left renal vein. In some cases it is easier to retract the vein cephalad to expose the artery. In others, caudal retraction of the vein provides better access.

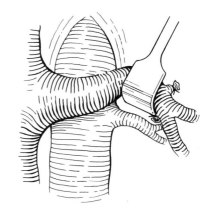

3a

Division of gonadal and adrenal veins

3a–c The gonadal and adrenal veins which enter the left renal vein must be ligated and divided to facilitate exposure of the artery. Another frequent tributary is a lumbar vein that enters the posterior wall of the left renal vein and is easily avulsed unless special care is taken in mobilizing the renal vein. After dividing the left adrenal and gonadal veins, the entire length of the left renal artery can be visualized behind the renal vein. Similarly, by dividing one or two sets of lumbar veins, the proximal right renal artery can be widely visualized.

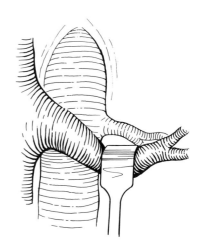

3b

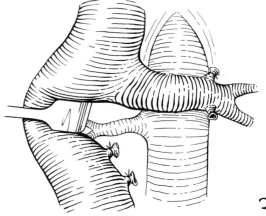

3c

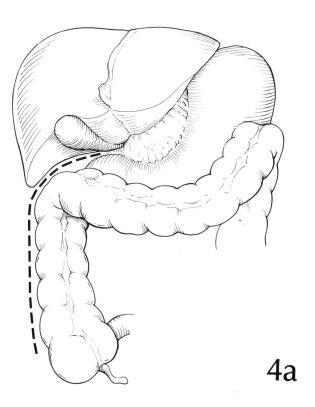

4a

Exposure of right renal artery

4a, b The proximal right renal artery can be exposed through the base of the mesentery by ligating two or more pairs of lumbar veins and retracting the vena cava to the patient's right and the left vein cephalad. The distal right renal artery is best exposed, however, by mobilizing the duodenum and right colon medially. The right renal vein is mobilized and is usually retracted cephalad to expose the artery. In some patients there is an accessory right renal artery which arises from the anterior wall of the aorta about 2.5 cm above the origin of the inferior mesenteric artery. This artery is unusual in that it courses anterior to the vena cava and then over the lower pole of the right kidney, as opposed to the retrocaval course of the right renal artery. It can be easily injured if the surgeon is unaware of its presence.

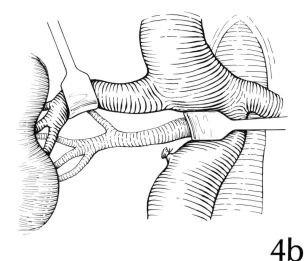

4b

Simultaneous bilateral exposure

5a–c When bilateral simultaneous procedures such as bilateral endarterectomies are performed we routinely mobilize the aorta to a level above the superior mesenteric artery for supramesenteric aorta crossclamping. Division of the diaphragmatic crura as they wrap around the aorta facilitates this exposure. Similarly, total mobilization of the right colon and small bowel with placement of these viscera onto the chest wall provides the wide exposure to enhance visualization of the entire area of the juxtamesenteric and juxtarenal aorta.

Incision begins at the base of the mesentery and continues around the caecum and up the right lateral mesocolon peritoneal reflection. Using this technique, the entire small bowel and right colon is eviscerated to expose the entire juxtarenal aorta and both renal arteries.

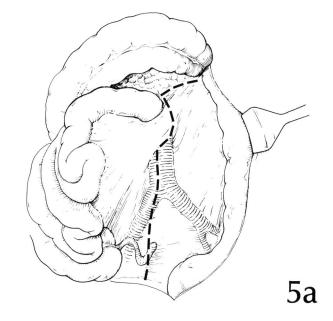

5a

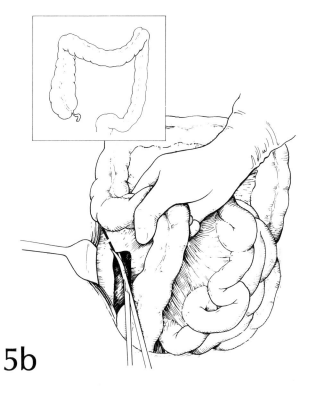

5b

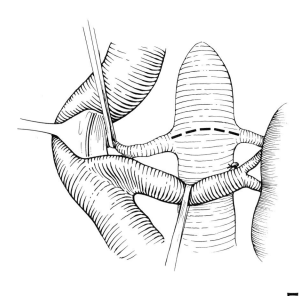

5c

AORTORENAL BYPASS

Technique

Three types of graft are usually available for aortorenal bypass: autogenous saphenous vein, autogenous hypogastric artery and synthetic prostheses. Arterial autografting using hypogastric artery has great theoretical appeal in that autogenous tissue is utilized, which matches in size and consistency the affected renal arteries. Despite these advantages, however, the added risk of pelvic dissection and the fact that the hypogastric artery itself may be atherosclerotic or the source of important collateral flow to the intestines seem to militate against its widespread use.

Expanded polytetrafluoroethylene (6 mm in diameter) has been our preferred material when a synthetic prosthesis is preferred. We have found it to be technically superior to Dacron in regard to the ease of suturing to small vessels. Although long-term studies are not available to assess its durability, we believe it compares favourably to Dacron in this regard. Nevertheless, we have limited our use of such grafts to instances of proximal atherosclerotic lesions where the distal renal artery is large (4 mm in diameter).

Although circumstances may require the use of these other graft materials, autogenous saphenous vein has emerged as the preferred graft material donor in most centres. It can be used for bypass in atherosclerotic disease and fibromuscular dysplasia. The advantages of autogenicity and flexibility allow the use of very fine suture for direct anastomosis to branch vessels, if necessary. Further, the procurement of a short segment of saphenous vein through a separate groin incision adds little to either operative time or postoperative morbidity. Nevertheless, if the saphenous vein is small (less than 4 mm in diameter) or if it has been previously sacrificed, other sources of graft material must be used. Although gonadal and iliac veins have been suggested as alternative sources, these intra-abdominal veins withstand aortic pressure poorly and should not be employed as arterial substitutes.

6a–c After the renal artery and infrarenal aorta have been mobilized, the vein graft is prepared. Mild distension with heparinized saline allows identification of adventitial bands, which should be divided. Extensive removal of the adventitia or distension under high pressure, however, is unnecessary and potentially detrimental to the long-term function of the vein graft. In end-to-side renal artery bypass, the renal artery–vein graft anastomosis should be performed first. Since this is generally the most difficult anastomosis, it is much easier if the graft is completely mobile. After an adequate exposure is obtained, small Silastic slings can be used to occlude the renal artery distally. This method of vessel occlusion is especially applicable to this procedure. In contrast to vascular clamps, these slings are essentially atraumatic to the delicate renal artery. The absence of clamps in the operative field is also advantageous. Further, when tension is applied to the slings, they lift the vessel out of the retroperitoneal soft tissue for more accurate visualization.

The length of the arteriotomy should be at least three times the diameter of the renal artery to guard against late suture line stenosis. Before the anastomosis is created, each of the branches of the renal artery is gauged with renal artery dilators. Since branch stenosis in patients with fibromuscular dysplasia may be missed on angiography, this manoeuvre may be diagnostic as well as therapeutic. A 6/0 or 7/0 monofilament polypropylene (Prolene) suture material is employed with loop magnification. A continuous suture line is used to allow the greatest exposure for the placement of sutures at the distal end of the arteriotomy. Greatest emphasis is placed on the placement of these four or five sutures. If these are placed deeply or with an inappropriate advancement, a stenotic outflow for the graft is created and there is the risk of later graft thrombosis.

After the renal artery anastomosis is complete, heparinized saline is injected and the suture line is checked for leaks. The occluding clamps and slings are then removed from the renal artery and an atraumatic small bulldog clamp is placed across the vein graft adjacent to the anastomosis. The aortic anastomosis is then performed.

The aorta is cross-clamped below the renal arteries and a wedge of aortic wall is excised to create a large orifice for the vein graft. This is especially important if the aorta is thickened or calcified by extensive atherosclerosis. Again, the anastomotic diameter should be at least three times the vein graft diameter to prevent later suture line stenosis and subsequent thrombosis. The graft is usually brought behind the renal vein on the left and behind the vena cava on the right. However, there are instances in which the anatomy of the renal arteries is such that a course anterior to the left renal vein or to the vena cava on the right seems more appropriate.

In contrast to the end-to-side bypass technique, we usually first construct the proximal (aortic) anastomosis

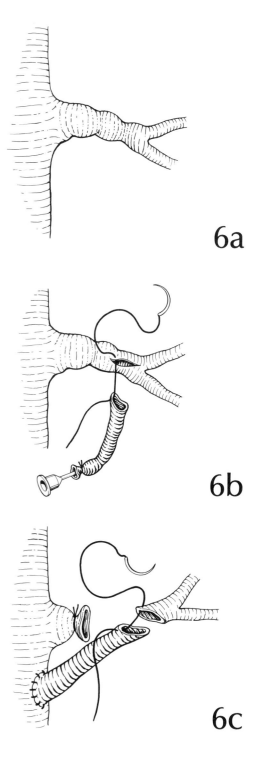

6a

6b

6c

when performing an end-to-end renal artery bypass. After the proximal anastomosis is completed the renal artery is ligated proximally and transected. The renal artery and graft are then spatulated to provide an anastomotic diameter at least three times the diameter of the renal artery. Again, a continuous suture line using 6/0 or 7/0 monofilament polypropylene is employed for this anastomosis.

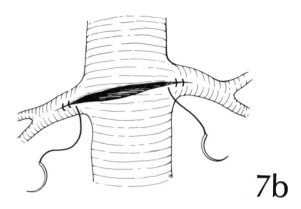

7a

THROMBOENDARTERECTOMY

Transaortic technique (transverse incision)

7a–c In some cases of bilateral atherosclerotic occlusions of the renal artery origins, simultaneous bilateral endarterectomy may be the most applicable procedure. Although transaortic endarterectomy is occasionally used we prefer a transverse incision in most instances. This arteriotomy is carried across the aorta and along the renal artery to a point beyond the stenosis. With this method, the distal intima can be assessed directly and tacked down with mattress sutures under direct vision if necessary. Following completion of the endarterectomy, the arteriotomy is closed. In most patients this closure is performed with a vein patch to ensure that the proximal renal artery is left widely patent.

7b

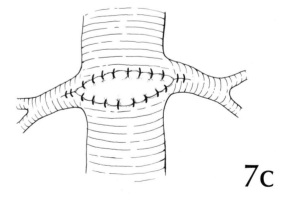

7c

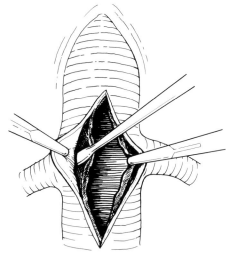

8a

Transaortic technique (longitudinal incision)

8a–c The use of transaortic endarterectomy is limited in this unit to patients with multiple renal arteries involved with orificial stenoses. In this instance we will proceed with a longitudinal aortotomy and endarterectomy of the aorta and renal arteries. It is important to have adequate mobilization of the renal arteries to allow eversion of the vessel into the aorta to visualize the distal component of the renal artery endarterectomy.

Duplex ultrasonography is used to examine the end point after completion of the endarterectomy.

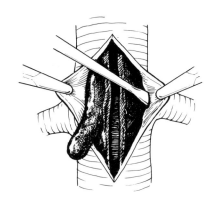

8b

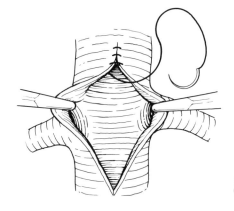

8c

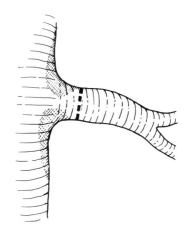

9a

RENAL ARTERY REIMPLANTATION

9a, b Many patients will have a somewhat redundant renal artery after it has been dissected from the surrounding retroperitoneal tissue. When renal artery stenosis is limited to its origin and the vessel is redundant, the renal artery can simply be transected and reimplanted, after spatulation, into the aorta at a slightly lower level. Occasionally this can even be done in small children and thereby abolish the necessity of using a graft.

Renal reimplantation is performed by suture ligation of the origin of the renal artery after transection. After excising a button of aorta just below the renal artery, the renal artery is spatulated and reattached to the aorta using 6/0 monofilament polypropylene sutures.

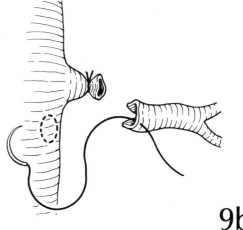

9b

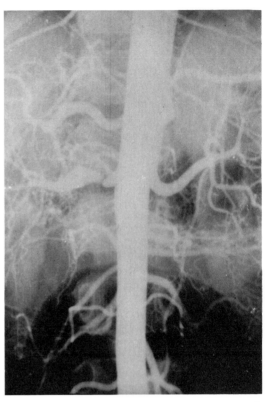

10a

Postoperative evaluation

10a, b We believe that it is imperative to obtain information to prove technical success after completion of the procedure. For many years we relied on pre-hospital discharge aortography for this assessment. More recently, however, we have used intraoperative completion duplex ultrasonography to confirm technical success. Its greatest value is for confirm technical success. Its greatest value is for assessment of main renal artery reconstructions. We continue to use postoperative aortography to evaluate success of *ex vivo* multiple branch vessel reconstructions.

References

1. Dean RH. Indications for operative management of renovascular hypertension. *J S C Med Assoc* 1977; 73: 523–5.

2. Dean RH. Operative management of renovascular hypertension. In Bergan JJ, Yao JST, eds. *Surgery of the Aorta and its Body Branches*. New York: Grune & Stratton, 1979: 377–407.

3. Dean RH, Foster JH. Criteria for the diagnosis of renovascular hypertension. *Surgery* 1973; 74: 926–30.

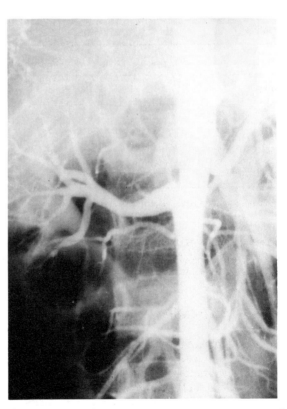

10b

Visceral artery aneurysms

James S. T. Yao MD, PhD
Magerstadt Professor of Surgery, Division of Vascular Surgery, Department of Surgery, Northwestern University Medical School, Chicago, Illinois, USA

Principles and justification

Visceral artery aneurysms are uncommon, approximately 3000 splanchnic artery aneurysms having been reported in the literature[1]. The incidence has been increasing in recent years due to the judicious use of arteriography and infusion computed tomography (CT) scanning in the diagnosis of abdominal complaints. These aneurysms may cause abdominal pain or rupture, leading to a catastrophic event.

The most common site for aneurysm formation is the splenic artery, followed by (in order of decreasing involvement) the hepatic, superior mesenteric, coeliac, gastric and gastroepiploic, small intestinal, pancreatico-duodenal, pancreatic, and gastroduodenal arteries (*Table 1*).

Table 1 Incidence of aneurysms in various parts of the intestinal circulation

Artery	Incidence (%)
Splenic	60
Hepatic	20
Superior mesenteric	5.5
Coeliac	4
Gastric and gastroepiploic	4
Jejunal, ileal, colic	3
Pancreaticoduodenal or pancreatic	2
Gastroduodenal	1.5

Reproduced from ref. 1 with permission of the publishers.

The aetiology of these aneurysms includes atherosclerosis, media degeneration, mycotic origin, trauma, and as a manifestation of systemic arteritis.

Clinical presentation

Presenting symptoms range from vague abdominal pain to the sudden onset of abdominal catastrophe from rupture of the aneurysm. Splenic aneurysm is known to be commonly associated with multiple pregnancy[2-4] or portal hypertension[5]. Aneurysm rupture during pregnancy causes maternal and fetal mortality rates as high as 70%[3]. In contrast, men are twice as likely as women[1] to be affected by hepatic aneurysms. Most of these aneurysms are either atherosclerotic or show medial degeneration. One of the fatal presentations of hepatic aneurysm is haematobilia from rupture of the aneurysm into the biliary tract[6]. Because of the location, coeliac axis aneurysm may present with a pulsatile mass and can be mistaken for abdominal aortic aneurysm. Gastro-duodenal and pancreatic aneurysms may result from pancreatitis.

Erosion of the artery from the inflammatory process of the pancreas often presents with a surgical challenge for treatment of an aneurysm in this location[7]. In systemic necrotizing arteriditis, multiple aneurysms involving jejunal, ileal, or colic branches are not uncommon clinical features[8].

Diagnosis

Both infusion CT scanning and arteriography help to establish the diagnosis. Arteriography is important to evaluate the blood supply and collaterals to the visceral organs.

Indications

Indication for surgical intervention depends on symptoms and the size of the aneurysm. In general, a small aneurysm (less then 2.0 cm) discovered during incidental examination should be left alone. The exception to this rule is the splenic aneurysm in women of childbearing age. A large aneurysm, especially with evidence of embolization, should be treated by surgery. Surgical intervention is also needed in those aneurysms with symptoms thought to be due to the aneurysm.

Preoperative

In most patients, routine preoperative evaluation for fitness for surgery is sufficient. In elderly patients with aneurysm due to atherosclerosis, evaluation of cardiac and pulmonary status is necessary.

Operations

COELIAC ANEURYSM

1 Unless the coeliac aneurysm is exceptionally large, most visceral aneurysms can be managed through a midline abdominal incision.

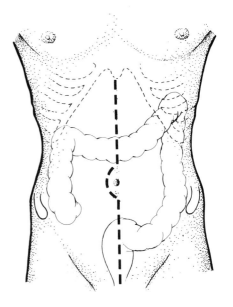

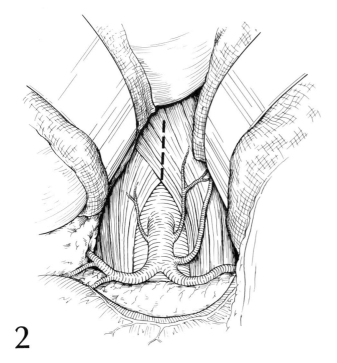

2 Resection of the coeliac aneurysm requires supra-coeliac control. The supracoeliac aorta is exposed by entering the lesser sac. With the left lobe of the liver retracted, the right crus of the diaphragm is divided, which allows the exposure of the supracoeliac aorta. Circumferential dissection of the aorta is seldom necessary.

3 Exposure of the lateral wall of the aorta is all that is needed for placement of the clamp. Once the supracoeliac aorta is exposed, the coeliac aneurysm is dissected free from the surrounding structure, exposing the hepatic, left gastric, and splenic arteries. These arteries are then circled with Silastic tape. The distal aorta is exposed in a similar manner.

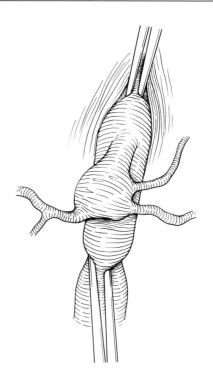

3

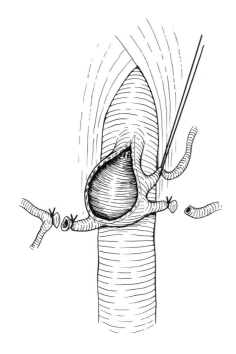

4

4 After proximal and distal control is achieved, the aneurysm is entered and the main hepatic artery is clamped and transected. In a large aneurysm the coeliac axis origin should be sutured closed from inside the aneurysm. The left gastric artery is then ligated. The splenic artery may be sutured from inside the aneurysm or ligated from the origin. After transection, the splenic artery is prepared for reanastomosis to the vein graft.

5 Long saphenous vein is harvested from the thigh and prepared for bypass. The vein graft is anastomosed first to the supracoeliac aorta (end-to-side) and then to the hepatic artery (end-to-end). Once the anastomosis is completed, the splenic artery is reanastomosed end-to-side to the vein graft.

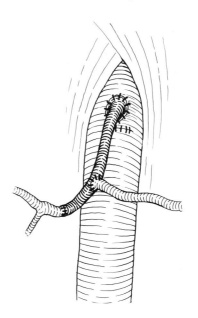

5

HEPATIC ARTERY ANEURYSM

6a, b Exposure of a hepatic aneurysm follows the same procedure as for the coeliac axis, but it is not necessary to expose the supracoeliac aorta. The hepatic aneurysm is resected and an interposed saphenous vein graft used to restore perfusion to the liver.

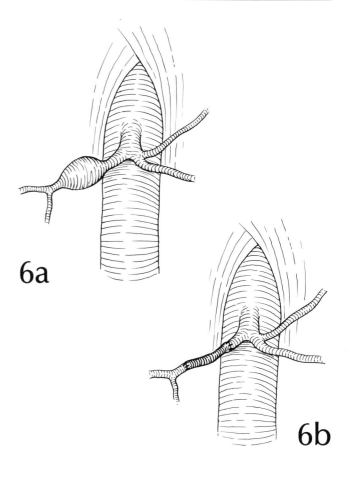

6a

6b

SUPERIOR MESENTERIC ANEURYSM

7 The transverse colon is retracted upward, a retroperitoneal incision is made over the aorta and the aorta is dissected free. The superior mesenteric artery is approached via the medial aspect of the intestinal mesentery. Palpation of the artery will locate the aneurysm, which is then dissected free from the surrounding structure.

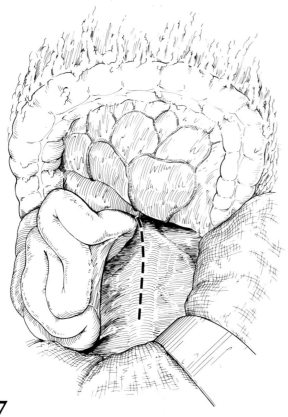

7

8a, b The aneurysm is resected and an interposed vein graft is used to restore the perfusion. If the origin of the superior mesenteric artery is intimately involved in the process, it may be necessary to perform a vein graft from the coeliac axis by repeating the manoeuvre used for exposure of the coeliac axis. For an aneurysm involving the distal part of the artery, ligation may be all that is needed because of the richness of the collaterals.

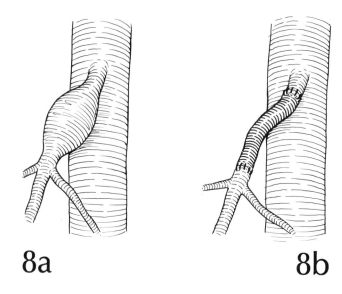

8a   8b

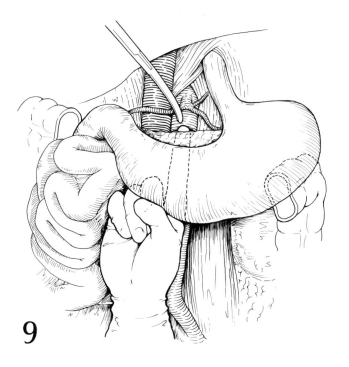

9

9 If a vein graft is needed, a retropancreatic tunnel is made.

10 The vein graft is passed behind the pancreas.

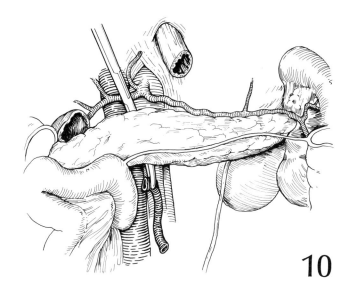

10

11 The vein graft is first anastomosed to the coeliac axis and then to the remaining superior mesenteric artery.

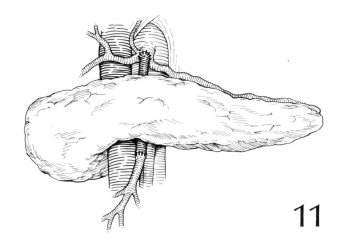

11

SPLENIC ARTERY ANEURYSM

The splenic artery is exposed along the inferior border of the pancreas. Preservation of the spleen and restoration of the flow should be considered. In general, the author prefers restoration of flow by end-to-end anastomosis or by a short interposed vein graft. Ligation of the splenic artery may be all that is needed, depending on the location of the aneurysm.

PANCREATIC ARTERY ANEURYSM

If the aneurysm forms because of pancreatitis, surgical treatment could be difficult. The inflammatory process surrounding the pancreas makes dissection difficult and resection of the aneurysm is often impossible. This type of aneurysm is best treated by entering the aneurysm sac and suturing the supplying artery tight with continuous suture.

ALTERNATIVE PROCEDURE

With the introduction of endovascular devices, some of these aneurysms may be treated by stent, coil placement, or embolization to enhance thrombosis with some success[9].

Postoperative care

Postoperative care is the same as that for patients undergoing laparotomy. The patency of a bypass graft can be assessed with duplex imaging or (more definitively) by arteriography. This assessment should be made before the patient is discharged from hospital, as a baseline for future follow-up studies.

References

1. Stanley JC. Aneurysms of the celiac and mesenteric circulations. In: Yao JST, Pearce WH, eds. *Aneurysms: New Findings and Treatment*. Norwalk, Connecticut: Appleton and Lange, 1993: (in press).

2. O'Grady JP, Day EJ, Toole AL, Paust JC. Splenic artery aneurysm rupture in pregnancy. A review and case report. *Obstet Gynecol* 1977; 50: 627–30.

3. Trastek VF, Pairolero PC, Joyce JW, Hollier LH, Bernatz PE. Splenic artery aneurysms. *Surgery* 1982; 91: 694–9.

4. Stanley JC, Thompson NW, Fry WJ. Splanchnic artery aneurysms. *Arch Surg* 1970; 101: 689–97.

5. Feist JH, Gajarej A. Extra- and intrasplenic artery aneurysms in portal hypertension. *Radiology* 1977; 125: 331–4.

6. Harlaftis NN, Akin JT. Hemobilia from ruptured hepatic artery aneurysm. Report of a case and review of the literature. *Am J Surg* 1977; 133: 229–32.

7. Hofer BO, Ryan JA Jr, Freeny PC. Surgical significance of vascular changes in chronic pancreatitis. *Surg Gynecol Obstet* 1987; 164: 499–505.

8. Selke FW, Williams GB, Donovan DL, Clarke RE. Management of intra-abdominal aneurysms associated with periarteritis nodosa. *J Vasc Surg* 1986; 4: 294–8.

9. Salam TA, Lumsden AB, Martin LG, Smith RB III. Nonoperative management of visceral aneurysms and pseudoaneurysms. *Am J Surg* 1992; 164: 215–19.

Mesenteric and coeliac arterial occlusion

C. W. Jamieson MS, FRCS
Consultant Surgeon, St Thomas' Hospital, London, UK

Restoration of the arterial circulation to the foregut and midgut may be necessary for chronic or, in very rare circumstances, acute occlusion.

Principles and justification

Chronic mesenteric ischaemia

These patients have an absolutely characteristic history: they show rapid, progressive and alarming weight loss accompanied by severe pain, which occurs very shortly after ingesting any food. The pain is so bad that they prefer not to eat rather than face it. In a minority of patients the symptoms are associated with a degree of diarrhoea and there is occasionally blood in the loose stools.

1a–d The physical signs are those of recent weight loss. There may be evidence of associated peripheral vascular disease, such as carotid bruits, loss of pulse and abdominal systolic bruits. The diagnosis is made by high-quality selective angiography; it is most important that films are taken of the abdominal aorta in the lateral plane because the origins of the coeliac axis and superior mesenteric artery are overlaid by the contrast medium in the aorta in the anteroposterior plane and a critical but short stenosis may be missed completely. These angiograms usually reveal the gross disease of both the coeliac and superior mesenteric artery with associated occlusion of the inferior mesenteric artery and the late films exhibit filling of the dilated, wandering and tortuous collateral vessels.

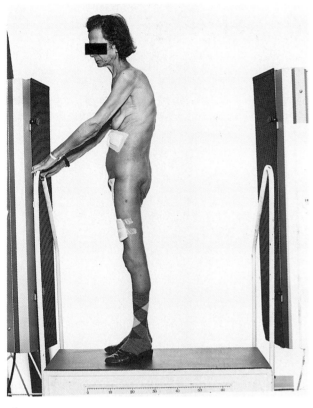

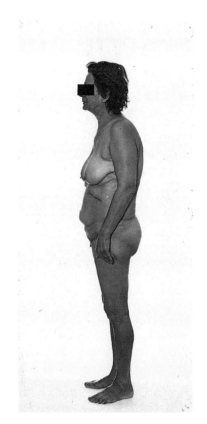

1a

1b

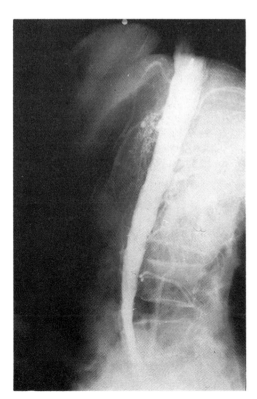

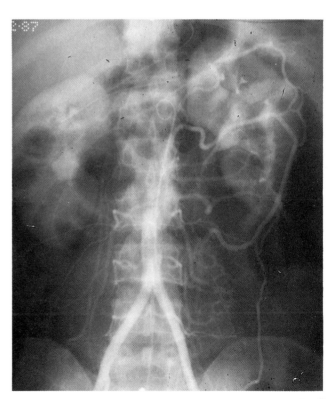

1c

1d

Acute mesenteric ischaemia

This disastrous emergency may arise spontaneously but is more frequently encountered following cardiac surgery, when a postoperative embolism from the heart into the mesenteric artery has occurred. The patients present with continuous abdominal pain related to movement, and abdominal distension. The pain may be insidious in onset and the patient is frequently *in extremis* before a definitive diagnosis of a disastrous intra-abdominal complication is made. A clue may be obtained from the rise in serum potassium which is associated with infarction of the bowel, but once this sign is present intervention is usually too late to save the patient. The diagnosis can only be made, therefore, with a high index of suspicion and a willingness to perform a laparotomy on any patient with abdominal distension and abdominal pain of sudden onset. Laparoscopy may make the diagnosis with less trauma. In late stages of the process gas in the portal circulation of the liver is diagnostic; however, patients exhibiting this radiological sign are doomed.

Preoperative

Once a diagnosis of chronic mesenteric ischaemia is made, the patient should be screened for other vascular disease and associated risk factors such as diabetes, polycythaemia, thrombocythaemia and hypercholesterolaemia. Two units of blood should be cross-matched.

Operations

SUPERIOR MESENTERIC AND COELIAC ARTERIAL BYPASS

Position of patient

The patient is positioned supine on the operating table. The whole abdomen is prepared, as is one thigh, to allow the saphenous vein to be harvested for use as a bypass.

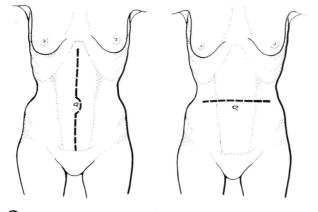

Incision

2 The recent weight loss in these patients makes access easy. A long midline incision or a transverse incision, centred 2 cm above the umbilicus, is used.

2

Exploration of the abdomen

The only other condition that can produce symptoms of ischaemia is a neoplasm; the pancreas and liver must be carefully palpated to exclude this diagnosis. The presence of mesenteric vascular disease is usually seen quite easily as the pulsation is lacking from the small branches of the mesenteric vessels and no pulse can be felt in the main trunk of the superior mesenteric artery when the base of the mesentery is gently pinched between finger and thumb. The coeliac axis, which is palpable through the gastrohepatic omentum just to the right of the gastro-oesophageal junction at the upper border of the pancreas, also has no detectable pulse.

Exposure of the vessels

3 The small intestine is reflected to the right and the parietal peritoneum opened along the line of the abdominal aorta, commencing distal to the inferior mesenteric artery and extending proximally to expose the left renal vein. Because of the considerable weight loss in these patients, the tissues are frequently so loose that it is possible to extend this dissection deep to the pancreas to expose the origin of the superior mesenteric artery.

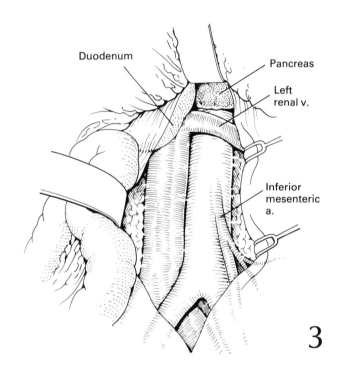

3

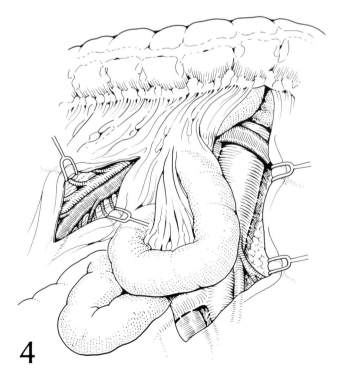

4

4 The superior mesenteric artery is best exposed in the root of the mesentery of the small intestine after it crosses anterior to the third part of the duodenum. The visceral peritoneum over the base of the mesentery is incised longitudinally on its left side. The superior mesenteric vein is encountered with the artery lying on its right side. Small branches are best controlled by metal clips.

5   The coeliac axis is exposed by dividing the gastrocolic ligament and reflecting the stomach superiorly, giving good access to the hepatic artery, left gastric artery and splenic artery arising from the common stem of the coeliac axis.

Provided that the vessels are soft and patent distally arrangements are made to harvest the saphenous vein for construction of the bypasses.

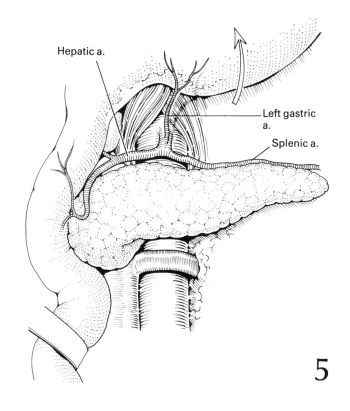

5

Harvesting the saphenous vein

A longitudinal incision is made in the thigh over the course of the saphenous vein and the whole saphenous vein harvested from its termination at the femoral vein to the knee. Tributaries are ligated with 2/0 silk as they are encountered, but the main vein should not be divided or clamped until heparin, 10 000 units (100 mg), has been administered intravenously and anticoagulation is satisfactory. The vein is then clamped and excised and placed in a swab soaked in heparin–saline. The wound in the thigh is loosely sutured to avoid development of haematoma and is sutured completely at the end of the operation.

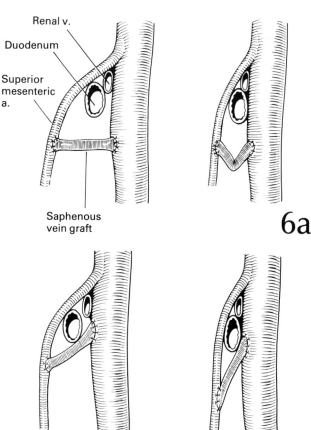

6a

Insertion of superior mesenteric artery bypass

6a, b   It is most important that the bypass should originate from the abdominal aorta as high as possible, just distal to the left renal vein. If it is placed more transversely, the bypass has a strong tendency to kink when the mesentery is returned to the abdominal cavity; this is avoided by placing the bypass proximally.

6b

7 A tape is placed around the abdominal aorta just distal to the left renal vein, avoiding the lumbar arteries, and the aorta controlled by two obliquely placed Crafurd clamps. A slightly oval window, 1 cm long, is then made in the anterior surface of the aorta using a No. 15 blade followed by fine scissors and the reversed saphenous vein is sutured obliquely end-to-side to this arteriotomy using a continuous 4/0 polypropylene suture.

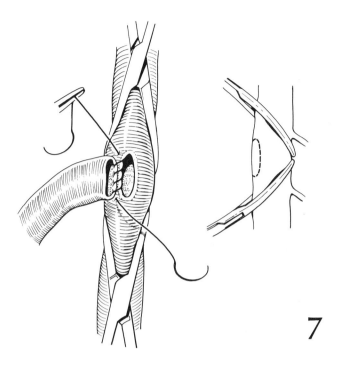

7

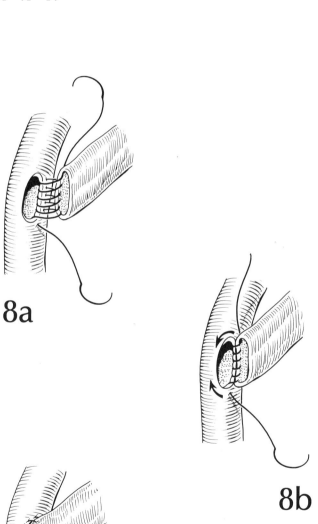

8a

8b

8c

— Vein graft

— Superior mesenteric a.

8a−c If the aorta is thick walled and diseased continuous suture may tend to stenose the origin of the bypass and interrupted sutures are more satisfactory. A suitable point in the superior mesenteric artery is selected and the artery proximal and distal to this area is controlled by small bulldog clamps. The length of vein used should be as short as possible, given the difficulty of suturing it in place with the mesentery extended. The vein is divided and sutured end-to-side to a 1-cm arteriotomy in the superior mesenteric artery, using a continuous 4/0 polypropylene suture.

The superior mesenteric artery is very thin walled and this anastomosis must be performed with great care. It is most easily accomplished using a posterior parachute suture which is drawn together only once the posterior layer is completed. The anterior suture is continued from both extremities of the parachute suture and tied in the centre of the anterior part of the anastomosis.

Oxycellulose gauze is then wrapped round both anastomoses. The proximal aortic clamps are removed first, to drive any retained air out of the bypass, followed by the distal bulldog clamps on the superior mesenteric artery. A good pulse should be restored on the superior mesenteric artery and this pulse should not be lost when the mesentery is returned to the normal position.

Coeliac artery bypass

Usually major disease of both vessels occurs, in which case both should be bypassed, to improve the mesenteric circulation to the maximal degree possible and secondly to act as an insurance should one bypass fail in the future. Haemodynamically only one bypass is necessary, as this seems to reverse the condition very satisfactorily, but it is not difficult to add a second bypass at this stage. The aortic clamps are re-applied, with the distal clamp at the level of the inferior mesenteric artery, and a 1-cm oval arteriotomy is made in the anterior surface of the aorta distal to the arteriotomy of the superior mesenteric bypass.

9, 10 Saphenous vein is then sutured in reversed fashion, end-to-side, to this arteriotomy using 4/0 polypropylene sutures. It is then led through the transverse mesocolon anterior to the pancreas to be sutured to the distal extremity of the trunk of the coeliac axis after the coeliac axis, the splenic artery, the left gastric artery and the hepatic artery are controlled with small bulldog clamps. The position of this bypass is less critical than the superior mesenteric bypass; indeed, it may be left slightly slack. It is technically easier to perform than the superior mesenteric artery bypass.

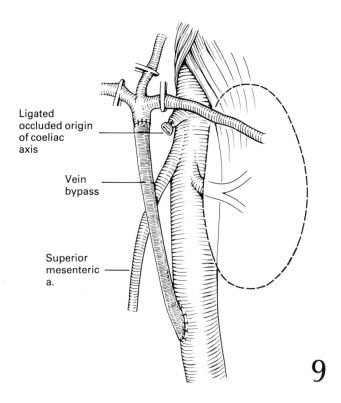

9

Inferior mesenteric artery reconstruction

This is very seldom necessary but there are occasions, particularly in Takayasu's disease, where extensive occlusion of the upper mesenteric vessels leaves the inferior mesenteric vessel as the major source of supply to the bowel and a stenosis develops at its origin. This may be treated by arteriotomy from the aorta into the inferior mesenteric artery, to be closed with a vein or Dacron patch, or by a short bypass from the aorta to the inferior mesenteric artery. This is a very rare situation and the author has never encountered a need for this procedure.

Wound closure

Following the establishment of good pulses in the mesenteric vessels the anticoagulation is reversed with protamine sulphate and, when complete haemostasis is secured, the abdomen is closed. These patients suffer from serious malnutrition and abdominal closure must be meticulous to avoid the risk of burst abdomen. The author's preference is for mass closure with 1/0 polyglycolic acid suture.

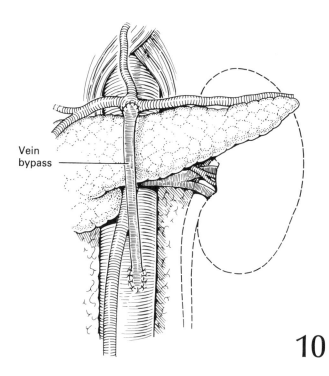

10

ACUTE MESENTERIC ISCHAEMIA

Position of patient

The patient is positioned as for treatment of the chronic disease.

Incision

The abdomen is explored through a midline or left paramedian incision. The diagnosis may be immediately apparent from the offensive smell of infarcted bowel. The area of infarction may be extensive, including the whole small intestine and proximal colon, in which case the patient's only chance of survival lies in major resection, although even this may be impossible and incompatible with life. Smaller lengths of infarcted bowel can be excised and thought must be given to acute revascularization at the same time as this operation.

Mesenteric embolectomy

11 Mesenteric embolectomy may be possible. The superior mesenteric artery is exposed in exactly the same manner as recommended for chronic mesenteric ischaemia; it may be soft or full of thrombus but will be pulseless. Following control of small branches with Ligaclips the artery is gently encircled with a snare, opened, and a short linear arteriotomy of approximately 1 cm is made. A transverse arteriotomy is less suitable, for, although it is easily closed should successful embolectomy be performed, it is not desirable if a bypass becomes necessary.

A 4-Fr Fogarty catheter is then passed proximally up the superior mesenteric artery; should the occlusion be due to an embolus it will pass into the abdominal aorta and withdrawal of the catheter will carry with it the embolus and restore normal flow. The artery is then clamped proximally and the catheter passed gently distally, withdrawing any propagated thrombus. If propagated thrombus is present the chances of successful embolectomy are slim. The arteriotomy is then closed using a 4/0 continuous suture.

If the catheter does not pass proximally an aortic to superior mesenteric artery bypass should be performed in the same manner as that recommended for chronic ischaemia. At the same time consideration should be given to a simultaneous aortic–coeliac axis bypass.

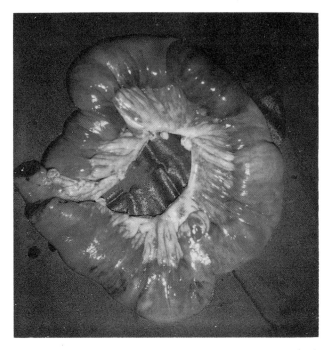

11

Reassessment of viability and resuscitation

Restoration of circulation to ischaemic bowel has profound systemic effects related to the release of vasodilator substances, endotoxin and potassium. The anaesthetist must be aware of this inevitable consequence which may prove fatal. Every attempt should be made to restore the blood pressure by support with dopamine and adrenaline, restore a normal pH by the administration of sodium bicarbonate, lower the sudden surge in serum potassium with glucose and insulin and cover with broad-spectrum antibiotics such as Augmentin (amoxycillin and clavulanic acid) and gentamicin.

It is most important that the operation should not be rushed at this stage. Obviously dead tissue should be resected promptly but no attempt should be made to restore continuity of the small intestine until the viability of the remaining tissue has been carefully assessed. It is extremely difficult to be sure whether intestine which has been profoundly ischaemic for some hours has the potential for survival and to heal an anastomosis. The presence of gas bubbles in the small veins at the junction of the intestine and mesentery is diagnostic of irreversible necrosis, as is thrombosis of these veins so that they fail to blanch upon pressure. A trial incision should produce bright red blood and there is usually vigorous peristalsis during the period of recovery from acute ischaemia. After about 1 h, during which the anaesthetic resuscitation proceeds apace, the surgeon is usually in a position to make a provisional assessment of the residual viability of the intestine. It is more important that the patient is left deficient to some extent in gastrointestinal function than to leave gangrenous tissue although loops of dubious viability may be exteriorized rather than resected. Some resection is frequently necessary.

Wound closure

Following the reversal of anticoagulation and completion of haemostasis, the abdomen is closed with a mass polyglycolic acid suture.

Postoperative care

The abdomen should be re-explored 24 h after surgery, to ensure that the intestine is fully viable. It is very common to find small areas of irreversible ischaemia which require resection, even in a patient who appears to be perfectly well. This 'second look' procedure is mandatory after any operation for acute mesenteric ischaemia in which there is some chance of the patient's survival.

Coeliac axis compression syndrome

C. W. Jamieson MS, FRCS
Consultant Surgeon, St Thomas' Hospital, London, UK

Principles and justification

Indications

The syndrome of severe epigastric pain related to ingestion of food has been highly suspect since its first description. It was originally described as a syndrome of epigastric pain occurring in relation to meals, associated sometimes with an epigastric bruit which changed pitch upon respiration; the finding on lateral angiography was of compression of the coeliac axis by the median arcuate ligament of the diaphragm[1]. Sceptics, however, have pointed out that this anatomical variation frequently exists in the absence of any symptoms, that the condition apparently never proceeds to acute or irreversible ischaemia of the intestine, therefore rendering the diagnosis of progressive ischaemia doubtful, and that even with surgical treatment there is a tendency for the symptoms to recur with time[2]. It seems, however, that there is possibly a small group of patients in whom there is a genuine symptomatic condition. The criteria necessary to make a provisional diagnosis are as follows:

1. A history as described above.
2. Definite severe constriction of the artery by the median arcuate ligament on lateral angiography.
3. Reduced pulse and pressure in the coeliac axis distal to the compression at laparotomy.
4. Total absence of any other abdominal condition on investigation and on laparotomy that would explain the symptoms[2,3].

Preoperative

Investigations

The patient must be investigated by gastroscopy, ultrasonography of the gallbladder and endoscopic retrograde cholepancreatography to exclude upper abdominal pathology, and the upper abdominal viscera must be carefully examined at laparotomy to confirm the negative investigations.

Operation

Incision

1 A longitudinal midline epigastric incision is made, through the linea alba, from the xiphisternum to the umbilicus.

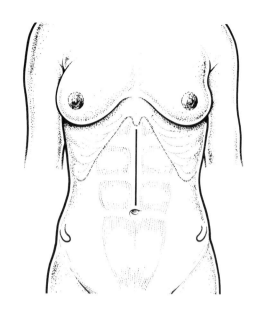

Exposure

2, 3 The lesser curve of the stomach is retracted downwards, the left triangular ligament of the liver is divided and the left lobe of the liver is reflected to the right, exposing the oesophageal hiatus. The coeliac axis is located on the upper border of the pancreas by following the left gastric artery to its origin or the hepatic artery. The axis is dissected free from the dense surrounding autonomic nerve tissue of the coeliac plexus. This dissection is tedious and time consuming, but eventually leads the surgeon posteriorly to the median arcuate ligament of the diaphragm.

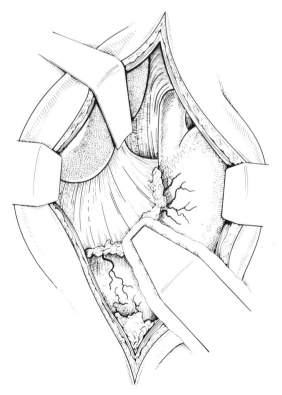

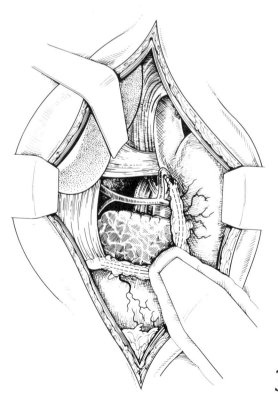

4 A Macdonald's dissector is gently inserted through the hiatus distal to the median arcuate ligament, which is divided with a size 15 blade, using the dissector to protect the artery. Great care must be taken not to damage the coeliac axis or, even more importantly, the underlying aorta. The first few millimetres of the dissection are the most difficult; after this the median arcuate ligament springs apart to expose the origin of the coeliac axis.

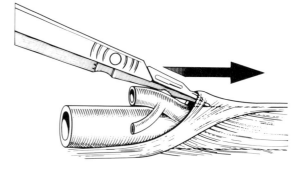

4

The stenosis is usually extravascular, but reports have appeared of a fibrotic stricture of the vessel which requires treatment by open arteriotomy and patching to restore its calibre. This has not been the author's experience.

Wound closure

After division of the median arcuate ligament a pulse is restored to the coeliac axis. The liver is allowed to return to position and the abdominal wall is closed in layers with polyglycolic acid sutures.

Postoperative care

After transperitoneal exploration of the coeliac axis there is usually a period of paralytic ileus lasting between 1 and 3 days, requiring intravenous fluid administration and nasogastric aspiration. There are no other specific postoperative measures.

It must be stressed that this operation should be reserved for patients in whom the pain is severe and refractory and no other cause has been found on careful and thorough investigation.

References

1. Harjola DT. A rare obstruction of the coeliac artery; report of a case. *Ann Chir Gynaecol Fenn* 1963; 52: 547–50.

2. Lord RSA, Stoney RJ, Wylie EJ. Coeliac axis compression. *Lancet* 1968; ii: 795–8.

3. Leading article. Compression of coeliac axis. *BMJ* 1971; 4: 378–9.

Surgery for sexual impotence

R. G. DePalma MD
Lewis B. Saltz Professor of Surgery, George Washington University School of Medicine, Washington DC, USA

Principles and justification

Surgery for sexual impotency involves correction of aortoiliac disease, penile and pudendal arterial bypass and venous interruptions for cavernosal leak syndrome. Large vessel reconstructions, i.e. aortoiliac or aorto-femoral bypass, aortoiliac endarterectomy and femoro-femoral bypass, aneurysm or limb ischaemia are modified specifically to prevent postoperative impotence. Internal iliac endarterectomy or bypass are employed for vasculogenic impotence. Small vessel microvascular reconstructions for impotence now comprise two procedures: bypasses into the dorsal artery or deep dorsal vein arterialization.

The diagnosis and treatment of vasculogenic impotence has progressed considerably in the past decade. Most patients are successfully treated medically with risk factor intervention such as smoking cessation, control of diabetes and change of blood pressure medication. Oral agents, such as isoxsuprine and yohimbine hydrochloride, and intracorporeal injections using papaverine, phentolamine or prostaglandin E_1 are used for conditions such as diabetes, neuropathy or hypertension[1]. After diagnosis and exclusion, the author estimates that about 4–5% of patients remain as candidates for vascular operations for impotence[2].

Large vessel reconstruction

Indications

The indications for large vessel reconstruction are aneurysm or occlusive disease. A procedure providing perfusion of both internal iliac arteries is selected whenever possible. One must avoid embolization into the internal iliacs and spare the neural axes about the aorta and iliac arteries.

Preoperative

Preoperative assessment and preparation of these patients is the same as that for aortoiliac disease. In all cases specific history of sexual activity should be obtained. Penile brachial indices and pulse volume recordings are measured along with pudendal and somatosensory evoked potentials before operation when the patient notes that sexual activity is important. The risk of postoperative impotence should be discussed with the patient.

Operations

AORTOILIAC RECONSTRUCTION

1 Exposure for aortoiliac reconstruction for occlusive and aneurysmal disease is a standard midline incision approaching the aortoiliac segment from the right side and sparing the nerves. Minimal dissection is needed and an extra limb can be added when necessary for internal iliac artery perfusion.

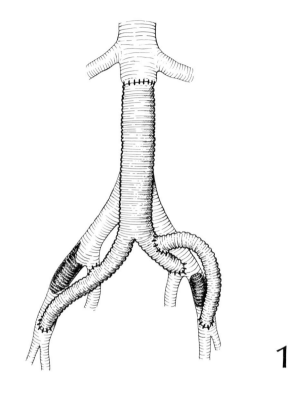

1

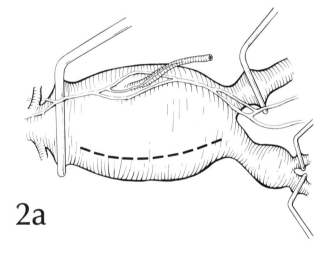

2a

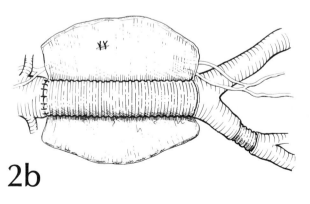

2b

AORTIC ANEURYSM RESECTION

2a, b In cases of aortoiliac aneurysm, perfusion of the internal iliac arteries is assured by using the inlay technique illustrated. The aneurysm sac is incised well to the right, avoiding interruption of the periaortic nerve plexus. The inferior mesenteric artery is sutured within the aneurysmal sac.

INTERNAL ILIAC ARTERY ENDARTERECTOMY

Indications for this procedure include buttock claudication and impotence in men with a chief complaint related to localized disease in the arterial distribution.

3a, b
A retroperitoneal approach developed for kidney transplantation is used to expose the distal internal iliac artery and its anterior and posterior divisions. A longitudinal incision is made along the edge of the rectus muscle and the peritoneum is reflected medially. As illustrated, the internal iliac artery is exposed and can be reconstructed either by endarterectomy or bypass.

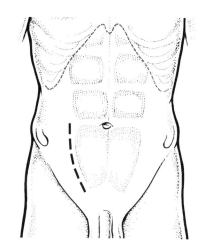

3a

Postoperative care

Postoperative antibiotics are given for a period of 5–7 days when graft material is used or until all catheters are removed. The patient is not fed until flatus or bowel movement occurs. Peripheral pulses are monitored. At the first postoperative visit, penile blood pressures and pulse volume recording are repeated to confirm maintained or improved function. The outcome of potency after aortoiliac correction in the author's experience is shown in *Table 1*. Note that postoperative sexual function appears to be age-dependent. Beyond the age of 65 years, men who are impotent before operation are more likely to remain impotent afterwards.

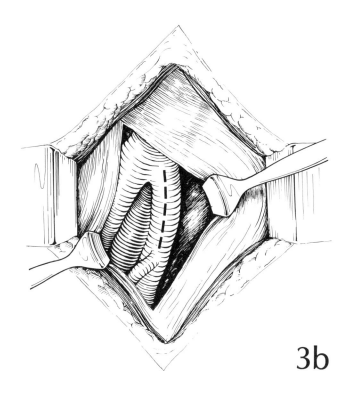

3b

Table 1 Three-year follow-up of erectile function after modified nerve-sparing aortoiliac operations (1990)

Before operation	After operation	Number	Mean (range) age (years)	Comments
Potent	Impotent	4	51.72	Two emergencies, two internal iliac aneurysms
Impotent	Impotent	53	64.6 (49–79)	Three found on screening for impotence
Potent	Potent	30	57.0 (39–71)	Failure of orgasm in one
Impotent	Potent	38	58.0 (38–69)	All elective procedures, including three aneurysms involving internal iliac arteries

Small vessel reconstruction

Small vessel reconstructions were initially attempted a decade or more ago with direct arterialization of the corpus cavernosum. These either produced priapism or failed because of fibrosis at the distal anastomoses. These procedures have now evolved into two types of operations: microvascular bypass into the dorsal artery and bypasses into the deep dorsal vein, using the inferior epigastric artery or a vein graft from the femoral artery. The author prefers the inferior epigastric artery as an inflow source whenever possible.

Preoperative

All patients undergoing these operations require careful screening. Preoperative non-invasive neurovascular tests help to select patients for further invasive studies. Diagnostic procedures have recently been summarized by DePalma *et al.*[3]. If there is failure to respond to increasing doses of intracorporeal vasoactive agents, candidates are studied by dynamic cavernosography and measurement of cavernosal artery occlusion pressure after injection of papaverine/phentolamine mixtures. In all of these patients it is important to perform dynamic cavernosography and cavernosometry as well as highly selective pudendal arteriography. About 12% of candidates for venous surgery will have undetected arterial disease. For dynamic infusion cavernosography a full dose of papaverine/phentolamine is injected to provoke erection if possible and to define sites of venous leak. For arteriography lower doses are used to provide tumescence to visualize the distal arterial tree better. A full erection will not allow study of the distal vessels.

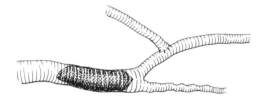

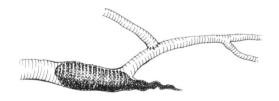

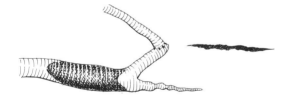

4 Appropriate candidates with communication between the dorsal and cavernosal arteries can only be selected with careful visualization.

4

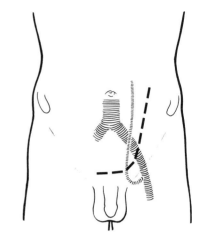

5a

Operations

DORSAL ARTERY BYPASS

5a, b General anaesthesia is used for dorsal artery bypass. The incision is started transversely at the base of the penis and continued upward at the reflection of the rectus sheath to just above the umbilicus. Both penile dorsal arteries and the dorsal vein are dissected as far proximally as possible beneath the arch of the pubic symphysis. The incision is then carried upward along the lateral edge of the rectus muscles. The inferior epigastric artery is harvested, ligating side branches and turning it down for microvascular anastomosis with the appropriate dorsal artery. The author has not used vein grafts from the femoral arteries.

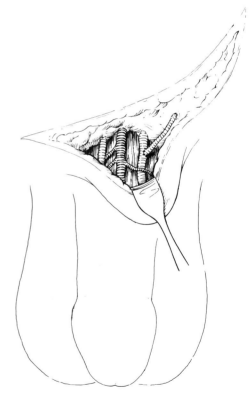

5b

DEEP DORSAL VEIN ARTERIALIZATION

6   In this operation the deep dorsal vein is isolated as far proximally as possible beneath the arch of the pubic symphysis. A microvascular anastomosis between the inferior epigastric artery and the deep dorsal vein is performed. Side branches are spared. The circumflex veins probably provide perfusion, mainly to the corpus spongiosum.

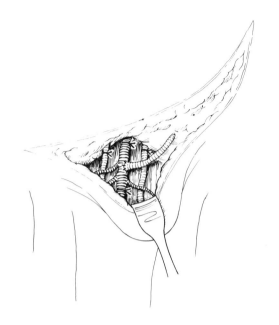

6

Postoperative care

Broad-spectrum antibiotics begun before operation are continued for 2–3 days. Urethral catheterization is optional. The one serious specific complication to deep dorsal vein arterialization is glans hyperperfusion. Management requires exploration of the veins just proximal to the corona. Any veins perfusing the glans are divided. The incidence of this complication has been reduced by performing the anastomosis as far proximal as possible and ligating the dorsal vein proximally and distally.

VENOUS LIGATION

The author's approach to venous ligation employs both direct ligation of the dorsal vein in appropriately selected cases and proximal embolization of draining veins, using Gianturco coils inserted by the invasive radiologist. At times an introducing catheter can be inserted directly via the deep dorsal vein, using an appropriate sheath. The exposure used is similar to that described for deep dorsal vein arterialization.

Postoperative care

Specific complications of small vessel reconstructions include penile oedema and tenderness. Intercourse is contraindicated until these subside. Nerve damage is a serious complication and must be avoided by careful neurovascular dissection with magnification. Parenteral antibiotics are continued for 2–3 days after operation.

Outcome

These are evolving procedures, and their long-term results have yet to be evaluated objectively. In properly selected patients, improved function can be obtained in 50–70%. Objective documentation of postoperative function includes repeat intracorporeal injection with similar doses of vasoactive agents. At times men who were non-responsive before operation become responsive to these agents and can function. We recommend dynamic cavernosography and cavernosometry at 3 months in all cases of venous ligation to rule out sham effect[4]. At this time additional embolization for new leaks can be done. With these combined procedures about 70% of men have regained erectile function or now function with intracorporeal injection.

References

1. DePalma RG, Schwab FJ. Vasculogenic impotence. In: Young JR, Graor RA, Olin TW, Batholomew TR, eds. *Peripheral Vascular Surgery*. St Louis: Mosby Year Book, 1991: 395–400.

2. DePalma RG, Schwab FJ, Emsellem HA *et al*. Vascular interventions for impotence. Effect of a screening sequence. *Int J Impot Rev* 1990; 2: 358–9.

3. DePalma RG, Schwab FJ, Emsellem HA, Massarin E, Bergsrud D. Noninvasive assessment of impotence. *Surg Clin North Am* 1990; 70: 119–32.

4. Yu GW, Schwab FJ, Melograna F, Miller HC, DePalma RG. Objective assessment of venous ligation for impotence. *Int Impot Res* 1990; 1: 379–80.

Illustrations by Joanna Cameron

Femorodistal *in situ* bypass

R. W. H. van Reedt Dortland MD
Consultant Vascular Surgeon, Department of Surgery, Section of Vascular Surgery, Utrecht University Hospital, The Netherlands

B. C. Eikelboom MD
Professor of Vascular Surgery, Department of Surgery, Section of Vascular Surgery, Utrecht University Hospital, The Netherlands

History

In 1906, in Madrid, José Goyanes performed the first successful human *in situ* bypass. After resection of a popliteal aneurysm, a defect of the artery was bridged with *in situ* popliteal vein. Despite many reports on successful venous grafting of femoral arteries published during the second decade of this century in German journals, this method did not gain general acceptance until Jean Kunlin reported his pioneering work in 1949. He used a reversed saphenous vein to bypass an occlusion of the superficial femoral artery. Reversed vein bypass procedures gradually became more popular during the late 1950s and the early 1960s. The first successful vein graft to an infrapopliteal vessel was carried out by Palma in 1960, and 6 years later Baird and collaborators reported bypass grafting to the arteries at the malleolar level. The experience reported by Darling and Linton (1962) and Mannick (1967) showed that autogenous vein grafts remained patent even in patients with only fair or poor outflow tracts. Today, autologous great saphenous vein is generally considered to be the graft material of choice for infrainguinal arterial reconstructions. It is usually available, accessible, expendable, and generally of adequate length and diameter. It is histologically similar to an artery and its historical and continued superior performance are responsible for this acceptance.

The concept of using the great saphenous vein *in situ* to bridge an occluded femoral artery can be attributed to Karl Victor Hall who, while working with Charles Rob at St Mary's Hospital in London in 1959, suggested that the saphenous vein bypass might be expedited if the vein were left in place and the valves rendered incompetent. Hall's first attempts to ablate the venous valves to obtain unobstructed distal flow using the blunt end of a varicose vein stripper – by introducing it proximally and advancing it distally – were unsuccessful because of the vascular wall injuries that occurred during this manoeuvre. On his return to Oslo, Hall subsequently used direct excision of the valve leaflets through transverse phlebotomies and reported the successful use of the saphenous vein *in situ* as an arterial bypass in 1962. Initially, there was some scepticism towards the performance of the *in situ* bypass concept, perhaps because of its tedious, time consuming and meticulous surgical technique. Further development of this technique has practically been identical with the advances made in the atraumatic destruction of venous valves and the evolution of instruments necessary for this procedure. In 1968 Hall introduced an efficient, rapid and relatively atraumatic technique for valve destruction. He developed a venous valvulotome and reported promising results. Hall's valvulotome was later slightly modified by Gruss (Insitucut). Using this improved instrument the superior results obtained have been attributed to the intrinsic properties of the *in situ* vein bypass. Properly performed, this bypass has been shown to give satisfactory results, especially when used as a long bypass to tibial vessels in cases of critical ischaemia. Its current popularity probably depends on the modification of the technique of valve ablation in which the vein is sutured to the common femoral artery *before* the valve disruption renders the valves tense and more easily destroyed.

Principles and justification

Autogenous vein is the graft material of choice for infrageniculate arterial reconstruction. What is still not known is whether the *in situ* bypass is the optimal graft. Porter[1] has stated that any vein suitable for *in situ* bypass can be used in reversed fashion, but the *in situ* technique has practical and theoretical advantages over the reversed vein bypass.

Practical advantages

The basic idea behind the *in situ* method is logical. The wider, proximal portion of the great saphenous vein is anastomosed to the wide common femoral artery and the narrower distal portion of the infrageniculate popliteal artery or one of the tibial arteries, which is about equal in diameter. The conical tapering form of the graft accelerates blood flow within the vein in a distal direction, thus improving haemodynamics at both anastomoses. Veins less than 4 mm in diameter (suggested minimal size for reversed vein bypass) can be used, thus allowing greater vein utilization with added length for more distal anastomoses at the ankle and foot.

Because of the easier accessibility for graft survey or graft repair the subcutaneous position of *in situ* bypass is also preferred. The *in situ* method of vein preparation also has the added advantage that a branch of the saphenous vein may be used for bifurcated bypass (inverted Y graft) with sequential distal anastomoses. Thus it is possible to improve total graft flow and increase perfusion to the distal calf and foot without constructing an extra anastomosis in the vein.

Theoretical advantages

Unlike the reversed vein, which is removed from its vascular bed, the *in situ* vein vasa vasorum are not disrupted. Preservation of the vasa vasorum may lead to reduced medial and intimal fibrosis and should reduce the incidence of graft stenosis. However, vasa vasorum preservation is not complete and both ends, the most vital areas of the graft, are denuded to facilitate construction of the anastomosis. It is also believed that an almost completely intact endothelial monolayer should protect against immediate or early thrombosis. It has been shown that prostacyclin, an active inhibitor of platelet function and a very effective peripheral vasodilator, is produced in significantly larger quantities by a vein that is left *in situ*[2]. In contrast, thromboxane, the primary activator of platelet adhesion and aggregation and a potent peripheral vasoconstrictor, is produced by the damaged wall of the excised and reversed vein. Arterialization of the *in situ* vein and exposure of its luminal surface to oxygenated blood may result in almost complete preservation of the endothelium when pulsatile arterial flow is established before distal transection, and even after the vein is subsequently mobilized from the surrounding tissue for construction of the distal anastomosis[3].

The technique of *in situ* bypass has remained controversial and certainly does not replace the traditional approach of reversing the vein, but it has distinct advantages when performing reconstructions to arteries below the knee.

Indications for surgery

The indication for *in situ* bypass is the same as for a reversed femoropopliteal or femorotibial vein bypass. In our opinion the *in situ* technique is not indicated in stage II disease with a segmental occlusion between the femoral bifurcation and the adductor canal where the popliteal artery is normal and there is a good run-off. It is in reconstructions below the knee, and particularly distal to the trifurcation of the popliteal artery, that this technique has most impact. Infrageniculate arterial reconstructions are performed primarily for chronic limb-threatening ischaemia (clinical stages III and IV). The objectives are to relieve rest pain, heal ulcers, promote healing of toe and forefoot amputation sites, and restore or maintain patient mobility. The combination of a long graft, low flow and a narrow lumen at the distal anastomosis results in very high failure rates when prosthetic materials are used.

In situ bypass, by its nature, is only applicable to those patients who have an ipsilateral intact saphenous vein. Veins with small diameters (2.5–4.0 mm) which would normally be discarded might give acceptable results with the *in situ* technique.

Preoperative

Preoperative assessment and preparation for an *in situ* bypass procedure is identical to that for classic reversed venous reconstructions. Preoperative evaluation of the patient involves complete assessment of both arterial and venous anatomy.

Patient selection

An important aspect in the selection of patients for this procedure is their general health as most are elderly, smokers and usually unfit. Elderly patients do not fare well with amputation and the result is usually long-term geriatric care. Femorodistal reconstruction should not be offered unless the patient has useful function in the limb. Thus, those patients already confined to bed for reasons other than limb ischaemia are excluded for arterial reconstruction, as are those with low output cardiac failure.

Arteriography

Biplane arteriograms are mandatory and should include the ankle and foot to help differentiate the tibial vessels from each other, to determine the true extent of the disease, and to select the proper side of distal anastomosis. Given patency of all three tibial arteries, the posterior tibial artery is preferred because it requires the least amount of mobilization of the distal vein and offers direct perfusion of the foot; the anterior tibial artery – with the exception of the most distal part at ankle level – and the distal two-thirds of the peroneal artery are less favourable since they require a relatively long segment of mobilized distal vein. If only one of these two arteries is patent it is preferable to use the reversed vein technique using an extra-anatomical lateral route.

In general, for limb salvage, all occlusions should be bypassed for maximal direct flow into the foot. With adequate angiography, virtually all patients are candidates for *in situ* bypass; isolated segments, pedal arteries and distal tibial vessels are all adequate outflow vessels.

Assessment of venous anatomy

In addition to adequate arteriography, preoperative evaluation of the saphenous vein has proved to be valuable in defining its variable anatomy. Knowledge of saphenous vein anatomy has the potential to reduce operation time, decrease the dissection required and is necessary for safe use of the venous valvulotome.

Simple physical examination is useful in thin patients, but in the majority of patients it does not provide adequate information. Venography and duplex scanning are two definitive methods available. Although preoperative or intraoperative venography was performed for several years with minimal complications, duplex scanning is now the method of choice. It is non-invasive and provides a map of the saphenous vein (with regard to the tributaries) that can be drawn on the overlying skin with a surgical marker pen.

During the examination the patient's leg should be dependent. The vein is then imaged from the groin to the ankle and major tributaries, double systems, varices or sclerotic valves should be noted. Venous anomalies have been encountered in approximately one-third of the saphenous vein systems studied so far.

Duplex scanning or venography is not a reliable predictor of the calibre of the vein. This can only be determined by exposure and intraoperative measurement of the vein before spasm occurs. A minimal external diameter of 2.5 mm (8-Fr) is still adequate.

Anaesthesia

The anaesthetic management of patients considered for femorodistal reconstruction is complicated by a variety of significant problems connected with their age and arteriosclerotic involvement. In general, continuous intrathecal, epidural or general endotracheal anaesthesia can be used. Frequently, intrathecal or epidural anaesthesia is preferred because it provides stable analgesia and blockage of the sympathetic nervous system, thus causing peripheral vasodilatation and reduction of peripheral arterial resistance.

Operation

Preparation of the saphenous vein for its use as an arterial bypass entails a few important steps:

1. Removal of valvular obstructions.
2. Control of the tributaries.
3. Mobilization of the ends for construction of the anastomosis.

The objective is to accomplish this with minimal operative manipulation of the vein.

The operation technique itself contains nine essential steps:

1. Assessment of the venous anatomy.
2. Selection of the site of distal anastomosis.
3. Distal exposure of the vein and host artery.
4. Excision of the saphenofemoral complex.
5. Construction of the proximal anastomosis.
6. Venous valvulotomy.
7. Interruption of the tributaries.
8. Construction of the distal anastomosis.
9. Final completion arteriography.

Position of patient

1 The patient is placed supine. Skin preparation is circumferential from the groin to the ankle and over the lower abdomen. The leg is rotated externally and must be completely free so that during the course of the operation it is possible to manoeuvre it. A pillow is placed behind the knee, thus allowing easy access to the groin, the full length of the great saphenous vein and the lower part of the popliteal fossa. The foot is draped in a sterile transparent bag to observe its circulation.

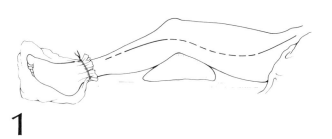

1

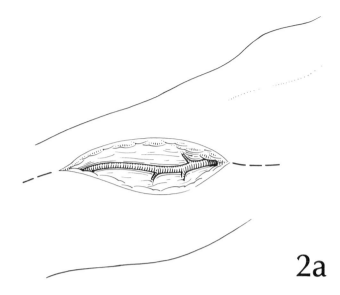

2a

Assessment of vein and host artery

2a−c The first step is to determine the suitability of the great saphenous vein. A longitudinal incision is made along the tibia at the level of the expected site of the distal anastomosis. The saphenous vein is identified, exposed and inspected without touching it. If the calibre of the vein is judged adequate (up to 3 mm for grafting of the popliteal artery, and up to 2.5 mm for the peripheral lower leg arteries), the distal host artery is exposed next at the level of the proposed anastomosis to ensure its accessibility.

Exposure of the infrageniculate popliteal artery (*Illustration 2b*), tibioperoneal trunk, posterior tibial (*Illustration 2c*) or peroneal artery can be achieved through the usual medial surgical routes.

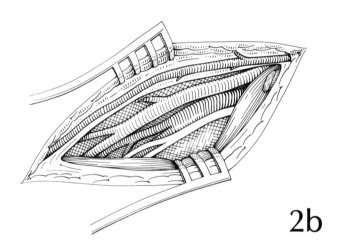

2b

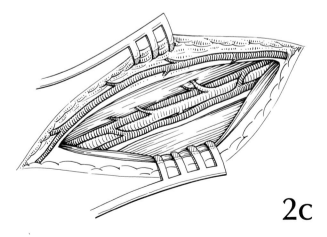

2c

Groin incision

3 The proximal segment of the saphenous vein is exposed and its entry into the deep femoral vein. A C- or S-shaped incision in the groin extends from the upper outer part of the inguinal region, across the inguinal ligament, downwards to the medial and anterior side of the thigh. By this incision the femoral bifurcation can also be exposed and, if required, extended proximally or distally.

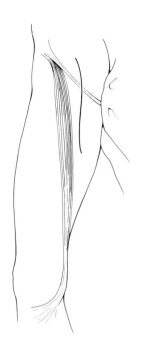

3

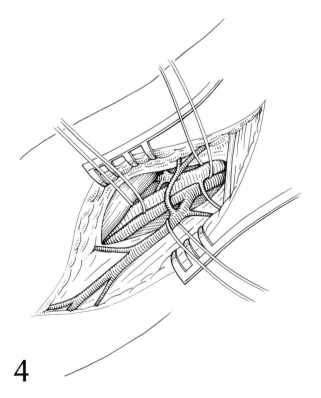

4

Groin dissection

4 The proximal segment of the great saphenous vein is identified in the subcutaneous fat and followed proximally to its entry into the deep femoral vein. The lymph nodes are retracted laterally and an incision is made in the deep femoral fascia. The vein is dissected carefully from the surrounding fat and a rubber tape passed around it for manipulation. It is important to dissect the inferior epigastric vein over a length of about 2–3 cm. The vein is an entrance into the saphenous vein and should be used for intraoperative angiography. The other proximal tributaries are ligated and divided. The femoral arterial bifurcation is exposed as usual. Tapes are placed around the superficial, common and deep femoral arteries.

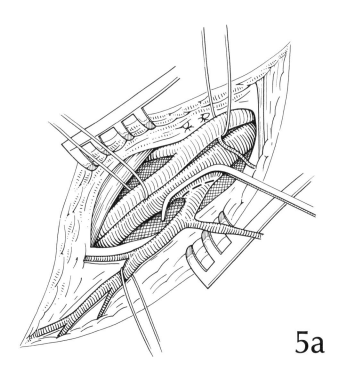

5a

Excision of saphenofemoral complex

5a, b The simplest and least traumatic method of rendering the bicuspid venous valves incompetent is to cut the leaflets in their major axis while they are held in a functionally closed position by pressure from above. This is the essence of the valve incision technique. Therefore, the excision of the saphenofemoral junction is started with the purpose of performing the proximal anastomosis. The saphenofemoral junction is invariably at the level of the common femoral bifurcation and a portion of the anterior aspect of the common femoral vein should be removed in continuity with the saphenous vein. Before the saphenofemoral junction is clamped the patient is given 30–35 units/kg intravenous heparin, which is supplemented every 2 h thereafter with 1000 units if necessary during the operation.

The saphenofemoral junction is occluded parallel to the long axis of the great saphenous vein with a small double curved vascular clamp (Satinsky) and divided tangentially just above it, using a pair of Potts' or Haimovici scissors. The femoral vein is repaired with a continuous 5/0 monofilament (polypropylene) suture.

Finally, the valve at the saphenofemoral junction is excised, removing only the transparent portion of the leaflets.

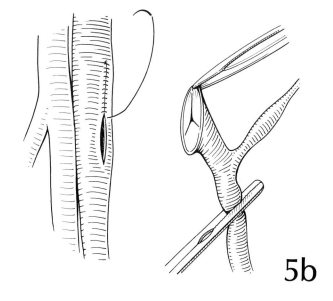

5b

Construction of proximal anastomosis

6a, b After the arterial blood flow has been interrupted with vascular clamps, a longitudinal arteriotomy is made in the femoral bifurcation. The arteriotomy is kept relatively short and is usually 1.5–2 times the diameter of the vein. To avoid late stenosis of the superficial femoral segment it is advisable to perform the anastomosis only end-to-side at the femoral bifurcation with inclusion of the common femoral artery. The pelvic arteries, the deep femoral artery and the superficial artery (if patent) are filled with heparinized saline solution. If localized stenosis or calcifications of the common femoral artery or of the ostium of the deep femoral artery are present, open thromboendarterectomy is necessary. It is helpful to place traction sutures in the middle of each side of the arteriotomy. A central horizontal mattress stitch is placed at the lower corner of the arteriotomy, and this passes from the outer side of the vein to its intimal surface and then from the intimal side of the artery to its outer side. A parachute technique with a double monofilament polypropylene 6/0 suture is preferred (*Illustration 6a*). The stitch is continued as a simple over-and-over everting stitch. After the first four or five stitches on both sides a second suture is started at the upper corner of the arteriotomy. The edges are also sutured with a continuous over-and-over stitch from the vein to the artery and, finally, the upper sutures on both sides are tied to the lower sutures. After removal of all occluding clamps and restoration of arterial blood flow, a strong pulse must be palpable at the proximal end of the vein to the first competent valve (*Illustration 6b*). If necessary, gentle pressure is applied directly over any bleeding points in the anastomosis for a period of approximately 5 min.

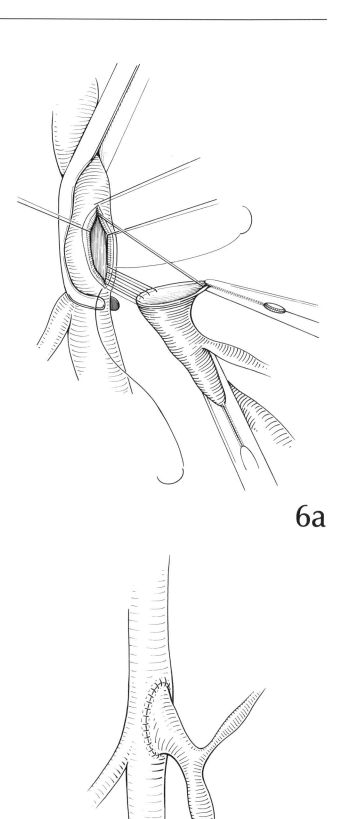

6a

6b

Venous valvulotomy

7a–c A modified Hall valve cutter (Insitucut) is preferred for venous valvulotomy. This instrument consists of two metal cylinders mounted on a rigid wire. There is a short distance between these two cylinders and the upper cylinder has blunt edges in a negative image of a venous valve (*Illustration 7a*). The cutter is introduced distally into the vein and advanced proximally to the saphenofemoral anastomosis, and is then slowly withdrawn. During this manoeuvre the vein is distended and stretched by the first cylinder, so that the second cylinder hooks into the valve leaflets. Resistance is felt as the cutter encounters each valve side and cuts the leaflets (*Illustration 7b*).

The great saphenous vein is dissected circumferentially and incised transversely for a few centimetres distally to the expected side of the distal anastomosis. The graft is flushed with heparinized saline solution and slightly dilated by careful injection of heparinized saline solution.

A valve cutter that just fits through the lumen of the vein is introduced and advanced proximally (*Illustration 7c*). During this manoeuvre no resistance whatsoever must be overcome. After palpation of the valve cutter in the proximal segment of the graft, it is withdrawn slowly. Each venous valve can be identified by a slight resistance or sudden tug. The instrument is then re-advanced carefully, rotated through 180° and withdrawn again, thus cutting the remaining leaflets. Thereafter it is usually possible to introduce a valve cutter of the next size and to repeat the manoeuvre. The graft ought to be flushed once again with heparinized saline solution and its distal end occluded with a bulldog clamp. Usually weak pulsations are now palpable in the distal segment.

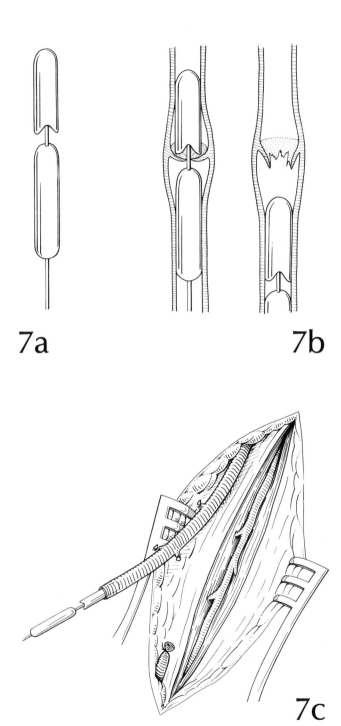

7a

7b

7c

Interruption of tributaries

8a, b After the proximal anastomosis has been completed and the venous valves destroyed, the venous branches should be localized and interrupted. We prefer to perform a so-called 'null flow' procedure. A sterile Doppler probe should be used to assess flow through the proximal vein. This probe must be placed upon the proximal segment of the vein. Occasionally there will be a continuous high-flow signal from the Doppler owing to the presence of significant fistulae. By occluding the vein manually in the upper thigh an occluded signal will be obtained. After the vein has been occluded more distally, a high flow signal will be detected, revealing the location of the most proximal fistula. This fistula can be exposed through a short incision and interrupted at the level of its entry with a metal clip or ligature. This manoeuvre must be repeated until all fistulae have been located and interrupted. At this point a good pulse at the distal segment and an occluded Doppler signal (null flow) in the proximal segment are obtained. Since this manoeuvre allows exact localization of venous branches, only short additional incisions are needed along the medial side of the thigh and the lower leg. Thus, circumferential dissection and complete denudation of the great saphenous vein can be avoided. Branches which have been overlooked and left *in situ* can eventually be identified by final completion arteriography, performed after the distal anastomosis has been completed.

9 An alternative method that can be used to identify venous branches is intraoperative phlebography. After the proximal anastomosis is completed and the venous valves are destroyed, radio-opaque markers (mosquito clamps or injection needles) are placed alternately along the medial surface of the leg at intervals of 10 cm. A blunt needle or intravenous catheter is inserted into the epigastric vein in the groin. Full strength ioxitalamic acid (Telebrix 350) is injected manually as rapidly as possible. After 15–20 ml has been infused the phlebogram is exposed. For long bypasses two films will be necessary to image the entire graft. Large perforating veins are filled over their entire length whereas all afferent venous branches are shown as far as the first closed valves. Exposure and interruption of the tributaries is as described earlier.

When the procedure is complete, there should be a strong, continuous flow exiting through the distal transected end of the vein. Weak flow or pulsation is indicative of a proximal stenosis or persistent fistula; there will be a palpable pressure drop at this point. In case of a missed valve the valvulotome should be re-advanced and withdrawn until this valve is destroyed; otherwise, the vein should be opened over the stenosis and either patched or replaced segmentally (if caused by endothelial injury).

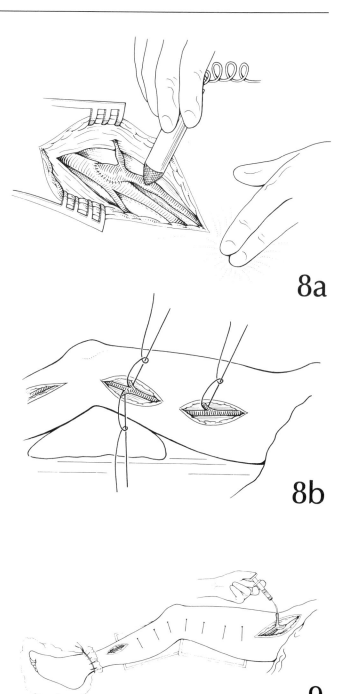

8a

8b

9

Construction of distal anastomosis

10a–d
After interruption of the tributaries and disruption of the venous valves the next step is the construction of the distal anastomosis. As stated earlier, the *in situ* technique has most impact when grafting to an infrageniculate artery. This artery should be exposed through the usual medial route with the site for anastomosis determined.

Pneumatic tourniquet control of the lower leg has proved helpful as an adjunct, particularly in those operations involving calcified arteries. Using this control it is not necessary to mobilize and to clamp the host artery, thus avoiding damage of artery wall and/or venae comitantes. When the distal artery is exposed, the operator can estimate the length of vein that remains to be prepared. A longitudinal arteriotomy approximately twice the vein diameter is made (*Illustration 10b*).

In the popliteal artery, the anastomosis may be performed either obliquely end-to-side or end-to-end depending on the anatomical situation; on a tibial artery the distal anastomosis is always end-to-side. If a distal end-to-side anastomosis on a small calibre artery is performed, the most difficult step is the stitches at the upper corner. Therefore it is advisable to start at the upper corner, employing a double continuous monofilament suture with a parachute technique again (*Illustration 10c*). To prevent narrowing at this site only very small bites of the venous wall should be taken. If the popliteal artery is anastomosed, 6/0 polypropylene sutures are used, whereas 7/0 or 8/0 sutures are used if the tibial artery is involved.

An end-to-end anastomosis seems preferable if a proximal trifurcation causes a sharp angulation of the graft on its course from the subcutaneous tissue to the popliteal artery. In such a case the popliteal artery is ligated as far proximally as possible and divided; its peripheral part is then mobilized to the vein graft and an oblique end-to-end anastomosis is made, using the rotation technique.

After completion of the anastomosis, flow through the distal artery is restored and assessed with the Doppler probe (*Illustration 10d*).

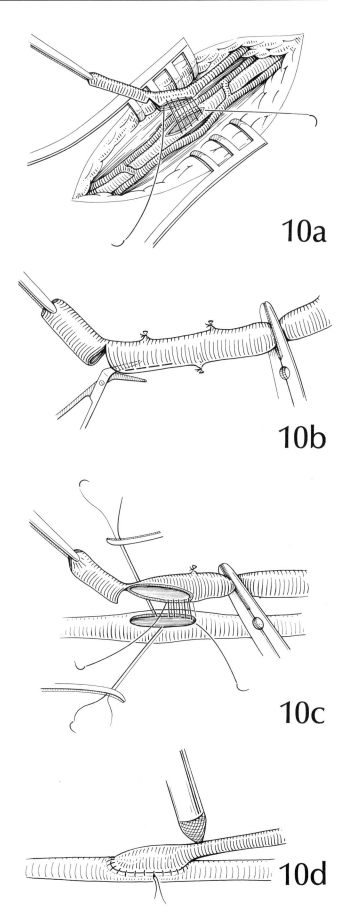

Final completion arteriography

11 A final completion arteriogram is mandatory. This allows accurate assessment of the graft and shows the location of any overlooked arteriovenous fistulae as well as any unsuspected technical errors in the *in situ* conduit or distal anastomosis. Fifteen to 20 ml full strength contrast medium (Telebrix 350) is injected by hand through the epigastric vein as described earlier. The arteriogram should be interpreted during operation and technical or anatomical imperfections, if present, should be corrected immediately. If the arteriogram and the Doppler examination are normal, the incisions are closed.

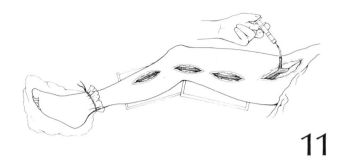

11

Postoperative care

All patients who have no contraindications undergo anticoagulation with dicoumarol preparations for life. Patients in whom this medication is contraindicated are given acetylsalicylic acid (aspirin) daily. A poor general circulation with long hypotensive periods and external compression of the graft should be avoided.

Postoperative patency is assessed by nursing personnel by simple palpation of the graft, preferably on a solid surface at the level of the knee joint. Before discharge from hospital, non-invasive tests should be used to determine that the haemodynamic results which were expected are, in fact, present. These include not only palpation of distal pulses, but also measurement of ankle pressures and/or duplex ultrasound study of the graft.

Complications

Immediate occlusion

The most common significant early complication of *in situ* arterial repair is graft thrombosis. An immediate occlusion can have four causes:

1. Excessively high resistance to run-off because of a poor outflow tract.

2. Poor general circulation owing to cardiac failure.
3. External compression of the graft.
4. Technical imperfections.

The first three causes are rare because blood flow through an *in situ* graft is usually maintained, even if blood pressure is reduced and the run-off is limited. Technical imperfections are the most common causes of an early graft thrombosis. The following list of imperfections specific to *in situ* bypass should be considered:

1. Endothelial or vein wall damage.
2. Incomplete valve destruction.
3. Persistent large perforating veins.
4. Imperfections of mobilized segment of vein.
5. Technical imperfections at the distal anastomosis.
6. Intimal dissection distal to the anastomosis.

To correct the occlusion, the most distal incision is reopened, the distal anastomosis exposed and the graft opened by a longitudinal phlebotomy at the anastomosis. A thrombectomy of the bypass is performed using a Fogarty balloon catheter, with the balloon softly inflated to avoid disruption of the intima or venous wall. Disobliteration is very simple. As soon as pulsatile blood flow is restored, the graft is filled with heparinized saline solution. It is advisable to repeat intraoperative angiography to detect the cause of graft thrombosis.

Endothelial or vein wall damage

12a, b Abrasion of the endothelium by instrumentation causes very rapid deposition of platelets. It can be readily detected by operative angiography as a characteristic foamy irregular filling defect within the vein. The most effective procedure is a longitudinal graft incision over the length of platelet deposition, complete removal of all platelet aggregates, and closure of the venotomy with a vein patch. A longer segment of damaged vein wall is best treated by excision and interposition of an excised vein segment.

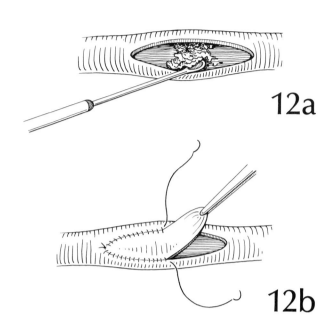

12a

12b

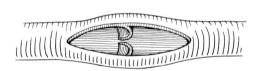

13a

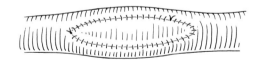

13b

Incomplete valve destruction

13a, b Incomplete valve destruction will cause bypass failure or may result in decreased ankle pressures. The mechanism of a functioning venous valve after valvulotomy can be explained as follows: advancing the valvulotome proximally into an arterialized vein may result in a displaced valve and a temporary unobstructed forward flow. This valve will eventually snap close and become obstructive. A balloon catheter can also produce this effect. If is therefore necessary to confirm an intact functioning valve during operation by allowing unrestricted flow through the open end of the vein for a short period of time. An intermittent or diminished flow after a few spurts is indicative of a proximal obstruction. Readvancement and withdrawal of a valvulotome of the largest possible size is required to ablate the remaining valve leaflets. Repeated intraoperative angiography provides a means of detecting persistent venous valve cusps. When valve leaflets are particularly stiff or fibrotic, it is best to open the vein longitudinally, excise the valve directly, and close the resulting venotomy by means of a vein patch angioplasty.

Persistent large perforating fistulae

14 Large perforating fistulae which are left *in situ* pose an additional risk in the long term. These veins can cause a steal phenomenon whereby arterial blood flow is shunted directly into the deep venous system and may lead to distal thrombosis of the graft. All large persistent fistulae that communicate with the deep venous system should therefore be ligated.

After graft failure because of large perforating fistulae, detection and interruption as described earlier is mandatory.

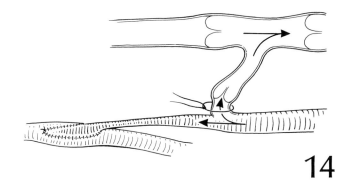

14

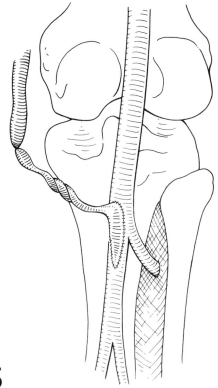

15

Imperfections of mobilized segment of vein

15 Peripheral graft imperfections can be a cause of graft failure. If the peripheral pulse disappears soon after the leg is extended, it is probably due to kinking of the vein at the margin of the crural fascia. Other causes are kinking of the distal part because of too long a segment of vein, anastomosis too far proximal on the popliteal artery thus causing an unfavourable angulation, and/or torsion of the mobilized segment of vein which was unexpected or which the surgeon did not deem severe enough for correction.

After thrombectomy of the graft these imperfections, if present, should be corrected.

Technical imperfections at distal anastomosis

16a, b The construction of the distal anastomosis takes precise surgical technique. This has to be done with as much care as any part of the operation. This anastomosis is frequently the source of postoperative problems. Its upper corner creates the most difficulty and a parachute technique with use of the tourniquet method is therefore highly recommended. After completion of the anastomosis its adequacy should be ascertained with use of Doppler ultrasonography and a completion angiography. If significant stenosis is present after restoration of blood flow, immediate correction by incorporation of a short autogenous vein patch should be performed during the same operation.

Failure to correct a stenosis will, in fact, result in ultimate jeopardy of the bypass.

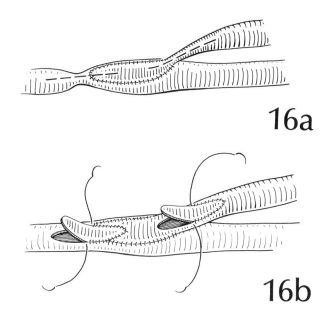

Intimal dissection distal to anastomosis

17 Thromboendarterectomy at the peripheral artery–graft junction should be avoided if possible. Intimal dissection is a frequent disorder which often causes graft thrombosis. This usually develops only after blood flow has been restored for a considerable time and is thus often overlooked during intraoperative completion angiography. Dissected intima should be removed and the remaining intima tightly opposed to the media. Two or three double-ended monofilament sutures (polypropylene 7/0) can be used to tack the intima to the media and be tied on the outside of the artery wall.

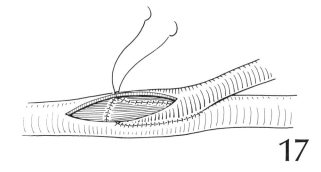

Superficial arteriovenous fistulae

A serious problem connected with the *in situ* technique is the presence of multiple arteriovenous fistulae. In the first week after operation painful inflammation and pulsating swelling like cellulitis may occur along the course of the vein graft on the medial side of the thigh and lower leg. Diagnosis and therapy are simple. The smaller superficial fistulae which exit mainly into the subdermal areas generally undergo spontaneous thrombosis by the development of phlebitis, so treatment is not necessary. The larger fistulae risk production of painful skin necrosis with the danger of infection.

Auscultation over these spots reveals a typical continuous machine-like murmur and a noticeable thrill can be palpated. Digital examinations of the vein combined with Doppler ultrasonography may detect the exact site of these fistulae, which can, if necessary, be interrupted in the postoperative period on an outpatient basis under local anaesthesia.

Late graft stenosis and occlusion

Longitudinal studies[4–6] have emphasized the importance of on-going graft surveillance to detect impending graft closure. An acute graft occlusion beyond the sixth postoperative month will usually result in a complete ischaemic syndrome of the extremity and should be treated, if possible, within a few hours. After thrombectomy, the cause of occlusion is to be discovered and the type of surgical reconstruction can be determined accordingly. Correction of graft defects result in much improved secondary patency and limb salvage.

When a late or neglected thrombosis of an *in situ* bypass occurs, the bypass wall becomes thick and oedematous and the lumen string-like. It is not possible to remove the thrombus and the use of a balloon catheter will usually result in splitting of the wall and its destruction. Surgical correction will almost always fail at this point.

Graft surveillance

Graft surveillance is performed in this clinic by duplex scanning using an ATL Ultramark IX scanner to prevent graft thrombosis. All patients are first examined at the time of discharge from the hospital. Follow-up intervals are gradually extended to 1 year. If a significant stenosis is present it is relieved using a short autologous vein patch or a balloon angioplasty.

Outcome

Properly performed, the *in situ* bypass can deliver excellent results, especially when used as a long bypass to infrageniculate vessels. *In situ* bypasses to the above-knee popliteal artery are probably no better than reversed vein bypasses as there is little vein actually left *in situ* in this situation. However, excellent graft patency rates are not achieved without constant graft surveillance and a high reoperation rate as evidenced by the marked difference between primary and secondary graft patencies.

Recently published data[4–6], as listed in *Table 1*, indicate the need for a graft surveillance programme with duplex scanning. Thus, excellent patency results and corresponding limb salvage rates can be achieved.

As with any surgical technique, there is undoubtedly a learning phase for *in situ* bypass. This procedure requires great care, patience, attention to detail and meticulous surgical technique. It should not be undertaken without appropriate training. In experienced hands, *in situ* bypass is a valuable technique, especially when performed in patients with critical ischaemia.

Table 1 Overall cumulative primary and secondary patency for critical limb ischaemia

Author	Year	Primary		Secondary	
		1	3	1	3
Bandyk et al.[4]	1987	74	58	86	80
Shanik et al.[5]	1989	74	70	86	83
Donaldson et al.[6]	1991	81	76	86	83

Values are percentages

References

1. Porter JM. *In situ* versus reversed vein graft: is one superior? *J Vasc Surg* 1988; 7: 79–80.

2. Bush HL, Graber JH, Jakubowski JA, Hong SL, McCabe M, Deykin D et al. Favourable balance of prostacyclin and tromboxane A2 improves early patency of human *in situ* vein grafts. *J Vasc Surg* 1984; 1: 149–59.

3. Leather RP, Karmody AM, Corson JD, Shah DM. The saphenous vein as a graft and as an *in situ* arterial bypass. In: Sawyer PN ed. *Modern Vascular Grafts*. New York: McGraw-Hill, 1987: 133–52.

4. Bandyk DF, Kaebnick HW, Stewart GW, Towne JB. Durability of the *in situ* saphenous vein arterial bypass: a comparison of primary and secondary patency. *J Vasc Surg* 1987; 5: 256–68.

5. Shanik GD, Moore DJ, Feeley TM. The value and limitations of *in situ* bypass: realistic expectations. In: Veith FJ, ed. *Current Critical Problems in Vascular Surgery*. St Louis: Quality Medical Publications 1989: 34–9.

6. Donaldson MC, Mannick JA, Wittemore AD. Femoro-distal bypass with *in situ* greater saphenous vein. Long-term results using the Mills valvulotome. *Ann Surg* 1991; 213: 457–65.

Femorodistal reversed vein bypass

D. Bergqvist MD, PhD
Professor, Department of Surgery, University Hospital, Uppsala, Sweden

T. Mätzsch MD, PhD
Associate Professor, Department of Surgery, Lund University, Malmö General Hospital, Malmö, Sweden

History

Reconstructive surgery for femoropopliteal occlusive disease, most commonly caused by arteriosclerosis, is the most commonly performed procedure in peripheral vascular surgery. A great step forward was taken by Kunlin[1], who used autologous vein as a bypass graft for superficial femoral artery occlusions, although reversed vein grafts had already been used after trauma during World War I. For many years the use of reversed vein dominated, but since the mid 1970s the *in situ* technique has increasingly been performed. Both techniques have pros and cons, and discussion of them can be vivid and aggressive. Few randomized studies have compared *in situ* and reversed vein bypass, and with the use of optimal techniques for both there seems to be little difference in outcome in terms of long-term patency. This discussion will not be further addressed here, and for analysis of results the reader is referred to Taylor and Porter[2] and Calligaro *et al*[3]. In addition to being used by some surgeons as first choice of treatment, knowledge of the reversed technique is needed when it is impossible to perform an *in situ* bypass.

Principles and justification

Whenever possible, the authors' preference is the *in situ* technique. The choice of whether to use the *in situ* technique or a reversed autologous vein grafting procedure depends on several factors. If the ipsilateral vein is missing because of previous variceal or other surgery, is unsuitable due to extensive varicosities, or is too small in calibre, the need for alternative conduits arises.

If the procedure aims at reconstruction on a crural level, i.e. below the popliteal artery, the reversed vein bypass is less suitable because of difficulties in harvesting a sufficiently long conduit and of discrepancies in luminal size between the proximal reversed vein segment and the small calibre arterial vessels in the lower leg.

Indications

The main clinical indications are intermittent claudication, chronic critical leg ischaemia, acute chronic ischaemia and popliteal aneurysm.

Intermittent claudication is a somewhat controversial indication. Some surgeons are fairly liberal, while others are very conservative and perform femorodistal bypass surgery only occasionally when the claudication is disabling. An argument supporting the more conservative approach is the often benign natural course, with increasing walking distance after training and stopping smoking.

Chronic critical leg ischaemia is defined on the basis provided by the Ad Hoc Committee[4] or the Second European Consensus document on chronic critical leg ischaemia[5]. Clinically, this means patients with rest pain, ischaemic ulcers, or frank gangrene.

Acute on chronic ischaemia must be differentiated from embolic disease, where embolectomy often is sufficient. On the other hand, an attempt with a Fogarty catheter in patients with acute on chronic ischaemia will often fail or aggravate the condition. In many cases, thrombolysis and balloon angioplasty will solve the problem; in others a bypass procedure is necessary.

Preoperative

Assessment and preparation

In addition to measurements of ankle–brachial index and toe pressure, preoperative assessment should always include angiography. Attention is directed towards acceptable run-in and run-off conditions. A poor run-in with significant atherosclerotic lesions in the suprainguinal segment will jeopardize the patency of the bypass, as will an inadequate run-off. Assessment of the run-off must be made with caution, as at times the arteries distal to an occlusion and the continuity of the pedal arch may not be visualized on the arteriogram due to poor contrast filling of the vessels if proper care is not taken during arteriography. A 'blind' popliteal segment, however, is not a contraindication to this type of operation.

Assessment of the vein is also important. Gross varicosities constitute a contraindication, but limited variceal sacculae can be accepted and corrected during operation. A vein less than 4 mm in diameter is less suitable for use as a bypass. If doubts concerning the quality of the vein arise, mapping with duplex ultrasonography can be helpful. Preoperative investigation of the vein should always be performed with the patient standing in order to achieve sufficient filling of the vein.

The patient should be prepared with a whole body scrub using a chlorhexidine-containing soap in order to minimize the risk of infection that is increased whenever performing a groin incision. For this reason, antibiotic cover is also provided. The antibiotic chosen should be active against *Staphylococcus epidermidis*, as this is the most commonly encountered organism in graft infections. If the extremity has overt gangrene, it has been recommended that antibiotics should be chosen according to the organisms identified in cultures of the gangrenous area.

Anaesthesia

General, spinal or epidural anaesthesia can be used.

Operation

Position of patient

The lower abdomen, groin and both legs are prepared
and draped. The foot is placed in a sterile plastic bag in
order to make inspection possible during the operation.
A small cushion under the knee allows easier access to
the popliteal artery. Special attention is directed
towards the heel of the foot; during the operation and
for as long as epidural or spinal analgesia is provided, a
pad should be in place to prevent pressure necrosis.

Skin incision

1a, b For exposure of the proximal saphenous
vein and common femoral artery, a
laterally convex incision lateral to the vessels is
preferred in order to minimize damage to the lymphatic
vessels. For exposure of the popliteal artery proximal to
the knee, the incision is placed just above the femoral
epicondyle and two fingerbreadths behind the femur
along the anterior border of the sartorius muscle. For
exposure of the distal popliteal artery, the 10–15-cm
incision is placed just behind the tibial margin.

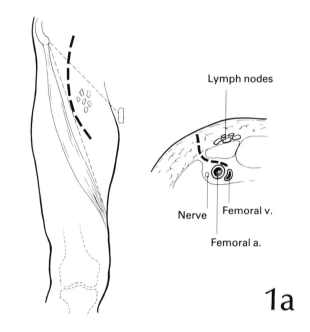

Lymph nodes

Nerve   Femoral v.

Femoral a.

1a

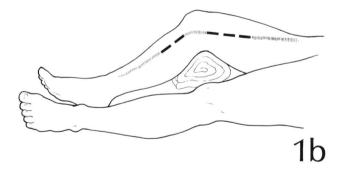

1b

Groin dissection

2   A slightly arched incision just lateral of the femoral artery is preferred to a vertical one above the artery in order to avoid damage to the lymph nodes or vessels, which could lead to prolonged lymphorrhoea or infection. A separate fascial incision over the saphenous vein at the foramen ovale about one fingerbreadth below and lateral to the pubic tubercle also helps to maintain the lymphatics intact. Utmost care must be taken not to create undue skin flaps in order to minimize risk of skin edge necrosis and infection, which may be disastrous for the reconstruction, the leg and the patient.

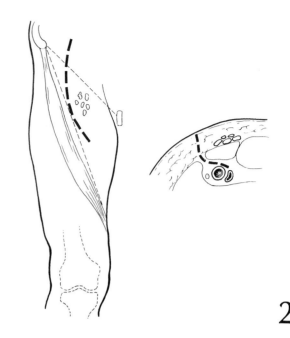

2

3a, b   The femoral artery and its branches are exposed, controlled and taped.

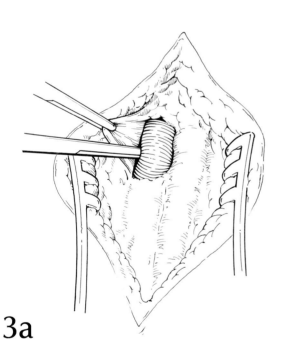

3a

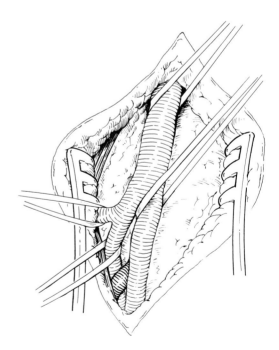

3b

Preparing the site of distal anastomosis

4a—d Before the vein is freed and prepared, the recipient artery should be dissected and checked for patency and suitability for anastomosis. If the distal anastomosis is to be placed at the proximal popliteal artery, an incision just above the femoral epicondyle and behind the medial edge of the femur is chosen. This is usually also the location of the saphenous vein, so care must be taken not to injure it during dissection. The incision is extended through the adductor fascia, and the artery is gently mobilized and held with soft rubber tapes. Major branches are preserved.

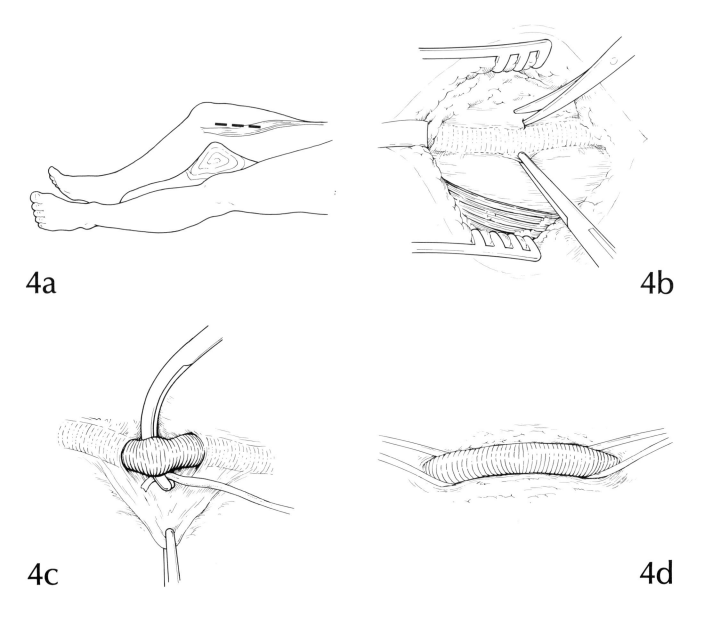

4a

4b

4c

4d

5a, b If the distal anastomosis is to be at the distal popliteal artery, an incision behind the tibial margin is chosen. The saphenous vein runs in close proximity to this incision and is easily injured if care is not taken. The fascia is divided 1–2 cm behind the tibial edge and the gastrocnemius muscle is retracted backwards. The tendons of the hamstring muscles must sometimes be divided, which can be done without risk. The popliteal artery, vein and nerve are found in the fatty tissue of the popliteal fossa. Usually there are two veins with the artery in between, which makes careful dissection necessary in order to avoid troublesome bleeding. The approach is made easier if a cushion is placed under the distal thigh. The artery should be mobilized to the point where it enters the soleus muscle and branches off into the tibiofibular trunk, and the anterior tibial artery. It is secured with rubber tapes and checked for suitability as a recipient artery.

Access to the crural vessels is described in detail on page 49.

6a, b The saphenous vein is divided and the proximal stump suture ligated at its junction with the femoral vein. All small tributaries are ligated with 4/0 non-resorbable material near the vein and with resorbable material on the peripheral side.

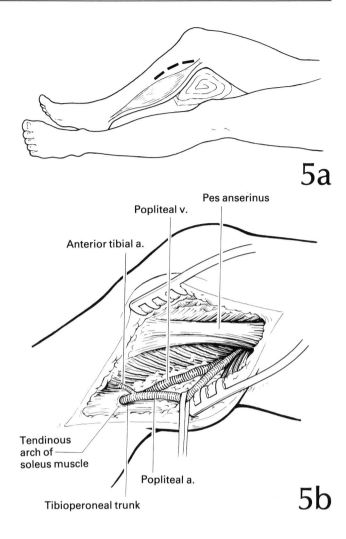

5a

Pes anserinus

Popliteal v.

Anterior tibial a.

Tendinous arch of soleus muscle

Popliteal a.

Tibioperoneal trunk

5b

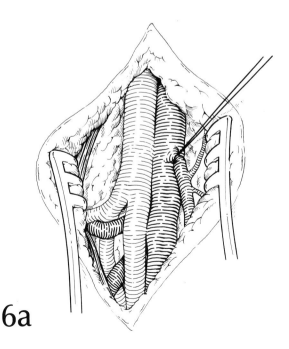

6a

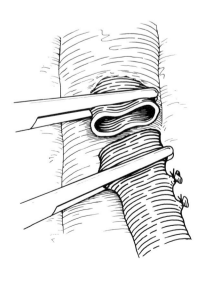

6b

7 The ligatures should be placed neither too near the saphenous vein nor too peripheral in order to avoid narrowing of the vein lumen or blind stumps where thrombosis will occur, which can ultimately progress and cause acute graft occlusion or distal embolization.

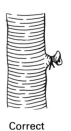 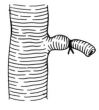 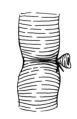

Correct   Wrong – too long   Wrong – too close

7

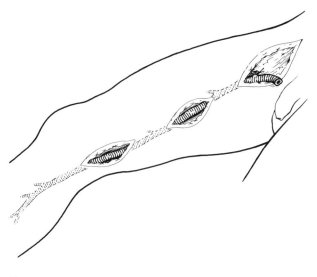

Freeing the vein

8 Using either multiple short incisions or one continuous incision along the vein, it is dissected free with all branches tied off and divided as described. Creating flaps or superficially undermined areas must be avoided at all times and hence a continuous incision that is sequentially extended distally with respect to the course of the vein is preferred. This method also minimizes the risk of undue tension on the vein, which must be avoided. The vein should be handled with utmost care at all times and desiccation prevented by frequent irrigation.

8

Use of short saphenous vein or arm veins

In cases where the long saphenous vein is absent due to earlier surgery or unsuitable as a conduit, the short saphenous vein or arm veins can be used as alternatives.

Harvesting the short saphenous vein

Ideally, the patient is placed in the prone position while the vein is dissected. This necessitates repositioning of the patient during operation, which can be cumbersome. With adequate assistance it is not very difficult to make the dissection with the patient supine. By flexion and inward rotation of the hip joint with the knee joint flexed it is also possible to gain access to the vein.

9 The vein is located just behind the lateral malleolus. When freeing the vein, care must be taken not to injure the sural nerve which runs in very close proximity to it.

After locating the vein and the nerve, the incision is extended along the vein up the calf. About halfway between knee and ankle, the vein penetrates the muscular fascia and runs underneath it. All branches are carefully ligated and divided.

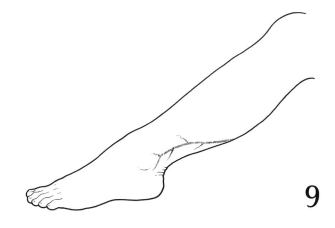

9

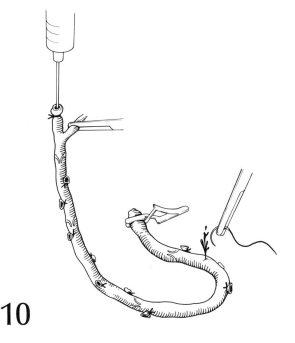

10

10 The short saphenous vein is particularly prone to spasm, which may be counteracted by irrigation with a solution of papaverine.

When harvesting the short saphenous vein, it is particularly important not to create any undermined skin flaps, in order to avoid skin edge necrosis. After having freed the vein for a sufficient length it is ligated, divided and handled as described for the long saphenous vein on page 318. The skin incision should be closed immediately.

Harvesting arm veins

11a–d If no other options for obtaining an autologous vein are available, the veins of the arm can be utilized. For this purpose, the patient's arm must be prepared and draped so that it can be moved freely. A separate table supporting the arm is preferable.

The cephalic vein can be harvested from the radial side of the wrist to the confluence with the subclavian vein in the deltoid–pectoral triangle. The basilic vein is less suitable for harvesting as it disappears underneath the fascia shortly above the elbow. Techniques have been described for using both the cephalic and the basilic vein as one conduit[6].

The main drawbacks of using arm veins as conduits are the great anatomical variations in size and conformation and the abundant branches. The arm veins are also very adherent to the skin, making dissection more difficult. The use of arm veins however, should always be considered if no other possibilities exist for obtaining an autologous vein graft.

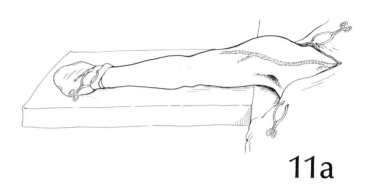

11a

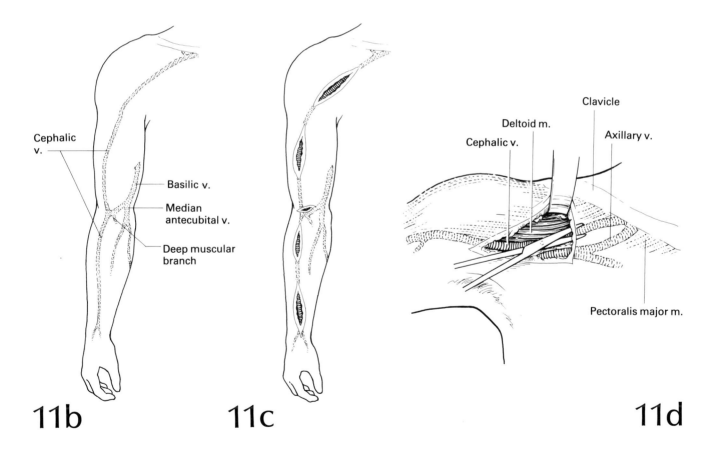

11b   **11c**   **11d**

Distension of vein and checking for leakage

12a, b After the vein has been dissected free it is curved through 180° and flushed (preferably) with cold heparinized blood. Pure saline solution is not optimal, but balanced salt and albumin solutions containing heparin and papaverine may be used as an alternative. In order to avoid damage to the endothelium the vein should never be distended above a pressure of about 200 mmHg – a pressure that is very easily achieved with a syringe if care is not taken. If papaverine has been used for relaxation of a contracted vein, it is particularly vulnerable to increased pressure.

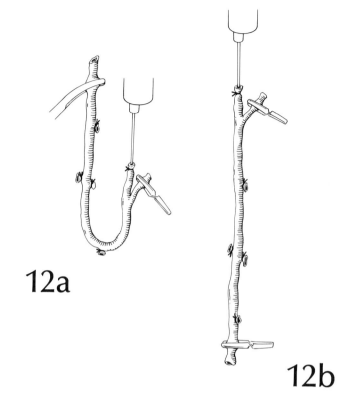

12a

12b

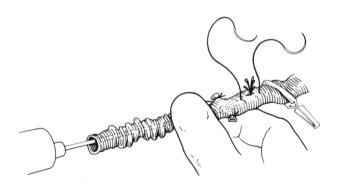

13

13 The vein is checked for points of leakage from divided and missed branches which, if present, are carefully sutured with a fine (8/0) monofilament. Luminal narrowing must be avoided. Magnification glasses (2.5 ×) are very useful for this step.

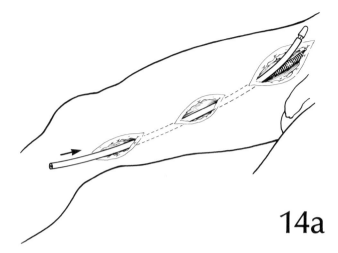

14a

Tunnelling

14a–c The vein is placed in a tunnel, preferably along the superficial femoral artery or subcutaneously. The tunnel is created with a tunneller, a curved steel tube containing a rod with has a coned end. The tunneller is passed from the point of the distal anastomosis subfascially to the groin incision. If the distal anastomosis is below the knee, care is taken to ensure that the tunneller is passed laterally to the medial tendons of the gastrocnemius. The end of the vein is attached to a pair of long grasping forceps after the rod has been removed, and pulled through the steel tube. Utmost care must be taken in order not to twist the vein as it is passed through the tube. The tunneller is then removed.

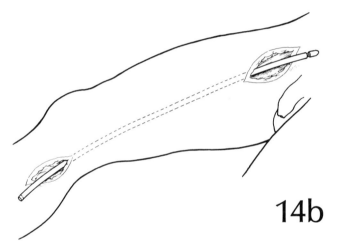

14b

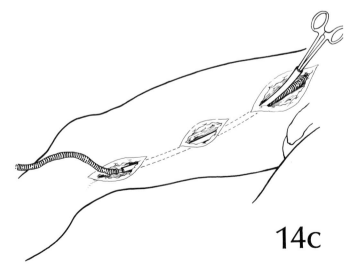

14c

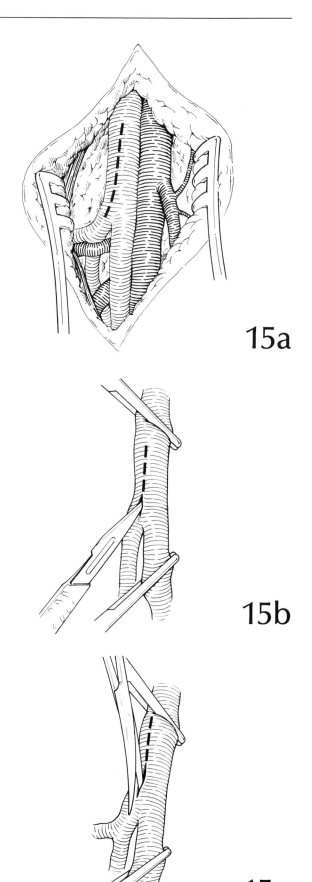

15a

Preparing the artery for anastomosis

15a–c Following systemic heparinization, the exposed common, superficial and deep femoral artery in the groin are clamped with vascular, atraumatic clamps. An arteriotomy is made as a stab incision in the common femoral artery with a number 11 scalpel blade. The intima of the posterior wall must be carefully avoided so as to eliminate the risks of intimal dissection and occlusion. The incision is extended with angled Pott's scissors. The distal end of the arteriotomy is placed so that it can be easily extended down into the deep femoral artery if there is a stenosis of the orifice.

15b

15c

Anastomosing the vein to the common femoral artery

16a–e
The end of the vein is cut obliquely to fit the arteriotomy without tension. The suture always begins at the heel with double-ended monofilament sutures. The authors prefer polytetratfluoroethylene (PTFE), which appears to be superior to the stiffer polypropylene sutures in handling. The sutures are always placed from the inside of the artery outwards in order to avoid separation of the thickened intimal layer. The first suture is tied down and the next is placed from the outside of the vein to the inside of the artery to form a continuous suture. Great attention is paid to avoid causing narrowing of the heel. This is avoided if the first two stitches are placed along the axis of the artery. A continuous suture is inserted for about half the length of the arteriotomy, and the same procedure is repeated on the other side. A second suture is then passed from the inside through the vein and artery at the toe of the arteriotomy, tied down and completed continuously to join the other two sutures where it is tied.

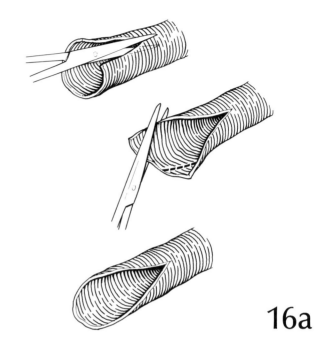

16a

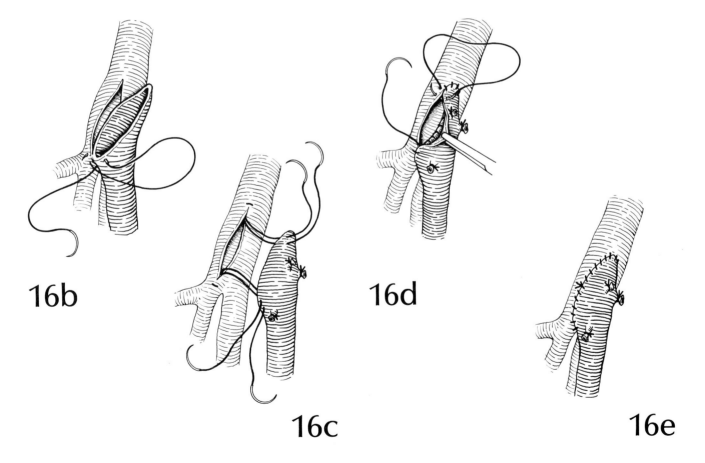

16b

16c

16d

16e

Completion of the anastomosis

17 Before the anastomosis is completed and the last two or three sutures are placed, adequate back-flow and down-flow are checked by briefly opening the clamps. The anastomosis is then irrigated with heparinized saline (5000 units in 0.51 sodium chloride). The anastomosis is completed and the flow in the artery re-established while the vein is clamped just distal to the anastomosis. Minor bleeding from the anastomosis will mostly stop after applying a dry swab for a few minutes.

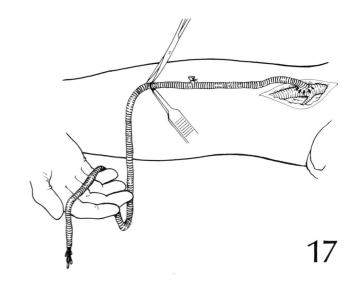

17

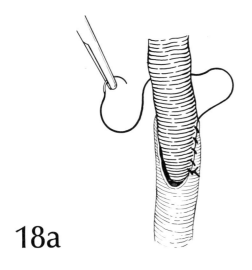

18a

Distal anastomosis

18a, b After an arteriotomy in either the above-knee or below-knee popliteal artery, the vein is trimmed and cut to fit the length of the arteriotomy having extended the knee fully to measure the required length. The anastomosis is performed using the same method as for the proximal anastomosis. Here, care must be taken to avoid narrowing of the distal end of the recipient vessel. If the vessel is of small calibre, three separate sutures should be placed at the toe and tied separately.

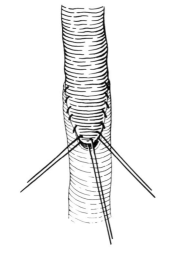

18b

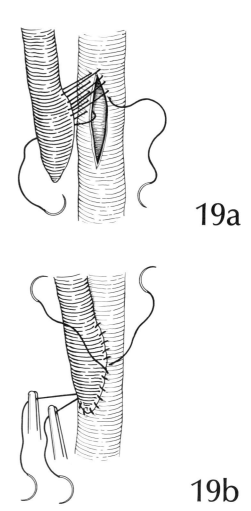

19a

19b

19a, b Alternatively, and if the vessel is located deep with a difficult approach, a parachute or sliding technique may be used for the distal anastomosis at the heel. The first stitch is made slightly below the corner of the proximal edge of the arteriotomy. Without tying, the next suture is placed proximal to the first and then the next around the corner of the heel, whereafter it is gently pulled down. Polypropylene monofilament sutures are better suited for this kind of technique than PTFE sutures, as they allow more sutures to be placed before approximation. The sutures may have to be tightened one by one using a nerve hook. In this way every suture can be placed exactly under visual control, even under difficult conditions.

Just before completion of the anastomosis, back-flow and on-flow are tested and the anastomosis is rinsed and irrigated as previously described.

Completion angiography

If there is any question about the function of a distal anastomosis, angiography is performed. This can often be done using a branch that has been saved for this purpose. Contrast medium, 20 ml, is injected and films are taken over the distal anastomosis and distal to it to ensure adequate filling of the recipient vessel.

Wound closure

After haemostasis has been ensured, the skin wounds are closed. The skin edges must be handled gently in order to avoid necrosis and infectious complications.

Errors and complications

Several technical errors are possible during dissection, harvesting and preparation of an autologous vein as a bypass conduit. Most of them will lead to acute or early graft occlusion and must thus be avoided at all times. Some of the most commonly encountered faults and complications and how to avoid them will be summarized.

Pitfalls during dissection and harvesting

20a, b Incorrectly tied branches will lead to either narrowing of the lumen or creation of blind stumps that can act as the origin of progressing thrombosis. The branches should be tied 1–2 mm away from the vein wall or oversewn if too short. One branch near the proximal anastomosis should be kept longer for use when performing completion angiography and tied correctly afterwards.

Rotation of the vein in excess of 90° will cause flow impairment, thrombosis and acute graft failure. This can be prevented by, for example, marking the vein with dye before the tunnelling procedure. Gentle filling of the vein with heparinized blood will also help to reveal any twists.

Undue traction and distension of the vein will cause damage to the endothelium, thus causing denuded and thrombogenic areas.

If the vein is too short it can be lengthened by using either the short saphenous vein or arm veins. If no other alternatives exist, a composite graft can be created by anastomosing a thin-walled 6-mm PTFE graft for the proximal part to the autologous vein graft that is used to make the critical distal anastomosis and to bridge the knee joint. The synthetic graft should be as short as possible. If only a short distance has to be gained, a thromboendarterectomy of the most proximal part of the superficial femoral artery may be enough, making it possible to anastomose the vein more distally than to the common femoral artery.

Numerous errors are possible when performing the anastomosis and in order to avoid these, the reader is referred to the chapter on pp. 51–58. At all times it must be remembered that the key to successful bypass surgery is meticulous technique.

Intraoperative prophylaxis against clot formation

When cross-clamping it is important to avoid blind segments as far as possible and, if such segments occur, to rinse them with heparinized saline and to check that they are free from clots before unclamping. Intravascu-

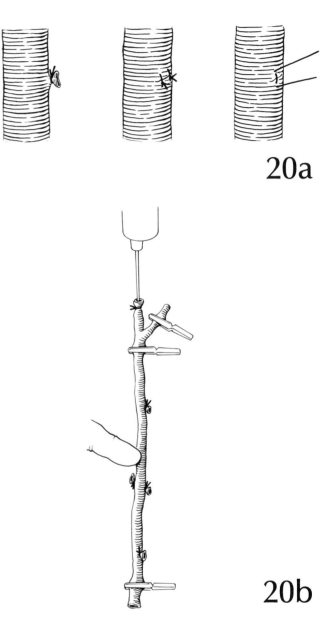

20a

20b

lar clots can be prevented with either dextran or heparin. Dextran, 500 ml, is given as an intravenous infusion during surgery, and this is repeated daily for 2–4 days after operation[7]. In addition to influencing platelet adhesion and clot formation, dextran also has beneficial rheological properties. Most vascular surgeons use heparin given by one of several regimens. Either 5 000 units or a total of 100 units/kg body weight is given at cross-clamping. Some surgeons recommend reversal with protamine sulphate after restoration of flow, using 1–2 mg/100 units heparin.

Postoperative care

Adjuvant therapy

Postoperative graft occlusion is a multifactorial process, and therefore it has proved difficult to study the pharmacological prevention of graft occlusion. The scientific background for practical recommendations is thus rather weak. There seems to be no doubt, however, that continuing smoking increases the risk of graft occlusion. Although difficult, it is important to motivate patients to stop smoking. Various antiplatelet drugs have been tried which appear to be beneficial when started preoperatively, at least in technically difficult femorodistal bypasses. Increasing patency with oral anticoagulants has not been proved. Both oral anticoagulant and antiplatelet drugs seem to increase patient survival.

Follow-up

During the hospital stay, the circulation is frequently checked with pulse palpation and/or Doppler ultrasonography. Routine surveillance after departure from hospital is still a matter of debate, but most vascular surgeons have some form of surveillance programme. Since the introduction of duplex scanning it has become clear that postoperative development of asymptomatic stenotic lesions occurs in both the inflow and outflow tracts and also within the graft, often at the site of the valve cusps. Simple measurement of the ankle–brachial index is not sensitive enough to detect these stenoses at an asymptomatic stage, and the presence of stenoses indicates an increased risk of graft occlusion. The majority of graft stenoses develop during the first year, and there are data indicating that it is possible to increase the overall patency of infrainguinal vein grafts by a systematic surveillance programme with reintervention at the stenotic sections of the graft[8]. Duplex scanning (or digital subtraction angiography) is recommended at least every 3 months during the first year with the first examination performed 3–6 weeks after the operation.

Complications

Early occlusion

Besides poor run-in and run-off, early occlusion of reversed vein grafts (within 30 days) is most often due to technical problems. If some form of measurement of flow or resistance has been made intraoperatively and there is an indication of a high-resistance, low-flow outflow tract, amputation is a reasonable choice following occlusion. If not, a revision procedure is indicated, thereby increasing secondary patency. If occlusion occurs during hospitalization, a technical failure should be suspected. The patient should immediately undergo catheter thrombectomy, followed by mandatory angiography or angioscopy to identify the cause of occlusion and then correct it. If occlusion occurs after 14 days or more, local thrombolysis is probably the most gentle technique that avoids destroying the vein. Thrombolysis is followed angiographically and again revision with either percutaneous angioplasty or a surgical procedure (patch or short-jump bypass) is directed to the cause of the graft occlusion. The longer the time lapse after the primary bypass the more likely it is that balloon angioplasty will succeed. Early in the postoperative course a graft stenosis will be too elastic and recur immediately. Simple Fogarty catheter thrombectomy is not often very successful in vein graft occlusions, which is one reason for instituting an aggressive surveillance programme to detect stenoses before occlusion occur.

References

1. Kunlin J. Le traiment de l'artérite oblitérante par la greffe veineuse. *Arch Mal Coeur* 1949; 42: 371–2.

2. Taylor LM, Porter JM. Reversed *vs in situ*: is either the technique of choice for lower extremity vein bypass? *Perspect Vasc Surg* 1988; 1: 35–55.

3. Calligaro KD, Friedell ML, Rollins DL, Semrow CM, Buchbinder D. A comparative review of *in situ* versus reversed vein grafts in the 1980s *Surg Gynecol Obstet* 1991; 172: 247–52.

4. The Ad Hoc Committee on Reporting Standards, Society for Vascular Surgery. Suggested standards for reports dealing with lower extremity ischemia. *J Vasc Surg* 1986; 4: 80–94.

5. Second European Consensus Document on Chronic Critical Leg Ischemia. European Workshop Group on critical leg ischemia. *Circulation* 1991; 84(Suppl 4): 1–26.

6. LoGerfo FW, Paniszyn CW, Menzoian Y. A new arm vein graft for distal bypass. *J Vasc Surg* 1987; 5: 889–91.

7. Rutherford R, Jones DN, Bergentz S-E *et al.* The efficacy of dextran 40 in preventing early postoperative thrombosis following difficult lower extremity bypass. *J Vasc Surg* 1984; 1: 765–73.

8. Harris P. Follow-up after reconstruction arterial surgery. *Eur J Vasc Surg* 1991; 5: 369–73.

Polytetrafluoroethylene (PTFE) femorodistal bypass

John H. N. Wolfe MS, FRCS
Consultant Vascular Surgeon, St Mary's Hospital, and Honorary Senior Lecturer, Royal Postgraduate Medical School, Hammersmith Hospital, London, UK

History

When polytetrafluoroethylene (PTFE) became available many surgeons turned to the 'graft on the shelf' from the more demanding vein harvesting techniques. For many years there were proponents for both extended PTFE grafts and vein but there is now conclusive evidence that vein grafts have a better patency rate when the distal anastomosis is below the knee. In fact, prosthetic grafts perform so poorly in the infrapopliteal segment (10–60% 12-month patency, average 40%[1]) that many surgeons believe these operations should probably not be attempted in the absence of vein[2]. Unfortunately, patients requiring bypass grafts may have already lost the long saphenous vein during previous coronary or peripheral arterial surgery. Many authorities have emphasized the fact that there is now good evidence to suggest that arm and short saphenous veins are useful alternatives to the long saphenous vein[3]. Indeed, some claim that with such a policy it is never necessary to insert a prosthetic graft to the infrapopliteal arteries. There are, however, many surgeons who are unable to find sufficient lengths of vein to perform a femorocrural graft in some of these patients with end stage arterial disease and multiple previous reconstructions. In patients with critical ischaemia the current primary amputation rate at the author's hospital is 3% and one-third of reconstructions are to the crural arteries; 20% of the patients no longer have adequate lengths of autologous vein. There is therefore a great need to develop techniques that might improve the results of femorocrural grafts with extended PTFE.

The reasons for the discrepancy between vein and prosthetic graft patency at the crural level are complex and controversial, but must include the increased thrombogenicity of the prosthetic material. Anastomosing the rigid, large diameter PTFE to a small diameter tibial vessel is also difficult. If these were the only explanations for the increased rate of failures it might be expected that all prosthetic graft failures would occur in the perioperative period rather than the months following operation. However, several centres have identified that the rate of formation and incidence of stenotic myointimal hyperplasia in the distal vessel is greater with PTFE than with vein grafts[4].

Principles and justification

Indications

Only patients with critical ischaemia should be considered for femorocrural grafting with PTFE. In the presence of critical ischaemia, however, there are rarely technical contraindications. Providing there is a segment of healthy crural artery, reconstruction should be considered. While the presence of a pedal arch is of great benefit, its absence does not preclude successful surgery. The major decision for the surgeon is whether a successful bypass will improve the quality of life and mobility of the patient, as some patients are already totally dependent upon nursing support.

Preoperative

It is particularly important to evaluate the other major vascular beds in these patients (i.e. cerebral, coronary and renal), as patients with severe femorodistal disease frequently have widespread atherosclerosis. When considering the leg itself, clinical evaluation supported with Doppler pressures can be performed at the bedside and pulse generated run-off can be of assistance when no signal can be found in any of the three vessels. These data will support the information obtained from a good angiogram, which must not only show the vessels in the full length of the calf, but also in the foot. Inadequate angiography has been the cause of failure to revascularize legs in many patients.

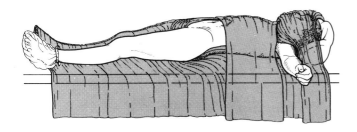

1

1 Areas of ulceration and gangrene should be cleansed as far as possible and the patient started on antibiotics with the premedication (cefuroxime 750 mg three times daily with the addition of metronidazole if there is skin breakdown is used by the author). General anaesthesia is usually the most appropriate. The patient is then draped so that the aorta and iliac arteries can be exposed should an unexpected proximal procedure be required. The full leg is exposed with the foot in a transparent bag so that the effects of revascularization are immediately apparent.

Operation

Exposure of vessels

Principles of vessel exposure

When performing an anastomosis to a crural vessel minor technical errors can result in disaster. The vessel should be dissected out under magnification with extreme care. The venae comitantes can be dissected and teased off the artery and then tied or clipped with a Ligaclip. Diathermy should not, however, be used since this can damage the artery indirectly. The author considers that a long arteriotomy is an essential feature for a successful PTFE bypass at this level and therefore a sufficiently long length of artery must be exposed. This will almost certainly necessitate the dissection of small perforating branches. These should not be tied or damaged because they may be an important contribution to 'run-off'. Once the vessel has been exposed, 1 ml of papaverine (20 mg) should be dripped onto the artery and left while proceeding with other aspects of the operation. The surgeon will hopefully then find that the crural artery has dilated considerably when the time comes to perform the arteriotomy for the distal anastomosis. No clamps should be applied to these crural arteries and slight traction on a Silastic loop is sufficient to control the blood flow. An endarterectomy should never be performed and dilators should never be used, because these will inevitably destroy the intima. For the same reason great care should be taken never to insert catheters of any type except under very specific circumstances.

Exposure of femoral artery

The femoral artery is exposed as described on pp. 41–43 in the chapter on 'Exposure of major blood vessels'.

Exposure of the posterior tibial artery

The proximal third of the posterior tibial artery is easily approached by a low popliteal fossa incision (see pp. 49–50 in the chapter on 'Exposure of major blood vessels'). By taking down the tibial head of the soleus the tibioperoneal trunk is exposed and thus the posterior tibial artery beyond it. The middle third of the posterior tibial artery is deep within the calf musculature and its exposure is not advisable unless this is the only healthy segment of artery. It can be a deep and damaging dissection for the calf muscles. The author's preference is to dissect out the posterior tibial artery in the lower third of the calf where it is close to the surface between flexor digitorum longus muscle anteriorly and flexor hallucis longus muscle posteriorly. In the lower third of the calf this is a simple exposure but with any of the crural arteries great care must be taken with the venae comitantes.

Exposure of the anterior tibial artery

The origin of the anterior tibial artery in the lower popliteal fossa is readily exposed by taking down the tibial head of the soleus. Anastomosis to this segment of the artery is, however, difficult and fraught with problems, as the arteriotomy cannot be extended more distally because the artery disappears beneath the tibia and through the tibioperoneal membrane. The artery can be exposed in its proximal third in the anterior compartment through an incision one finger's breadth lateral to the tibia by dissecting between the tibialis anterior and extensor digitorum longus muscles. The middle third of the artery is again rather deep behind the musculature and, for preference, is exposed in the tendinous lower third of the leg where it lies between the tendons of extensor digitorum longus and tibialis anterior muscles. At this level the exposure is simple but the same proviso pertains to the venae comitantes.

Exposure of the peroneal artery

2, 3 The peroneal artery can be readily exposed from the medial side of the lower third of the calf but this is not the exposure of choice when using a PTFE graft. The best approach is laterally. An incision is made over the fibula and deepened until the bone is exposed. A periosteal elevator is then used to strip the periosteum from the bone, taking great care to ensure that the instrument remains in the correct layer, because otherwise the underlying peroneal artery can be damaged. The segment of fibula is then resected using a ring bladed rib cutter. Following this the peroneal vessels are visible in the wound and the artery should be carefully dissected from the surrounding venae comitantes (which are particularly troublesome around the peroneal artery).

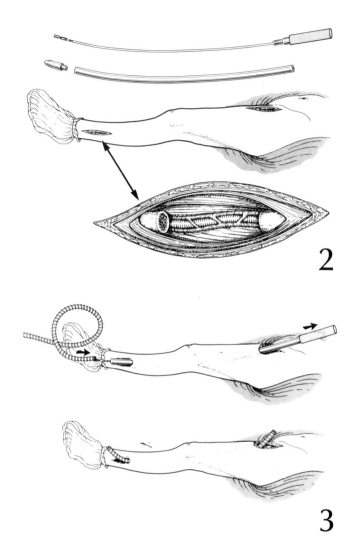

2

3

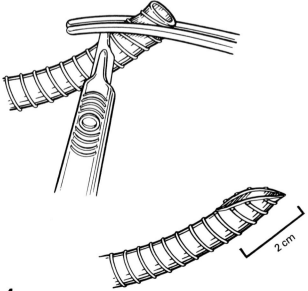

4

Proximal anastomosis

4 The proximal anastomosis should be straight-forward. The PTFE is cut obliquely; in order to cut it cleanly rather than crushing it with scissors, forceps can be applied and a scalpel used to shave the PTFE along the forceps.

5a, b

A 5/0 polypropylene suture is then used to perform a parachute technique anastomosis, starting and finishing at the widest diameter of the arteriotomy.

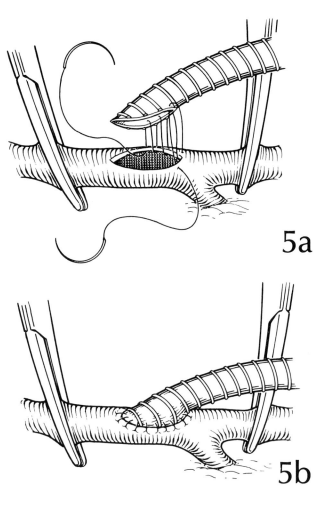

5a

5b

Distal anastomosis

Various techniques have been used for this and the author's opinion of their merits and problems is presented here.

Direct PTFE to artery anastomosis

When PTFE is anastomosed directly to artery there is inevitable distortion of the artery by the rigid PTFE[5]. Furthermore, intimal hyperplasia occurs between PTFE and the small recipient crural artery and these two factors probably lead to the very high occlusion rate when this technique is used in crural arteries.

Composite PTFE vein graft

This technique overcomes the problems at the distal anastomosis but the data suggest that myointimal hyperplasia occurs between the PTFE and vein. Since this is an oblique end-to-end anastomosis between the PTFE and vein there is no capacious conduit to accommodate the inevitable myointimal hyperplasia, which might explain why these grafts are little better than PTFE alone in the experience of most surgeons.

Linton patch

6

This technique has been used by many surgeons in the past and is useful on larger calibre vessels. In the author's experience, however, it is a difficult and inadequate technique when used on a 1.5–2.0-mm crural vessel. Having patched the vessel, it is difficult to incise the vein patch and anastomose the PTFE onto this without producing a technical error. Furthermore, the distance between the PTFE–vein anastomosis and vein–artery anastomosis is extremely small.

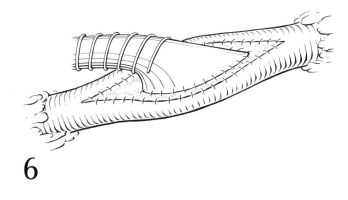

6

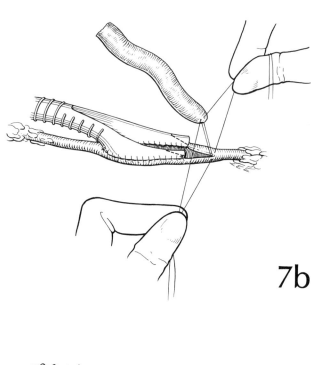

7a

Taylor patch

7a–c This has been shown to be an extremely successful technique which can be attributed to both the compliant vein segment and the length of the anastomosis in the crural artery (greater than 2 cm). It does not, however, address the problem of intimal hyperplasia developing at the heel where PTFE abuts directly onto the small recipient artery. When an anastomosis is performed to a crural vessel the proximal flow into the calf vessels and collaterals is an essential component of success, and if this back flow is low the peripheral resistance may increase sufficiently for the graft to fail.

7b

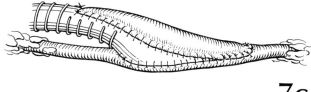

7c

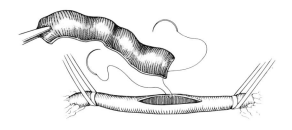

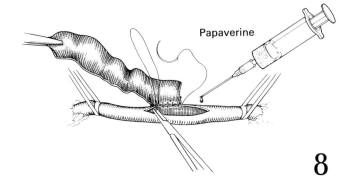

Papaverine

8

Miller collar

8, 9 The author has used this technique with some
success for PTFE grafts running the full length
of the leg to the ankle but the collar is an oval cushion
and lacks the haemodynamic elegance of the Taylor
patch. The considerable turbulence in the collar
probably predisposes the graft to medium-term failure.

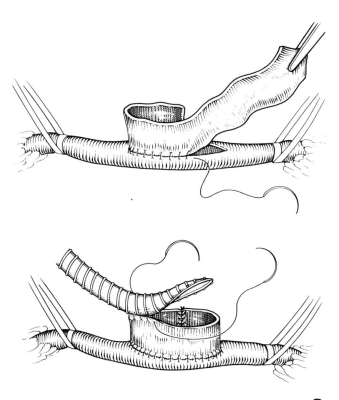

9

NEW PROSTHETIC VENOUS BOOT ANASTOMOTIC TECHNIQUE COMBINING THE BEST OF OTHER PROCEDURES

10 A segment of vein is used to form a long interposition boot between PTFE and artery. A 5–6-cm length of vein is harvested from a suitable site (frequently it is necessary to use arm vein if all other available vein has been previously used). This segment of vein is then slit down its longitudinal axis to yield a venous rectangular sheet.

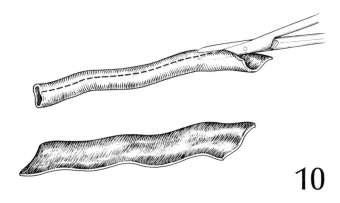

10

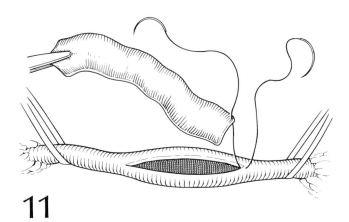

11

11 An arteriotomy is performed in the crural vessel which should be at least 2 cm in length – the length of this incision may be part of the reason for the success of this procedure. There should be an excess of vein available so that mosquito forceps can be applied to one end in order to anchor and control the vein segment while the anastomosis is being performed. Magnification loupes are essential when performing an accurate anastomosis. The distal edge of the vein is anastomosed to the apex of the arteriotomy using a 7/0 polypropylene suture. The distal edge of the vein is then anastomosed to one side of the arteriotomy using the shorter end of the double ended suture.

12 The far edge of the venous sheet is then draped around the arteriotomy and sewn down with the longer end of the double ended suture. Great care must be taken to ensure that there is no nipping at the heel of the suture line, as proximal flow is as important as distal flow in these very distal grafts. By positioning the mosquito forceps (which are holding the distal edge of the venous sheet) correctly it is possible to align the anastomosis without difficulty so that the assistant can concentrate on the anastomosis itself.

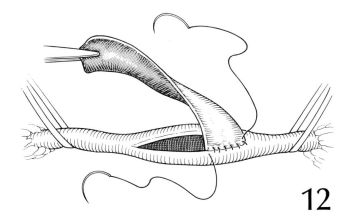

12

13 The venous sheet is then anastomosed along the anterior edge until eventually the sutures meet the first corner of the graft. Redundant vein is resected using a pair of Potts scissors. At this stage it is essential that the two suture ends are tied in order to secure the suture line between vein and artery. The shorter end is then cut and the longer suture used to sew the vein boot to itself.

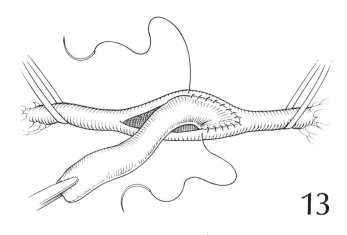

13

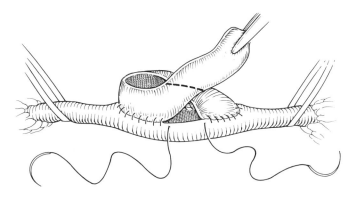

14

14, 15 The boot is then completed by cutting back the heel in order to allow the PTFE graft to be anastomosed to the collar at a 30° angle to the artery.

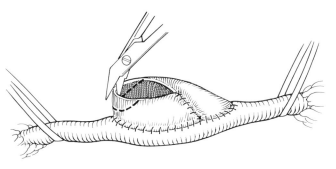

15

16 With magnification and a set routine this anastomosis becomes straightforward. It also has the advantage that the completed anastomosis can be readily inspected to ensure that it is technically satisfactory. Once the boot is complete the anastomosis between PTFE and vein is quite simple.

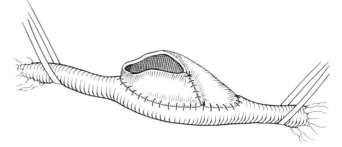

16

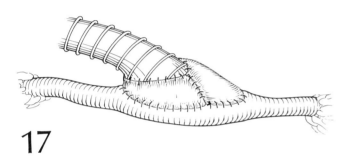

17

17 There is the theoretical risk that a weak vein will blow out, but this has only occurred on one occasion in the author's experience and he is happy to use arm veins for the venous boot. The sheet of vein should be kept under slight tension while the anastomosis is being performed – if it is allowed to contract too much then the collar is too baggy under arterial pressure. It is important that the PTFE is cut to the correct length because any tension between vein collar and PTFE (as with any anastomosis) would lead to tearing of the vein at the anastomosis. This technique does, however, have the slight advantage that there is a very small amount of play between PTFE and the venous boot so that any slight movements resulting from changes in the leg position do not affect the artery directly.

Myointimal hyperplasia eventually starts to develop between PTFE and vein collar but spares the distal artery so that the graft continues to function.

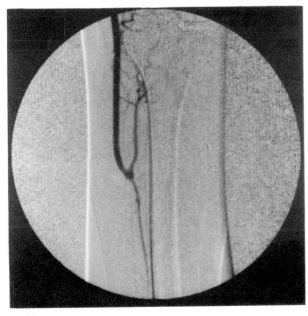

18

18 An intravenous angiogram of a venous boot patch on a bypass to the anterior tibial artery is shown.

Postoperative care

After the operation the wound should be dressed with soft dressings and Netelast; no sticky tape should be used. The patient can be mobilized after 24 h and should remain on subcutaneous heparin (5000 units twice daily) while in hospital. Following this either long-term aspirin or long-term anticoagulation with warfarin is given, depending on the patient's ability to comply with an anticoagulant regime.

References

1. Michaels JA. Choice of material for above-knee femoropopliteal bypass graft. *Br J Surg* 1989; 76: 7–14.

2. Bell PRF. Are distal vascular procedures worthwhile? *Br J Surg* 1985; 72: 335.

3. Stipa S. The cephalic and basilic veins in peripheral arterial reconstructive surgery. *Ann Surg* 1972; 175: 581–7.

4. DeWeese JA. Anastomotic intimal hyperplasia. In: Sawyer PN, Kaplitt NJ, eds. *Vascular Grafts*. New York: Appleton-Century-Crofts, 1978: 147–52.

5. Tyrrell MR, Chester JF, Vipond MN, Clarke GH, Taylor RS, Wolfe JHN. Experimental evidence to support the use of interposition vein collars/patches in distal PTFE anastomoses. *Eur J Vasc Surg* 1990; 4: 95–101.

Illustrations by Mark Iley

Composite sequential bypass graft

William H. Pearce MD
Associate Professor of Surgery, Division of Vascular Surgery, Department of Surgery, Northwestern University Medical School, Chicago, Illinois, USA

Walter J. McCarthy MD
Assistant Professor of Surgery, Division of Vascular Surgery, Department of Surgery, Northwestern University Medical School, Chicago, Illinois, USA

William R. Flinn MD
Associate Professor of Surgery, Division of Vascular Surgery, Department of Surgery, Northwestern University Medical School, Chicago, Illinois, USA

James S. T. Yao MD, PhD
Magerstadt Professor of Surgery, Division of Vascular Surgery, Department of Surgery, Northwestern University Medical School, Chicago, Illinois, USA

History

The composite sequential bypass is one of a number of surgical options for the treatment of limb-threatening ischaemia of the lower extremity. While it is generally agreed that an all-autogenous venous distal bypass is superior to other techniques, vascular surgeons frequently face situations in which the saphenous vein is inadequate[1-3]. These situations occur after failed previous venous bypasses of the lower extremity, coronary artery bypass surgery and venous disease. In these cases the choice is between an all-prosthetic bypass or a composite graft. Several series report disappointing long-term patency with all-prosthetic bypasses to tibial vessels. In the Veterans Administration Cooperative Study the 2-year patency for femoro-tibioperoneal bypasses was 30%, and in the multicentre study by Veith *et al.* the 4-year patency for femorotibial polytetrafluoroethylene (PTFE) grafting was 12%[4-6]. Chronic anticoagulation may increase patency. However, no randomized study has yet been performed.

A composite graft offers a potential alternative to an all-prosthetic bypass. The critical bending area of the knee is crossed by a venous conduit better able to tolerate low flow. The composite graft may be constructed either by a direct end-to-end anastomosis between the prosthetic graft and the vein, or as a composite sequential in which the prosthetic graft is initially sewn to the native vessel with a jump graft to the distal tibial vessel. A straight composite femoro-popliteal graft has had variable long-term patency

ranging from 16% to 63% (6 years)[7-9]. This experience is limited to femoropopliteal bypasses and does not include tibial vessels. In comparison with an all-prosthetic bypass there is no statistical difference in patency[7].

In 1971 DeLaurentis and Friedmann first described the composite sequential bypass by grafting to an open popliteal vessel with a saphenous vein jump graft to the distal patent vessel[10]. Later, enthusiasm for this bypass was reported by Bliss and Fonseka[11] and Flinn *et al.*[12]. In a recent review by McCarthy *et al.* the 4-year patency of a composite sequential bypass was 40% at 4 years, with a limb salvage of 70% without anticoagulation[13]. In this detailed review there was no difference in the long-term patency of grafts whether the intermediate popliteal anastomosis was above or below the knee. While this did not reach statistical significance, there was an apparent difference in patency of 72% for an intermediate anastomosis above the knee compared with 46% for those patients with anastomoses below the knee. In addition, this review also points out the utility of the short saphenous vein. In this series of 67 patients the short saphenous vein was used in ten patients and segments of the long saphenous vein in 57 patients. As Rutherford *et al.* have pointed out, many long segments of patent long saphenous vein may be present in limbs where a partial harvest has been performed[14]. Duplex venous mapping before surgery is helpful in locating usable vein segments.

Principles and justification

The composite sequential bypass is indicated in all patients with limb-threatening ischaemia who do not have sufficient vein for an all-autogenous bypass to the tibial vessels. Every attempt should be made to avoid a long prosthetic tibial bypass. Upper extremity veins may be harvested and used for lower extremity bypasses[15]. Multiple segments of long saphenous, short saphenous and upper extremity veins may be spliced together to form conduits long enough for femorotibial bypasses. Alternative inflow sites will shorten the length of graft required. In selected patients the deep femoral, superficial femoral or popliteal artery may provide adequate inflow for a distal bypass[16, 17]. Finally, a bypass to an isolated popliteal segment may restore sufficient distal arterial flow to relieve the rest pain and potentially heal small arterial ulcers[18, 19]. The composite sequential bypass is indicated because it is difficult to assess the adequacy of collateral outflow from an isolated popliteal segment and predict with any degree of accuracy the healing of larger ulcers. Instead of relying upon the geniculate collaterals to reconstitute the tibial vessels, a direct bypass is made from the prosthetic graft to the tibial vessels providing pulsatile arterial flow to the foot.

Operation

Standard operative exposures are used for the common femoral, popliteal and tibial arteries. All grafts are placed in anatomical locations rather than in subcutaneous tunnels.

Above-knee anastomosis

1 If the popliteal artery is patent, the authors' preference is to use the above-knee popliteal segment for the intermediate anastomosis so that the venous conduit will cross the knee to the tibial anastomosis.

Below-knee anastomosis

2 An alternative configuration if the above-knee segment of the popliteal artery is occluded is illustrated. An external supported PTFE graft may be used in this location. Occasionally, a popliteal artery endarterectomy is needed to enhance outflow, but is not recommended for occluded vessels.

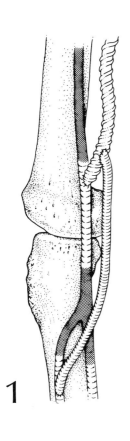

1

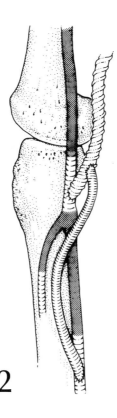

2

Harvesting short saphenous vein

3 The short saphenous vein is often suitable for the distal segment of the composite sequential graft. It is harvested from the ipsilateral leg. The vein is identified midway between the lateral malleolus and the Achilles tendon; with the leg elevated by the assistant, the vein is dissected to the popliteal fossa. Occasionally the vein continues into the mid-thigh. In the authors' experience it is unnecessary to place the patient prone to remove the vein. As it is difficult to assess the short saphenous vein on physical examination, it is mapped before surgery in all patients considered for a composite sequential bypass.

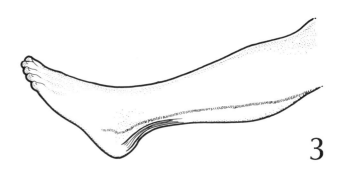

3

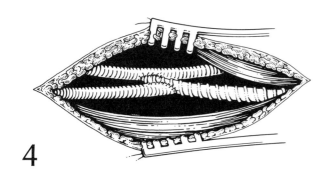

4

Intermediate anastomosis

4 After heparinization the proximal and distal anastomoses are completed simultaneously by separate operating surgeons. The intermediate popliteal anastomosis is constructed using a standard end-to-side technique. The venous–PTFE anastomosis is performed as close to the popliteal anastomosis as possible. A small portion of the PTFE graft is excised and a long venous hood is placed directly over the previous prosthetic popliteal artery anastomosis. This location of the venous–prosthetic anastomosis maximizes arterial flow through the prosthetic segment, much as is described for axillofemorofemoral bypasses. It is important to extend the leg to determine the length of the venous graft.

At the completion of the procedure angioscopy and arteriography are performed. The distal and intermediate anastomoses may be visualized with a single femoral injection of contrast medium. Rarely, the venous limb is not visualized because flow may be directed preferentially into the popliteal artery. By clamping the prosthetic graft distal to the venous anastomosis, the distal venous anastomosis is visualized. Surprisingly, while most of the blood may flow into the popliteal artery, flow in the vein graft can be demonstrated with either a Doppler or magnetic flow probe.

Outcome

The experience at Northwestern University McGaw Medical Center comprised 67 consecutive composite sequential bypasses in 62 patients. Indications were: rest pain, 57%; ulceration, 27%; and gangrene, 16%. The composite sequential bypass was the primary procedure in 30 patients and the secondary procedure in the remainder; 53% of the patients were maintained on chronic warfarin anticoagulation. The intermediate anastomosis was to the above-knee popliteal artery in 44 cases and below-knee in 23 cases. The venous graft was harvested from the short saphenous vein in ten patients and from portions of the long saphenous or other veins in the remainder. The follow-up ranged from 1 month to 91 months (mean 33 months). Using life table analysis primary patency was 72% at 1 year, 64% at 2 years, 48% at 3 years, and 40% at 4 years. Overall limb salvage was 84% at 2 years and 70% at 4 years. There were no operative deaths and two significant wound infections. In analysing a variety of different factors, including run-off score, vein diameter and coagulation status, none appeared to affect long-term patency. There was no statistical difference in the patency of above-knee and below-knee intermediate anastomoses, but there was clearly a trend (72% *versus* 46%).

In summary, the composite sequential bypass for long leg bypasses appears to be a durable solution in patients with inadequate venous conduit. The authors' preference remains the use of an all-autogenous vein bypass, when possible, to revascularize the tibial vessels. However, when long venous segments are not available the composite sequential bypass is used. In order to perform this procedure an open popliteal segment, either above the knee or below the knee, is required. Satisfactory long-term patency and limb salvage is achievable.

References

1. Leather RP, Shah DM, Chang BB, Kaufman JL. Resurrection of the *in situ* saphenous vein bypass: 1000 cases later. *Ann Surg* 1988; 208: 435–42.

2. Taylor LM, Edwards JM, Porter JM, Phinney ES. Reversed vein bypass to infrapopliteal arteries: modern results are superior to or equivalent to *in situ* bypass for patency and for vein utilization. *Ann Surg* 1987; 205: 90–7.

3. Calligaro KD, Friedell ML, Rollins DL, Semrow CM, Buchbinder D. A comparative review of *in situ* versus reversed vein grafts in the 1980s. *Surg Gynecol Obstet* 1991; 172: 247–52.

4. Brandt B, Corson JD, Curl GR, Jamil Z, Person PF, McKaroun M. Comparative evaluation of prosthetic, reversed, and *in situ* vein bypass grafts in distal popliteal and tibial–peroneal revascularization. *Arch Surg* 1988; 123: 434–8.

5. Veith FJ, Gupta SK, Ascer E, White-Flores S, Sanson RH, Scher LA. Six-year prospective multicenter randomized comparison of autologous saphenous vein and expanded polytetrafluoroethylene grafts in infrainguinal arterial reconstructions. *J Vasc Surg* 1986; 3: 104–14.

6. Bergan JJ, Veith FJ, Bernhard VM, Yao JST, Flinn WR, Gupta SK. Randomization of autogenous vein and polytetrafluoroethylene grafts in femoral–distal reconstruction. *Surgery* 1982; 92: 921–30.

7. LaSalle AJ, Brewster DC, Corson JD, Darling RC. Femoro-popliteal composite bypass grafts: current status. *Surgery* 1982; 92: 36–9.

8. Dale WA, Pridgen WR, Shoulders HH. Failure of composite (Teflon and vein) grafting in small human arteries. *Surgery* 1962; 51: 258–62.

9. Scribner RG, Beare JP, Harris EJ, Sydorak GR, Tawes RL, Brown WH. Polytetrafluoroethylene vein composite grafts across the knee. *Surg Gynecol Obstet* 1983; 157: 237–41.

10. DeLaurentis DA, Friedmann P. Arterial reconstruction about and below the knee: another look. *Am J Surg* 1971; 121: 392–7.

11. Bliss BP, Fonseka N. 'Hitch-hike' grafts for limb salvage in peripheral arterial disease. *Br J Surg* 1976; 63: 562–4.

12. Flinn WR, Flanigan DP, Verta MJ Jr, Bergan JJ, Yao JST. Sequential femoral–tibial bypass for severe limb ischemia. *Surgery* 1980; 88: 357–65.

13. McCarthy WJ, Pearce WH, Flinn WR, McGee GS, Wang R, Yao JST. Long-term evaluation of composite sequential bypass for limb-threatening ischemia. *J Vasc Surg* 1992; 15: 761–70.

14. Rutherford RB, Sawyer JD, Jones DN. The fate of residual saphenous vein after partial removal or ligation. *J Vasc Surg* 1990; 12: 422–8.

15. Harris RW, Andros G, Dulawa LB, Oblath RW, Salles-Cunha SX, Apyan R. Successful long-term limb salvage using cephalic vein bypass grafts. *Ann Surg* 1984; 200: 785–91.

16. Veith FJ, Gupta SK, Samson RH, Flores SW, Janko G, Scher LA. Superficial femoral and popliteal arteries as inflow sites for distal bypasses. *Surgery* 1981; 90: 980–90.

17. Veith FJ, Ascer E, Gupta SK, Flores SW, Sprayregen S, Scher LA. Tibiotibial vein bypass grafts: a new operation for limb salvage. *J Vasc Surg* 1985; 2: 552–7.

18. Brewster DC. Bypass to isolated popliteal artery segment. In: Bergan JJ, Yao JST, eds. *Evaluation and Treatment of Upper and Lower Extremity Circulatory Disorders*. Orlando: Grune and Stratton, 1984: 337–49.

19. Veith FJ, Gupta SK, Daly V. Femoropopliteal bypass to the isolated popliteal segment: is polytetrafluoroethylene graft acceptable? *Surgery* 1981; 89: 296–303.

Reoperations for failed bypass grafts below the inguinal ligament

F. J. Veith MD, FACS
Division of Vascular Surgery, Montefiore Medical Center, Albert Einstein College of Medicine, New York, USA

Principles and justification

Arterial reconstructions for limb ischaemia include axillofemoral and femorofemoral procedures and infrainguinal bypass grafts. All these bypass grafts may fail because of thrombus or progressive atherosclerosis. As a result of graft failure, many patients will develop disabling or limb-threatening ischaemia. Appropriate management of this condition has become an important aspect of vascular surgery, and a committed vascular surgeon needs to be familiar with the various techniques available to reverse the ischaemia. This chapter discusses strategies of management with a specific emphasis on repeated vascular surgery.

Indications

In general, arterial reconstructions should rarely be performed for intermittent claudication[1]. This attitude, however, is not universal and present practice accepts 'truly disabling' claudication as an indication for primary arterial reconstruction to at least the popliteal level. In contrast, almost all vascular surgeons would currently tend to avoid secondary arterial operations for intermittent claudication. Thus gangrene, a non-healing ischaemic ulcer or severe rest pain should be the indications for most *secondary* arterial reconstructions, especially those below the inguinal ligament.

Aetiology

Early failure (within 30 days)

The original operation can thrombose or fail within the early postoperative period. Generally this is because of a technical flaw in the operation or the poor choice of inflow or outflow sites. In addition, thrombosis may occur for no apparent reason, presumably because of the inherent thrombogenicity of the graft in a low flow setting. Usually this occurs only with polytetrafluoroethylene (PTFE) and other prosthetic grafts, but rarely it can also occur with a vein graft. A transient fall in cardiac output, hypotension or increased coagulability can contribute to such unexplained thrombosis. Additionally, the original operation, although technically satisfactory and associated with a patent bypass graft, can fail to provide haemodynamic improvement sufficient to relieve the patient's symptoms. This, in turn, can be because of the choice of the wrong operation, e.g. the performance of an aortofemoral bypass in a patient whose femoral artery pressure was normal and who actually needed a femoropopliteal bypass. Such haemodynamic failure could also occur in the presence of multisegment disease and extensive foot gangrene or infection. In this setting, uninterrupted arterial circulation to the foot may be required and a primary or secondary sequential bypass may be indicated.

Late failure (after 30 days)

Delayed failure can be due to some of the factors already mentioned. However, it is usually due to the development of some flow-reducing lesion within the bypass graft or its inflow or outflow tract. Intimal hyperplasia is a prominent cause of failure and graft thrombosis. When this does occur, it usually produces infrainguinal graft failure between 2 and 18 months after operation[2]. It can involve any portion of a vein graft in a focal or diffuse manner and either the anastomosis of the vein or prosthetic grafts. Because the lumen of the distal artery is smaller, this site is most vulnerable to flow reduction by this process. Progression of the atherosclerotic disease process involving the inflow or outflow tract of the arterial reconstruction becomes the predominant cause of failure and graft thrombosis and often accounts for graft failure over the 18-month period.

After 3–4 years a variety of other degenerative lesions can also afflict autogenous and umbilical vein grafts[3]. These processes, which are rare in autogenous but extremely common in umbilical vein grafts, can lead to wall changes and aneurysm formation with thrombosis or embolization.

Recurrent ischaemic signs and symptoms can occur because of haemodynamic deterioration in patients with a previous arterial reconstruction without concomitant thrombosis of the bypass graft[4–6]. We have referred to this condition as a 'failing graft' because, if the lesion is not corrected, graft thrombosis will almost certainly occur. The majority of these failing grafts are vein grafts,

but approximately one-third are PTFE or Dacron grafts. Invariably the corrective procedure is simpler than the secondary operation that would be required if the bypass went on to thrombose. Many lesions responsible for failing grafts could be remedied by percutaneous transluminal angioplasty, although some require vein patch angioplasty, a short bypass of a graft lesion or a proximal or distal graft extension.

Operations

Early failure (within 30 days of operation)

If the primary operation was for limb salvage indications, early graft failure or thrombosis will always be associated with a renewed threat or even a worse threat to the limb. If the original preoperative arteriogram was satisfactory, repeat arteriography is not performed. The patient is given intravenous heparin and returned to the operating room as expeditiously as possible. Since vein grafts can be injured by the ischaemia associated with intraluminal clot and since it may be more difficult to remove solid thrombotic material from these grafts, a patient with a failed autogenous vein graft requires reoperation more urgently than a patient with a PTFE graft. In any event, reoperation should be undertaken within 12 h of the detection of failure. Even greater urgency is required if calf muscle tenderness or neurological changes are associated with graft failure.

REOPERATION ON OCCLUDED VEIN GRAFTS

The distal incision of the arterial reconstruction is reopened. The graft thrombosis is confirmed by palpation. Control of the artery proximal and distal to the distal anastomosis is obtained and a full anticoagulating dose of intravenous heparin (7500 units) is given.

Distal anastomosis

1 A linear incision is made in the hood of the graft to visualize the interior of the distal anastomosis.

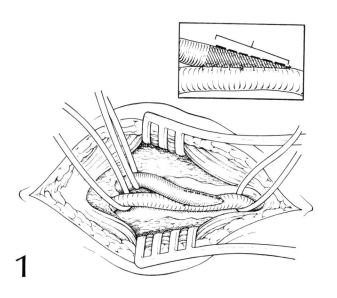

1

Thrombectomy

2   Balloon catheters are gently passed retrograde in the graft to remove clot. If necessary, clot is removed from the proximal and distal adjacent host artery in a similar manner and any visualized anastomotic defect is repaired.

Proximal anastomosis

Valves in the vein graft may prevent retrograde passage of the catheter or it may be impossible to restore adequate normal prograde arterial flow through the graft. In either event the proximal incision is opened and the same procedures performed at the proximal anastomosis. With flow restored and all openings in the graft closed with fine running monofilament sutures, an intraoperative arteriogram is performed to visualize the graft and the outflow tract. If no defect is seen, adequacy of the reconstruction and the inflow tract is demonstrated by direct arterial pressure measurements which should reveal no gradient in excess of 15–20 mmHg between the distal end of the graft and the brachial or radial artery. Any gradient in excess of 25 mmHg should be localized to the inflow tract or the graft by appropriate needle placement. If there is a gradient in

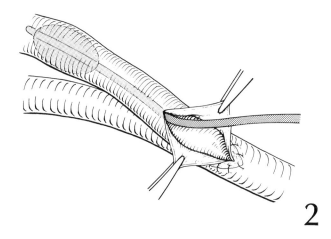

2

the vein graft, it should be eliminated by revision. If this is impossible, the graft should be replaced by a prosthetic PTFE graft. Often such unexplained gradients can be because of recanalized, thrombophlebitic segments of vein. Unless removed, such segments will cause recurrent failure. If an inflow gradient is present, it should be eliminated by a suitable inflow bypass (aortofemoral, femorofemoral or axillofemoral), or occasionally by an intraoperative or postoperative balloon angioplasty.

Graft extension

3   If disease in the outflow tract is detected and is the presumed cause of graft failure, this is generally best treated by an extension to a more distal, less diseased segment of the same or another outflow artery.

If no defect is detected by arteriography or pressure measurements, the procedure is terminated. Despite previous evidence to the contrary, an occasional vein graft will undergo early failure for no apparent reason and will remain patent indefinitely after simple thrombectomy. Unexplained thrombosis may perhaps be because of undetected decreased cardiac output with hypotension and decreased arterial flow.

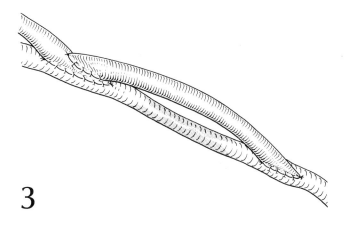

3

Patch angioplasty

4   Stenosis just distal to the anastomosis can be caused by an unrecognized atherosclerotic lesion. This can be corrected by extending the graft incision distally across its apex and down the recipient artery until its lumen is no longer narrowed. A patch of PTFE or vein is then inserted across the stenosis to widen the lumen. Similar treatment is appropriate for intimal hyperplasia which may cause late graft occlusion.

REOPERATIONS FOR OCCLUDED PTFE AND OTHER PROSTHETIC GRAFTS

Early thrombosis of PTFE grafts is managed in essentially the same fashion as already described for early failure of vein grafts. Differences include the almost complete freedom from graft defects as a cause of failure, although occasionally a PTFE graft will be compressed, kinked or twisted because of poor tunnelling technique and malpositioning around or through some of the tendinous structures in the region of the knee. In addition, graft thrombosis for no apparent reason is more common with PTFE grafts than vein grafts. Simple thrombectomy of the graft using the techniques described above has resulted in patency rates in excess of 50% after 3 years, if no other defect was found and if the distal end of the graft was above the knee joint[2, 7].

Late failure (1 month or more after operation)

Patients with presumed late graft failure should undergo a standard transfemoral or translumbar arteriogram with visualization of all arteries from the renal arteries to those of the forefoot. If a failing graft is found, it is urgently treated with reintervention as already discussed. If a failed or thrombosed graft is present, the patient is not subjected to reinterventional treatment unless the limb is unequivocally threatened. Patients with recurrent severe ischaemia, however, require reoperation. The standard surgical approaches to arteries in patients who have undergone previous failed bypasses are often rendered more difficult or even impossible to use because of surgical scarring and/or infection. For this reason a variety of surgical approaches to all the infrainguinal arteries have been developed which allow these vessels to be approached through unoperated tissue planes[8]. These approaches can be helpful in avoiding scarred standard access routes and can be essential if a previous operation has been complicated by infection.

Preparation

The availability of remaining autogenous veins such as short saphenous vein, cephalic vein or accessory great saphenous vein can be assessed by duplex scanning.

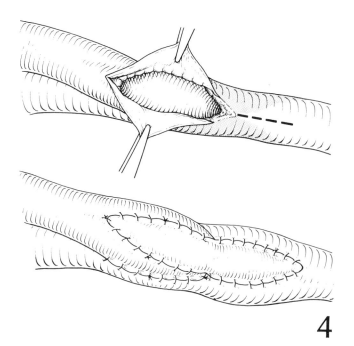

4

Duplex ultrasonography can also be helpful in predicting the length and diameter of usable upper or lower extremity venous segments. Venography is also indicated before surgery in patients who have previously undergone a prosthetic bypass. Often the greater saphenous vein in such cases has been damaged at the first operation or by scarring.

REOPERATION FOR INFLOW

The deep femoral artery has been widely advocated as an outflow site for aortofemoral or axillofemoral bypasses when disease makes the common femoral artery unsuitable. The deep femoral artery has also been used as a site of origin for more distal bypasses when the common femoral artery is diseased or scarred or when autogenous vein length is limited. The standard surgical technique for exposing the deep femoral artery uses a groin incision to identify its origin from the common femoral artery. After the large crossing veins that are frequently present are divided, the deep femoral artery is traced distally as far as necessary.

In the course of caring for a large number of patients requiring secondary arterial reconstructions after failure of one or more previous vascular operations, we realize that gaining surgical access to the common femoral artery and proximal few centimetres of deep femoral artery can be extremely difficult or impossible because of scarring or residual infection. Because of this, and because the more distal portions of the deep femoral artery appear relatively disease-free in many of these patients, we have developed methods to approach the distal parts of this artery directly without the use of a groin incision.

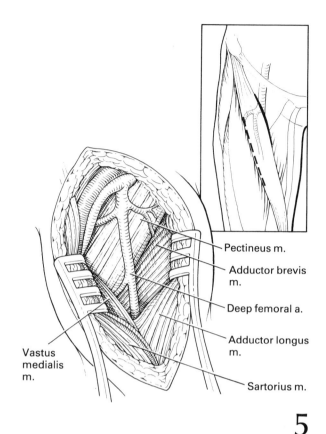

Exposure of distal deep femoral artery

5 An incision is made parallel to either the medial or lateral border of the sartorius muscle. An effort is made to make this incision inferior to any previous surgical scar or infection in the groin. In general, the anteromedial approach along the medial border of the sartorius muscle has been used to access the upper middle zone of the artery. The more anterior approach lateral to the sartorius muscle has been used to access the lower middle and distal zones of the artery. This anterior approach is particularly valuable in patients with postoperative scarring or infection on the medial aspect of the middle third of the thigh. The anterior approach also makes it possible to preserve the blood supply of the sartorius muscle which enters by way of its medial border.

Vastus medialis m.

Pectineus m.

Adductor brevis m.

Deep femoral a.

Adductor longus m.

Sartorius m.

5

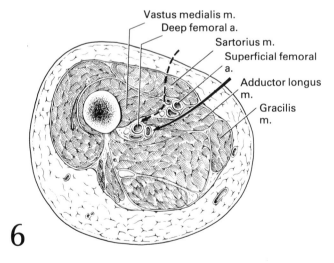

Vastus medialis m.
Deep femoral a.
Sartorius m.
Superficial femoral a.
Adductor longus m.
Gracilis m.

6

6 The incision is deepened beyond the sartorius muscle, and the superficial femoral vascular bundle is mobilized and reflected medially in the anterior approach (dashed arrow) or laterally in the anteromedial approach (solid arrow). This exposes the fibrous connection or dense fascial union between the sheaths of the long adductor and vastus medialis muscles. Incision of this fibrous union for several centimetres exposes the underlying deep femoral vascular structures. Usually a vein is the most superficial of these and bulges forth when the fibrous union between the long adductor and the vastus medialis muscles is incised. Deep to the vein is the deep femoral artery which can be carefully dissected free, avoiding injury to the many small friable branches that arise from this vessel. Self-retaining retraction methods can be helpful in holding apart the deeper layers of the wound to provide adequate exposure.

If the deep femoral artery is not pulsatile, it can easily be located by identifying venous branches deep to the incised fascial junction of the long adductor and vastus medialis muscles. Tracing of these branches to one of the main deep femoral veins will permit localization of the adjacent artery even when it is pulseless and soft. Because the surgeon is working in unoperated tissue planes and with previously undissected vessels, the described approaches to the two distal zones of the deep femoral artery can be accomplished in 5–15 min.

REOPERATION FOR OUTFLOW ARTERY FOR DISTAL ANASTOMOSIS

Lateral approaches to the popliteal artery

Above-knee popliteal artery

7 The popliteal artery above the knee joint is approached with a lateral incision between the iliotibial tract and the biceps femoris muscle. By deepening the incision in the lateral intermuscular septum the popliteal space is entered and the neurovascular bundle can be palpated within the popliteal fat. The popliteal artery is easily isolated from the adjacent popliteal vein or veins, taking care not to injure the common peroneal nerve. After the popliteal artery has been dissected from these structures, gentle traction with silicone vessel loops can elevate it to close to the skin level, where surgical manipulation and anastomosis can be carried out with the same ease as is usual through the standard medial approach.

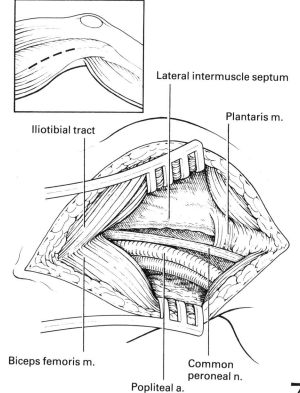

Lateral intermuscle septum

Plantaris m.

Iliotibial tract

Biceps femoris m.

Common peroneal n.

Popliteal a.

7

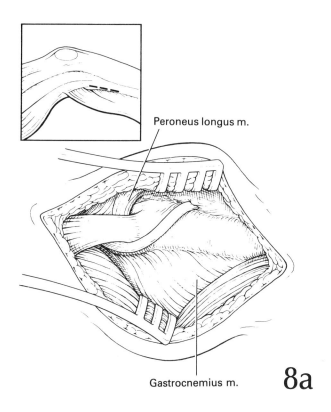

Peroneus longus m.

Gastrocnemius m.   8a

Below-knee popliteal artery

8a, b This is approached by a lateral incision over the head and proximal fourth of the fibula. The incision is deepened through the subcutaneous tissue and superficial muscular attachments to the fibula, taking care to identify the common peroneal nerve as it courses around the neck of this bone. This nerve is dissected free so that it can be retracted and protected from injury. The biceps femoris tendon is divided. The ligamentous attachments of the fibula head are incised and the upper fourth of the fibula freed bluntly from its muscular and ligamentous attachments, staying as close to the bone as possible. A retractor is placed deep to the fibula to protect the underlying structures, and one or two holes are drilled in this bone at its proposed site of transection. With such holes, a rib shears can cleanly transect the bone without leaving sharp spicules. After the bone has been divided, any remaining deep attachments can be exposed and cut. With the upper fibula removed the entire below-knee popliteal artery, tibioperoneal trunk, anterior tibial artery, and the origins of the peroneal and posterior tibial arteries lie just deep to the excised bone and can easily be dissected from their adjacent veins. After mobilization, these arteries are more superficial in the wound than by way of standard medial approaches, and surgical manipulation and anastomotic suturing can be performed with greater ease.

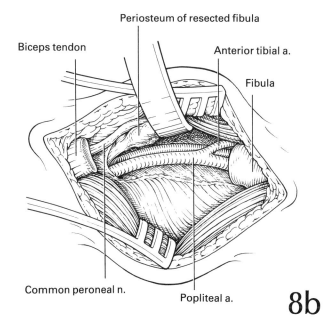

Biceps tendon   Periosteum of resected fibula   Anterior tibial a.   Fibula

Common peroneal n.   Popliteal a.   8b

Tunnelling for grafts

9 To conduct grafts to or from a popliteal artery that is approached laterally, tunnels are constructed in a subcutaneous plane. For grafts from the femoral arteries approached by way of a standard groin incision, the course should be across the anterior aspect of the mid-thigh and then down the lateral aspect of the lower thigh to the popliteal fossa. If the external iliac artery, the axillary artery, or the thoracic aorta provides graft inflow, the tunnel follows a gradual curve from the inflow artery to the lateral aspect of the thigh and then inferiorly to the popliteal fossa.

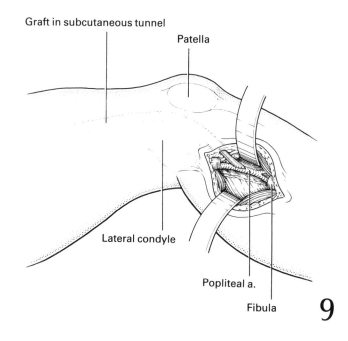

9

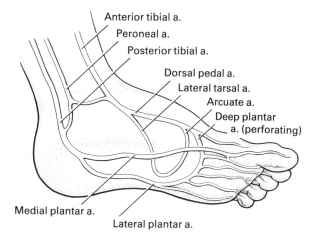

10

Approaches to inframalleolar arteries

10 In the past decade, as more patients have required reoperation with very limited lengths of remaining autogenous vein, we have been forced to perform a variety of bypasses to inframalleolar arteries[9]. These include the posterior tibial and dorsal pedal (dorsalis pedis) arteries below the ankle joint and their main terminal branches. These consist of the medial and lateral plantar branches of the posterior tibial and the lateral tarsal and deep plantar or deep metatarsal arch branches of the dorsal pedal artery.

Exposure of the lateral and medial plantar branches

11a, b The lateral and medial plantar branches are the continuation of the posterior tibial artery in the foot. The lateral plantar artery ends in the main or deep plantar arch and is usually larger than its medial counterpart. The medial branch gives off small collateral vessels to the intrinsic muscles of the first, second and third toes. However, when the lateral branch is occluded the medial branch may enlarge and conjoin with the plantar arch through collateral vessels. The initial skin incision is made sufficiently long to permit exposure of the retromalleolar portion of the posterior tibial artery. It extends inferiorly and laterally onto the sole. After the posterior tibial artery is isolated, the dissection is progressively extended across the sole. A direct approach to the individual branches is not advisable for several reasons. First, the skin of the sole is not easily retracted. Therefore, adequate exposure is difficult to obtain when the incision does not follow the exact course of the arterial branch. Second, these plantar branches tend to lie deep within the foot, and this, coupled with their small diameter, further hinders their localization. Finally, the dissection of the bifurcation of the posterior tibial artery is recommended because it can aid in distinguishing the lateral from the medial plantar branch. Exposure of the proximal 2–3 cm of the plantar branches is accomplished by incision of the flexor retinaculum and transection of the abductor muscle of the great toe. If necessary, more distal exposure of these branches can be obtained by division of the medial border of the plantar aponeurosis and the short flexor muscle of the toes.

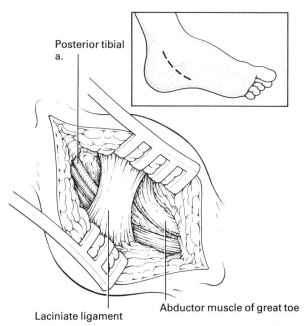

Posterior tibial a.

Laciniate ligament

Abductor muscle of great toe

11a

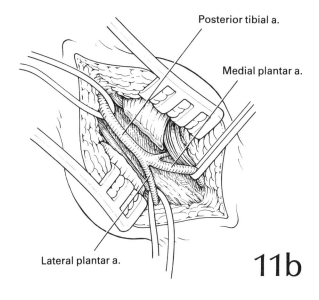

Posterior tibial a.

Medial plantar a.

Lateral plantar a.

11b

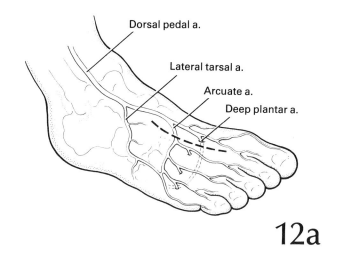

Exposure of the deep plantar or deep metatarsal arch branch

12a–d

The deep plantar branch is the main extension of the dorsal pedal artery. It originates at the metatarsal level, where it descends into a foramen bounded proximally by the dorsal metatarsal ligament, distally by the dorsal interosseous muscle ring, and medially and laterally by the base of the first and second metatarsal bones. As the deep plantar branch exits from this tunnel it connects with the lateral plantar branch to form the deep pedal arch.

A slightly curvilinear longitudinal 3–4-cm incision over the dorsum of the midportion of the foot permits the dissection of the dorsal pedal artery down to its bifurcation into the deep plantar and first dorsal metatarsal branches. The short extensor muscle of the great toe is retracted laterally, or transected if necessary, and the dorsal interosseous muscle ring is split to allow better exposure of the proximal portion of the deep plantar branch. The periosteum of the proximal portion of the second metatarsal bone is then incised and elevated. A fine-tipped rongeur is used to excise enough of the metatarsal shaft to allow for ample exposure of the deep plantar branch.

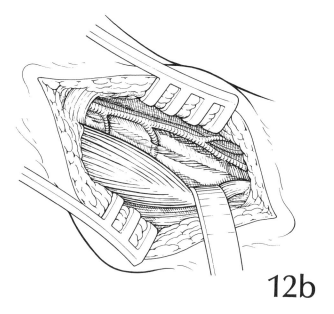

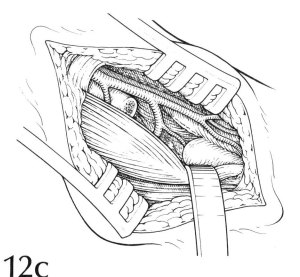

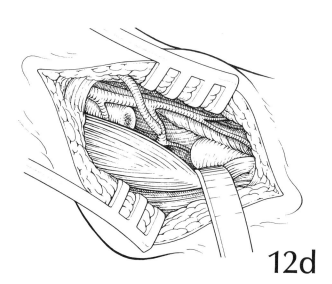

Exposure of the lateral tarsal branch

The lateral tarsal artery arises from the dorsal pedal artery at the level of the navicular bone and runs laterally towards the fifth metatarsal bone and under the short extensor muscle of the toes. This branch is an important source of blood supply to the dorsal aspect of the foot and anastomoses with the arcuate artery of the foot.

To expose the lateral tarsal artery, the dorsal pedal artery is dissected at the level of the ankle joint after division of the inferior extensor retinaculum. Dissection is then continued distally to the origin of the lateral tarsal branch. Further mobilization of the latter artery can be achieved by lateral retraction of the long extensor tendons of the toes and partial incision of the short extensor muscle of the great toe. If additional exposure of the lateral tarsal branch is necessary, division of the first and second long extensor tendons of the toes may be performed.

FEMOROFEMORAL GRAFTS

When failure of femorofemoral grafts occurs, the inflow tract of the graft should be examined with angiography. If significant inflow disease is found, it may be corrected by percutaneous transluminal angioplasty or a new bypass from an alternative site must be performed. If, for example, inflow iliac disease has caused failure of a femorofemoral graft, it can be corrected by percutaneous transluminal angioplasty or an aortobifemoral bypass, or an aortic limb can be brought to the thrombectomized femorofemoral graft.

The same arteriogram should also seek evidence of progression of outflow disease and should define patent distal segments that can be used to bypass such outflow disease if necessary. An example of this would be progression of deep femoral artery disease in a patient for whom that vessel was providing outflow for femorofemoral bypass. In this circumstance the popliteal artery should be evaluated angiographically and thrombectomy of the graft should be followed by a profundaplasty or graft extension to the undiseased deep femoral or popliteal artery.

After suitable arteriographic examination, the patient is subjected to a secondary operation. The graft is opened over the hood or hoods of the distal anastomoses so that the interior of the distal anastomosis can be inspected. In this way a single opening in the graft permits thrombectomy of prosthetic graft, thrombectomy of arteries in one groin, and diagnosis and correction of anastomotic problems at one distal anastomosis. Although occasionally successful, the practice of blind balloon catheter thrombectomy of any distal anastomosis via an opening in the graft remote from the anastomosis is to be condemned. The chance of damage to the anastomosis, intimal injury or plaque disruption in the adjacent artery is too great. While it is true that the anastomosis and its adjacent arteries must be dissected free and controlled and that this procedure may be difficult because of scar, it is clearly worth the effort. If distal anastomotic intimal hyperplasia is detected as the cause of graft failure, it is treated by a graft extension or by incising across the hyperplastic lesion and inserting a patch graft. In the latter circumstance the incision and patch are usually placed across the origin of the deep femoral artery.

If no cause of failure is found on preoperative arteriography or intraoperative inspection, an intraoperative arteriogram is performed. If no defects or partially obstructing lesions are found, as is often the case with these grafts, the reoperative procedure is terminated and good results can be expected.

An alternative approach, which is particularly useful if multiple failures have occurred, is to perform a totally new bypass using undissected arteries. In this regard, the aorta is approached retroperitoneally or the iliac arteries are useful options to provide inflow. The distal portions of the deep femoral artery and the popliteal artery lateral approach are good options to provide inflow.

Acknowledgements

This work was supported by the Manning Foundation and the New York Institute for Vascular Studies.

References

1. Veith FJ, Gupta SK, Samson RH, Scher LA, Feu FC, Weiss P *et al.* Progress in limb salvage by reconstructive arterial surgery combined with new or improved adjunctive procedures. *Ann Surg* 1981; 194: 386–401.

2. Veith FJ, Gupta SK, Daly V. Management of early and late thrombosis of expanded polytetrafluoroethylene (PTFE) femoro-popliteal bypass grafts: favorable prognosis with appropriate reoperation. *Surgery* 1980; 87: 581–7.

3. Szilagyi DE, Elliott JP, Hageman JH, Smith RF, Dall'Olmo CA. Biologic fate of autogenous vein implants as arterial substitutes: clinical, angiographic and histopathologic observations in femoro-popliteal operations for atherosclerosis. *Ann Surg* 1973; 178: 232–46.

4. Veith FJ, Weiser RK, Gupta SK, Ascer E, Scher LA, Samson RH *et al.* Diagnosis and management of failing lower extremity arterial reconstructions prior to graft occlusion. *J Cardiovasc Surg* 1984; 25: 381–4.

5. O'Mara CS, Flinn WR, Johnson ND, Bergan JJ, Yao JST. Recognition and surgical management of patent but hemodynamically failed arterial grafts. *Ann Surg* 1981; 193: 467–76.

6. Smith CR, Green RM, DeWeese JA. Pseudoocclusion of femoro-popliteal bypass grafts. *Circulation* 1983; 68 (Suppl): II88–II93.

7. Ascer E, Collier P, Gupta SK, Veith FJ. Reoperation for polytetrafluoroethylene bypass failure: the importance of distal outflow site and operative technique in determining outcome. *J Vasc Surg* 1987; 5: 298–310.

8. Veith FJ, Ascer E, Nunez A, Wengerter KR, White-Flores S, Gupta SK. Unusual approaches to infrainguinal arteries. *J Cardiovasc Surg* 1987; 28: 58 (Suppl).

9. Ascer E, Veith FJ, Gupta SK. Bypasses to plantar arteries and other tibial branches: an extended approach to limb salvage. *J Vasc Surg* 1988; 8: 434–41.

Illustrations by Mark Iley

Adjuvant arteriovenous fistula

P. L. Harris MD, FRCS
Consultant Vascular Surgeon, Royal Liverpool University Hospital, Liverpool, UK

Principles and justification

Some grafts to small distal vessels may fail because occlusive disease in the recipient artery and peripheral vascular bed impedes the run-off from the graft to an excessive degree. In these circumstances there is a very small volume of flow through the graft and if, as a consequence, blood velocity is reduced below a threshold level, thrombosis will occur. The 'thrombotic threshold velocity'[1] varies according to the type of graft and is higher for prosthetic than for autologous materials. The purpose of an adjuvant arteriovenous fistula constructed at or close to the distal anastomosis is to increase the velocity of blood flow through the graft above thrombotic threshold levels.

Disadvantages

The pressure in the deep veins is increased only slightly by the presence of an adjuvant fistula provided that there is no proximal venous obstruction. Nevertheless, this may be sufficient to accentuate oedema occurring after reconstruction. In addition, there is a possibility that high velocities of blood flow in the graft itself and across the anastomosis may promote greater turbulence and an increased risk of subintimal fibrous hyperplasia in the recipient artery. The interposition of a vein cuff between the graft and the recipient vessels may help to offset this effect, although so far this contention remains unproved.

Indications

Critical limb ischaemia

Construction of an adjuvant arteriovenous fistula is appropriate for patients with critical ischaemia for whom major amputation is the only alternative.

Long prosthetic grafts

Its usefulness is confined mainly to long prosthetic grafts anastomosed to a single tibial vessel. Occasionally it may be considered beneficial to employ an adjuvant fistula with an autologous vein graft, particularly in an attempt to salvage the graft after early postoperative thrombosis.

Poor run-off in the recipient artery or pedal vessels

This may be determined by:

1. Angiography, undertaken either before or during operation.
2. Preoperative pulse-generated run-off measurements[2].
3. Intraoperative measurement of peripheral resistance[3].
4. Direct observation of the vessels at operation.
5. Failure of the bypass despite an adequate inflow and perfect operative technique.

Contraindications

Occluded recipient arteries

Some arterial run-off is essential. Attempts to salvage critically ischaemic limbs by creation of an arteriovenous fistula alone or arterialization of veins have proved unsuccessful.

Occluded deep veins

The deep venous system must be patent and free from postphlebitic change. Superficial veins must not be employed, because to do so leads to localized venous hypertension, impaired wound healing and ulceration.

Restricted inflow

It is essential to ensure that inflow into the graft is unrestricted. Failure to do so results in the development of a pressure gradient under high-flow conditions and impaired peripheral perfusion. Aortoiliac stenosis must therefore be identified by appropriate angiographic or haemodynamic studies and eliminated by balloon angioplasty or open surgery.

Heart failure

It is not advisable to employ an adjuvant arteriovenous fistula in a patient with severely impaired myocardial function, because of the risk of inducing or aggravating heart failure.

Operations

Preparation of the vessels

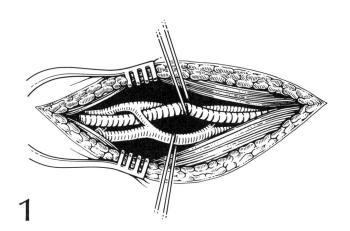

1

1 The selected tibial artery and its largest concomitant vein are carefully dissected out and controlled with narrow latex slings. Clamps must not be applied to these delicate vessels.

COMMON OSTIUM ARTERIOVENOUS FISTULA[4, 5]

2 Longitudinal incisions approximately 15 mm in length are made in the adjacent artery and vein. Small, round-ended atraumatic catheters (not shown) are inserted proximally and distally in the artery and in a proximal direction in the vein to control bleeding and to act as stents during suturing. Adjacent walls of the artery and vein are then sutured together with 7/0 polypropylene to form the common ostium.

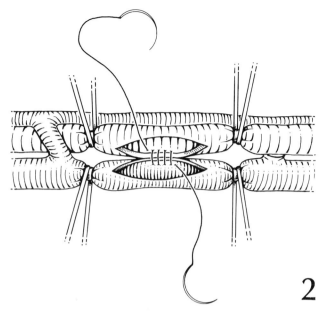

2

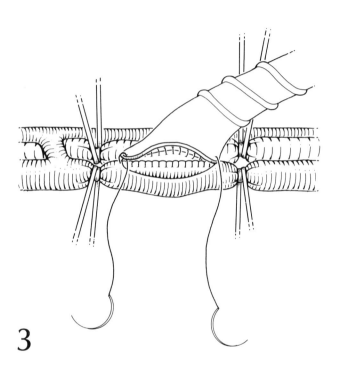

3

Anastomosis of the graft

3 The distal end of the graft is anastomosed to the margins of the common ostium. The intraluminal catheters are removed just before completion, and the anastomosis is thoroughly irrigated with heparinized saline to wash away blood clots.

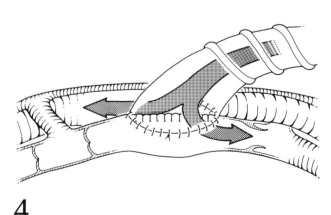

4

4 On restoration of blood flow the presence of a palpable thrill over the anastomosis confirms satisfactory functioning of the fistula. A further check can be made by measuring blood flow through the graft with a Doppler or electromagnetic flow probe. A mean flow in excess of 200 ml/min is to be expected. Experimental studies indicate that normally less than 20% of the flow passes distally into the peripheral arteries[6], the rest being shunted into the veins. There is no evidence that the presence of a fistula in this situation ever 'steals' blood away from the foot.

On-table angiography following completion of the procedure is essential to ensure that all relevant channels are patent. Some surgeons ligate the vein just distal to the fistula to reduce the risk of venous hypertension developing in the distal part of the limb, but there is no objective evidence that this is beneficial.

MODIFIED COMMON OSTIUM ARTERIOVENOUS FISTULA

5 By reducing the size of the venotomy relative to that of the arteriotomy, the size of the fistula may be reduced in order to limit the volume of flow through it. Flows in excess of 750 ml/min are likely to be detrimental[6]. In practice, it is the calibre of the vessels involved rather than the aperture of the fistula that determines flow rates in the case of a common ostium fistula. This modification does, however, simplify the graft-to-artery anastomosis at the toe and heel and may for this reason be beneficial.

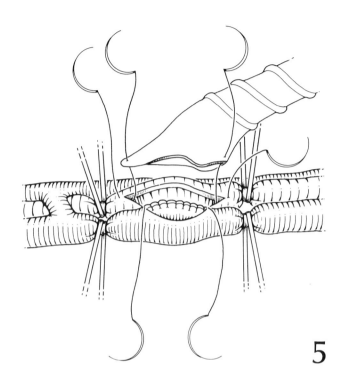

5

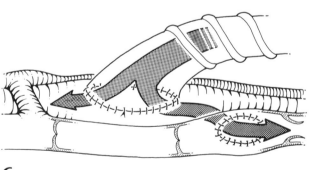
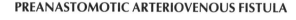

6

PREANASTOMOTIC ARTERIOVENOUS FISTULA

6 The construction of a side-to-side arteriovenous fistula at a point 5–10 mm proximal to the graft-to-artery anastomosis confers the following potential advantages: (1) the intervening segment of natural artery provides resistance to effectively limit the volume of flow through the fistula; (2) the graft-to-artery anastomosis is simplified; (3) the simple form of construction may promote better flow characteristics at the graft-to-artery junction, with less turbulence and a lower risk of myointimal hyperplasia. In practice, the results following common ostium and preanastomotic fistulae are similar.

REMOTE POSTANASTOMOTIC ARTERIOVENOUS FISTULA

7 An arteriovenous fistula that is constructed distal to the graft-to-artery anastomosis has the effect of drawing a larger flow of blood into the artery than the other methods. The major disadvantage is that the perfusion pressure in the vessels distal to the fistula itself is likely to be greatly reduced. For this reason, a fistula of this type should be situated as remotely as possible in the limb. A second problem with this technique is that it may not achieve the primary aim of accelerating blood flow in the graft above thrombotic threshold levels.

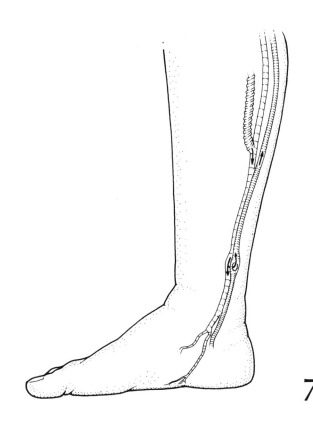

7

Postoperative care

Anticoagulation, which is commenced at operation with a bolus dose of heparin before interruption of blood flow, is maintained after surgery by continuous perfusion. The average dose is 1000 units/h but the dose for specific patients is determined by monitoring appropriate coagulation tests. This regimen is continued for 5 days and in the absence of specific contraindications is followed by long-term oral anticoagulation with warfarin. The addition of low-dose aspirin to reduce the risk of platelet-induced thrombosis may be beneficial and can be given safely in combination with warfarin provided that its potential effect is taken into account when calculating the dose of warfarin. Aspirin therapy is commenced at least 48h before operation and maintained continuously after operation.

The presence of an arterial vein fistula may increase slightly the amount of oedema following the reconstruction. This usually subsides within a period of approximately 8 weeks and during this time the patient should rest frequently with elevation of the limb.

References

1. Sauvage LR, Walker MW, Berger K, Robel SB, Lischko MM, Yates SG *et al*. Current arterial prostheses: experimental evaluation by implantation in the carotid and circumflex coronary arteries of the dog. *Arch Surg* 1979; 114: 687–91.

2. Scott DJA, Beard JD, Farmilo RW, Poskitt KR, Evans JM, Skidmore R. Non-invasive assessment of calf vessels by pressure generated run-off. *Br J Radiol* 1988; 61: 543–4.

3. Ascer E, Veith FJ, Morin L, Lesser ML, Gupta SK, Samson RH *et al*. Components of outflow resistance and their correlation with graft patency of lower extremity arterial reconstructions. *J Vasc Surg* 1984; 1: 817–28.

4. Dardik H, Sussman B, Ibrahim IM, Kahn M, Svaboda J, Mendes D *et al*. Distal arteriovenous fistula as an adjunct to maintaining arterial and graft patency for limb salvage. *Surgery* 1983; 94: 478–86.

5. Harris PL, Campbell H. Adjuvant distal arteriovenous shunt with femorotibial bypass for critical ischaemia. *Br J Surg* 1988; 70: 377–80.

6. Campbell H, How TV, Harris PL. Experimental evaluation of arterial steal in *in-vitro* models of femoro-tibial bypass with adjuvant arteriovenous shunt. *Clin Phys Physiol Measure* 1984; 5: 253–62.

Illustrations by Patrick Elliott

Deep femoral reconstruction

Robert J. Lusby MD, FRCS, FRACS
Professor of Surgery, Department of Surgery, Sydney University, Concord Hospital, Sydney, Australia

Principles and justification

Deep femoral reconstruction effectively opens a stenotic or occluded deep femoral artery with restoration of flow to the main collateral blood supply to the leg. Revascularization of the deep femoral artery can be critical to limb salvage when the superficial femoral artery is occluded. The deep femoral artery, being a supply artery to the thigh, is relatively spared of extensive atheromatous disease. In up to 75% of patients stenosis is limited to the proximal 1–2 cm, often being the result of a continuation of a common femoral artery plaque. In the remaining patients the disease may extend to the next major branch, commonly the lateral circumflex, or first perforating branches. Occasionally, the plaque extends to the second or third perforating branches, so correction requires more extensive exposure and repair.

Indications

Deep femoral reconstruction is commonly performed as an adjunct to a proximal inflow procedure, such as aortofemoral, femorofemoral, or axillofemoral bypass, or to an outflow procedure, such as femoropopliteal bypass or *in situ* femorodistal bypass. Localized procedures are usually limited to high-grade stenotic lesions or short segment occlusions of the common femoral and deep femoral origin. Balloon angioplasty of the iliac and superficial femoral arteries may also be combined with operative deep femoral reconstruction. Stenotic lesions may develop at the distal aortofemoral anastomosis requiring revision surgery with extension of the anastomosis from the common to the deep femoral artery. Occasionally, if graft infection occurs, bypass via an extra-anatomic route to the deep femoral artery may be the most appropriate way to revascularize a lower limb.

Contraindications

The presence of digital or forefoot gangrene is a contraindication to deep femoral reconstruction alone. Limb salvage generally requires the addition of a bypass to the infragenicular vessels. In patients with diabetes, deep femoral reconstruction for distal ischaemia is also unlikely to lead to success.

Preoperative

Investigations

Angiography is essential to show the proximal inflow and the extent of deep femoral involvement, and to delineate the distal collateral and run-off vessels. Tight nipping of collateral vessels where they join the popliteal artery or marked occlusive disease of the popliteal run-off vessels indicate a low likelihood of success. Duplex scanning demonstrating tight deep femoral stenosis can be of help, particularly if only uniplanar angiograms are available. Doppler segmental pressure measurements are of value not only in establishing baseline pressures but also in predicting outcome.

The deep femoral–popliteal collateral index may be obtained by dividing the difference between above-knee and below-knee Doppler pressures by the above-knee pressure; an index below 0.5 indicates good potential for deep femoral reconstruction, while a high index suggests little benefit from opening the deep femoral collateral network.

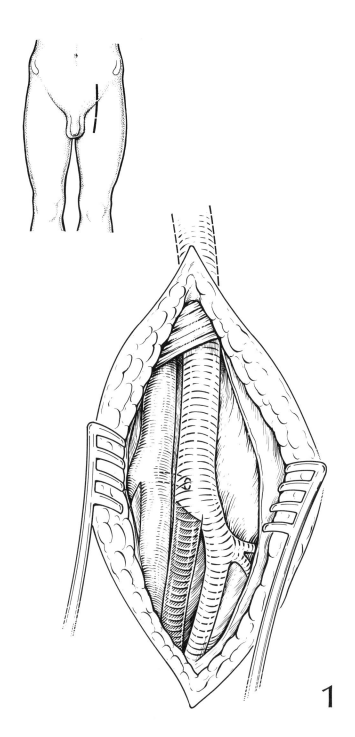

Operations

Incision

1 A 10–15 cm incision is made in the groin in the line of the common, femoral artery, so that the proximal portion extends over the inguinal ligament. Care is taken not to divide lymph nodes and to ligate lymphatic vessels. The incision is deepened through the femoral fascia to expose the common, superficial and deep femoral arteries. The proximal extent of the dissection is usually carried back under the inguinal ligament to a point where the external iliac artery is suitable for clamping.

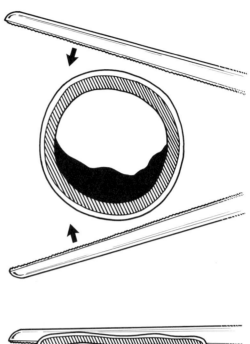

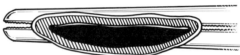

2

2 As most plaque at this site is on the posterior wall, a clamp applied from the soft anterior to the harder posterior wall will avoid cracking the plaque. Side-to-side clamping may crack the plaque and lead to its lifting with thrombus formation.

Distally the artery is exposed for 1–2 cm beyond the palpable plaque. Division of the circumflex femoral vein is necessary to enhance the deep femoral artery exposure. The surgical anatomy of the common and deep femoral arteries may vary considerably, and care is taken to mobilize the entire common femoral artery and identify branches, including the superficial and deep circumflex iliac arteries and the larger circumflex femoral arteries which may arise from either the common or deep femoral arteries.

OPERATION FOR LOCALIZED LESIONS

3 Following the intravenous administration of heparin, 5000 units, careful definition of the plaque is made by digital palpation. A longitudinal arteriotomy is made from the common femoral artery and carried down the lateral aspect of the deep femoral artery, away from the crotch of the femoral bifurcation, to a point approximately 1 cm distal to the palpable end of the plaque.

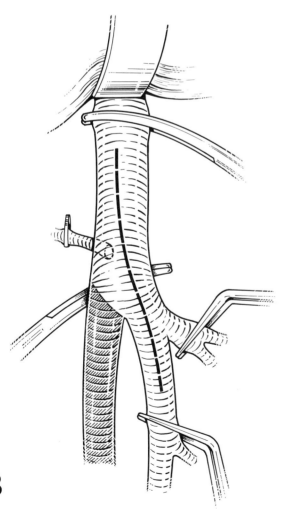

3

Endarterectomy

4a–e A uniform plane of dissection is developed within the outer layer of the media of the common femoral artery and extended circumferentially by advancing and spreading the Lahey right-angled forceps. The plaque is then lifted using a Lahey right-angled forceps and divided with scissors. The dissection plane is developed in a proximal direction within the artery. When the external iliac artery is reached just below the inguinal ligament, a suitable site is selected for external blunt disruption of the plaque. The Lahey forceps is then closed externally over the artery and the proximal end of the plaque is fractured. The proximal plaque is then removed by traction on the lower cut end.

Distal endarterectomy under direct vision will often result in a 'feathered' end in the proximal deep femoral artery. When the plaque extends to the first major branch, sharp dissection at the point of transition from plaque to more normal intima may be necessary.

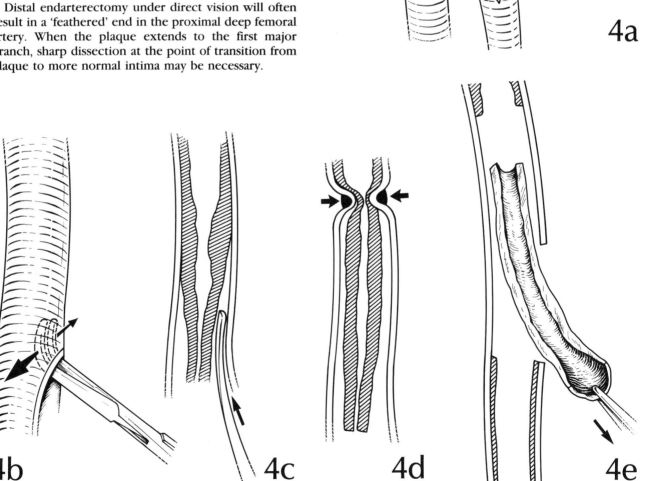

4a

4b

4c

4d

4e

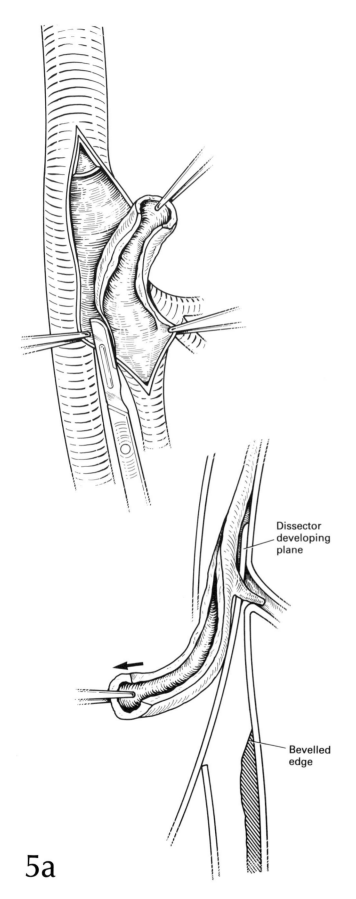

5a

Dissector
developing
plane

Bevelled
edge

5a, b
Using a beaver blade (number 64), the distal intima is incised obliquely to obtain a graded end with firm distal adherence of the intima. Very occasionally a distal tacking suture may be necessary to ensure that no flap develops. The arteriotomy should extend to just beyond the end of the plaque, so that patch closure will ensure that the edges of the end point are sutured and the distal end is widely open. After removal of the plaque, the vessel wall is cleared of any loose strands by circumferential stripping. Heparinized saline, 1000 units/500 ml saline, is used to flush the vessel and check that no loose tags remain.

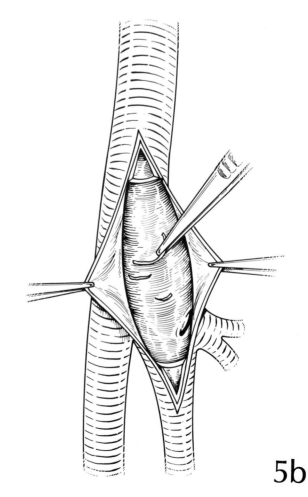

5b

ENDARTERECTOMY FOR EXTENDED DEEP FEMORAL RECONSTRUCTION

Extension of the plaque distal to the lateral circumflex branch, often to the second or third perforators, requires careful dissection to avoid damage to these small collateral branches and branches of the femoral nerve. The deep femoral artery passes beneath the adductor longus muscle 15–20 cm from its origin. Added exposure can be achieved by bending the knee or, very occasionally, dividing the muscle.

In extended procedures, a 'natural' cleavage plane or end point is not always found. The deep femoral artery is mobilized to beyond the disease or to a point that is beyond the major stenotic lesions. The distal graded end is achieved using a beaver blade, and the plaque is shelled out, taking care to extract elements of the plaque extending into the side-branch origins.

BALLOON ANGIOPLASTY COMBINED WITH DEEP FEMORAL RECONSTRUCTION

6a–c

Localized disease of the common and deep femoral arteries may be associated with iliac or superficial femoral stenosis suitable for balloon angioplasty. Balloon dilatation may then be combined with local endarterectomy and patch angioplasty.

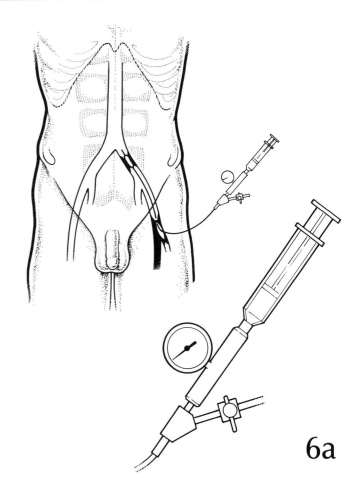

6a

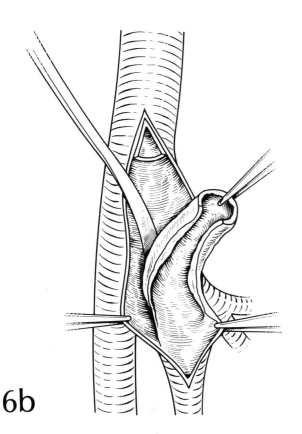

6b

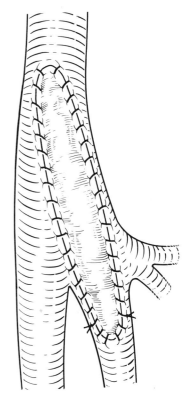

6c

Closure of arteriotomy

Inflow graft–deep femoral closure

7a, b The distal end of the inflow graft is cut to match the shape of the arteriotomy and to ensure a widely patent deep femoral artery. A continuous 4/0 suture is used to perform an end-to-side graft-to-vessel anastomosis. When an extended arteriotomy is used, a tongue of the inflow graft can be taken distally to achieve closure without tension.

Before final closure, the lumen is flushed with heparinized saline. The distal deep femoral clamps are released temporarily to ensure back-bleeding, and the inflow is also flushed to ensure that no clots feed into the anastomosis. A final flush with heparinized saline is done just before closure of the arteriotomy.

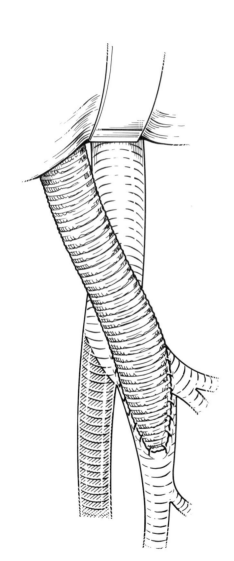

7a

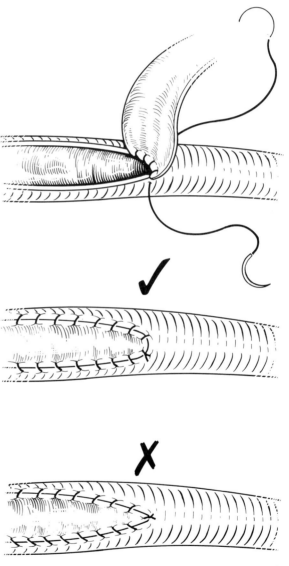

7b

Patch angioplasty

8 While a primary closure can occasionally be achieved after local endarterectomy of the deep femoral artery, in general a patch of autologous vein or occasionally endarterectomized superficial femoral artery is used to widen the deep femoral artery. The long saphenous vein should be preserved, but a tributary can often be found which is suitable. This will depend on the arteriotomy size. Care should be taken to gradually taper the patch, with rounding of the distal end to avoid narrowing the outflow. A double-ended 5/0 non-absorbable suture is used to secure the patch, suturing distally to proximally, to ensure a 'funnelled' distal end. Where no suitable vein is available, the superficial femoral artery can be detached and following endarterectomy and shaping may be used as a free patch. Occasionally also the superficial femoral artery can be left attached proximally but endarterectomized and advanced as a flap to close the deep femoral artery.

Care is again taken to flush the vessels and endarterectomy site with heparinized saline just before final closure of the arteriotomy. Perioperative angiography should be used to confirm the patency of the outflow tract.

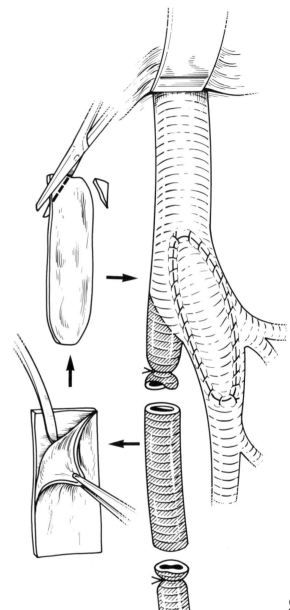

8

IN SITU BYPASS AND DEEP FEMORAL RECONSTRUCTION

9a–c With *in situ* bypass grafting the proximal vein anastomosis may be used to widen the origin of the deep femoral artery and increase flow to the limb collaterals. Occasionally, where the length of the proximal end of the vein graft is insufficient to reach the common femoral artery, it may be attached to the deep femoral artery distal to its origin. This may also be combined with deep femoral endarterectomy. Occasionally a tributary of the long saphenous vein may be used to add length to the proximal vein and extend it to the level of the common femoral artery.

Wound closure

Closure in multiple layers to minimize the dead space is important in the groin because of the risk of lymphatic leakage or haematoma formation.

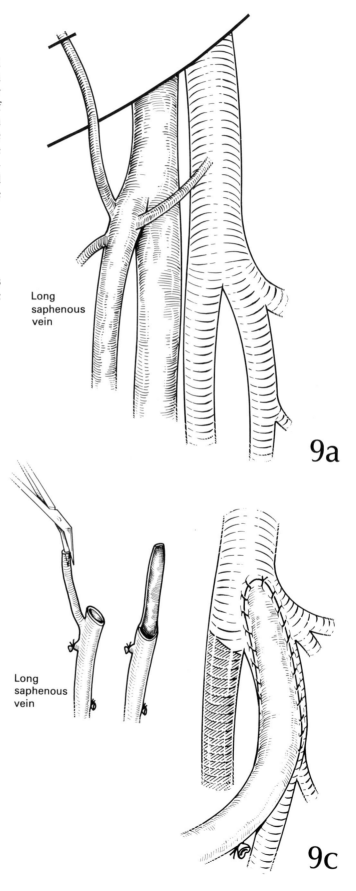

Long saphenous vein

9a

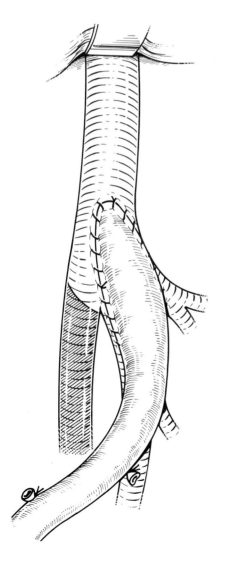

9b

Long saphenous vein

9c

Postoperative care

Complications

Haemorrhage should be dealt with by applying local pressure initially, with re-exploration to evacuate any haematoma and control bleeding points. The additional dissection associated with deep femoral reconstruction can lead to an increase in the incidence of lymphatic complications. Lymphocoele formation can be reduced by meticulous ligation of divided lymph ducts and avoidance of cutting through lymph nodes. A prolonged discharge may be treated with bed rest and frequent dressing changes. Culture of the fluid is needed to ensure that no infection is associated with the discharge.

Povidone–iodine or a similar cleansing fluid should be applied to the wound and appropriate antibiotic cover given, particularly if synthetic material has been used in the reconstruction. Skin staples should be left in until the wound has completely healed.

Superficial wound infections should be treated with appropriate antibiotics and opening of the superficial layers, with frequent dressing changes to allow drainage. Deep wound infection needs careful management and a variety of approaches depending on the circumstances.

Obturator bypass

Paolo Fiorani MD
Chief, Department of Vascular Surgery, University of Rome 'La Sapienza', Rome, Italy

Maurizio Taurino MD
Assistant, Department of Vascular Surgery, University of Rome 'La Sapienza', Rome, Italy

Francesco Speziale MD
Associate Professor, Department of Vascular Surgery, University of Rome 'La Sapienza', Rome, Italy

Ivano Paolo Renzi MD
Resident, Department of Vascular Surgery, University of Rome 'La Sapienza', Rome, Italy

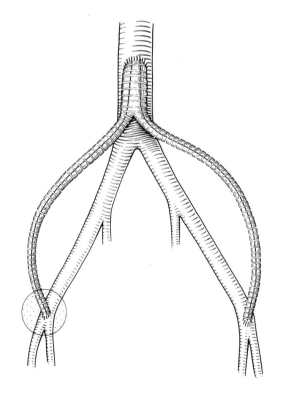

1

History

1 Obturator bypass was first proposed in 1962 by Shaw and Baue for three patients affected by infection of a previously implanted aortofemoral prosthesis in the groin[1].

Since then, obturator foramen bypass has been utilized in lower limb revascularization when direct exposure of femoral vessels in the groin is not possible because of infection in a previously implanted prosthetic graft, septic necrotizing arteritis, or mycotic aneurysm[2-4].

This technique has also been employed in lower limb revascularization in the presence of crushing injuries of the groin, diffuse malignancies and ionizing radiation arteritis.

Principles and justification

Indications

Major indications for obturator bypass are groin infections, as in cases of graft infection of a previously implanted aortofemoral graft, septic arteritis in drug addicts and mycotic aneurysm[1-4]. In these cases, it is mandatory to avoid graft implantation in infected sites.

Obturator bypass is preferable to other extra-anatomical techniques such as axillopopliteal bypass in these circumstances, having the advantages of a shorter prosthesis, located in a deeper position not at risk of extrinsic compression.

Preoperative

Assessment

Preoperative assessment includes standard thoracic radiography, electrocardiography, routine haematology (renal and hepatic function, coagulation factors, red and white blood cell counts, haemoglobin, packed cell volume and platelet count).

In the presence of a groin infection, it is useful to perform a labelled leucocyte scintigraphic scan, which will detect labelled cells binding to the site of infection, at the level of either the distal (groin) or the proximal (abdominal aortic) anastomosis. When the information gained from this technique is equivocal or positive, a more accurate anatomical evaluation is needed. Computed tomography (CT) can be useful in defining the presence of periprosthetic gas or fluid collections in abdominal or inguinal sites.

Positive bacteriology in fluid from a discharging sinus or from CT-guided fine-needle aspiration represents the gold standard. The identification of a specific bacterium enables treatment with an appropriate antibiotic to be given.

Preoperative angiography is of critical importance to define occlusive aortoiliac lesions and reveal false aneurysms.

Patient preparation

Patient preparation for surgery includes placing one or more intravenous catheters to administer fluids and drugs. Pulse rate and arterial blood pressure are monitored continuously. A bladder catheter is inserted to allow monitoring of intraoperative urinary output. Intra-arterial radial catheterization may sometimes be useful for the measurement of blood gases.

Anaesthesia

Obturator bypass is usually performed under endo-tracheal anaesthesia which allows adequate muscle relaxation, enough time to prepare the donor vessel (aorta or iliac vessels), and completion of possibly complicated surgery.

Operation

Position of patient

2 The patient is placed in the supine position, with the lower limb externally rotated, abducted and flexed to relax the thigh muscles. When an exposed graft is present at the inguinal level, the groin sinus or dehiscence must be carefully covered with an adhesive drape.

Incision

Exposure of the aorta and iliac vessels can be obtained through a transperitoneal midline incision, or by a retroperitoneal route through a paramedian or transverse incision. If angiography demonstrates patency of the iliac vessels, a retroperitoneal approach is preferable.

In the presence of a groin infection of an aortobifemoral graft, the new graft must be as proximal as possible. The safety level is determined by the upper limit of labelled leucocyte uptake or fluid collection identified by CT.

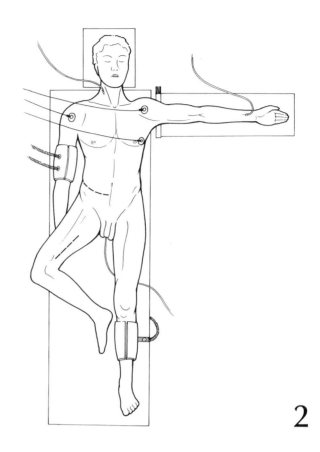

2

Insertion of the graft

The graft may be anastomosed to the common iliac artery, the terminal aorta, or the graft limb, which requires careful mobilization taking into account the location and possible adhesions of the ureter.

3 After determining the proximal anastomosis site, the obturator foramen is identified. On digital palpation, the foramen is identified at the superior apex of the obturator fossa and can be recognized by its relationship to the obturator artery, nerve and vein.

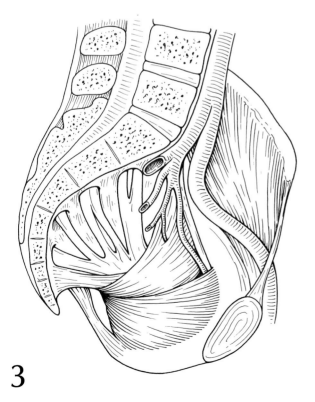

3

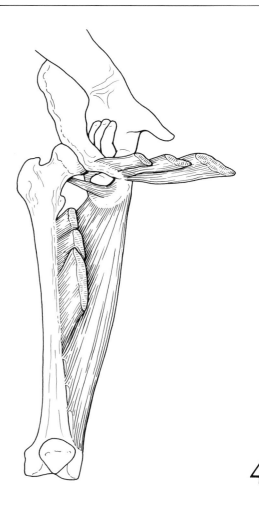

4 The obturator artery usually arises from the hypogastric artery and lies posterolaterally to the nerve on the anterolateral side of the obturator fossa.

It is then necessary to identify the avascular area of the obturator membrane where the graft is to be located medial to the obturator vessels and nerve, taking care not to damage them. The graft thus lies superiorly anteriorly to the internal obturator vessel, posteriorly inferiorly to the pubic branch, and medially to the obturator vessels and nerve.

A conventional tunnelling instrument is passed through the obturator membrane, which is a tough sheet of fascia. Here the graft lies above the external obturator vessel and, after crossing the ischial branch, passes anteriorly to the adductor magnus muscle.

Through a vertical incision on the anteromedial thigh, the superficial femoral artery is exposed and the site of distal anastomosis is selected. If necessary, this can be at the popliteal level.

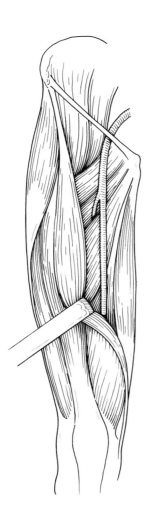

4

5 The adductor tunnel is prepared. The sartorius muscle is retracted laterally, and the adductor longus muscle is identified.

The tunnelling instrument is felt deeply, coming from the upper site below the pectineus, the adductor longus and the adductor brevis muscles, superiorly to the adductor magnus muscle. An additional short transverse incision can be made at the femoral (Scarpa's) triangle, where the adductor longus muscle crosses the gracilis muscle. To achieve an adequate tunnel, the surgeon's finger reaches from below to touch another finger coming from above.

The tunnelling instrument then carries the graft up to the superficial femoral artery close to the adductor magnus tendon; here the adductor muscles are located between the graft and the femoral artery.

5

Completion of anastomosis

If a previous aortofemoral graft is present, the anastomosis is performed end-to-end.

6 When the iliac artery is utilized, the anastomosis is end-to-side.

At the superficial femoral or popliteal artery level, the anastomosis is usually end-to-side, taking care to avoid possible back-bleeding at the inguinal level.

Dacron, polytetrafluoroethylene (PTFE), autologous reversed saphenous vein, non-reversed translocated saphenous vein, or human umbilical vein can be employed as the prosthetic material in this procedure[5,6].

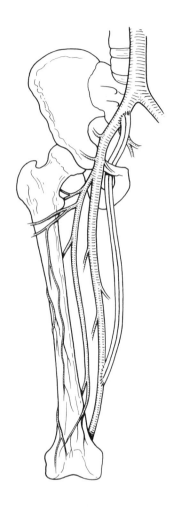

6

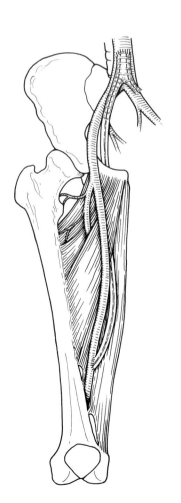

7

Wound closure

After declamping, the peritoneum is reflected, vacuum drains are positioned, and both the abdominal and thigh incisions are closed.

7 If a groin infection from a previously implanted aortofemoral graft is present, the distal limb of the graft must be excised with wide debridement of surrounding tissues.

A lateral running suture or a vein patch is used to eliminate back-bleeding at the femoral bifurcation.

When possible, the surgical wound is closed after positioning drains for continuous washing with antiseptic solutions, otherwise it is left open for delayed healing.

Postoperative care

No particular postoperative problems are encountered, other than those common to all operations for direct revascularization of the lower limbs, and the risk of secondary haemorrhage from the groin wound.

In patients with multilevel arterial lesions and poor run-off, postoperative anticoagulant therapy is sometimes needed. If so, it is initiated with heparin and continued with oral anticoagulants.

A continuous wave Doppler examination is helpful to evaluate the immediate patency of the graft.

Outcome

Late results, evaluated in a literature review of 3-year follow-up, are good[7, 8]. The patency rate is about 75% when distal anastomosis is performed above the knee; however, when the distal anastomosis is below the knee, the patency rate is only 50%.

References

1. Shaw RS, Baue AE. Management of sepsis complicating arterial reconstructive surgery. *Surgery* 1963; 53: 75–86.

2. VanDet RJ, Brands LC. The obturator foramen bypass: an alternative procedure in ileo-femoral artery revascularization. *Surgery* 1981; 89: 543–7.

3. Tilson MD, Sweeney T, Gushberg RJ, Stansel HC. Obturator canal bypass graft for septic lesion of femoral artery. *Arch Surg* 1979; 114: 1031–3.

4. Patel KR, Semel L, Clauss RH. Routine revascularization with resection of infected femoral pseudoaneurysms from substance abuse. *J Vasc Surg* 1988; 8: 321–8.

5. Panetta T, Sottiurai VS, Batson RC. Obturator bypass with nonreversed translocated saphenous vein. *Ann Vasc Surg* 1989; 3: 56–62.

6. Nevelsteen A, De Leersnijder J, Suy R. Aorto(ilio)popliteal grafting by the obturator route using the human umbilical vein graft. *Acta Chir Belg* 1985; 85: 115–20.

7. Nevelsteen A, Mees U, De Leersnijder J, Suy R. Obturator bypass: a sixteen year experience with 55 cases. *Ann Vasc Surg* 1987; 1: 558–63.

8. Rawson HD. Arterial grafting through the obturator foramen. *Aust NZ J Surg* 1986; 56: 127–30.

Management of peripheral arterial aneurysms

Kenneth Ouriel MD
Associate Professor of Surgery, University of Rochester School of Medicine and Dentistry, Rochester, New York, USA

James A. DeWeese MD
Professor of Surgery and Chief Emeritus of Cardiothoracic and Vascular Surgery, University of Rochester Medical Center, Rochester, New York, USA

Principles and justification

Peripheral arterial aneurysms occur most commonly in the popliteal, femoral and visceral locations. In contrast to the haemorrhagic complications of aortic aneurysms, peripheral aneurysms are generally associated with thromboembolic phenomena. The patient's life is thus seldom compromised by peripheral aneurysms; rather limb or end organ ischaemic events represent the most frequent complications.

Peripheral aneurysms may be categorized into: (1) true aneurysms, with representation of all three layers of the arterial wall; and (2) false aneurysms, with a wall composed of adventitial or fibrotic components only. False aneurysms occur most frequently in the femoral position. They are almost always iatrogenic, secondary to catheterization procedures or subsequent to breakdown of a femoral graft anastomotic suture line. Repair of a true aneurysm is advisable when the diameter reaches twice the diameter of the normal artery, if the patient will tolerate the procedure. All false aneurysms are generally repaired, irrespective of size.

Femoral artery aneurysms

Aneurysms of the common femoral artery may be atherosclerotic in origin, in which case they are usually associated with aortic aneurysms. Alternatively, the aneurysm may be a false aneurysm, involving the anastomosis of an aortofemoral or femoropopliteal bypass graft. A second aetiology of femoral false aneurysms is represented by those occurring after catheterization procedures; such aneurysms are becoming increasingly frequent with the proliferation of coronary angioplastic and fibrinolytic techniques.

Popliteal artery aneurysms

Two distinct types of popliteal aneurysm are encountered. The first presents as a diffuse sausage-shaped dilatation of the superficial femoral and popliteal vessels, generally 2–3 cm in diameter. The second form presents as a localized saccular dilatation of the popliteal artery at the knee level and frequently achieves a diameter in excess of 4 cm. Both types of popliteal aneurysm are associated with distal embolization; the saccular form is also associated with acute thrombosis and compression of the surrounding neurovenous structures.

Operations

ATHEROSCLEROTIC FEMORAL ANEURYSMS

Incision

1   Atherosclerotic aneurysms may be limited to the common femoral artery or may also extend into the proximal portions of the deep and superficial femoral arteries. Although these aneurysms may attain great size, rupture is rare and when complications occur they are usually a result of thrombosis or distal embolization. The aneurysm is best approached through a longitudinal groin incision, achieving proximal control through gentle dissection immediately beneath the inguinal ligament. When the aneurysm is very high or very large, proximal control may be achieved through a separate retroperitoneal flank incision. Distal control of the superficial femoral artery is obtained at the caudal aspect of the groin incision.

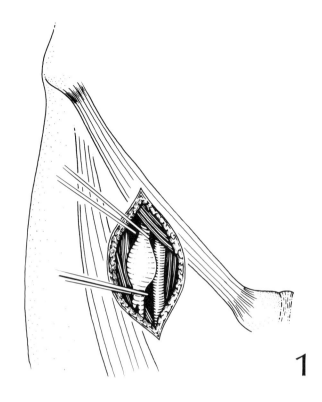

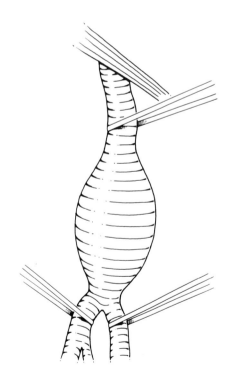

Proximal and distal control

2   Control of the deep femoral artery is obtained with gentle medial retraction of the common and superficial femoral vessels. Control of this artery is most important, as the back-bleeding from it is always vigorous. The back-bleeding may be controlled with a balloon catheter placed in the orifice of the deep femoral artery, after opening the aneurysm in instances where dissection is difficult, but the large proximal branches of the artery render complete control of back-bleeding unusual with the balloon technique.

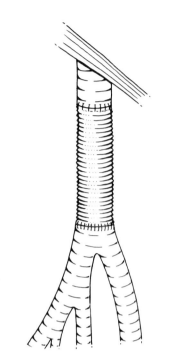

3

Graft replacement

3 The three vessels are clamped after systemic anticoagulation. The aneurysm is resected in its entirety if it is relatively small, and vascular continuity is restored with proximal and distal end-to-end anastomoses. Dacron or polytetrafluoroethylene grafts are appropriate, although a large saphenous vein may be used as well.

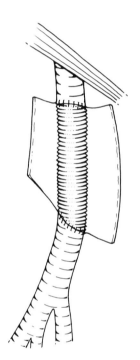

4 When large, the aneurysm is opened longitudinally and is not resected. The graft is then sewn from within the aneurysm cavity in a manner analogous to the common technique of abdominal aortic aneurysm repair. The aneurysm sac may then be closed over the graft to provide an additional layer of protection between the graft and the skin.

4

Treatment of extensive femoral aneurysms

5 Involvement of the proximal deep and/or superficial femoral vessels requires transection of the vessels beyond the dilated area. The two orifices may then be sewn together, using the new conjoined lumen for the distal anastomosis. Alternatively, the distal anastomosis may be performed in an end-to-end fashion to the superficial femoral artery, with anastomosis of the deep femoral vessel to the side of the graft.

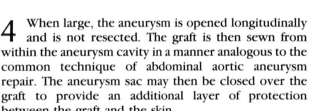

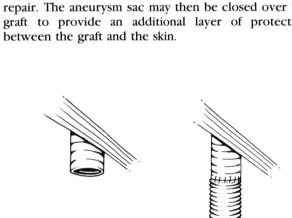

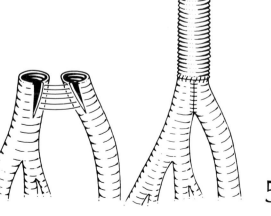

5

FEMORAL FALSE ANEURYSMS

Arterial defect

6 Femoral false aneurysms occurring as a result of catheterization procedures are approached in a manner identical to that of true aneurysms. The defect is frequently at the junction of the deep and superficial femoral arteries, and closure may be effected with several interrupted sutures. Large defects and defects occurring in heavily diseased arteries may require patch angioplasty in order to avoid compromise of the vessel lumen. Vein is preferred as the patch material, as bacterial contamination is frequent after prolonged femoral catheterization.

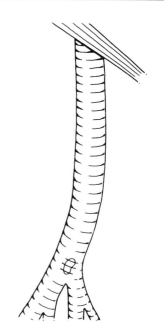

6

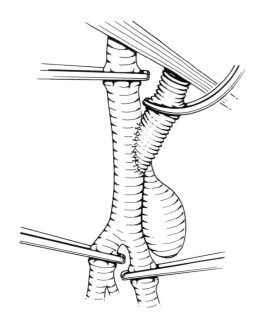

7

Anastomotic aneurysm

7 Aneurysms occurring secondary to disruption of femoral anastomoses are approached with control of the three native vessels as well as the prosthetic conduit. Proximal control of the common femoral vessel is occasionally difficult because of its location beneath an aortofemoral graft limb, and in these instances intraluminal balloon control can be advantageous.

Graft replacement

8 In the absence of an infectious aetiology, an extension of the old graft with anastomosis distally to the most distal common femoral artery is indicated. When infection is thought likely, extra-anatomic reconstruction is appropriate, with an obturator or laterally positioned bypass to the distal superficial or deep femoral artery.

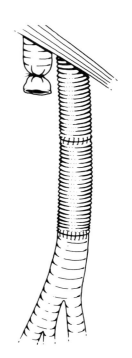

8

POPLITEAL ARTERY ANEURYSMS

Diffuse aneurysm

9 Therapy of the diffuse form of popliteal aneurysms is directed at preventing distal embolization. Rupture and compression of surrounding structures do not occur and resection of the aneurysm is therefore unnecessary. A standard autogenous vein femoro-popliteal bypass is accomplished, followed by exclusion of the aneurysm from the arterial circulation. Exclusion can be achieved with ligation of the popliteal artery just proximal to the distal anastomosis, or with interruption of the superficial femoral artery at its origin. The latter technique is favoured as it maximizes blood flow through the bypass graft.

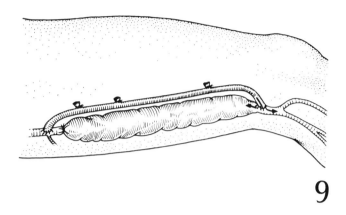

9

10

Skin incisions

10 Saccular popliteal aneurysms should be resected, if possible, because proximal and distal ligation has been associated with continued expansion from collateral flow. Autogenous conduits using end-to-end or end-to-side anastomoses are most appropriate for bypass after the aneurysm has been resected. The posterior approach using an S-shaped incision has the advantage of ease of dissection, although care must be exercised with respect to the frequently adherent popliteal veins and tibial nerves. The medial approach has the advantage of the accessibility of the long saphenous vein, but resection of the aneurysm is difficult, requiring division and forceful retraction of the medial head of the gastrocnemius muscle. Exclusion of the aneurysm with proximal and distal ligation may be all that is possible with the medial approach.

UNUSUAL PERIPHERAL ARTERIAL ANEURYSMS

Extracranial carotid aneurysms

Most pulsatile masses in the neck represent tortuous, folded common carotid arteries rather than aneurysms. This distinction can frequently be made with a duplex scan but arteriography is occasionally necessary. True aneurysms of the carotid bifurcation are rare, but when they are encountered they should be resected to prevent embolic complications.

Vein graft replacement

11 Reconstruction is accomplished with a venous bypass graft, using end-to-end anastomoses to the common carotid artery proximally and internal carotid artery distally. The external carotid artery is usually ligated. Electroencephalography or internal carotid stump pressure measurement may be used to predict the need for shunt placement during the cross-clamp period, as well as to determine the safety of distal internal carotid ligation when revascularization is impossible in the case of a very high aneurysm.

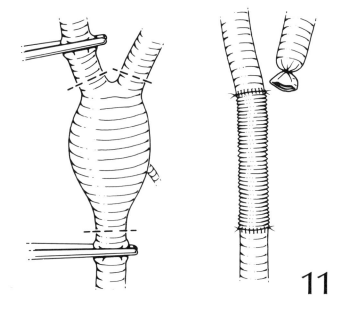

11

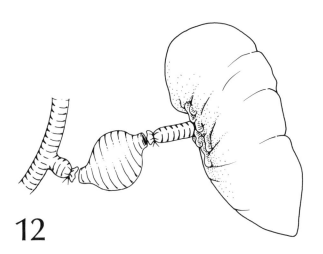

12

Splenic artery aneurysms

12 Splenic artery aneurysms are the most common variety of visceral aneurysm and are frequently encountered in multiparous females. Most aneurysms are asymptomatic and remain so, though an increased incidence of rupture is found in pregnant women. Resection without revascularization is indicated for large aneurysms or those in women of child-bearing age. Proximal aneurysms are removed without splenectomy, while those located at the splenic hilum are removed with the spleen.

Hepatic artery aneurysms

13 Hepatic artery aneurysms are most frequent in the common hepatic artery but may also be intrahepatic. Symptoms include right upper quadrant pain, jaundice, and haemobilia from rupture of the aneurysm into the bile duct. Treatment comprises resection and reconstruction for common hepatic artery aneurysms and angiographic embolization for intraparenchymal aneurysms.

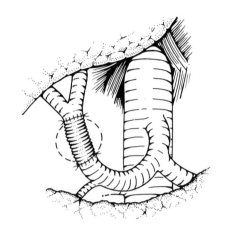

13

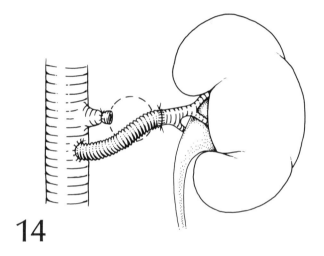

14

Renal artery aneurysms

14 The management of renal artery aneurysms is somewhat controversial and indications for operation are not clear-cut. Once the decision to resect the aneurysm has been made, several options are feasible. First, the aneurysm may be resected and arterial continuity restored with a graft from the aorta to the distal renal artery. A second option is to reimplant the distal renal arterial stump onto the aorta, after complete mobilization of the kidney. Finally, aneurysms involving the hilum of the kidney are best dealt with using an *ex vivo* bench procedure.

Coeliac and superior mesenteric artery aneurysms

15 These rare aneurysms are best managed with resection and restoration of arterial flow with aortomesenteric or aortocoeliac bypass. Both autogenous vein and prosthetic grafts are appropriate conduits. It is frequently easiest to exclude the aneurysm with proximal and distal ligation, followed by bypass to a more distal vessel, for example to the hepatic artery in the case of an aneurysm involving the coeliac axis.

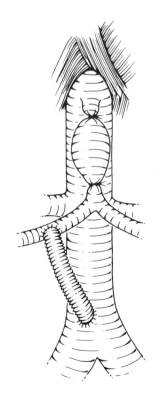

15

Femoral and popliteal embolectomy

C. W. Jamieson MS, FRCS
Consultant Surgeon, St Thomas' Hospital, London, UK

Principles and justification

Patient assessment

About 50% of patients presenting with acute ischaemia with no previous history of intermittent claudication do not have acute ischaemia due to embolism; the ischaemia is caused by an acute exacerbation superimposed upon chronic atheromatous disease. This large subgroup of patients presents a considerable challenge in clinical management, much greater than that of an embolus, and every attempt must be made to differentiate the two groups before embarking upon treatment.

The presence of acute on chronic ischaemia rather than acute ischaemia alone may be suspected if the degree of ischaemia does not correspond to the loss of pulse. A patient losing a femoral pulse as a result of acute ischaemia usually has signs of critical ischaemia of the lower limb extending above the knee, with motor and sensory loss, but in the presence of some degree of collateral development these signs are lessened and the level of ischaemia may be lower. The patient should have a potential cause for an embolus, i.e. atrial fibrillation or recent myocardial infarction, if an embolus is to be diagnosed, otherwise it is unlikely. The patient should have normal pulses in the contralateral limb and no evidence of chronic vascular disease: if these criteria are not met the patient should be assessed by emergency angiography to assess the state of the arterial supply of the affected limb and of the contralateral side.

The vascular surgeon faced with a patient with acute critical ischaemia must act promptly if the limb is to be saved and has two modes of therapy: direct surgical thrombectomy or embolectomy and emergency intra-arterial fibrinolysis. The latter mode is reasonable if the degree of ischaemia is not profound and particularly if the cause of the acute ischaemia is in doubt, as clearance of the arterial tree by fibrinolysis may reveal the cause of the occlusion and the degree and quality of run-off. However, this policy is unsafe in the presence of acute and severe motor and sensory loss or ischaemia of considerable duration, as in the time taken to achieve lysis the chance to prevent irreversible tissue damage may be missed. If there is doubt over the cause of the acute episode, but revascularization must be achieved with all possible speed, the artery should be explored thoroughly as for acute on chronic ischaemia.

Indications

Thrombectomy

A patient with no pulses in the lower limb and the possibility of acute on chronic ischaemia should undergo emergency angiography, but this may not be helpful if there has been thrombosis with secondary occlusion of the run-off, in which case little or no arterial supply to the limb may be demonstrated. However, it will at least reveal the height of the occlusion and the presence of other arterial disease, particularly in the contralateral limb and in the aorta and iliac arteries.

Femoral embolectomy

When an aortic, iliac or femoral embolus does appear to be the cause of the acute ischaemia the operation may be performed under local or general anaesthesia. Permission should be sought for a bypass (should it prove necessary) and for fasciotomy.

Fasciotomy

Any patient with substantial motor or sensory loss should be treated by prophylactic fasciotomy of the anterior compartment of the leg and, if severe, by simultaneous fasciotomy of the posterior compartment, immediately following embolectomy. The classic signs of muscle ischaemia, such as contracture and hardness, are those of irreversible ischaemia and to wait until they develop before fasciotomy is performed is disastrous: it is far better for a prophylactic fasciotomy to prove unnecessary than to risk irreversible ischaemia.

Popliteal embolectomy

Occasionally an embolus lodges in the distal popliteal artery or part of an embolus is removed satisfactorily from the common femoral artery, but some remains in the distal popliteal artery.

The patient with a distal popliteal embolus has acute ischaemia of the leg to the mid-calf level but has a normal, bounding popliteal pulse. The diagnosis is confirmed by femoral arteriography.

Operations

THROMBECTOMY AND ASSESSMENT OF ACUTE ON CHRONIC ISCHAEMIA

The patient's consent for whatever procedure may be necessary should be obtained, and he or she should be prepared to permit exploration of the arterial circulation of the whole lower limb plus access for an axillofemoral graft should it prove to be necessary.

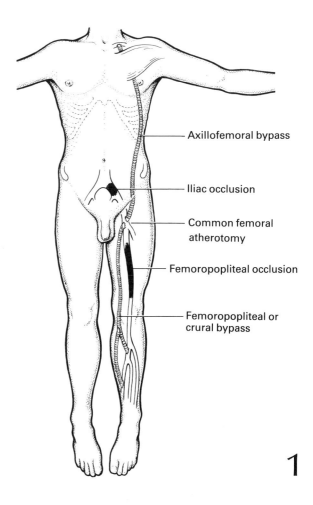

- Axillofemoral bypass
- Iliac occlusion
- Common femoral atherotomy
- Femoropopliteal occlusion
- Femoropopliteal or crural bypass

1

1 The degree of atheroma of the femoral artery is assessed and it is then explored and opened. If there is no evidence of atheromatous disease in the common femoral artery a transverse arteriotomy should be performed, as this facilitates thrombectomy and is easily closed without stenosis. Should the femoral artery be thickened a linear arteriotomy is more appropriate for an eventual bypass. A Fogarty catheter, 4 or 5 Fr, is then passed proximally. If it passes easily into the abdominal aorta and its withdrawal is followed by a good downflow and the release of a typical brown, hard thrombus of an embolus, all is well. Failure to restore good flow to the groin indicates the need for an axillofemoral bypass.

The catheter is then passed distally. Frequently it will arrest somewhere in the superficial femoral or popliteal artery. The catheter must be passed gently; it is very easy to dissect the artery or dislodge an atheromatous plaque and accentuate the problem. If the catheter passes easily to the foot thrombectomy should be performed and an operative arteriogram obtained,

following closure of the femoral arteriotomy, to check the completeness of thrombectomy.

If the catheter will not pass to the popliteal artery this must be explored. If the popliteal artery is diseased it may be possible to explore the posterior tibial artery or the dorsal artery of the foot distally, but it is unlikely that these efforts will be successful. If the popliteal artery is healthy but pulseless and thrombosed it should be opened, local thrombectomy performed and a catheter passed proximally to the distal extremity of the occluding lesion. Given a successful thrombectomy of the popliteal artery the limb may be rescued by a femoropopliteal bypass or occasionally by a femoro-crural bypass.

Thus the acute operative management of a patient with acute on chronic ischaemia may require all the expertise of an experienced vascular surgeon. It is most important that this is borne in mind when patients present.

FEMORAL EMBOLECTOMY

Incision

2   The femoral artery is exposed through a longitudinal incision in the groin, curved slightly laterally to avoid the lymphatic vessels, and extended distally in the line of the saphenous vein.

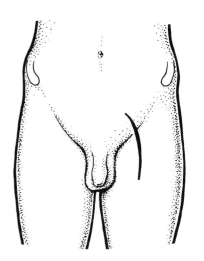

2

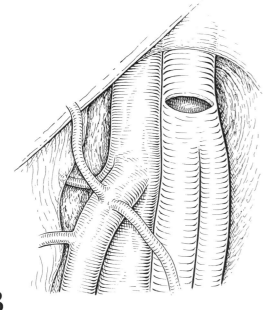

3

3   The artery is assessed and if it proves to be atheromatous the procedure outlined above should be followed. If it is healthy but occluded a transverse arteriotomy is made and a 4-Fr or, in large vessels a 5-Fr, Fogarty catheter passed proximally without its guide-wire into the abdominal aorta and gently withdrawn until good, audible downflow is re-established. The snare around the artery is lifted and an arterial clamp is gently applied. At this stage the patient should be fully anticoagulated with systemic heparin, 10 000 units (100 mg), and a little heparin–saline instilled proximally into the clamped artery to prevent thrombosis in the static column of blood in the thrombectomized segment.

4 A 4-Fr Fogarty catheter is passed proximally then distally through the popliteal artery, using the marks on the catheter to indicate when it has passed beyond the distal popliteal artery, the surgeon using one hand to withdraw the catheter and the other to regulate the pressure in the bulb by feeling the tension on the barrel of the syringe to avoid damage to the artery. The catheter must be passed gently; it may dissect or dislodge an atheromatous plaque and on occasion may transgress the arterial wall with disastrous consequences – when it is withdrawn in its inflated form the injury to the arterial wall is aggravated. Once the main femoral and popliteal arteries are cleared using the 4-Fr Fogarty catheter, a 3-Fr catheter should be passed distally into the foot to clear the crural vessels. This may not be possible, in which case exploration of the popliteal artery is required.

Following extraction of all possible thrombus 100 ml of heparin–saline should be injected into the femoral arteriotomy, pinching the artery with finger and thumb. The ease with which this injection is performed gives some indication of the adequacy of clearance of the run-off.

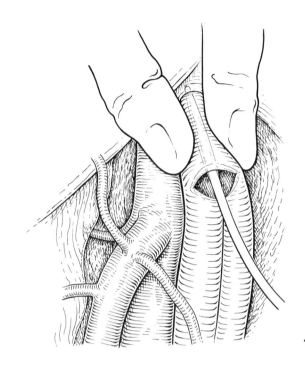

4

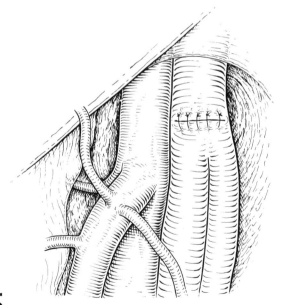

5

5 The femoral artery is then closed with interrupted 4/0 polypropylene sutures, following repeated flushing of downflow from the iliac artery to make sure that further static thrombus has not developed during clearance of the distal vessels.

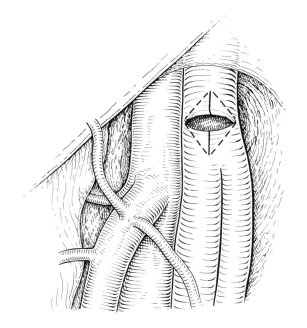

6

6, 7 Operative arteriography is then performed to check the adequacy of thrombectomy and further treatment taken as appropriate. Should embolectomy prove to be impossible and a bypass be necessary the transverse arteriotomy may be converted to a diamond arteriotomy which can then be closed with the extremity of a bypass.

Wound closure

The wound is then closed over a suction drain. The heparin treatment is not reversed.

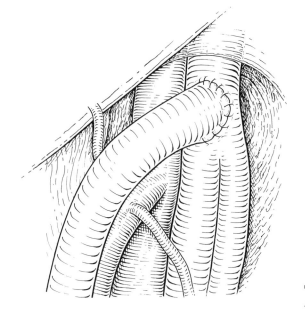

7

SADDLE AORTIC EMBOLUS

The management of a saddle embolus, in which the patient presents with sudden ischaemia of both lower limbs, is very similar to that of a unilateral femoral embolus. Immediate anticoagulation with heparin is undertaken, and the patient taken as soon as possible to the operating theatre.

Position of patient

The patient is placed supine on the operating table with the whole abdominal wall and both groins prepared and draped.

Incision

Bilateral incisions are made, as for femoral embolectomy. Both femoral arteries are dissected free, including the origin of the deep and superficial femoral arteries. The common femoral arteries and their two major branches are then clamped and opened with linear arteriotomies.

Embolectomy

A 6-Fr Fogarty catheter is passed proximally from each femoral arteriotomy into the aorta. The bulb is inflated and the catheter withdrawn. Almost invariably good downflow is restored.

Occasionally the catheter cannot be passed proximally into the aorta and downflow cannot be obtained. This may be because: (1) the arteries are so tortuous that the catheter will not pass, and yet the acute ischaemia is still due to an embolus; (2) the acute ischaemia is due to acute on chronic atheromatous occlusion; (3) very occasionally there is thrombosis of a proximal aortic aneurysm. The best procedure, if the patient's condition will permit, is direct exploration of the aortoiliac system with local treatment of the condition found – aortoiliac endarterectomy or, more commonly, an aortofemoral bifurcation graft. An axillo-femoral graft plus a crossover femoral bypass is indicated in a sick patient.

Good downflow is usually restored by passage of a catheter proximally, and smaller Fogarty catheters are then passed distally until the clot is withdrawn.

Wound closure

The femoral arteriotomies are closed with a running continuous suture. Both femoral wounds are closed over suction drains.

POPLITEAL EMBOLECTOMY

The popliteal artery may be exposed directly and opened, but this operation is quite delicate and is not to be recommended for an inexperienced vascular surgeon. It is worth attempting to remove the embolus from above via an arteriotomy in the common femoral artery using a Fogarty catheter passed from that level before attempting direct exploration of the artery. However, this embolectomy often fails to extract all the embolus, which can be confirmed by operative arteriography, and therefore some form of direct attack upon the embolus in the distal popliteal artery must be made because the limb will almost certainly be lost if distal popliteal occlusion persists, even though all embolic material has been removed from the more proximal arterial tree.

A compromise can occasionally be reached between simple popliteal embolectomy via the femoral route and popliteal embolectomy via an arteriotomy in the distal popliteal artery with its attendant difficulties of dissection, suture and closure with a vein patch.

Exposure of popliteal artery and 'closed' embolectomy

8 The popliteal artery is exposed via an incision along the posterior subcutaneous border of the tibia through the deep fascia which permits exposure of the artery between the bone and the medial head of the gastrocnemius muscle. This exposure is simple and, under direct vision, the Fogarty catheter may be directed from the femoral artery into each individual branch of the popliteal artery and manipulated with precision.

This technique is often successful and the embolus may be moved from above without opening the distal popliteal artery. It may be necessary to achieve direct exposure of the origin of the anterior tibial artery to ensure that the catheter enters that vessel.

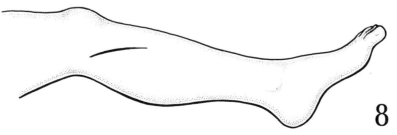

8

Direct embolectomy

9 The popliteal artery is exposed as above and dissected free from its surrounding veins, which are divided between fine ligatures. It is important to expose the origin of the anterior tibial artery by dividing the anterior tibial vein and the tibioperoneal trunk between ligatures. The separate division of the tibioperoneal trunk into the posterior tibial and peroneal arteries is often 2–3 cm distal and need not be exposed.

The patient is administered heparin as described above, and the distal popliteal artery, anterior tibial artery and tibioperoneal trunk are snared, clamped and a short linear arteriotomy made in the most distal centimetre of the popliteal artery. This is almost always the site at which the embolus is lodged, where the calibre of the artery changes.

The embolus is removed and Fogarty catheters are passed proximally up the superficial femoral artery and distally into the tibioperoneal trunk and anterior tibial artery under direct vision. It is not possible to ensure that the catheter has passed down both the posterior tibial and the peroneal arteries, but it may be encouraged to enter each one if a slight bend is placed upon the catheter tip, which is first inserted to point towards the medial posterior tibial artery and then rotated through 180° to point laterally towards the peroneal artery.

Great care must be taken that the bulb of the catheter is not over-inflated in small, delicate calf arteries. Rupture of these arteries has been reported, in which case the limb is usually lost.

10 When no more thrombus is obtained and downflow is satisfactory, the popliteal arteriotomy is closed using a small patch of saphenous vein or one of its tributaries and 4/0 or 5/0 polypropylene sutures.

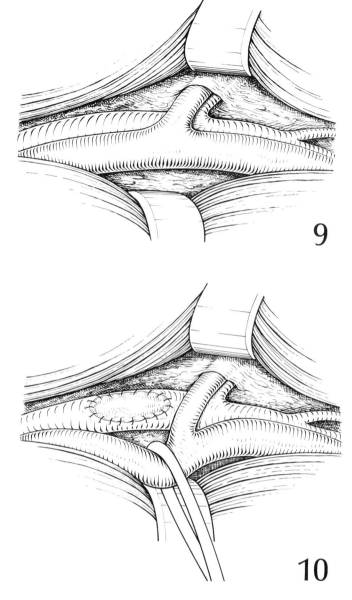

Wound closure

The deep fascia is closed over a suction drain and the skin is closed with interrupted nylon sutures.

Postoperative care

Femoral embolectomy has a high mortality rate (approximately 18%), which reflects the general condition of the patients who suffer embolism. Postoperative anticoagulation is continued and the patient is simultaneously given oral warfarin, 10 mg daily for 3 days, after which prothrombin time estimation should be performed to assess the dose required in long-term management.

Care must be taken to support the patient in general, particularly the cardiovascular status. In a limb which has been severely ischaemic there is considerable release of potassium, haemoglobin and vasodilator substances once the circulation is restored. Renal output must be preserved by administration of diuretic and renal support doses of dopamine. Acidosis may need to be reversed and the cardiac status must be carefully monitored.

The limb must be protected during the critical re-establishment of adequate circulation by avoiding pressure under the heel in the 1 h or so taken for the circulation to recover fully.

The patient must be assessed frequently and further thrombosis must be investigated promptly by emergency angiography and the appropriate surgical treatment instigated if the chances of a successful outcome are to be maximized.

Fasciotomy

C. W. Jamieson MS, FRCS
Consultant Surgeon, St Thomas' Hospital, London, UK

Principles and justification

Indications

The muscles of the lower and upper limb are enclosed in a rigid fascial envelope. If circulation is restored after a period of acute ischaemia, there is a tendency for increased capillary permeability which results in a transudation of fluid from the capillaries into the postischaemic muscle with a rise in extracellular pressure. This is reflected by a rise in pressure in the whole deep compartment, which may impair the circulation and cause muscle necrosis[1]. Fasciotomy must therefore be considered after any restoration of circulation in acute and severe ischaemia, particularly if that ischaemia was associated with motor or sensory loss. The classical signs of muscle necrosis (contractures, induration and erythema of the overlying skin) develop only after irreversible muscle damage has taken place and are therefore not indications for fasciotomy.

Fasciotomy is indicated in any patient in whom there has been severe or prolonged acute ischaemia associated with paralysis of muscle, and particularly if there is any muscle tenderness or the slightest induration[1]. Fasciotomy must be radical and prompt if it is to be successful. It is also indicated in the later case of acute ischaemia presenting with classical muscle induration, but is unlikely to save the bulk of muscle in this circumstance.

Fasciotomy may be conveniently divided into three operations in the lower limb – semi-closed fasciotomy, open fasciotomy and fibulectomy – and semi-closed and open fasciotomy only in the upper limb. Semi-closed fasciotomy is almost never indicated; its only value might be in the patient in whom the surgeon feels the ischaemia is so minimal that an open fasciotomy is not justified. In general, once the decision to perform a fasciotomy has been made, an open fasciotomy is infinitely preferable.

Operations

SEMI-CLOSED FASCIOTOMY

1 The whole lower limb is prepared and towelled. A small incision, approximately 6 cm long, is made over the proximal part of the anterior compartment of the leg.

The deep fascia is divided through this incision and a pair of scissors or a fasciotome is passed down subcutaneously, dividing the fascia. The diagnosis is confirmed by the muscle bulging through the defect in the fascia and it is usually then apparent that the overlying skin still causes compression, in which case the operation must be converted immediately to a full open fasciotomy (*see* below). The wound in the skin is left open and dressed with paraffin gauze; it is obviously important that no constricting bandage is applied to the limb.

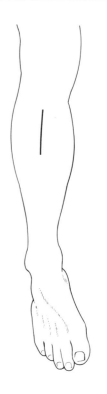

1

OPEN FASCIOTOMY

2a, b The limb is prepared and towelled. An extensive longitudinal incision is made over the whole length of the affected compartment; this may be the anterior compartment alone but, more frequently, incisions in the calf and peroneal muscles are also necessary. The oedematous muscle bulges through the incisions and a large defect is left. The exposed areas of muscle are covered with paraffin gauze and the wound is lightly dressed. The wounds are left to heal by secondary intention, which is surprisingly rapid if the circulation has been restored adequately.

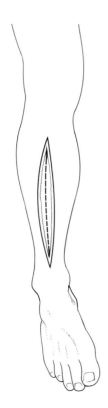

2a

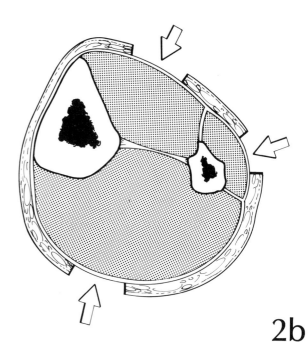

2b

FIBULECTOMY

This procedure is indicated in cases of severe acute ischaemia after restoration of circulation, particularly if it has been associated with blunt trauma causing direct muscle damage[2]. The lower limb consists of several fascial compartments: the anterior compartment, the peroneal compartment, the superficial, intermediate and deep posterior compartments, all of which are contained in fascial envelopes. The lateral extremity of all these fascial planes is attached to the fibula and an extraperiosteal excision of the fibula therefore opens them all.

Incision

3 The limb is prepared and towelled. A longitudinal incision is made over the cutaneous surface marking of the fibula, taking great care to avoid the lateral popliteal nerve which winds round the neck of the fibula immediately distal to the proximal tibiofibular joint.

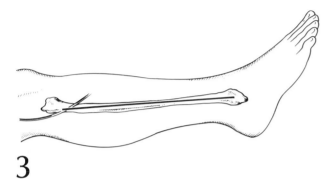

3

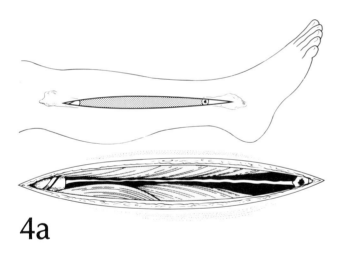

4a

4a, b This incision is extended through the deep fascia and the peroneal muscles and the fibula are then excised extraperiosteally, including division of the interosseous membrane between the tibia and fibula. The fibula is divided proximally at the level of the lateral popliteal nerve, again taking great care to avoid any damage to the nerve, and distally immediately proximal to the distal tibiofibular joint.

This dissection is fairly traumatic and causes considerable minor bleeding which must be controlled with diathermy or under-running fine catgut sutures. The muscles bulge into the wound and the skin gapes widely.

The wound is dressed with paraffin gauze and a loosely applied dressing with no constricting bandage. The patient is encouraged to exercise the limb as much as possible. Healing takes place by secondary intention but may be assisted, if necessary, by a split skin graft performed 10–14 days after the operation, although this leaves a more obvious scar than allowing healing by secondary intention and is probably undesirable.

References

1. Parent NF, Bernhard VM. Acute ischaemia. In: Bell PRF, Jamieson CW, Ruckley CV, eds. *Surgical Management of Vascular Disease*. London: Saunders, 1992: 427–8.

2. Kelly RP, Whitesides TE. Transfibular route for fasciotomy of the leg. *J Bone Joint Surg [Am]* 1967; 49-A: 1022–3.

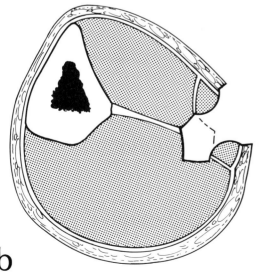

4b

Management of vascular injuries

M. O. Perry MD
Professor and Chief of Vascular Surgery, Texas Tech University Health Sciences Center, Lubbock, Texas, USA

Principles and justification

Mechanisms of injury

Although major vascular injuries can be encountered in any civilian setting, the highest incidence is in urban areas where violence is endemic. Penetrating wounds caused by knives and bullets are usually seen, but accidental stab wounds caused by shards of glass or metal also occur. The damage produced by knives or bullets travelling at a low velocity is mainly confined to the wound tract, but high-velocity bullets are associated with blast injury. As the blast cavity collapses, a suction effect is generated which can draw skin, dirt and bits of clothing into the wound. Secondary missiles (bullet fragments or bone splinters) can produce further damage. Such destructive effects may not be suspected from inspection of the skin where, in some cases, rather small wounds are present[1, 2].

Motor vehicle accidents are important causes of vascular trauma and victims frequently have multiple injuries. Direct vascular trauma occurs, but often these wounds are the result of fractures and dislocations. This is especially likely to occur near joints where the vessels are relatively fixed. Dislocations of the knee, for example, are particularly prone to injure the popliteal artery, and similar episodes can damage the brachial or axillary vessels.

Lacerations are seen most often with knife wounds, but contusions, punctures and transections are also encountered. Stretching, angulation and subsequent occlusion are more often seen with fracture dislocations, but the concussive effects of high-velocity missiles can cause such wounds. Immediate vessel disruption and bleeding may not occur, but delayed thrombosis or haemorrhage can lead to ischaemia or false aneurysm formation.

Clinical evaluation

Most arterial injuries can be identified readily because of external haemorrhage or large haematomas. Ischaemia distal to the injury is uncommon with isolated vascular injuries except for wounds occluding the popliteal or common femoral arteries. Moreover, distal pulses may be intact in up to 20% of patients with acknowledged arterial wounds, although weak or absent distal pulses are important findings[2]. The indications for operative exploration of a suspected vascular wound are as follows:

1. Diminished or absent distal pulse.
2. Persistent arterial bleeding.
3. Large or expanding haematoma.
4. Ischaemia.
5. Bruit at or distal to the suspected site of injury.

Most patients can be readily identified by a combination of clinical features, but in some patients adjunctive diagnostic methods are helpful. If the patient has an ankle:brachial blood pressure index greater than 0.9, it is unlikely that there is a significant injury of a major axial artery. This does not rule out injury to other vessels such as the deep femoral or deep brachial arteries, but it is unusual to find a major arterial injury when patients have normal ankle blood pressures[2].

In other patients duplex ultrasonography may be helpful in excluding or detecting arterial injuries. In patients who do not have firm indications for operation, yet there is some question as to the presence or absence of an injury, and there are equivocal or marginal ankle:brachial indices, then duplex ultrasonography may disclose an arterial wound. In other patients duplex studies may demonstrate that the artery and adjacent structures are intact, and suggest that no significant injury exists. None of these tests is sufficiently reliable that it can be used without a careful clinical evaluation and follow-up. The patient must be followed carefully to be certain that the diagnosis is correct.

Arteriography can be very useful in the evaluation of potential arterial injuries, especially in patients with multiple pellet wounds, fractures and penetrating injuries of the neck and thoracic outlet. If high-grade biplane films can be obtained, arteriography presents reliable, although not infallible, evidence regarding the presence or absence of an arterial wound. In some patients surgical management can be improved by identifying the location and extent of the vascular damage, especially when specialized incisions or other adjunctive therapeutic manoeuvres are required.

Preoperative

Most patients with major vascular wounds require immediate operation, and if haemodynamically unstable they should be taken directly to the operating theatre. If the patient is stable, further diagnostic manoeuvres can be undertaken.

Bleeding is controlled with direct pressure (tourniquets are avoided) and two large-bore intravenous lines are secured. Balanced salt solutions are given intravenously while type-specific and matched blood is obtained. General anaesthesia is preferred, and special precautions must be taken to avoid extending the damage or dislodging clots in patients with cervical and thoracic wounds. Wide operative fields are prepared because it may be necessary to enter the abdomen or chest.

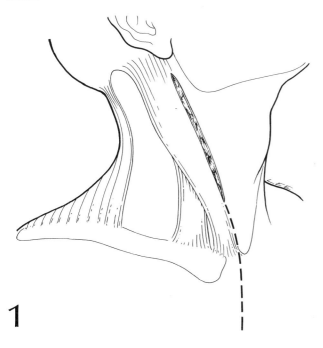

1

General principles of operation

Incisions

1 Vertical incisions are favoured for exposing vascular wounds; they can be extended easily in either direction along the course of the vessel and are parallel to other neurovascular structures. A vertical incision into the anterior cervical triangle to expose the carotid artery can be extended into a midline sternotomy, for example, or lateral supraclavicular incision as needed. Similarly, a midline abdominal incision can be extended into the sternum or across the costal margin to enter the chest.

Exposure

If the haematoma is large, it is often best to expose the vessels proximally and gain control where the artery is clearly seen. Latex tubing or soft vascular tapes are passed around the vessel and vascular clamps selected. Usually the vascular wound can then be approached safely and the bleeding controlled with direct digital pressure. With multiple injuries, and especially if large veins are involved, temporary proximal and distal vascular occlusion and vigorous suction may be required.

Debridement

Lacerations or punctures of larger vessels can be treated by lateral repair, but it is best not to make a firm decision until debridement is concluded. Most civilian wounds are inflicted by knives or low-velocity missiles and wide debridement is unnecessary; however, blunt trauma and high-velocity bullets cause more extensive damage.

If debridement is needed it is usually required only to excise the portion of the vessel that appears to be damaged. If, on the other hand, the patient has sustained an injury from a high-velocity missile it is prudent in many cases to resect an additional 4–5 mm of the vessel to be certain that all of the injured artery is removed before reconstruction is undertaken[2].

Graft interposition

Resection and end-to-end anastomosis is usually preferred to repair injured arteries, but if this cannot be done without tension, graft interposition is indicated. Autogenous grafts (saphenous vein, cephalic vein, autogenous artery) are favoured, but prosthetic grafts made of polytetrafluoroethylene (PTFE) have been used successfully, and plastic grafts are required for the large vessels of the aortoiliac system. Although Dacron fabric grafts have been used in trauma patients, it is now believed that PTFE grafts may be more resistant to infection.

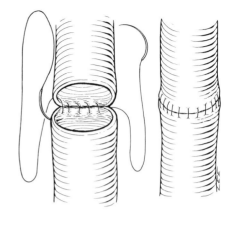

2

Anastomoses

2,3 After debridement has been performed in a vessel that is more than 4 or 5 mm in diameter, a simple end-to-end anastomosis is constructed using continuous monofilament sutures. Many surgeons favour loupe magnification, but in vessels of this size the anastomosis can be fashioned without difficulty. In smaller vessels, those less than 4 mm in diameter, it is helpful to spatulate the artery to construct an oblique suture line that is larger than can be obtained with a simple end-to-end anastomosis. In children and for small arteries, interrupted suture techniques are favoured to permit enlargement of the artery as the child grows.

Anticoagulants

Systemic heparin is often given to patients with isolated vascular wounds, but many trauma surgeons believe that full doses of heparin are contraindicated in patients with multiple injuries, and in those with damage to the central nervous system and eyes[1,2]. Local irrigation of the damaged vessel with a solution containing 100 units of heparin per 10 ml saline is helpful in removing debris and retarding local thrombosis. Anticoagulants are not used after operation in most patients, although those in whom plastic grafts have been used may benefit from antiplatelet agents, e.g. one 325-mg aspirin tablet each day during the immediate postoperative period.

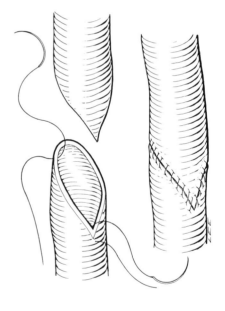

3

Determining patency

A diligent search for distal clots is mandatory despite what may appear to be adequate back-bleeding. The presence of collateral systems, such as in the superficial femoral and brachial arteries, may permit what appears to be brisk back-flow, yet there may be clots further distal in the limb. Many surgeons routinely pass a Fogarty catheter in both directions before completing the repair to be certain that there are no residual clots. This is a helpful manoeuvre, but it must be done carefully to avoid damage to the endothelium; this is likely to predispose to thrombosis. If distal pulses and normal flow are not readily obtained, an event likely to be seen in patients who are hypovolaemic or whose body temperature is lower than normal, adjunctive diagnostic methods are necessary. The intraoperative use of Doppler ultrasonography may disclose distal pressures and flow which are deemed adequate even when palpable pulses are not present. If the surgeon is uncertain as to the adequacy of normal blood flow, completion arteriography is indicated to be certain that no residual clots are present.

To illustrate the application of these principles, the management of three of the more common vascular injuries is described: a penetrating wound of the carotid artery, a stab wound of the inferior vena cava, and a gunshot wound of the femoral artery.

CAROTID ARTERY INJURIES

Sites of injury

4 It is the author's practice to explore all penetrating wounds of the anterior triangles of the neck which pierce the platysma muscle, but this is a controversial indication for surgery[3]. Recent studies have suggested that in patients in whom there are suspected injuries in zones I and III arteriography, endoscopic procedures and contrast radiological procedures may satisfactorily demonstrate the absence of an injury. In such patients careful observation has been successful when there were no other indications for operation. The management of carotid artery injuries is assisted by dividing the neck into three zones: zone I extends inferiorly from the superior surface of the clavicle to include the thoracic outlet; zone II extends from zone I to the angle of the mandible; and zone III includes the area from the angle of the mandible to the base of the skull. In patients with suspected wounds of the carotid artery in zones I and II, preoperative arteriography is especially helpful. Special procedures may be required to expose and control the great vessels at the root of the neck. In zone III exposure of the carotid artery may be somewhat difficult and mandibular subluxation or mandibular osteotomy may be required to see the carotid as it enters the foramen at the base of the skull. These manoeuvres require the preoperative placement of dental wires and appliances.

Exposure of the carotid artery is begun by a standard incision placed parallel to the sternocleidomastoid muscle in the anterior triangle of the neck inferiorly extending from just behind the angle of the mandible below the area of suspected injury. The platysma muscle is divided and allowed to retract with temporary pressure control of bleeding while the investing layer of the deep cervical fascia is incised. The carotid artery is then approached directly by retracting the sternocleidomastoid muscle and jugular vein laterally, preserving the descending and hypoglossal nerve branches. The common carotid artery in the proximal third of the neck is controlled first. The wound in the artery is not

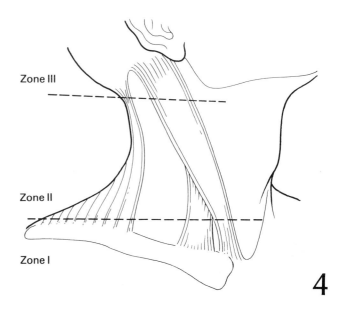

Zone III

Zone II

Zone I

4

disturbed and the clot is not removed until proximal control has been obtained. In some cases it may be possible to obtain control of the internal and external carotid arteries before an injury of the bulb is exposed. In patients who have injuries of the distal internal carotid artery, proximal control can be obtained easily. If the wound is near the base of the skull it may be possible, via a small transverse arteriotomy in the common carotid artery, to advance a latex balloon catheter beyond the area of injury and temporarily control the back-flow from the internal carotid artery. Throughout the course of this dissection it is important to preserve the major cervical nerves in the area: the hypoglossal and its branches, the vagus and the glossopharyngeal, and the superior and recurrent laryngeal nerves.

Zone II injuries (common carotid)

5 The mid-cervical carotid artery is exposed through an incision anterior to the sternocleidomastoid muscle. The common carotid artery proximal to the wounds is encircled first, and distal control is then obtained if feasible. Bleeding is initially controlled with gentle finger pressure, then vascular clamps are applied. If simple suture is impossible, patch graft angioplasty or resection and anastomosis are undertaken.

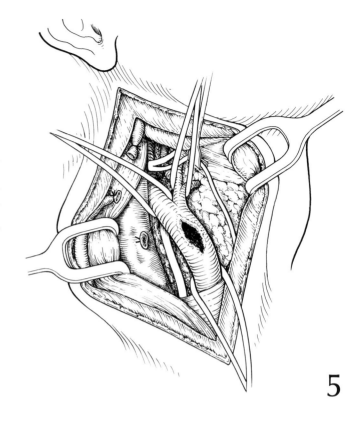

5

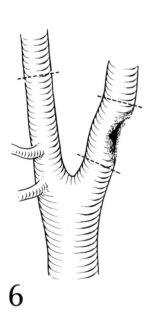

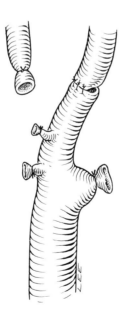

6

Zone II injuries (internal carotid)

6 If the proximal portion of the internal carotid artery is severely injured and cannot be repaired by simple resection and end-to-end anastomosis, then the external carotid artery may be substituted in continuity as illustrated. Small monofilament interrupted sutures are usually employed to restore continuity.

Graft interposition

7a–c
If the damage to the internal carotid artery is extensive and there is scanty back-bleeding from the distal artery, an autogenous saphenous vein graft is threaded over a 10-Fr shunt and interposed between the ends of the artery.

Zone I and III injuries

Patients who have suspected injuries of the common carotid artery in zone I may require median sternotomy for control of bleeding. If the patients are stable many of them will have had preoperative arteriography to determine if there are wounds in the great vessels in the thoracic outlet; this is helpful in deciding about incisions.

In patients who have injuries of the carotid artery at the base of the skull (zone III), exposure may require division of the digastric muscle and excision of the styloid process. If this is inadequate, anterior subluxation of the mandible or a mandibular osteotomy may also be needed. These are specialized procedures and the assistance of an oral surgeon is helpful.

At completion of the repair, intraoperative Doppler techniques can be used to detect the characteristic signals of prograde flow in the internal carotid artery. Duplex ultrasonography may also be helpful in ensuring distal patency. If there is any question about the accuracy of the repair, completion arteriography is indicated.

The patients must be followed carefully after operation, with frequent evaluation of neurological status and physical examination of the vascular system. Doppler techniques can help to document continued patency of the artery.

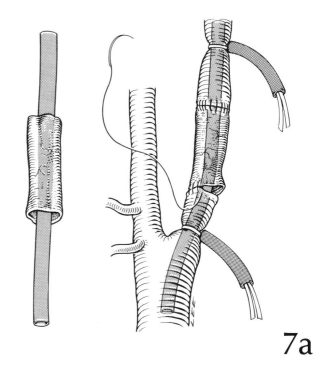

7a

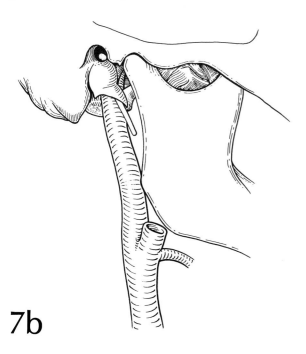

7b

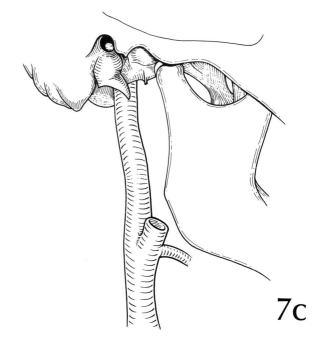

7c

INFERIOR VENA CAVA INJURIES

It has been reported that one in every 50 gunshot wounds and one in every 300 knife wounds of the abdomen damages the inferior vena cava[4]. One-third of victims die before reaching the hospital and half of the remainder die during treatment. Multiple wounds of other organs are common; over three-quarters of these patients have damage to other retroperitoneal structures[4].

Most patients obviously have a serious injury, usually a bullet wound of the lower chest or abdomen, and shock. There are few laboratory data of diagnostic value

and it is best to take unstable patients directly to surgery.

Exposure

The abdomen is opened through a midline incision from xiphoid to pubic symphysis, the extent of the damage assessed, and priorities set. All centrally located retroperitoneal haematomas above the pelvis that are caused by penetrating trauma are explored.

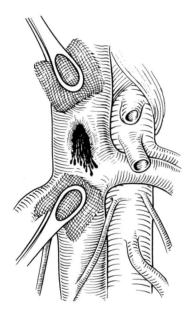

Control of bleeding

8 Bleeding is initially controlled with finger pressure or sponge sticks.

Sometimes small lacerations and punctures can be closed with simple sutures passed beneath an occluding finger, or the edges of the inferior vena cava can be held together with vascular forceps.

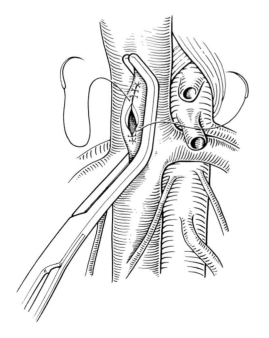

9 More often, a partially occluding vascular clamp (Satinsky) is needed to permit accurate repair. Occasionally clamp application may be too difficult and a balloon catheter (Foley or Fogarty) can be inserted to plug the wound and stop the bleeding.

Through-and-through injuries

10 Wounds which pierce both anterior and posterior walls of the inferior vena cava can be closed by lateral repair after mobilizing the vena cava by ligating and dividing one or two sets of lumbar veins. Alternatively, the anterior wound can be enlarged and the posterior laceration closed from within the inferior vena cava. The anterior wall is then repaired.

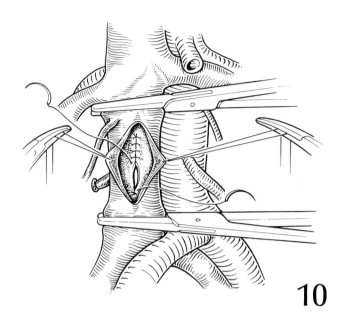

10

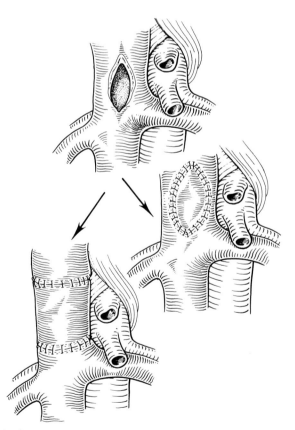

11

Suprarenal cava injuries

11 More extensive suprarenal damage to the inferior vena cava may require a vein graft (the left renal vein or the common iliac vein is preferred) or a patch graft. For the infrarenal cava, in unstable patients with multiple injuries, ligation is recommended if direct repair cannot be accomplished.

Division of the hepatic ligaments and anterior and medial rotation of the right lobe of the liver will usually permit repair of the suprarenal cava and hepatic veins (one major hepatic vein or any small accessory hepatic vein can be ligated safely).

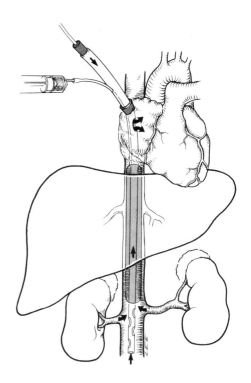

12, 13 If prolonged inferior vena cava occlusion is necessary for repair or if bleeding is so brisk as to obscure vision, a transatrial intracaval shunt (Madding–Kennedy) is inserted. The right atrium is reached by extending the abdominal incision into a midline sternotomy. This manoeuvre is not often required, however.

In the majority of patients control of bleeding can be successfully accomplished by left medial rotation of the liver with exposure of the retrohepatic vena cava. In many patients the decision to place a transatrial intracaval shunt is not made until the patient is already in haemorrhagic shock; in such a case the outcome is likely to be unfavourable. If a transatrial shunt is required it should be put in place before the patient is in irreversible shock. Even in busy trauma centres this procedure is rarely used, and there are few surgeons who have experience with insertion of these shunts. Once in place the shunts offer adequate control of bleeding from the retrohepatic cava, but it is also helpful to occlude the aorta temporarily at the aortic hiatus, and place a clamp across the portal structures, thus occluding the hepatic artery and portal vein while adequate exposure is being obtained. Once the retrohepatic cava and the hepatic veins are seen and the injuries adequately controlled, repair is usually performed utilizing continuous techniques with a monofilament suture. One of the hepatic veins may be ligated safely, but it is prudent not to ligate all three major veins.

12

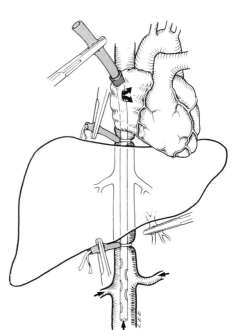

13

GUNSHOT WOUND OF FEMORAL ARTERY

Femoral artery wounds constitute approximately 20% of all arterial injuries[5]. These are serious problems. Haemorrhage is often profuse and acute ligation of the common femoral artery results in amputation rates near 50%, only slightly less than that following acute occlusion of the popliteal artery[2].

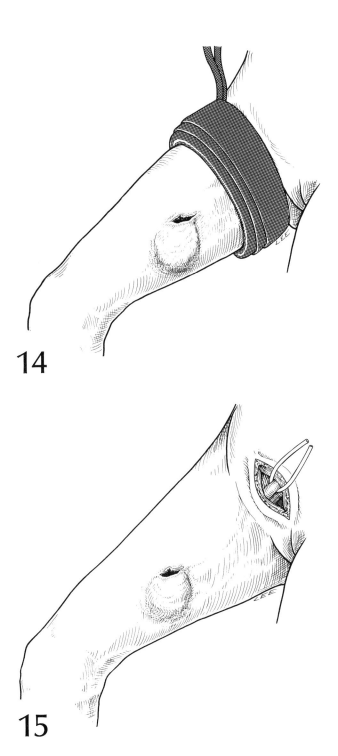

14

15

Most patients with penetrating arterial trauma have severe haemorrhage or large haematomas; the injury is obvious and immediate surgery is required. If arteriograms are needed to visualize the deep femoral or popliteal–tibial systems, they can be obtained in the operating theatre.

Compression control

14 Bleeding can usually be stopped with finger pressure, but if there are multiple wounds or large haematomas it is prudent to place an orthopaedic pneumatic cuff proximally before draping the limb. Troublesome bleeding can be arrested quickly by inflating the cuff.

In the event that the injury is too close to the inguinal ligament and femoral triangle to permit the placement of a proximal cuff, the arteries can be approached directly for proximal and distal control as described earlier in this chapter. Vertical incisions are employed and extended over the inguinal ligament. The ligament itself may be divided if necessary to obtain control of the artery at the junction of the external iliac and the common femoral arteries over the pubic ramus. The standard vertical incision is carried down through the superficial layer of fascia, and the femoral artery is exposed after opening the femoral sheath in the usual fashion. If the wound involves the superficial or deep femoral arteries, the common femoral artery can be exposed and encircled with latex tubing for proximal control. In most instances distal exposure is not necessary because local control of bleeding can be obtained until the wound is exposed and clamps placed immediately adjacent to the injury. If there is a large haematoma it may be appropriate to expose the superficial femoral artery in the mid-thigh and obtain control at this level before the clots are evacuated.

Proximal control

15 If there is insufficient room to place a proximal tourniquet, the external iliac artery can be exposed through a muscle-splitting extraperitoneal incision above the inguinal ligament, and then encircled with a vascular tape.

Direct control

16 Once proximal control is secured, the haematoma is evacuated and vascular clamps are applied. Although punctures can be repaired with simple sutures, resection and anastomosis is needed in most situations. If this is not possible without tension a saphenous vein graft is inserted.

After direct control is obtained repair of the artery is accomplished either by direct suture as described on page 54 or grafted if necessary to avoid tension. If the saphenous vein is not available a segment of cephalic vein can be used. If the wound is clean and there is no evidence of bacterial contamination, and there are no suitable autografts available, a short segment of PTFE graft can be used to re-establish continuity. The anastomoses are performed in the usual fashion, utilizing 5/0 or 6/0 monofilament sutures in a continuous over-and-over method.

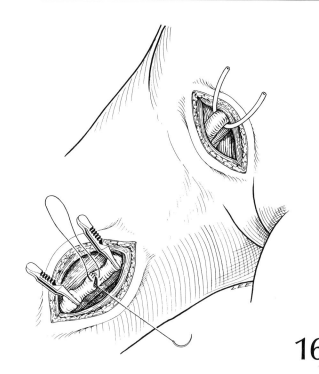

16

Determining patency

17 Before completion of the repair a Fogarty catheter is passed to ensure a patent system free of clots. Major vein injuries are repaired with simple suture techniques, or resection and anastomosis if this does not prolong the operation unduly. Grafts are needed only on rare occasions (popliteal vein).

Postoperative management

After operation the distal pulses and limb blood pressures are followed, and a regular evaluation of neuromuscular function is essential. Any deterioration in the perception of light touch or motor function is a firm indication for further studies, usually arteriography, regardless of skin colour or temperatures, distal pulses or limb blood pressure[1,5].

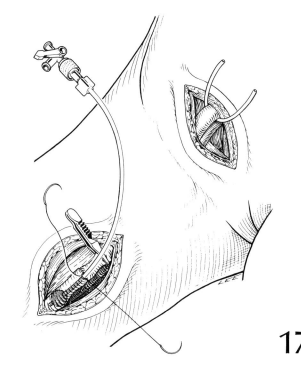

17

References

1. Perry MO. *The Management of Acute Vascular Injuries*. Baltimore: Williams and Wilkins, 1981.

2. Rich NM, Spencer FC. *Vascular Trauma*. Philadelphia: WB Saunders, 1978.

3. Thal ER, Snyder WH, Hays RJ, Perry MO. Management of carotid artery injuries. *Surgery* 1974; 76: 955–62.

4. Perry MO. Metabolic response to trauma. In: Schwartz SI, ed. *Principles of Surgery*, 3rd edn. New York: McGraw-Hill, 1979: 223–6.

5. Snyder WH, Thal ER, Perry MO. Vascular injuries of the extremities. In: Rutherford RB, ed. *Vascular Surgery*, 3rd edn. Philadelphia: WB Saunders, 1989: 613–37.

Illustrations by Marc Donon

Treatment of iatrogenic vascular injuries

R. M. Green MD, FACS
Associate Professor of Surgery, Chief, Section of Vascular Surgery, University of Rochester School of Medicine, Rochester, New York, USA

C. G. Rob MChir, FRCS, FACS
Professor of Surgery, Uniformed Services University of the Health Sciences, F. Edward Hebert School of Medicine, Bethesda, Maryland, USA

History

The first descriptions of iatrogenic vascular injuries were made by William Hunter[1,2]. The injuries described were caused by barbers performing therapeutic phlebotomy and occurred between the brachial artery and vein. Any artery or vein may be injured by a therapeutic procedure. Vascular injuries may cause haemorrhage or thrombosis, a false or dissecting aneurysm, or an arteriovenous fistula. The most common causes of vascular injuries today are cardiac catheterization, invasive angiography, invasive monitoring devices, intra-aortic balloon pumps, umbilical artery catheters in neonates and various surgical procedures[3]. Since these injuries occur in a hospital or doctor's surgery they should be promptly recognized and treated to minimize serious potential sequelae.

Principles and justification

Arterial injuries should be repaired if at all possible as ligation is associated with a predictable risk of ischaemic complications[4].

The risk of stroke after ligation of the neck arteries is as follows: common carotid, 20%; internal carotid, 40%; and vertebral, 8%.

The risk of amputation with ligation of upper extremity arteries is as follows: subclavian, 30%; axillary, 43%; brachial (above elbow), 55%; brachial (below elbow), 25%; radial, 5%.

The risk of amputation with ligation of lower extremity arteries is as follows: common iliac, 53%; external iliac, 46%; common femoral, 80%; superficial femoral, 55%; popliteal, 73%.

The problems a surgeon encounters when dealing with an iatrogenic vascular injury are numerous and may be unique to the artery or vein involved. Illustrated examples describing the management of a variety of different situations will serve to illustrate the basic principles of repair of the iatrogenic vascular injury which can then be applied to the specific situation.

Procedures

THROMBOSIS OF BRACHIAL ARTERY AFTER CORONARY ANGIOGRAPHY

This is currently the most common iatrogenic vascular injury and is the most common cause of arterial insufficiency in the upper extremity[5]. This problem occurs in approximately 1–2% of patients undergoing cardiac catheterization through the brachial approach. Factors contributing to this problem include 'redo' punctures, catheter change, improper closure, failure to use heparin, brachial artery atherosclerosis, prolonged catheter time, female patients and the experience of the cardiologist. These injuries are best repaired at the time of catheterization with thrombectomy and venous patch angioplasty or resection of the injured segment and end-to-end repair. Delay may require a more complex reconstruction with an interposition vein graft.

Exposure of occluded artery

1a, b Local infiltration anaesthesia with 1% lignocaine is used. A longitudinal incision is made medial to the biceps muscle centred over the puncture site. If the incision must cross the elbow crease it is done in an S fashion. A reasonable length of artery is exposed above and below the puncture site. The patient is heparinized and a bulldog clamp is placed proximally if a satisfactory pulse is present. If not, no occluding clamp is applied at this point. No clamp is applied distally because a bulldog may fracture the occluding thrombus. If intact, a recent thrombus can be extracted completely with a forceps. Since it is difficult to visualize the intima in a vessel this size through a transverse arteriotomy, a longitudinal cut is made through the puncture site. The clot usually begins to extrude when the artery is opened.

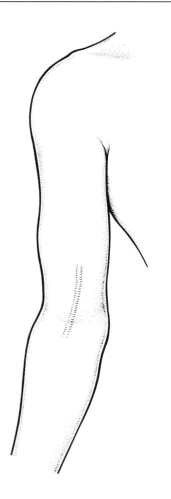

1a

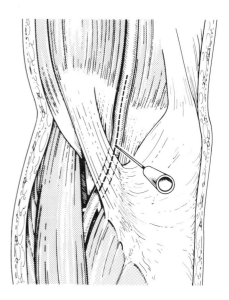

1b

Removal of thrombus and any damaged intima

2a, b Thrombus can often be completely removed with forceps, suction and irrigation and, if inflow is pulsatile, catheterization of the artery is not required. A bulldog clamp is placed on the distal vessel when backflow occurs. The intima is inspected and loose flaps are debrided. A common finding is an intimal elevation posteriorly. If extensive, the segment of artery should be resected. A no. 2 or 3 Fogarty catheter may be passed distally to remove any residual thrombus and, if possible, both the radial and ulnar vessels should be thrombectomized. It is important to remember that thrombectomy catheters can do damage themselves and should always be used with caution and only when necessary.

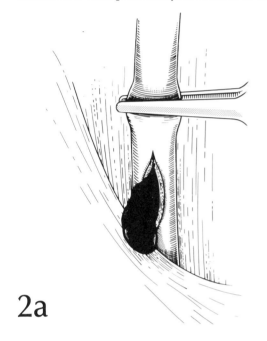

2a

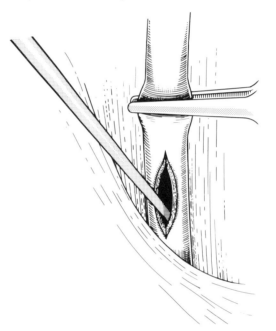

2b

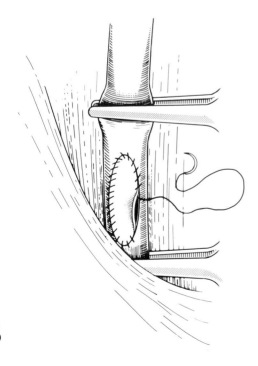

3

Closure with venous patch graft angioplasty

3 If the back wall of the vessel is intact and the anterior surface can be debrided the artery can be closed with a venous patch angioplasty. A length of cephalic vein is harvested and opened along its length. The vein is sutured to the artery with 6/0 polypropylene. The use of a patch will prevent postoperative thrombosis which would more than likely follow primary closure in this setting. If palpable pulses do not return at the wrist, an intraoperative arteriogram is performed to identify the cause of the problem. When the artery has been extensively damaged and closure with a patch is not possible, two alternatives exist. The artery can be mobilized over a sufficient distance to perform an end-to-end anastomosis after the involved segment has been excised, or, if a sufficient length of artery cannot be obtained, an interposition graft of cephalic vein can be inserted. The wound is closed primarily without drainage. The patient is placed on antibiotics for several days because these injuries often occur in less than ideal sterile conditions. Aspirin (5 g) is given daily for 6 weeks.

REPAIR OF FALSE ANEURYSM OF FEMORAL ARTERY AFTER ARTERIOGRAPHY

Patients may present with a painful, pulsatile mass in the groin hours, days, weeks or months after retrograde catheterization. Often there is a history of excessive bleeding at the time of the procedure or repeated catheter exchanges. The diagnosis of a false aneurysm can usually be made at the bedside. Colour-flow duplex sonography is particularly helpful in distinguishing a haematoma from a false aneurysm[6]. Repair is recommended if there is flow seen outside the artery on the ultrasonographic examination. Immediate operation is not recommended if little or no flow is seen in the groin mass. These patients are observed and treated with antibiotics. If pain or fever occur the patient is then taken to the operating room for repair.

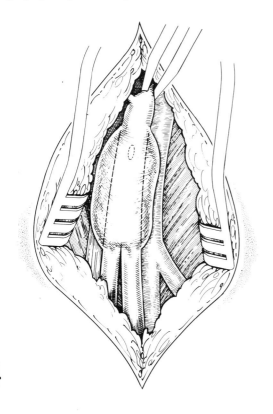

4

Incision and control of artery

4 These patients often have symptomatic coronary artery disease and every effort should be made to avoid significant blood loss and hypotension. This is complicated because the haematoma may be large and the tissue planes obscured. To facilitate the operation an incision to expose the femoral artery under the inguinal ligament is often necessary. This may be done with local infiltration of 1% lignocaine but in some cases, particularly in the obese patient, a general or regional anaesthetic is advised. Control of the femoral artery should be achieved before entering the haematoma. Repairing these injuries by premature entry into the haematoma and controlling the bleeding with a finger is a dangerous approach and should be avoided whenever possible. If the common femoral artery can be clamped under the inguinal ligament the haematoma can be entered and the bleeding point identified.

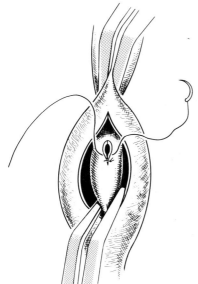

5

Repair of injury

5 Once proximal control has been obtained and the vessel clamped, the distal dissection is completed. These injuries are usually the result of tangential entry into the vessel, often at the femoral artery bifurcation. Two or three interrupted pledgeted sutures of 5/0 polypropylene are all that is required to repair most of these injuries. If the femoral artery is diseased, a patch closure may be required. When this injury occurs in a young child a patch of autogenous vein is applied.

The haematoma is evacuated. The wound is closed in layers with closed suction drainage. Antibiotics to cover Gram-positive cocci are given for 5 days.

ACCIDENTAL INJURY TO COMMON FEMORAL ARTERY DURING LIGATURE OF SAPHENOUS VEIN

This unfortunate injury must be recognized at once. It is likely to be caused by an operator unfamiliar with groin vascular anatomy. As with any vascular injury it is important that the situation is not made worse by blind attempts to stop the bleeding with haemostats. The correct manoeuvre is to control the bleeding with direct pressure, get help and then dissect out the artery proximal to the injury and deliberately control the injured vessel with a vascular clamp.

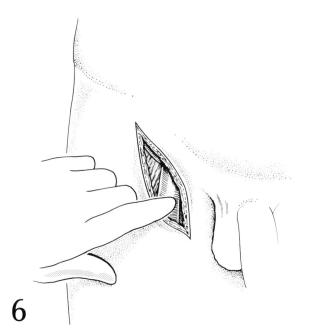

6

Rarely, a far worse situation develops. The surgeon mistakes the superficial femoral artery for the long saphenous vein, carefully dissects the superficial artery and clamps it. A stripper is then introduced into the artery and is passed distally to the ankle. The whole length of the main arterial system is then removed by stripping. The inevitable result is massive gangrene. This error can be avoided by always introducing the stripper into the long saphenous vein at the ankle and passing it proximally.

Control of arterial haemorrhage

6 The first step is to apply firm pressure over an area which is gradually reduced in size so that eventually only the actual bleeding point is compressed. The surgeon and his assistant then isolate the femoral artery proximal to the injury. The easiest approach to this is to reflect the inguinal ligament upwards and slip a vascular clamp around the distal external iliac artery. This allows the assistant to keep pressure on the injured vessel and reduces blood loss. When the proximal artery is clamped, heparin is given and the distal vessels are controlled. Depending on the site of arterial injury the deep femoral artery may be difficult to visualize. The pressure point on the bleeding segment can be further reduced in area and careful dissection is continued until all the branches are controlled with bulldog clamps or vessel loop occluders. The dissection must proceed in an orderly fashion to reduce the chance of further injury.

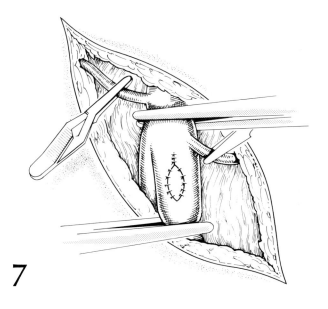

7

Repair of arterial wound

7 A clean surgical knife wound can be sutured primarily, but if haemostats have been used in an attempt to control bleeding the damaged wall must be excised and the artery repaired with a patch angioplasty. Care must be taken in selecting a suitable patch. A varicosed saphenous vein should not be used. Usually there are normal segments, even in a vein removed for varicosities.

AORTIC THROMBOSIS SECONDARY TO UMBILICAL ARTERY CATHETERS IN NEONATES

Umbilical artery catheters are essential in monitoring severely ill neonates but complications, including aortic thrombosis, can result from their use. If untreated this complication is invariably fatal[7]. Non-occlusive aortic thrombi have been seen by ultrasonographic imaging in as many as 60% of babies with umbilical catheters in place, and 95% of infants will have a fibrin sheath around the catheter at the time of removal. These non-occluding thrombi have some potential to do harm but are currently left alone.

Significant causative factors in the development of an aortic thrombus in the presence of an umbilical artery catheter include catheter composition (polytetrafluoroethylene (PTFE, Teflon) is worst, silicone rubber is safest), side-hole *versus* end-hole openings, low *versus* high aortic placement and hypertonic acidic solutions[8]. Lower extremity ischaemia is the most frequent clinical manifestation of aortic thrombosis. Some neonates will present with sudden congestive heart failure and hypertension. The diagnosis is best made with colour Doppler ultrasonography, acknowledging that this technique cannot provide precise anatomical details about the status of the major visceral branches. Infants with aortic thrombosis can be divided into those with non-occlusive thrombus and those with complete aortic occlusion. Neonates with adequate distal circulation and no evidence of visceral involvement can usually be managed without operation with anticoagulation if not contraindicated, antihypertensives and cardiac support. Those patients with limb-threatening ischaemia and any evidence of visceral involvement require aortic thrombectomy.

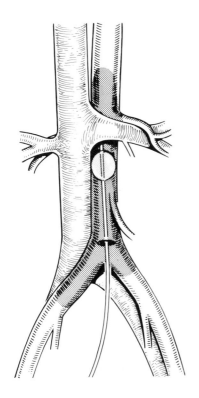

8

Aortic thrombectomy

8 The patient is heparinized and the aorta exposed through a midline incision. A transverse aortotomy is made just above the iliac bifurcation. A no. 2 Fogarty catheter is inserted and the occluding thrombus removed. The bulk of the thrombus will be in the aorta and care must be taken not to injure the fragile iliac arteries. The catheter should be inserted only far enough distally to remove any clot present. The proximal aorta usually measures 10–12 mm and is easily catheterized. The clot in the aorta often extends up to the renal arteries, and these should be protected with gentle bulldog clamps to prevent thrombus entry into both the renals and the inferior mesenteric artery as the balloon passes by. The aortotomy is closed with interrupted 6/0 polypropylene sutures once flow is established.

INJURY TO INFERIOR VENA CAVA OR COMMMON ILIAC VEINS DURING OPERATION ON ABDOMINAL AORTA

These injuries are best avoided by performing only the essential dissection necessary for control and suture. It is not necessary to encircle the proximal aorta or iliac arteries completely during aneurysmectomy and is certainly not necessary to remove the aneurysmal sac.

9

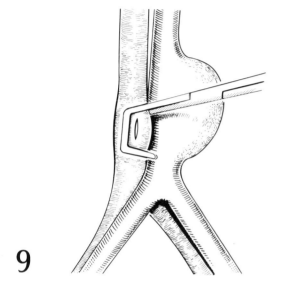

10

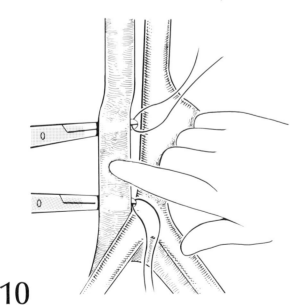

The aorta must be completely dissected during aortic reconstruction for occlusive disease, but this dissection should be performed above the level of the inferior mesenteric artery where adhesions of the diseased aorta to the vena cava are minimal.

Temporary control of haemorrhage

9 Once again the injury should not be made worse by inappropriate attempts at control by blind clamping or application of haemoclips. Such manoeuvres invariably worsen the problem. These injuries usually begin as small tears and the first step in control should always be direct pressure. The pressure point is gradually reduced in area until the surgeon identifies the injury and its extent. A suitable segment of the injured vein is dissected out and then controlled with a partially occluding Satinsky clamp. This injury is then easily repaired with vascular sutures.

Management of major defect which cannot be controlled with side clamp

10 If the injury is extensive a partially occluding clamp may not control the bleeding. In this situation bleeding is usually massive and the surgeon should realize that he is in a very difficult and possibly disastrous situation in which the patient could exsanguinate. The first step is again to control the bleeding with firm pressure. The surgeon then proceeds in a step-by-step manner. He confirms with the anaesthetist that adequate blood is available for immediate transfusion. A rapid infusion autotransfusion device is extremely useful in this setting as warmed blood can be returned to the patient very quickly. The surgeon then confirms with the operating room nurse that all instruments and supplies needed are ready, including instruments for clamping the vena cava, sutures for repair with pledgets and ligatures for the vena cava should repair fail.

While an assistant is applying firm pressure to control the bleeding, the surgeon dissects out the vena cava above and the iliac veins below the injury. This is preferable to attempting to control the haemorrhage with balloon catheters. Occluding clamps are then applied. Significant bleeding may still occur from lumbar veins which must be controlled with bulldog clamps or suture ligatures. If the bleeding has been extensive and rapid the surgeon should give the anaesthetist enough time to replace volume and stabilize the patient before attempting repair. This may require application of pressure for a long period but it is time well spent if the injury is safely repaired.

Ligature or repair of inferior vena cava

11 The surgeon now inspects the injured vena cava. If repair is possible it should be done if the patient is stable. Otherwise, ligation is required. Repair may consist of lateral suture or replacement with a prosthetic ringed PTFE graft. Once completed, the remainder of the original operation is completed. After operation, the patient is placed in elastic support stockings. No anticoagulation is given. Serial duplex ultrasonographic scans of the lower extremity are recommended to monitor for potential venous complications.

CORRECTION OF ARTERIOVENOUS FISTULA BETWEEN ABDOMINAL AORTA AND LEFT COMMON ILIAC VEIN OR INFERIOR VENA CAVA BECAUSE OF LUMBAR DISC OPERATION

This complication was first reported in 1945 by Linton and White[9]. This remains a rare but potentially fatal complication of lumbar disc procedures. It is most likely to occur when the patient is operated on in the prone position and when the annulus fibrosis is deficient so that the pituitary rongeur used slips through the disc space and inadvertently causes a fistula. A rush of blood follows which can be controlled by pressure. Once the diagnosis is established preparation for a major operation with significant blood loss is made. There is rarely time for an arteriogram. Colour flow Doppler may be sufficient to make the diagnosis. The level of the disc space operated on determines the site of the vascular injury[10]. Most injuries occur through the L4–L5 and L5–S1 interspaces. The common iliac vessels are most often involved. Direct aortocaval injury occurs through

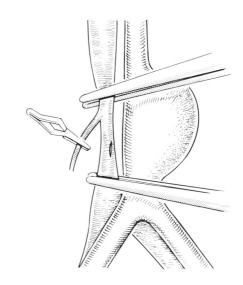

11

the L3–L4 interspace. In the absence of a precise anatomical diagnosis the midline abdominal approach gives the operator maximum flexibility.

When the injury is at the L3–L4 level, proximal and distal clamps on the aorta and vena cava are all that is required for repair. Injuries at the confluence of the iliac vessels at the L4–L5 interspace require control of all six major vessels. Unilateral iliac artery and vein control is sufficient for L5–S1 space injuries. Although there may be a small retroperitoneal haematoma, it may be deceptively small. It is important not to approach the arteriovenous communication until all the involved vessels are controlled. If the site is uncertain the aorta is controlled distal to the inferior mesenteric artery. The vena cava is controlled at the same level.

Control of iliac vessels

12 The right and left iliac arteries and veins are now isolated well away from the lesion and close to the bifurcation of the common iliac artery and the junction of the hypogastric and external iliac veins. The blood flow to the area of the arteriovenous fistula will now be under control except for the middle sacral artery and vein and sometimes a pair of lumbar arteries and veins. If possible, these vessels can be clipped before opening the vessels.

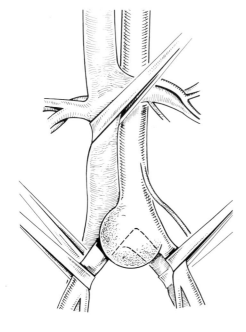

12

Exposure of arteriovenous fistula

13 The patient is heparinized and all the vessels are clamped. The distal aorta is opened, the fistula visualized and the aortotomy is then carried downward onto the involved iliac artery or upward onto the aorta itself. Bleeding from uncontrolled lumbar vessels is controlled with sutures from within. The venous defect is then identified through the cut in the artery.

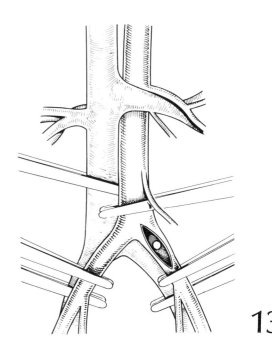

13

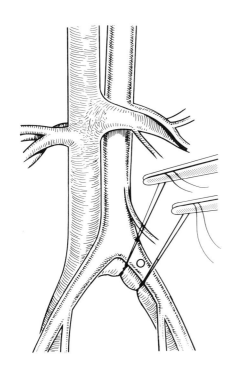

14

Ligature of common iliac vein

14 It is a mistake to attempt venous repair if the iliac vein is involved. Repair is difficult in an injury created by a rongeur. Instead, the iliac vein should be securely ligated proximal and distal to the injury. The vena cava can and should be repaired.

Repair of arterial injury

15 The artery is open on both its anterior and posterior aspects because of the injury which caused the problem. The posterior defect is closed first, a patch being required if the defect is large and irregular. The artery can be rotated to accomplish this or the closure can be done from within. The former is technically easier but does require more dissection. The anterior arteriotomy can often be repaired without a patch but one should not hesitate to use one if primary closure could narrow the vessel. If the injury cannot be repaired with a patch a prosthetic graft can be inserted. Heparin is reversed following repair. Antibiotics are administered in the operating room and continued for 5 days if prosthetic material is used.

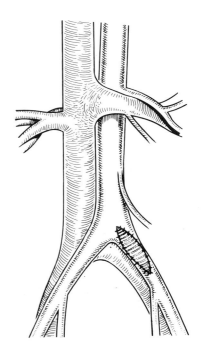

15

References

1. Hunter W. The history of an aneurysm of the aorta with some remarks on aneurysms in general. *Medical Observations and Inquiries* 1757; 1: 323–57.

2. Hunter W. Observations upon a particular species of aneurysm. *Medical Observations and Inquiries* 1762; 2: 390.

3. Mills JL, Wiedeman JE, Robison JG, Hallett JW Jr. Minimizing mortality and morbidity from iatrogenic arterial injuries: the need for early recognition and prompt repair. *J Vasc Surg* 1986; 4: 22–7.

4. Ehricks E. Major vascular ligations. In: Eiseman B, ed. *Prognosis of Surgical Disease*. Philadelphia: Saunders, 1980: 102–5.

5. McCollum CH, Mavor E. Brachial artery injury after cardiac catheterization. *J Vasc Surg* 1986; 4: 355–9.

6. Sheikh KH, Adams DB, McCann R, Lyerly HK, Sabiston DC, Kisslo J. Utility of Doppler colour flow imaging for identification of femoral arterial complication of cardiac catheterization. *Am Heart J* 1989; 117: 623–8.

7. Krueger TC, Neblett WW, O'Neill JA, MacDonell RC, Dean RH, Thieme GA. Management of aortic thrombosis secondary to umbilical artery catheters in neonates. *J Pediatr Surg* 1985; 20: 328–32.

8. Colburn MD, Gelabert HA, Quinones-Baldrich W. Neonatal aortic thrombosis. *Surgery* 1992; 111: 21–8.

9. Linton RR, White PD. Arteriovenous fistula between the right common iliac artery and inferior vena cava. Report of a case of its occurrence following an operation for a ruptured intervertebral disc with cure by operation. *Arch Surg* 1945; 50: 6–13.

10. Bernhard VM. Aortocaval fistulas. In: Haimovic H, ed. *Vascular Emergencies*. New York: Appleton-Crofts, 1982: 353–63.

Illustrations by Mark Iley

Amputations of the lower extremity

R. M. Green MD, FACS
Associate Professor of Surgery, and Chief, Section of Vascular Surgery, University of Rochester School of Medicine, Rochester, New York, USA

C. G. Rob MChir, FRCS, FACS
Professor of Surgery, Uniformed Services University of the Health Sciences, F. Edward Hebert School of Medicine, Bethesda, Maryland, USA

Principles and justification

Indications

Peripheral vascular disease due either to atherosclerosis and/or diabetes is the most common cause of amputation in the USA and Europe today. Curiously, the actual number of amputations has not decreased despite increasing use of arterial reconstructive procedures. Most major lower extremity amputations are performed only after failed femorodistal reconstructions[1]. Amputations are performed less often in the setting of acute arterial ischaemia where the ischaemic muscle mass becomes a metabolic threat to the patient. Finally, major amputations may be necessary in diabetic patients who may present with lower extremity infections that are beyond primary healing and may be life threatening when first seen[2].

Selection of amputation level

A combination of factors goes into determining the appropriate level of amputation. Clinical signs are subjective and experience which is often gained only by trial and error is necessary to predict the lowest possible amputation level accurately. Arteriography, which is essential in making a decision regarding arterial reconstruction, is imprecise and often misleading in predicting the proper level of amputation. Non-invasive testing is becoming increasingly more useful in defining the lowest level that will heal, particularly when used in conjunction with the clinical findings.

We have established certain clinical criteria that guide us in determining the proper amputation level. The presence of a palpable pulse at the ankle should ensure healing after a local excision of tissue, a transmetatarsal amputation or the removal of a toe and head of a metatarsal. These patients are usually diabetic with infection and neuropathy; ischaemia plays a lesser role. Diabetic patients with palpable pulses, neuropathy and gangrene of the first toe present a special problem. If only the great toe is removed the other toes are likely to become ulcerated and repetitive digital amputations are the rule. We often recommend that in this setting all the toes are removed. This allows the patient to wear a slightly modified shoe and be free of further problems of digital gangrene in the future. On the other hand, if one of the four small toes is gangrenous and the great toe is normal, only the gangrenous toe need be removed.

When gangrene or severe ischaemia extends proximal to the mid-foot, amputation at the level of the calf or thigh is indicated. In patients with peripheral arterial disease, the transmetatarsal and Syme amputations are rarely indicated because healing is unlikely unless the underlying perfusion defect is corrected, and this is often impossible. A decision regarding an above-knee or below-knee amputation can be difficult. We feel that primary wound healing can occur at the mid-calf level when the skin of the proximal calf is free from trophic changes and infection. The presence or absence of palpable pulses may be misleading but we believe that a patent deep femoral artery is essential for healing at the mid-calf level, and therefore we would not perform a below-knee amputation when the femoral pulse is absent. A palpable popliteal pulse is not required for healing below the knee. The presence or absence of bleeding and the status of the muscles when the flaps are cut are other factors which determine the fate of a below-knee amputation. The operator should not hesitate to move to a higher level if these are not satisfactory.

Non-invasive measurements of arterial pressures are not an absolute guide to proper site selection[3]. Although a below-knee amputation is likely to heal if the ankle pressure is 70 mmHg or greater, healing can and does occur at lower perfusion pressures. A very helpful finding, however, is the absence of an audible Doppler signal in the popliteal space. This is uniformly associated with failure of a below-knee amputation. The measurement of transcutaneous Po_2 is a more reliable laboratory predictor of amputation healing than are skin temperature measurements or arterial pressures. If the transcutaneous Po_2 reaches 10 mmHg or more after the inhalation of oxygen, healing is likely to occur[4].

The blood circulation in the toes can be measured by digital plethysmography even in the presence of the incompressible arteries of the diabetic patient[5]. A digital blood pressure above 10 mmHg predicts foot amputation healing in non-diabetics; in diabetics, 25 mmHg predicts healing.

Technical considerations

The following general principles apply to amputations at all levels:

1. The skin must not be traumatized. The instruments which should touch the skin are the knife and the needle.
2. Haemostasis must be complete.
3. There must be no tension on the skin flaps.
4. Drains should be used liberally.
5. A proper occlusive dressing should be applied.

Wound healing

Amputations of the toes and local excision of tissue for ischaemia are best left open; other amputations should be closed. This means that most amputations for infected or neuropathic gangrene in diabetic patients should not be sutured. When a satisfactory plantar flap is not available, an alternative to primary closure of a transmetatarsal amputation is the delayed application of a split-thickness skin graft.

Immediate casting and early ambulation

In the absence of severe infection, diabetic patients undergoing below-knee amputations should be fitted with a cast dressing in the operating room by a trained prosthetist[6]. The next morning a pylon device is put on the cast and physical therapy begins. Ambulation training without weight bearing continues for 7–10 days in some patients, when the cast is changed and the wound inspected. A new cast is then applied and the patient discharged to a rehabilitation unit. Another cast is applied 10 days later. A temporary prosthesis can be used 30 days after the amputation.

The benefits of the immediate-fit prosthesis result from the rigidity of the dressing and the prevention of oedema[7]. Wound immobilization may also limit postoperative pain and prevent knee contracture. Early ambulation reduces pulmonary complications, facilitates nursing care and increases the psychological well-being of the patient. Some surgeons feel that a plaster cast prevents access to the wound and recommend a Jobst air splint.

Operations

AMPUTATION OF ONE TOE FOR GANGRENE

Incision

1 Gauze is wrapped around the adjacent toes to provide retraction. A circular incision is made around the proximal phalanx 1 cm distal to the base so that the skin will be loose and fall together over the defect. It is important to remember that the skin will not be sutured unless the blood supply is excellent and this is rarely the case. The tendons are divided as high as possible and the digit removed through the metatarsophalangeal joint. Any bleeding vessels are secured and the head of the metatarsal is removed with fine-tipped rongeurs. A formal resection of the metatarsal head requires an extension of the incision which could compromise the circulation and should be avoided.

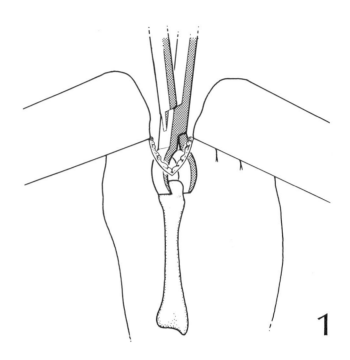

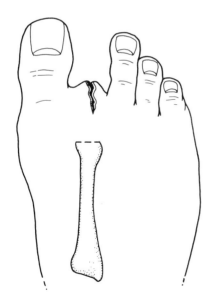

Removal of distal metatarsal

2 A small rongeur forceps is now introduced into the wound and the head of the metatarsal bone, together with the distal 2–3 cm of the shaft, is removed. Loose fragments of tendon and joint capsule are trimmed. The wound is irrigated with saline and a 0.25-inch rubber drain is inserted into the cavity if gross infection is present. Steristrips are applied to approximate the skin if the wound is not infected. A gauze dressing is applied to approximate the wound. These wounds should not be packed tightly with gauze.

AMPUTATION OF TOE AND METATARSAL BONE

In some patients with infective or neuropathic gangrene it may be possible to excise the toe and metatarsal bone, leaving the rest of the foot. As a good blood supply is essential for healing, this procedure is not indicated if the foot is ischaemic.

Incision

3 The incision is made around the base of the toe and extends along the plantar surface of the foot. It is deepened to expose the flexor tendons of the involved toe and the metatarsal bone.

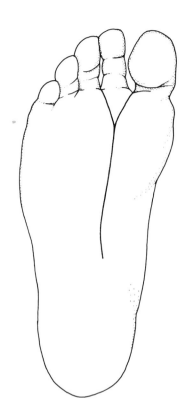

3

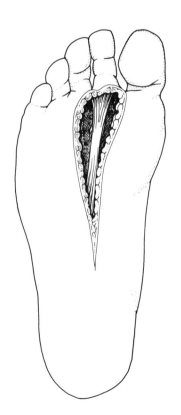

4

Removal of toe and metatarsal

4 The infected flexor tendons and fascia are divided as far proximal as possible and the base of the metatarsal bone is disarticulated. The metatarsal bone and extensor tendon are then freed from the dorsal skin. The wound is irrigated with saline and any additional necrotic tissue removed with scissors. Care must be taken not to enter tissue planes of adjacent metatarsals. The plantar aspect of the wound is sutured. A drain is brought out through the toe amputation site if the wound is infected. A light sterile dressing is applied to approximate the tissues.

AMPUTATION OF ALL TOES

Amputation of all the toes is superior to a transmetatarsal procedure and should be used when the condition of the skin permits. It should also be used in most diabetic patients with ischaemic, neuropathic or infective gangrene of the great toe even though the other four toes are still viable. Once the great toe has been removed in a patient with this type of gangrene, there is still considerable risk that the other toes will soon become deformed, ulcerated and eventually gangrenous.

5 The procedure is the same as that described for removal of one toe. Again it is stressed that the skin incision is circular and about 1 cm distal to the base of the proximal phalanx. The toe is removed through the metatarsophalangeal joint and the head and distal shaft of the metatarsal are then removed piecemeal with a rongeur. The skin is neither sutured not packed open, but liberal use of drains for infection is recommended. A light gauze dressing is applied to approximate the skin edges. The bridges of skin between the toe amputations hold the dorsal and plantar skin together.

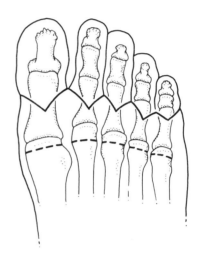

5

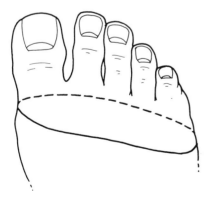

6

TRANSMETATARSAL AMPUTATION

We prefer to amputate the toes and distal metatarsal individually so that the remaining skin bridges facilitate healing. If the skin of the distal part of the dorsum of the foot between the toes is gangrenous, a transmetatarsal amputation is indicated. The advantage of this amputation is that the patient can wear a normal shoe with minimal orthotic adjustments.

Incision

6 The plantar skin incision is made as close to the digits as possible and the dorsal incision crosses the foot about 3 cm from the base of the toes. The plantar flap is fashioned by cutting close to the metatarsals and plantar tendons. The flexor tendons are divided individually.

Division of metatarsals

7 Each metatarsal is identified from the plantar surface and the shaft divided with bone-cutting forceps 2 cm from its base. After all five metatarsals have been transected the tendons and other soft tissues are sharply divided. Redundant fascia is removed, the area is irrigated and bleeding vessels are secured.

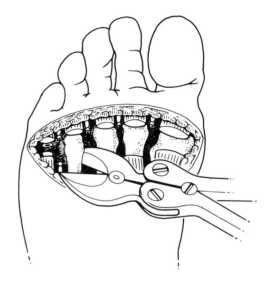

7

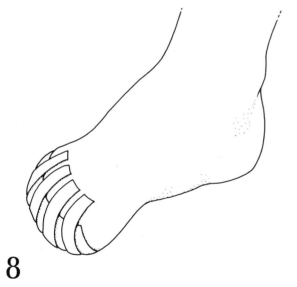

8

Skin closure

8 The skin flaps should be loose and under no tension. The skin must be treated very gently; it should not be picked up with forceps. When possible the deep fascia is closed with interrupted absorbable sutures. Drainage through a small stab incision in the plantar flap is recommended. The skin can be closed with Steristrips or sutures and the wound dressed with a light gauze wrap.

BELOW-KNEE AMPUTATION

Patients with lower extremity ischaemia often have serious cardiorespiratory problems. We prefer therefore to operate on these patients in the supine position under regional (preferably continuous epidural) anaesthesia.

Incision

9 Although equal anterior–posterior flaps may be cut, we prefer a short anterior and a long posterior flap containing gastrocnemius muscle for its protection and bulk. The anterior skin incision should be placed about 2 cm distal to the level of the bone section, which is four fingerbreadths from the tibial tubercle. The skin incision is made directly down to the periosteum. The posterior flap is cut about 14 cm distal to the level of the bone section. It is wise to cut the posterior flap longer than necessary to ensure that there is no tension on the closure.

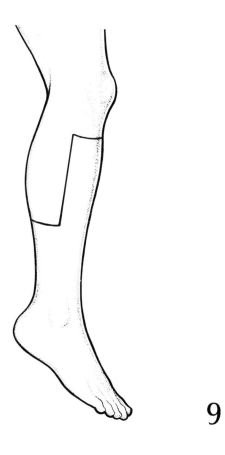

9

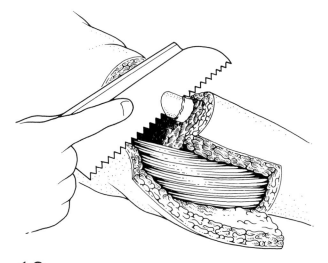

10

Division of anterior muscles

10 The fibrous attachments to the periosteum are raised with an elevator from the anteromedial surface of the tibia for a distance of 1 cm. This manoeuvre can devascularize the anterior skin so it should be done only to free enough periosteum for use in approximating the deep closure layer. The muscles of the anterior compartment are divided transversely. It makes no sense to cut the posterior skin or muscles until the bones are divided.

Division of bones and posterior flap

11 The tibia is cut at an angle of 45°. The fibula is freed with a periosteal elevator and divided with a right-angled bone cutter at least 2.5 cm above the tibial cut to avoid penetration of the flap. Irregularities of the bones are smoothed off with a rongeur. The calf muscles are now divided in an oblique fashion so that a smooth, tapered muscular posterior flap is created. Bleeding vessels are secured with either cautery or absorbable sutures. The popliteal artery and vein are suture ligated. The nerves are ligated with fine catgut and allowed to retract into the popliteal space. A tourniquet should never be used when this operation is performed for ischaemia.

Drainage and closure

12 The wound is thoroughly irrigated with saline to remove any bone debris. A closed suction drainage catheter is placed through a small lateral stab wound across the wound beneath the deep fascia. The fascia is closed with absorbable sutures. The central part of this suture line consists of the deep fascia of the posterior flap which is sutured to the periosteal flap anteriorly to cover the end of the tibia. The skin is closed with interrupted synthetic monofilament sutures. It is essential that the skin is touched only gently. A sterile elastic stump dressing is applied.

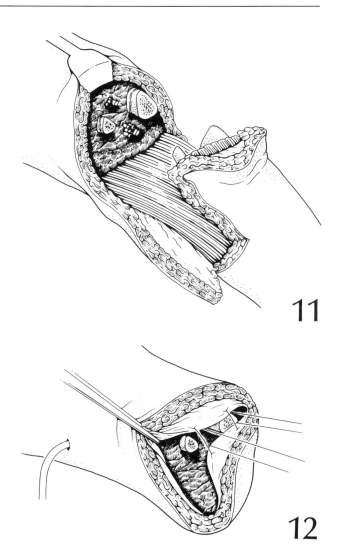

11

12

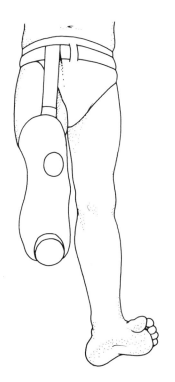

13

The plaster cast

13 The cast controls oedema, protects the stump from trauma and reduces postoperative pain. A dressing of this type should be applied to all below-knee amputations except those performed for foot sepsis.

The cast should be applied according to the method described by Burgess *et al.*[8]. Ambulation with partial weightbearing is encouraged early in the rehabilitation process. Full weightbearing on the amputation stump is not allowed until the permanent prosthesis has been applied.

ABOVE-KNEE AMPUTATION

Incision

14 To avoid skin flaps that are too short posteriorly, the skin incision is almost circular with the anterior incision placed at the upper border of the patella. This ensures that the skin flaps are loose and under no tension when closed. The skin incision should pass through the deep fascia. At this time the long saphenous vein may require ligation and division. The skin and deep fascia are then dissected proximally to create a flap length of about 4 cm.

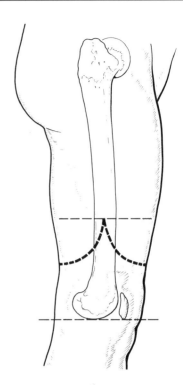

14

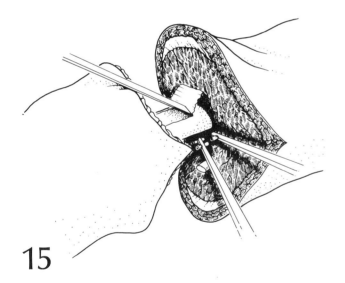

15

Division of soft tissues

15 The muscles are divided circumferentially at a level 2–3 cm proximal to the level of the skin incision. The femoral artery and veins are clamped and divided. The presence of clot in the vein should be noted. The sciatic nerve is gently pulled down, tied with fine catgut, divided and allowed to retract proximally. Posteriorly and laterally there may be branches of the deep femoral artery that require ligation and division.

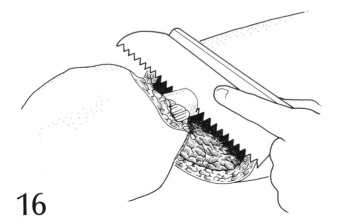

16

Division of femur

16 The periosteum is now divided. Ideally, the bone is divided at a level 22–28 cm distal to the tip of the greater trochanter. The muscles are protected with a gauze pack or a stump retractor as the bone is sectioned.

Wound closure

17a, b The wound is now thoroughly irrigated with saline to remove any loose debris. A closed drainage system is placed across the cut end of the femur and brought out through a separate stab high in the thigh so it can be removed without disturbing the dressing. The deep fascia is now closed with interrupted absorbable sutures over the drain. The skin is closed with monofilament suture and a light dressing is applied. We recommend that unless complications develop this dressing not be changed for 7–10 days when the sutures can be removed. Although a plaster cast offers the same potential benefits as in below-knee amputation, it is difficult to keep a cast on an above-knee amputation and we do not currently recommend its application.

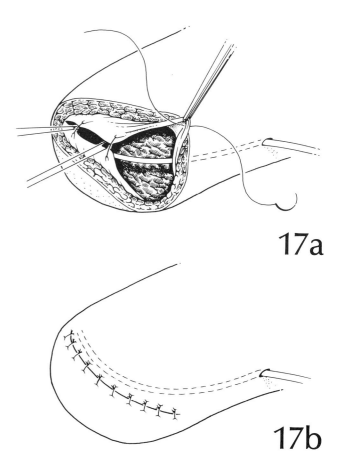

17a

17b

Postoperative care

Toe amputations

The wounds should be dressed as infrequently as possible. They should not be packed. If there was preoperative infection, appropriate antibiotics should be given. Patients should remain non-weightbearing and in bed for the first week or until signs of healing are present.

Transmetatarsal amputation

Antibiotics are continued if infection was present before operation. The drain is removed after 2–3 days. Full hip, knee and ankle exercises are encouraged but weight-bearing is prohibited for at least 7 days.

Below-knee amputations

A trapeze is attached to the bed of every patient with a major lower extremity amputation. Patients are placed prone at least three times a day for 20 min to avoid hip joint contractures. The patient is encouraged to stand by the bed on the evening of the operation or at least within the first 24 h. Patients walk between parallel bars and eventually with a walker as soon as possible.

Antibiotics and analgesic drugs are given as necessary. The closed drainage system is removed on the third postoperative day. The plaster cast is changed on day 7 unless it becomes very loose or the patient complains of extraordinary amounts of pain. If there is confusion, unexplained tachycardia, excessive serosanguineous drainage or fever the cast is removed and the wound

inspected. The sutures are removed at the 7-day cast change and another cast is applied. At this point the patient is transferred to a rehabilitation unit. Under ordinary circumstances patients are fully ambulatory with a permanent prosthesis within 3 months of operation. This is possible even in patients 75 years and older.

Above-knee amputations

The aim once again is early ambulation and, if possible, the patient should stand with assistance at the bedside within 24 h of operation. If there is excessive stump pain or evidence of a wound infection the dressing should be removed and the wound inspected.

The closed drainage system is removed on the third postoperative day. The rehabilitation process includes early walking between parallel bars with a walker and with crutches. Stump exercises are begun immediately, particularly the prone manoeuvres to prevent hip contractures. A temporary prosthesis is fitted as soon as possible, but full weightbearing is not allowed for some time.

Patients with an above-knee amputation often gain weight. The patient should have an early dietary consultation to discuss this important issue.

References

1. Stern PH. Occlusive vascular disease of lower limbs: diagnosis, amputation surgery and rehabilitation. A review of the Burke experience. *Am J Phys Med Rehabil* 1988; 67: 145–54.

2. Fearon J, Campbell DR, Hoar CS, Gibbons G, Rowbotham J, Wheelock FC. Improved results with diabetic below-knee amputations. *Arch Surg* 1985; 120: 777–80.

3. Barnes RW, Shanik GD, Slaymaker EE. An index of healing in below-knee amputation: leg blood pressure by Doppler ultrasound. *Surgery* 1976; 79: 13–20.

4. Oishi CS, Fronek A, Golbranson FL. The role of non-invasive vascular studies in determining levels of amputation. *J Bone Joint Surg* 1988; 70-A: 1520–30.

5. Barnes RW, Thornhill B, Nix L, Rittgers SE, Turley G. Prediction of amputation wound healing: roles of Doppler ultrasound and digit photoplethysmography. *Arch Surg* 1981; 116: 80–3.

6. Condon RE, Jordan PH Jr. Immediate postoperative prosthesis in vascular amputations. *Ann Surg* 1969; 170: 435–47.

7. Burgess EM, Romano RL, Zettl JH, Schrock RD. Amputations of the leg for peripheral vascular insufficiency. *J Bone Joint Surg* 1971; 53-A: 874–90.

8. Burgess EM, Romano RL, Zettl JH. *The Management of Lower Extremity Amputations,* 1969 (TRIO-6 available for $7.50 from Superintendent of Documents, US Government Printing Office, Washington DC 20402).

Surgical treatment of acquired and congenital arteriovenous fistulae

Calvin B. Ernst MD
Clinical Professor of Surgery, University of Michigan Medical School and Head, Division of Vascular Surgery, Henry Ford Hospital, Detroit, Michigan, USA

Daniel J. Reddy MD
Clinical Associate Professor of Surgery, University of Michigan Medical School and Senior Staff Vascular Surgeon, Henry Ford Hospital, Detroit, Michigan, USA

Principles and justification

More than 230 years have passed since William Hunter's classic description of chronic arteriovenous fistula (AVF) of the extremity. Although Hunterian quadrilateral ligation has been replaced by contemporary vascular reconstruction, the principles and justification for operation remain the same.

Acquired AVFs, in contrast to congenital AVFs, are curable. Acquired AVFs most often result from penetrating trauma but these lesions may also follow blunt trauma, particularly to an extremity or the neck. Percutaneous angiographic procedures, haemodynamic monitoring and other iatrogenic causes are becoming increasingly important in the pathogenesis of these lesions[1].

Congenital AVFs have been recognized since antiquity. While present from birth, they are often asymptomatic and may remain undetected for months or years. Most are best managed non-operatively. Operative treatment is reserved for symptomatic, small, accessible lesions or for complications of large lesions. While haemangiomas are thought to be arrests in the capillary network stage of embryological development, AVFs are due to arrests in the retiform stage of embryological development before the final stage of vascular formation[2].

Acquired AVF

The degree of physiological derangement is defined by the anatomical location and size of the fistula. Large central AVFs cause cardiac decompensation, whereas small peripheral ones do not. Small distal fistulae, because of low blood flow, may not require repair and they may also close spontaneously[3]. With a large fistula, systemic vascular resistance falls, with resulting increased arterial and venous blood flow proximal to the fistula, decreased arterial pressure distal to the fistula, and a corresponding increased distal venous pressure. The distal extremity, supplied with less arterial flow which may become reversed in the distal axial artery, may become ischaemic. Regional venous hypertension may result in obvious varicose veins. The potential systemic effects include increased heart rate, stroke volume, blood volume, and pulse pressure with cardiomegaly and high-output cardiac failure. A Nicoladoni–Branham sign, reflex slowing of the heart and increased diastolic blood pressure following compression of the fistula, is often present. With the uncommon aortocaval fistula, cardiac failure is rapid and can only be reversed by prompt recognition and emergency operative repair[4]. Late non-haemodynamic consequences of an acquired AVF include erosion or compression of adjacent structures, endovasculitis at the fistula, or bacterial endocarditis. An accompanying false aneurysm or aneurysmal degeneration of the proximal arterial system may also cause peripheral or pulmonary thromboemboli, or may expand and rupture.

Operative repair is indicated once the diagnosis is confirmed. Delay may make repair more difficult after collateral arterial and venous elements have enlarged or when scar tissue encasement makes dissection more difficult. Small or inaccessible AVFs, such as intrarenal or intrahepatic ones which develop following needle biopsies, are best managed by interventional radiological embolic techniques.

Congenital AVF

Congenital AVFs are classified as microfistulous and macrofistulous types according to their angiographic appearance. Clinically, the differences between haemangiomas and microfistulous AVFs are indistinct because approximately 70% of congenital AVFs are complex vascular malformations containing haemangiomatous elements[5]. Vascular malformations limited to the venous system are usually termed cavernous haemangiomas. Although sometimes confused with AVFs, they have no arterial connections and are not considered further.

Congenital AVFs predominate in the lower extremities but also occur in the upper extremities, pelvis, or head and neck. Even when an AVF is discovered in a young patient, symptoms may not develop for months or years.

Clinical presentation and prognosis vary greatly and depend on the location and extent of the AVF. AVF enlargement usually parallels growth of the patient but sudden enlargement may follow changes in blood pressure or hormonal modulation. Although bleeding is the most dramatic presentation, AVFs of the pelvis or extremity also exhibit skin discoloration, pain, palpable mass and limb hypertrophy. High-output cardiac failure is uncommon in congenital AVFs. Symptoms of venous hypertension with pulsatile veins, extremity oedema and stasis dermatitis may be noted. The Nicoladoni–Branham sign may be seen.

The diagnosis of a congenital AVF may be made by history and physical examination alone. Although non-invasive testing supports the diagnosis, such tests are practical only when the AVF involves an extremity. Examination by duplex ultrasonography may delineate abnormal flow patterns in major vessels, venous insufficiency, or thrombosis. Magnetic resonance imaging (MRI) and dynamic computed tomography are useful diagnostic modalities[6]. MRI has the advantage of not requiring intravenous contrast material and the anatomical extent of the lesion can be delineated.

Bleeding resulting from trauma is common in extremity AVFs and is an indication for urgent operation. Functional impairment or cosmetic deformity are relative indications for operation, as are discrepancies of limb length. Other indications for operation include uncontrolled pain, distal extremity ischaemia, and rarely, congestive heart failure.

Management of acquired AVF

Preoperative

Angiography is indispensable for diagnosis of an acquired AVF and for planning the operation. Thorough cardiac evaluation is required, particularly when cardiac symptoms are present. If the patient is hypervolaemic, preoperative phlebotomy with banking of the blood for future autotransfusion has proved helpful. Appropriate cannulae are placed for haemodynamic monitoring.

Preparation

1 A pneumatic tourniquet placed proximal to the AVF facilitates dissection and repair in a bloodless field. Since the tourniquet must not encroach upon the operative field, use is limited to lesions involving only the distal thigh and leg. The entire leg should be draped in a sterile field. The foot is placed in a transparent sterile plastic bag so that distal circulation may be monitored. The contralateral groin is also included in the sterile field in the event that a segment of saphenous vein is required for vascular reconstruction.

Anaesthesia

Regional anaesthesia is preferred when repairing AVFs of the lower extremities in adults. For AVFs other than those involving the lower extremities, and in children, general anaesthesia is required. Local anaesthesia is used only for very localized AVFs in which tourniquet occlusion is not anticipated. An example of a small, localized AVF suitable for local infiltration anaesthesia is the persistent fistulous communication following an infrainguinal *in situ* vein bypass graft.

Operation

Incision

2 An incision is made directly over the AVF which is localized by palpating the most intense site of the thrill. Collateral channels which may have developed in chronic lesions should be ligated and divided. Use of electrocautery is not appropriate to control large collateral vessels.

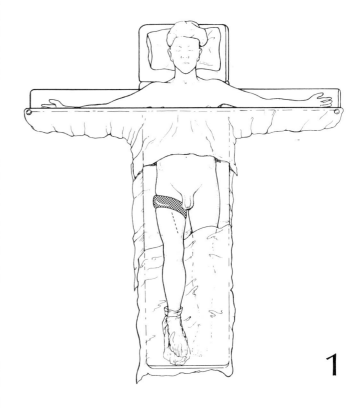

1

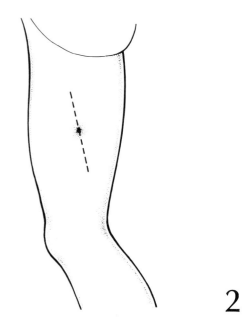

2

Vessel dissection

3 Scalpel dissection will often be required when dissecting the fistula and the involved artery and vein, as chronic post-traumatic lesions are often surrounded by dense scar tissue. Dissection of the proximal artery proceeds first, encircling it with a vessel loop. The artery distal to the AVF is then isolated and looped, and finally the proximal and distal venous elements of the AVF are mobilized and controlled.

Small arterial and venous branches must be ligated with non-absorbable sutures and divided with care lest the thin-walled venous branches are torn with ensuing haemorrhage. If the fistula is entered before adequate mobilization of the vessels and bleeding obscures the operative field, an occlusion balloon catheter passed through the defect provides temporary haemostasis while the involved vessels are dissected.

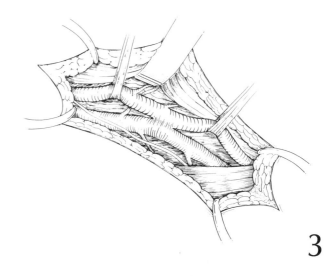

3

Repair of AVF

Several options are available for vessel repair depending on the size of the fistula, whether or not there is an associated pseudoaneurysm, and the vein involved. When a small fistula involves non-critical veins, the veins may be safely ligated. However, large axial veins such as the superficial femoral should be repaired, either by venorrhaphy or end-to-end anastomosis. The artery is then repaired by lateral arteriorrhaphy or end-to-end anastomosis after resecting the damaged segment.

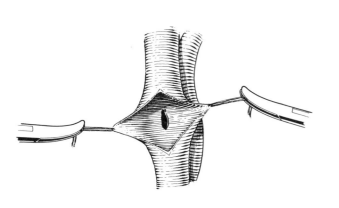

4 When the fistula results from a puncture wound between the artery and vein, such as following cardiac catheterization, transvenous suture repair of the small communication is appropriate. However, most surgeons are more comfortable with dividing the fistula and performing an arteriorrhaphy and venorrhaphy in order to preclude any possibility of recurrence, which is theoretically possible following transvenous repair.

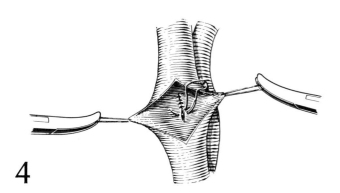

4

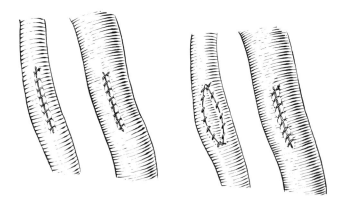

5

Patch angioplasty

5 The artery may require vein patch angioplasty to minimize narrowing. The patch may be obtained from any available vein in the operative field, provided the vein is not critical to the venous circulation.

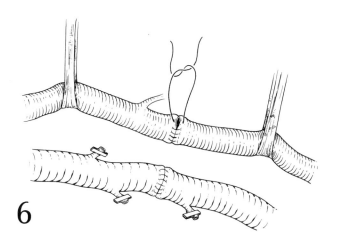

6

End-to-end repair

6 End-to-end arterial repair is preferred provided the artery may be adequately mobilized and debrided to allow a tensionless anastomosis. The proximal and distal arteries are spatulated and the anastomosis is constructed with 6/0 polypropylene sutures.

Interposed vein graft

7 When the fistula is large, a long segment of artery must be debrided, or an associated pseudoaneurysm excised, saphenous vein interposition grafting will be required. Ordinarily, in young patients the superficial femoral artery can be adequately mobilized to allow excision of a 1–1.5-cm segment and still permit tensionless end-to-end repair. However, following excision of a large segment of artery or when in the surgeon's judgement a tensionless primary anastomosis cannot be accomplished, interposition grafting will be required.

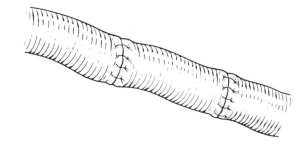

7

End-to-end anastomosis

8 The saphenous vein segment is harvested from the contralateral groin. It is gently distended with either cold heparinized crystalloid solution or cold heparinized blood and the branches are ligated with fine non-absorbable sutures. If the vein segment contains a valve, the vein is reversed. The vein ends are spatulated and end-to-end anastomoses to the artery are performed with 6/0 polypropylene sutures. When autogenous tissue is not available a chronic fistula may be repaired using a segment of 6-mm diameter polytetra-fluoroethylene graft. When managing an acute AVF, with the possibility of bacterial contamination, prosthetic material is contraindicated.

Wound closure

The incision is closed in layers without drains. When prosthetic material is used it is important to cover it with at least two layers of tissue, deep fascia and subcutaneous tissue.

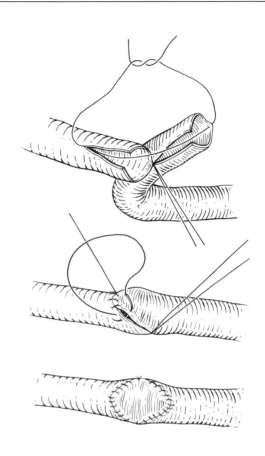

8

Postoperative care

Postoperative care is individualized and is dictated by the location and extent of the surgical procedure. Limb elevation, use of low molecular weight dextran, and pneumatic venous compression devices are valuable adjuncts following major venous repair. One must be alert to the consequences of postoperative hyper-volaemia as a result of the preoperative expanded vascular volume. In young individuals with normal cardiac function, postoperative cardiac failure rarely develops. However, in elderly patients with marginal cardiac reserve, cardiac failure may develop and appropriate monitoring is required employing central venous pressure measurements or, under unusual circumstances, Swan–Ganz catheter monitoring.

Outcome

Results following repair of acquired AVFs depend upon the size, chronicity and location of the fistula. Excellent results can be expected after repair of small fistulae of the extremities. Good results can also be expected following management of large fistulae provided the postoperative complications noted above are adequately anticipated and managed.

Of particular note is that longstanding chronic AVFs may be complicated by proximal arterial dilatation which may result in aneurysm formation. Therefore, extended regular follow-up is required to identify such aneurysms. Ultrasonographic and computed tomographic imaging studies are helpful adjuncts in identifying and following these lesions.

Management of congenital AVF

Operation is not the primary treatment for most congenital AVFs. Resectional therapy is often ineffective and may result in amputation or disfigurement, and feeder vessel ligation results in an unacceptable recurrence rate. External elastic compression is the mainstay of treatment when these lesions involve the extremities.

Although arteriography is important for assessment of congenital AVFs, the arteriographic appearance can be confusing. Selective arterial catheterization is often required to avoid superimposition of multiple overlying arteries and veins. Even with selective catheterization the multiple fistulae may not be visible if the AVF is of the microfistulous variety. Angiography is recommended before operation or embolization to define the flow characteristics of the lesion and delineate feeding arteries and draining veins.

When a congenital AVF requires operation because of progressive enlargement or other complications such as ulceration and bleeding, coordinated management involving the vascular surgeon and interventional radiologist is advised. With the development and refinement of transcatheter embolization techniques, operative therapy has assumed a secondary role. The goal of embolotherapy is to reduce abnormal shunting by occluding communicating vessels with embolic material such as autologous blood clot, Ivalon, Gelfoam, polyvinyl alcohol sponge, or isobutyl cyanoacrylate. Repeated embolization of multiple arterial segments may be required during follow-up.

Successful transcatheter embolization requires patent axial vessels feeding the AVF. Therefore, if an attempt at excision of the AVF is to be made it is important that the main vessels feeding the AVF are not ligated, unless the lesion can be completely excised, because large vessel ligation precludes subsequent transcatheter embolization.

Bleeding often poses a serious problem when resecting a congenital AVF and can be minimized with prior embolotherapy[7]. Moreover, reduction in the bulk of the AVF by preoperative embolization may facilitate resection. It is recommended that embolization be performed the day before operation to minimize recruitment of new collateral vessels and to avoid the inflammatory reaction that sometimes follows embolotherapy.

Operation

If operation is required, it is important that the operative field be widely prepared and draped. As these lesions may bleed massively an autotransfusion device is important for reinfusion of shed blood. In addition, as these procedures are elective and many patients are hypervolaemic, up to 3–4 units of blood should be deposited before surgery for replacement during operation, thereby minimizing the risks of blood-transmitted diseases.

As with acquired AVFs, pneumatic tourniquet occlusion has proved helpful when it can be employed. For excisional therapy to be successful, the entire microfistula must be excised. This may require removal of large segments of skin, subcutaneous tissue, and muscle. In so doing, vital blood vessels and nerves must be preserved in order to maintain a functional extremity. After excising the AVF the tourniquet is released and small bleeding vessels are ligated.

Closure of the incision may require split-thickness skin grafting. Occasionally, the assistance by a plastic surgeon is required, particularly when large segments of tissue must be excised which require innovative reconstruction techniques.

Outcome

Operation for congenital AVF requires lifelong follow-up. Recurrence following incomplete excision is predictable because, as collateral vessels are recruited, the residual AVF enlarges. Under such circumstances palliative control of an extremity AVF by continued use of external elastic support is required. When external elastic compression is unable to control symptoms or is not feasible, transcatheter embolotherapy may be the only available alternative. Ultimately, when all forms of therapy to preserve an extremity have been exhausted and the AVF persists, amputation may be the only practical treatment.

References

1. Skillman JJ, Ducksoo K, Baim DS. Vascular complications of percutaneous femoral cardiac interventions: incidence and operative repair. *Arch Surg* 1988; 123: 1207–12.

2. Szilagyi DE. Vascular malformations (with special emphasis on peripheral arteriovenous lesions). In: Moore W, ed. *Vascular Surgery: A Comprehensive Review*. 2nd edn. Orlando, Florida: Grune and Stratton, 1986: 773–90.

3. Shumacker HB Jr, Wayson EE. Spontaneous cure of aneurysms and arteriovenous fistulas, with some notes on intravascular thrombosis. *Am J Surg* 1950; 79: 532–44.

4. Shepard AD, Ernst CB. Aortoenteric and aortocaval fistulae. In: Bergan JJ, Yao JST, eds. *Vascular Surgical Emergencies*. Orlando, Florida: Grune and Stratton, 1987: 359–76.

5. Szilagyi DE, Elliott JP, DeRusso FJ, Smith RF. Peripheral congenital arteriovenous fistulas. *Surgery* 1965; 57: 61–81.

6. Pearce WH, Rutherford RB, Whitehill TA, Davis K. Nuclear magnetic resonance imaging: its diagnostic value in patients with congenital vascular malformations of the limbs. *J Vasc Surg* 1988; 8: 64–70.

7. Kadir S, Ernst CB, Hamper U, White RI. Management of vascular soft tissue neoplasms using transcatheter embolization and surgical excision. *Am J Surg* 1983; 146: 409–12.

Combined therapeutic embolization and surgery

J. E. Jackson MRCP, FRCR
Consultant Radiologist, Department of Diagnostic Radiology, Royal Postgraduate Medical School, Hammersmith Hospital, London, UK

D. J. Allison BSc, MD, MRCP, FRCR
Professor and Director, Department of Diagnostic Radiology, Royal Postgraduate Medical School, Hammersmith Hospital, London, UK

Principles and justification

Indications

Vascular embolization plays an increasingly important role in a large number of clinical conditions, particularly as an emergency procedure for the control of haemorrhage from abdominal viscera, either as a definitive treatment or as a means of stabilizing the patient before subsequent surgery. On the other hand, outside major trauma centres, the indications for vascular embolization in the peripheral vascular system are relatively few. There are several situations, however, where percutaneous vascular embolization and surgery may be usefully combined and these are best considered under the following headings:

1. Preoperative embolization.
2. Pre-embolization surgery to create vascular access for embolization.
3. Therapeutic embolization of postoperative complications.
4. Operative treatment of postembolization complications.
5. Complementary embolization and surgical procedures.

Each of these will be discussed in turn. Case histories will be used in several to illustrate specific points. Before dealing with each of these subject headings, however, some of the general technical aspects of angiography and vascular embolization and possible complications of these procedures will be described, and some of the more commonly used embolic agents will be discussed. Several of the points that are to be discussed in this section will be re-emphasized later in the chapter under the headings given above.

Arterial access

The route chosen for embolization depends to some extent upon the indication for the procedure. A common femoral arterial puncture is, however, the one most commonly used for arteriography, and should the arterial anatomy allow, embolization is usually performed via the same route. A surgical cut-down onto the brachial artery at the antecubital fossa or a direct puncture of the 'high' brachial or axillary artery are other less commonly used sites of access.

As will be discussed later, access to a lesion which requires embolization may occasionally be best achieved by a direct puncture into the abnormality itself, or into a vessel immediately adjacent to it.

Catheters

A variety of angiographic catheters is available for selective arterial catheterization; these differ in shape, size, internal and external diameter and composition. A full description of the large number of the more commonly used catheters lies outside the scope of this chapter and may be found elsewhere[1]. Those most commonly used are 5 Fr or 7 Fr and have a 0.035-inch (0.89-mm) or 0.038-inch (0.96-mm) diameter lumen. Coaxial catheters (i.e. catheters which pass through the centre of a conventional angiographic catheter) of 3 Fr or less may be used to achieve extremely selective positions in small and tortuous vessels, and are invaluable in certain vascular territories. Once a suitable position for occlusion has been achieved, embolic agents are introduced through the catheter lumen by careful injection under fluoroscopic control or, in the case of coils, by pushing them into the desired site using a guidewire.

Embolic agents

A large number of different materials has been used to occlude blood vessels. They range from autologous substances such as blood clot, fat and chopped muscle fragments to materials such as wool, silk, cotton, microfibrillar collagen, polyvinyl alcohol, absorbable gelatin sponge, steel coils, detachable balloons and liquids such as alcohol or acrylates. The agent that is chosen depends very much upon the nature of the abnormality being embolized and the indication for embolization. The purpose of embolization before operation is to help reduce operative blood loss. This is best achieved by central occlusion of the lesion and small particulate embolic agents such as polyvinyl alcohol or gelatin sponge are ideal agents for this purpose in most instances. The size chosen depends upon the size of vessel which requires embolization and the presence or absence of arteriovenous communications. Care must be taken when such communications are present that as little of the embolic agent as possible passes through into the venous side. A more proximal arterial occlusion may have to be performed in such instances when compared with that which would be possible when embolizing similarly sized arterial vessels supplying a lesion which does not contain significant arteriovenous shunts. Liquid embolic agents such as dehydrated alcohol, cyanoacrylate and sodium tetradecyl sulphate are powerful sclerosants and need to be used with extreme care because of the risk of non-target organ infarction. They are rarely required when embolization is performed before operation as the safer particulate agents described above are just as effective in reducing the vascularity of a lesion immediately before surgery in most instances. Embolic devices such as coils and detachable balloons allow proximal large vessel occlusion and are, therefore, of little use in the context of preoperative embolization; their use may, in fact, be detrimental to the patient's further management, as will be illustrated later.

Complications

The most frequently reported, but still fortunately uncommon, complications of vascular embolization are the inadvertent embolization of vessels other than those supplying the lesion being treated and the passage of emboli into the venous circulation. Non-target organ ischaemia or infarction may occur. Liquid embolic agents such as alcohol and cyanoacrylate are especially dangerous, and complications such as skin necrosis and neural damage may occur even in experienced hands. A postembolization syndrome, which consists of a variable combination of pain at the site of the lesion that has been embolized, pyrexia, leucocytosis and a general feeling of malaise, is common after the procedure. The condition generally lasts for only 24–48 h but may persist for a week or more before it disappears. Symptomatic treatment is usually all that is required.

The more serious complication of infection at the site of embolization is exceedingly rare but this should always be considered, particularly in the case of a severe or unduly prolonged postembolization syndrome. Blood cultures should be taken in any case featuring pyrexia and leucocytosis.

Basic principles

There are a few basic principles which must be adhered to during any embolization procedure:

1. A thorough knowledge of the normal arterial anatomy in the area being embolized is essential. The vascular anatomy of the lesion to be embolized must be precisely defined by good quality angiography so that all the communications between the normal and abnormal vessels are appreciated before the introduction of embolic material.
2. In no other area of interventional radiology is experience with selective and superselective vessel catheterization more important. Inappropriate catheter placement results in failed embolization and the possible occlusion of a contiguous normal vascular territory.
3. Non-opaque embolic agents must always be mixed with a contrast agent so that they are visible during injection.
4. The embolic agent being used must be injected in small amounts and under continuous fluoroscopy so that the inadvertent embolization of a normal vascular territory is avoided.
5. Reflux of emboli into other vessels occurs very easily as flow progressively diminishes in the vascular bed. Frequent contrast medium injections should be made between small aliquots of embolic material so that the progress of the procedure is continuously monitored.

Operations

PREOPERATIVE EMBOLIZATION

In the peripheral vascular territory there is a growing number of indications for preoperative vascular embolization. This procedure is most commonly performed to reduce the vascularity of the lesion which is to be resected in an attempt to limit perioperative blood loss. Occasionally, however, embolization is performed as a temporary measure to stabilize the patient before surgery.

To reduce vascularity before resection

Arteriovenous malformations

These relatively rare congenital vascular abnormalities are probably the lesions that the vascular surgeon and radiologist are most likely to treat together. A knowledge of their correct classification is of paramount importance. Unfortunately, there are numerous different classifications and these lesions are therefore known by a whole host of confusing terms which include angioma, pulsatile naevus, capillary or cavernous haemangioma, arteriovenous fistula and cirsoid aneurysm. In the authors' view the use of a single method of classification in this field is absolutely imperative, not least because it will lead to a better understanding of both the nature and treatment of these lesions.

Perhaps the simplest and most workable classification is that described by Mulliken[2]. A full description of this lies outside the scope of the present chapter and interested readers are strongly advised to refer to his text. The brief descriptions used below are based on his classification.

The term *haemangioma* should be restricted to a vascular tumour of infancy which passes through stages of rapid proliferation and subsequent spontaneous slow resolution. Active treatment is unnecessary in most cases. Haemangiomas which are particularly large, however, and which cause severe haemorrhage because of platelet trapping and subsequent profound thrombocytopenia (Kasabach–Merritt syndrome), or those which cause complications because of their position (e.g. those which interfere with the visual axis) may require treatment. Embolization is very rarely necessary.

Table 1   Angiographic findings in vascular malformations

Arteriovenous
  High-flow lesions
  Enlarged feeding arteries
  Rapid arteriovenous shunting usually present

Capillary
  Low-flow lesions
  Normal or slightly enlarged feeding arteries
  Often dense capillary blush
  Normal or slightly early venous return

Venous
  Low-flow lesions
  Normal arterial supply
  Dilated, tortuous veins which fill very slowly (may not fill
      completely from an arterial injection)
  No arteriovenous shunting

A *vascular birthmark*, or *vascular malformation*, on the other hand, is always present at birth (although it may not become apparent until later life if in a deep-seated location) and tends to grow commensurately with the patient. It may, however, grow more rapidly in response to certain stimuli such as trauma, puberty, or pregnancy.

These lesions can be subdivided according to the predominant vessel type which is abnormal and this can usually be determined clinically. Each of the various forms of vascular malformation has characteristic angiographic findings (*Table 1*).

The method of treatment of these lesions depends upon their location, associated symptoms and on the type of vessel which is predominantly affected. Cure can usually only be achieved by complete surgical excision, but, unfortunately, this is rarely possible because of the large size and diffuse nature of many of these lesions. For symptomatic malformations, therefore, embolization usually provides the mainstay of treatment. Small, localized lesions and those which are life-threatening and not controlled by embolization alone are often approached by a combined procedure of embolization followed by surgery.

Small localized arteriovenous malformations
It is important to realize that the primary objective of preoperative embolization in these patients is to reduce the vascularity of the lesion and not to reduce the extent of surgical excision. To achieve a permanent cure complete excision of the lesion, if this is possible, is essential.

Illustrative case history 1 (*Figure 1a–e*)

The patient was a young lady with a small and localized, but disfiguring, arteriovenous malformation involving the soft tissues overlying the left mandible. Preoperative angiography demonstrated a high-flow lesion overlying the angle of the mandible which derived its supply from a single branch arising from the left facial artery. There were no other arterial feeding vessels. In particular there was no supply from the contralateral external carotid artery branches across the midline and the ipsilateral internal carotid artery angiogram was normal.

The single feeding vessel to the malformation was catheterized and embolization was performed with polyvinyl alcohol with a particle size of 150–250 μm (Contour, International Therapeutics Corporation). The postembolization arteriogram demonstrated complete embolization of the lesion with no residual demonstrable abnormal vascularity, and preservation of the facial artery. Complete surgical excision was performed 24 h later with no blood loss and an excellent cosmetic result. The patient remains well 2 years later with no evidence of recurrence.

Several points regarding the above case merit further discussion. Firstly, it is imperative that a complete angiographic study is performed before embolization is commenced to define the full extent of the malformation. In lesions supplied predominantly by the external carotid artery, bilateral external carotid and ipsilateral internal carotid angiograms are mandatory. An internal carotid artery supply to a facial malformation (often via the ophthalmic artery) is not uncommon and, unless the presence of such a supply is appreciated, potentially catastrophic complications may occur because of the retrograde passage of embolic material into these vessels. Imaging of the full extent of a malformation and all of its potential arterial feeders is essential regardless of the vascular territory which it involves. If this lesion had been situated more posteriorly a vertebral artery study would also have been required.

Secondly, small particulate matter was used to embolize the central portion of the malformation without proximal vessel occlusion with permanent agents such as coils. The need to embolize the central portion of the malformation has already been mentioned and the importance of this cannot be overemphasized. Proximal occlusion alone would allow the development and enlargement of surrounding collateral vessels to the malformation and this process may occur with great rapidity, even within the short period before attempted surgical excision.

Thirdly, surgical excision should, if possible, be performed within 48 h of embolization. Thrombosis of the lesion will have occurred by this time and the surrounding fat planes will still be preserved. If excision is attempted at a later date (1–2 weeks), surrounding soft tissue inflammation, fibrosis and loss of the normal fat planes will make surgery more difficult. Larger

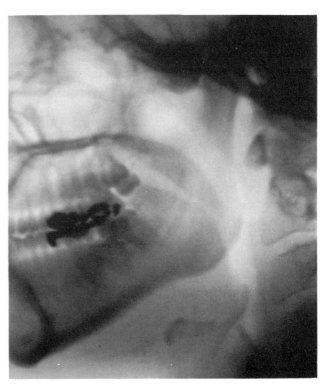

1a

Figure 1 *Preoperative embolization of localized high-flow arteriovenous malformation overlying left mandible. (a) Left external carotid arteriogram using a digital subtraction technique (lateral projection). (b) Abnormal collection of vessels seen overlying left mandible arising from hypertrophied left facial artery. (c) Left facial arteriogram (lateral injection). The abnormal tortuous vessels of the arteriovenous malformation are better visualized. (d) Selective catheterization of single vessel supplying arteriovenous malformation before embolization. (e) Selective left external carotid arteriogram after embolization. The arteriovenous malformation is completely occluded. Note preservation of the left facial artery*

lesions, however, may benefit from two or more embolization procedures spaced several weeks apart, with surgery being performed within 48 h of the final embolization.

Life-threatening arteriovenous malformations
Arteriovenous malformations may threaten the patient's life either because of high-output cardiac failure or because of severe haemorrhage. If these complications cannot be successfully controlled by embolization, heroic surgery may be required. Both preoperative and peroperative embolization may prove useful.

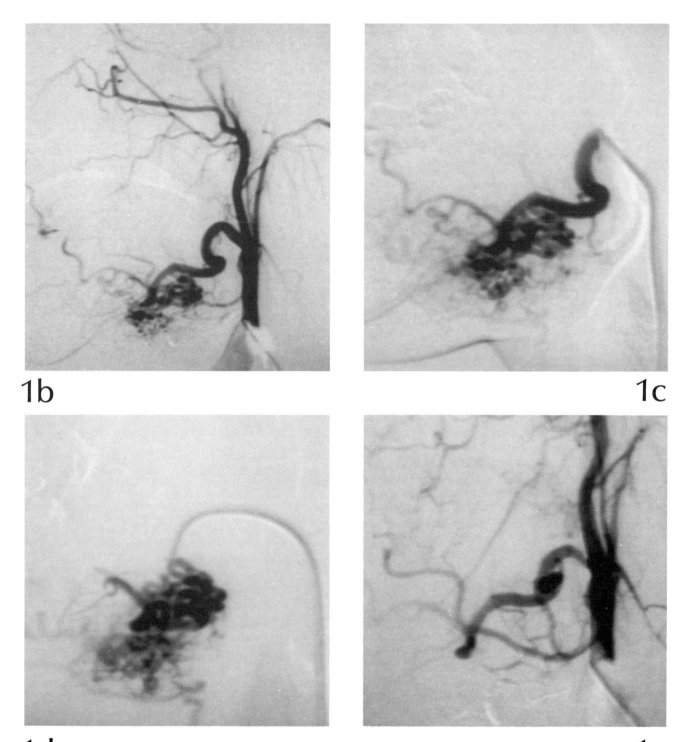

1b

1c

1d

1e

Illustrative case history 2 (Figure 2a–e)

The patient was a young man with a life-threatening mandibular arteriovenous malformation. He had initially presented 10 years before subsequent definitive treatment with a large pulsating mass involving the left side of his face from which he had occasional large intraoral haemorrhages. Angiography at this time demonstrated a massive lesion with extremely rapid arteriovenous shunting. The arterial supply was via lingual, facial and maxillary arteries bilaterally and there was also some supply from the left ophthalmic artery. The lesion was considered inoperable at this stage and embolization was therefore performed on many occasions over the next 10 years with reasonable control of episodes of haemorrhage. Despite this, however, there was a gradual deterioration in the lesion and several life-threatening haemorrhages in the space of a few weeks, which were not adequately controlled by further embolization, precipitated the need for emergency surgery. At this time, the teeth of the mandible were visibly moving because of the underlying pulsating malformation, and massively dilated and pulsatile veins were present within the left cheek.

Preoperative embolization of the feeding vessels to the malformation was performed. Subsequently, under cardiac bypass, the teeth of the lower jaw were all removed, together with the abnormal vessels coursing through the body of the mandible which was then packed with bone cement. The dilated veins in the left cheek were decompressed by intralesional sutures (after Popescu[3]) and sodium tetradecyl sulphate was injected into the 'compartmentalized' veins to induce thrombosis. The postoperative course was complicated by a transient hemiparesis. Two years later the patient is very well with an extremely acceptable cosmetic result and no evidence of recurrence of the malformation.

Venous malformations

Unlike the more aggressive arteriovenous lesions, venous malformations are rarely life-threatening and tend not to grow rapidly during the lifetime of the patient. They may, however, cause considerable deformity and thus necessitate treatment. These malformations are often much more extensive than clinical examination alone would suggest and thorough preoperative imaging is essential. Direct puncture venography may delineate the lesion well, but magnetic resonance imaging is proving extremely useful in this regard and is probably the investigation of first choice if any imaging study is necessary. Conventional intravascular venography is frequently disappointing or useless.

If a lesion is considered to be of a size amenable to surgical excision then a combination of percutaneous sclerotherapy and subsequent resection may prove useful. In very extensive lesions partial surgical excision combined with percutaneous sclerotherapy of residual venous spaces may be the only option.

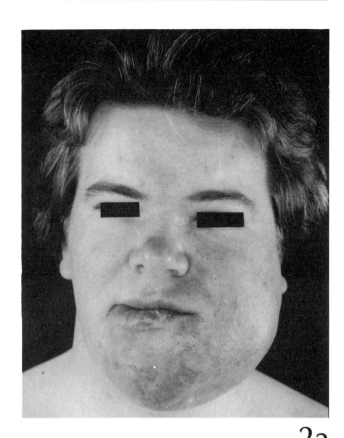

2a

Figure 2 Life-threatening mandibular arteriovenous malformation. (a) Clinical photograph before surgery. (b) Transaxial contrast-enhanced computed tomography scan at the level of the body of the mandible. Cavities are visible within the mandible owing to involvement by the arteriovenous malformation. Massively dilated veins are opacified by contrast medium in the soft tissues of the floor of the mouth and the left cheek. (c, d) Selective lingual arteriogram (lateral projection). Note the mandibular erosion caused by the arteriovenous malformation on the control film. A markedly hypertrophied lingual artery supplies the arteriovenous malformation in the mandibular ramus. Normal lingual arterial branches are seen superiorly. (e) Clinical photograph 6 months after surgery showing an excellent clinical and cosmetic result

Vascular soft tissue tumours

In much the same way as embolization and surgery can be usefully combined in the treatment of arteriovenous malformations, so they may also be successfully used together in the management of vascular soft tissue tumours. The same technique and basic principles of embolization apply, as described above. As with arteriovenous malformations, the proximal coil embolization of feeding vessels must be avoided if at all possible. This manoeuvre does not confer any additional benefit over the central embolization of tumour vessels with small particulate matter, and may obviate or hamper future access to the lesion for repeat embolization should this be required because of incomplete excision or tumour recurrence.

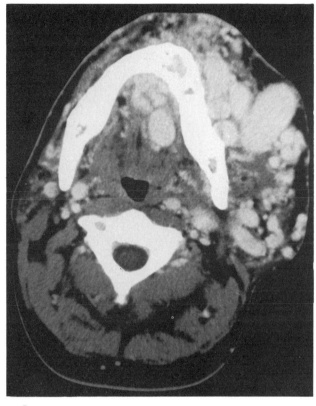

2b

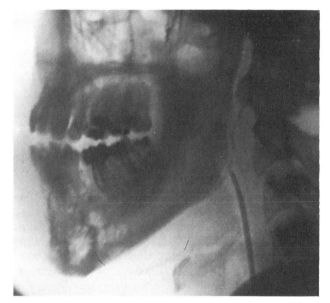

2c

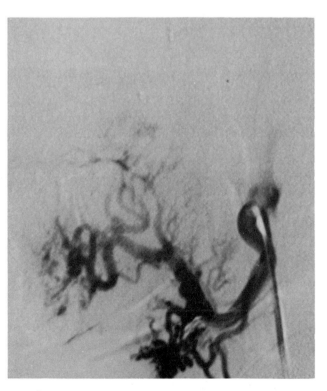

2d

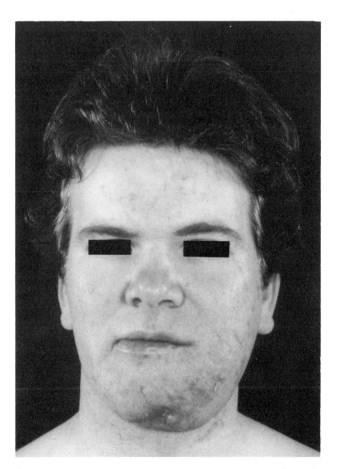

2e

Illustrative case history 3 (Figure 3a–h)

The patient was a young lady with a massive pelvic haemangiopericytoma. The diagnosis of a very large and extremely vascular haemangiopericytoma occupying the pelvis was initially made at laparotomy. Excision was considered impossible and, after a biopsy, the abdomen was closed. The vascularity of the lesion and the large number of vessels supplying it were demonstrated subsequently at angiography. The predominant arterial supply was via numerous branches arising from the anterior division of the left internal iliac artery but there were also significant feeding vessels from the right internal iliac, median sacral and inferior mesenteric arteries. Embolization of the internal iliac and median sacral arterial supply with polyvinyl alcohol (150–500-μm diameter particles) achieved an approximately 90% reduction in tumour vascularity. Successful excision was performed 48 h later with only moderate blood loss. Eighteen months later the patient remains well with no evidence of recurrent tumour.

The embolization performed in this case merits further comment. It was not felt possible to embolize the inferior mesenteric arterial supply to the tumour because of the large number of small vessels arising from the superior haemorrhoidal branches. Embolization with small particulate material in this situation would have carried a high risk of producing colonic/rectal ischaemia. Tumours often obtain a parasitic blood supply from surrounding organs and this may make complete embolization very difficult, if not impossible. If it is planned to remove the normal organ which is contributing its blood supply to the tumour at subsequent surgery, then embolization of all or part of this organ may also be performed to decrease the vascularity of the neoplasm further. If there is a possibility, however, that an attempt will be made to preserve the normal organ at surgery, then embolization is inappropriate even if this means that some arterial supply to the tumour remains.

3a

Figure 3 Preoperative embolization of massive pelvic haemangiopericytoma. (a–d) Pelvic arteriogram with catheter in the lower abdominal aorta, showing a highly vascular, well-defined tumour in the pelvis supplied predominantly by the left internal iliac artery. Note the hypertrophied inferior mesenteric and median sacral arteries. (e) Selective median sacral arteriogram before embolization. (f) Selective inferior mesenteric artery angiography demonstrates supply to the tumour from branches of the superior haemorrhoidal artery. (g) Selective internal iliac artery angiogram demonstrates predominant supply from this vessel. (h) Left common iliac artery angiogram performed after embolization. The supply from the left internal iliac artery has been largely obliterated

To stabilize the patient before later surgery

There are few instances in the peripheral vascular system when embolization is performed to stabilize a patient before later surgery. This is in contradistinction to the visceral arteries where control of haemorrhage is a major indication for embolization. The reason for this difference is that the surgical control of haemorrhage in visceral arterial bleeding is usually extremely difficult, not least because the source of haemorrhage is often not obvious and may be located deep within an organ such as the liver or kidney. The source of severe haemorrhage in the peripheral vascular system, however, is usually much more obvious and therefore amenable to definitive surgical treatment.

In the authors' experience only one patient satisfactorily fits into this category. This patient suffered from Behçet's disease and had a large inflammatory aortic pseudoaneurysm[4]. Coil embolization of the aneurysm was successfully performed during an acute inflammatory exacerbation of his condition to reduce the risk of fatal rupture. Once the patient's inflammatory indices had returned to normal with medical treatment the diseased aorta was resected and a graft inserted. This is obviously an unusual case but serves to demonstrate how embolization may be used to create time during which a patient can be made fit for surgery.

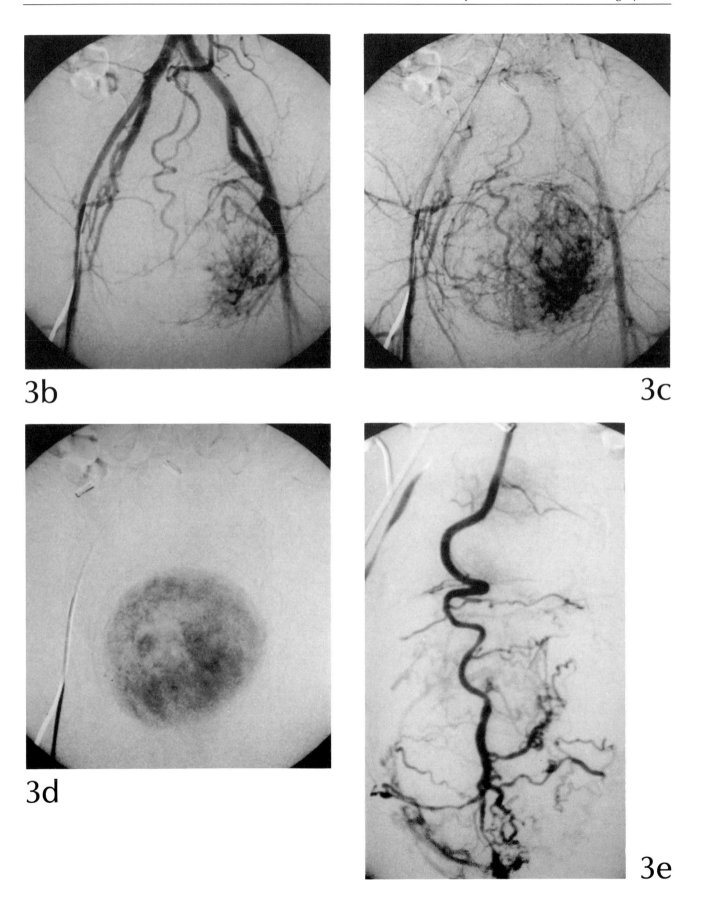

3b

3c

3d

3e

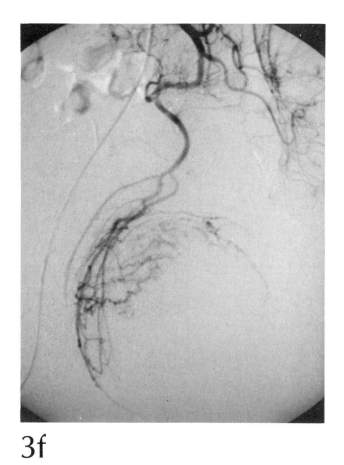

3f

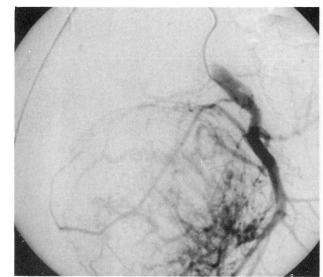

3g

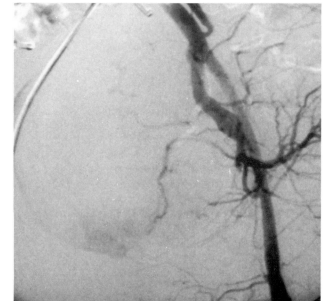

3h

SURGERY TO CREATE VASCULAR ACCESS FOR EMBOLIZATION

Surgical procedures may occasionally be very useful in creating an access route to a vascular territory for subsequent embolization. The authors' experience with this technique is confined to patients with arteriovenous malformations in whom the major feeding vessel to the malformation has been previously occluded, either surgically or by previous embolization[5].

In four patients treated at Hammersmith Hospital a surgical graft has been used to bypass a previously occluded vessel to allow further transarterial therapy. Surgery in these patients is likely to be difficult because of the vascularity of the lesion and the frequent history of previous surgery. Preoperative imaging, which will usually include angiography, and a close liaison between surgeon and radiologist are essential to ensure that the anatomy is clearly defined and that a satisfactory graft is inserted which will allow subsequent catheterization and embolization.

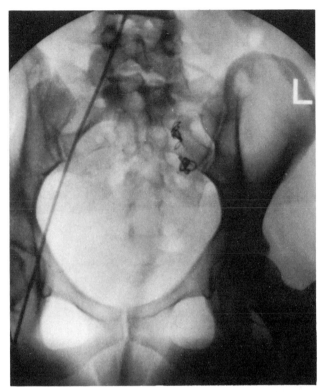

4a

Illustrative case history 4 (Figure 4a–g)

The patient was a young lady with a symptomatic and enlarging arteriovenous malformation involving her left buttock and pelvis. This case demonstrates the harm which may result from coil embolization (or indeed, surgical ligation) of the main feeding arteries to an arteriovenous malformation. She was referred to the authors' centre with a large left buttock and a pelvic arteriovenous malformation which had previously been embolized. Peripheral embolization of the malformation with particulate matter had been followed by occlusion of the main trunk of the left internal iliac artery with steel coils. The patient's symptoms returned after a relatively short-lived improvement. Angiography now demonstrated complete occlusion of the left internal iliac artery with numerous collateral vessels supplying the malformation arising from lumbar, median sacral, superior haemorrhoidal, inferior epigastric, contralateral internal iliac and deep femoral arteries.

As successful arterial embolization was no longer possible through all of these collateral vesels, a surgical graft was inserted between the left external iliac artery and the left internal iliac artery beyond the occluding coils. Embolization of the majority of the malformation with small particulate matter was then possible through the graft with good symptomatic benefit.

Maintenance of graft patency after embolization to allow subsequent embolization is desirable but not always possible. Preserved patency is more likely if

Figure 4 *Embolization of arteriovenous malformation through surgically placed access graft. (a) Control film showing metallic embolization coils overlying left side of sacrum. (b) Pelvic arteriogram with catheter in lower abdominal aorta. Occlusion of the left internal iliac artery by metallic coils is demonstrated. Enlarged left lumbar, inferior mesenteric and median sacral arteries are also seen. (c) The left internal iliac artery is reconstituted beyond the occluded coils by numerous collateral vessels. (d) Rapid venous filling is seen within the large high-flow arteriovenous malformation involving the left pelvis and buttock. (e, f) Selective catheterization of surgically placed graft which bypasses the occluding coils. The abnormal vessels within the arteriovenous malformation are visualized before embolization. (g) Postembolization arteriogram demonstrates occlusion of abnormal vessels*

some antegrade flow persists through the graft to normal vessels.

Very occasionally a vessel supplying a lesion which requires embolization cannot be catheterized because of its site of origin or because of extreme tortuosity. In such instances it may be possible to expose this vessel surgically and insert an angiographic catheter before transfer of the patient to the angiography department for embolization.

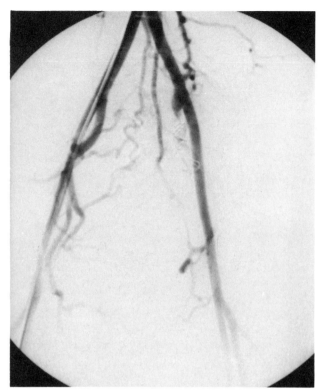

4b

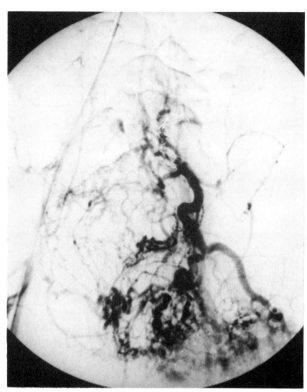

4c

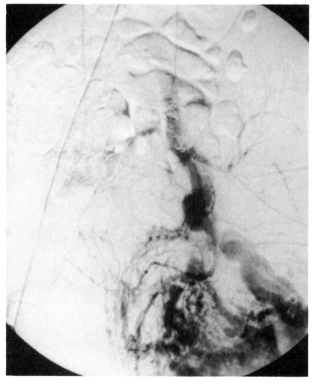

4d

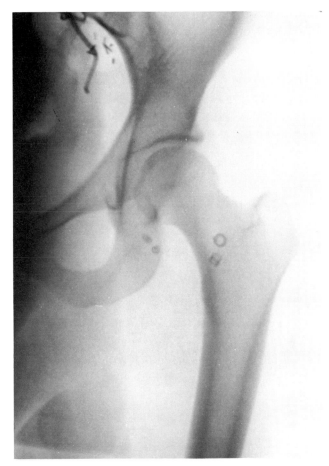

4e

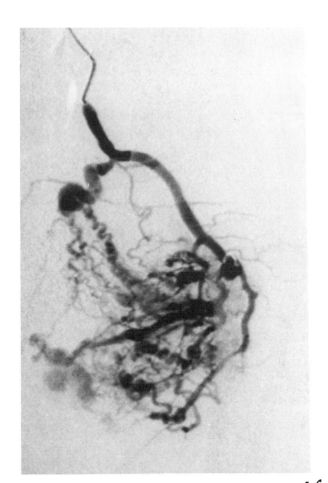

4f

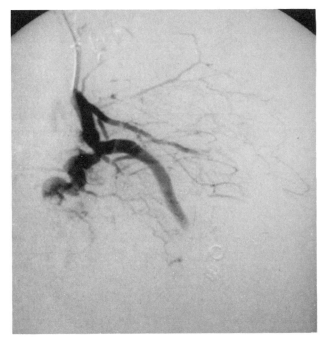

4g

EMBOLIZATION OF POSTOPERATIVE COMPLICATIONS

There is a variety of miscellaneous conditions where embolization procedures may be extremely useful to the surgeon. There have, for example, been a few case reports describing successful embolization of aortic aneurysms which, although surgically bypassed, have continued to expand or have ruptured[6, 7].

Postoperative haemorrhage or pseudoaneurysm formation owing to inadvertent arterial injury or a slipped ligature may often be treated successfully by percutaneous embolization techniques.

Illustrative case history 5 (Figure 5a–e)

The patient was an elderly gentleman with persistent haemorrhage from a wound site after revisional right hip surgery. Angiography demonstrated a large pseudoaneurysm arising from a branch of the right deep femoral artery. Embolization was performed by placing steel coils within the feeding vessel on either side of the 'neck' of the pseudoaneurysm, thus completely isolating it from the circulation. Immediate thrombosis occurred with resolution of the wound haemorrhage.

The techniques employed in the embolization of pseudoaneurysms deserve further discussion. The aim is to isolate the aneurysmal cavity from the circulation. It is therefore imperative that the vessel beyond the origin of the pseudoaneurysm is occluded to prevent continued supply through the 'back-door' via collaterals. Embolization across and proximal to the neck of the lesion is then performed. Coils or detachable balloons are the preferred embolic agents. An alternative embolization technique is to pack the aneurysmal cavity itself with embolic material. It must be remembered, however, that the pseudoaneurysm, by definition, lacks a true wall and packing it may result in its rupture. This method of embolization may, however, be the only option if the vessel from which the pseudoaneurysm arises has to be preserved. Embolization in such cases is not easy as it may be very difficult to obliterate flow into the cavity completely without encroaching upon the lumen of the normal artery.

Arteriovenous shunts are occasionally deliberately created surgically: for example, when performing a venous reconstruction to maintain its patency. Subsequent embolization of such shunts may be possible if required in certain instances.

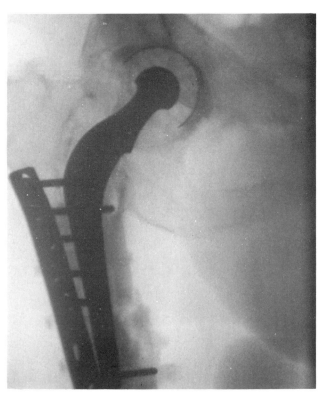

5a

Figure 5 Embolization of postoperative deep femoral pseudoaneurysm. (a–c) Right total hip replacement is present. Right femoral arteriogram demonstrates large pseudoaneurysm arising from a branch of the right deep femoral artery. (d) A selective arteriogram of the branch from which the pseudoaneurysm arises demonstrates the arterial defect and large pseudoaneurysm cavity. (e) Embolization of feeding vessel performed with steel coils positioned across the neck of the pseudoaneurysm (see text). There is complete occlusion of the feeding vessel and no further filling of the pseudoaneurysm

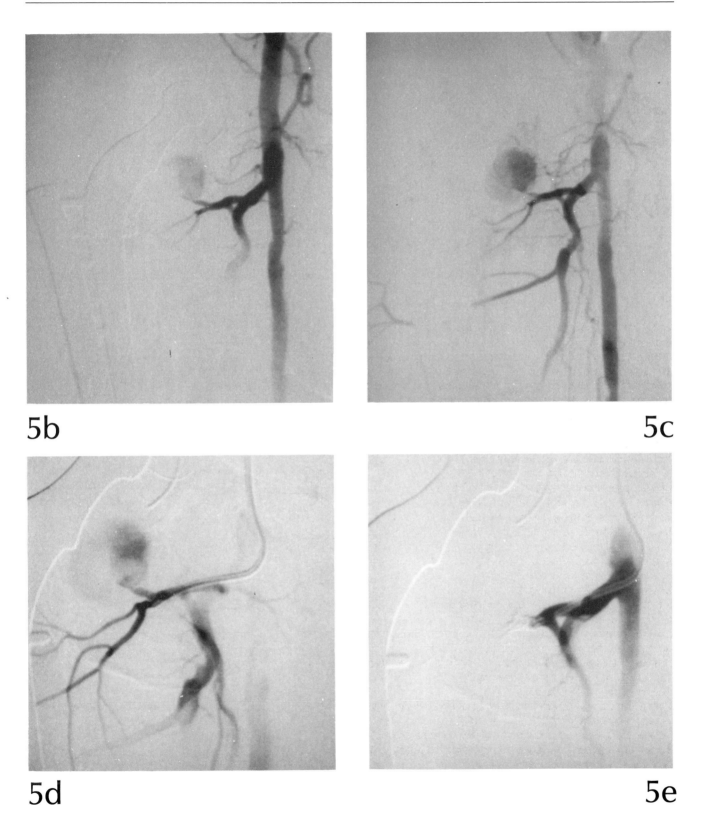

5b

5c

5d

5e

OPERATIVE TREATMENT OF POSTEMBOLIZATION COMPLICATIONS

Complications directly attributable to embolization are fortunately extremely uncommon and surgery is rarely required. Complications of angiographic catheterization, such as femoral artery pseudoaneurysm formation or femoral arteriovenous fistulae, are also very uncommon but when they do occur they are often relatively easily treated surgically. Many of the pseudoaneurysms, however, undergo spontaneous thrombosis and those that do not may sometimes be treated using compression Doppler ultrasonography[8].

Embolic agents such as coils and detachable balloons may very occasionally be misplaced and thereby occlude an important normal vessel. It is usually possible for the angiographer to remove or reposition these devices percutaneously with an appropriate retrieval device, but if this is not achieved then surgery may be necessary.

Tissue necrosis and abscess formation are fortunately also infrequent complications of embolization. The former is more likely if liquid sclerosants such as alcohol or cyanoacrylate are used for embolization. If a large area of skin or soft tissue necrosis does occur then surgical debridement and/or skin grafting may be required. Abscess formation has most frequently been described during visceral organ embolization (liver, spleen) and may necessitate percutaneous drainage. Surgery may occasionally be necessary.

COMPLEMENTARY EMBOLIZATION AND SURGICAL PROCEDURES

A combination of embolization and surgical techniques may be life-saving in the patient with multiple injuries. For example, an unstable patient with severe pelvic trauma is very difficult to treat surgically; angiography and embolization has been shown to be associated with considerably lower mortality and morbidity rates when compared with surgery and can be performed rapidly to stabilize the patient before surgical treatment of other injuries if required.

Conclusion

There is no doubt that a combination of embolization and surgery can be extremely useful in a variety of different circumstances. Preoperative embolization may not only make subsequent surgery considerably easier, it may also convert a potentially unresectable lesion into a resectable one by reducing or abolishing its blood supply.

In the peripheral vascular system arteriovenous malformations are perhaps the major indication for a combined embolization and surgical procedure, but other vascular soft tissue tumours may also be best treated in this way. What is most important is that there is a close liaison between surgeons and radiologists in the treatment of these conditions so that the combined procedure is used to its best advantage. In addition, either the surgeon or the radiologist may be helped by the other in the management of post-procedural complications.

References

1. Allison DJ, Machan LS. Arteriography. In: Grainger RG, Allison DJ, eds. *Diagnostic Radiology. An Anglo-American Textbook of Radiology*. 2nd edn. Edinburgh: Churchill Livingstone, 1991: 2205–75.

2. Mulliken JB. Classification of vascular birthmarks. In: Mulliken JB, Young AE, eds. *Vascular Birthmarks. Haemangiomas and Malformations*. Philadelphia: WB Saunders, 1988: 24–37.

3. Popescu V. Intratumoral ligation in the management of orofacial cavernous haemangiomas. *J Maxillofac Surg* 1985; 13: 99–107.

4. Smith EJ, Abulafi M, McPherson GA, Allison DJ, Mansfield AO. False aneurysm of the abdominal aorta in Behçets' disease. *Eur J Vasc Surg* 1991; 5: 481–4.

5. Vaughan M, Hennessy O, Jamieson C, Hemingway AP, Allison DJ. The preoperative embolization of vascular malformations. *Br J Radiol* 1985; 58: 717–20.

6. Mori H, Fukuda T, Ishida Y, Hayashi N, Hayashi K, Maeda H. Embolization of a thoracic aortic aneurysm; the straddling coil technique: technical note. *Cardiovasc Intervent Radiol* 1990; 13: 50–2.

7. Rowe PH, Ellis FG, Reidy JF. Transcatheter embolization of a suprarenal aortic aneurysm persisting after bypass surgery. *Br J Clin Pract* 1990; 44: 692–5.

8. Resar JR, Trerotola SO, Osterman FA, Aversano TR, Brinker JA. Ultrasound guided ablation of pseudoaneurysm following coronary artery stent placement: a preliminary report. *Cathet Cardiovasc Diagn* 1992; 26: 215–18.

Lumbar sympathectomy

John J. Ricotta MD

Professor of Surgery and Director, Division of Vascular Surgery, State University of New York at Buffalo, Buffalo, New York, USA

History

Periarterial sympathectomy was first performed for arterial occlusive disease by Leriche in 1913, with disappointing results. Lumbar sympathetic ganglionectomy was first reported by Diez in 1924[1] and was used extensively before the advent of arterial reconstruction. Over the last 20–30 years, this procedure has been supplanted by arterial reconstructive procedures and is now seldom performed. There are specific instances, however, in which lumbar sympathectomy may be useful.

Principles and justification

Sympathectomy increases blood flow to the limbs by causing vasodilatation of both arterioles and precapillary sphincters. This can produce large increases in blood flow to normal limbs, but its effect may be attenuated in patients with arterial ischaemia because maximal vasodilatation is often already present. Similarly, patients with advanced diabetes and neuropathy often exhibit 'autosympathectomy'. Much of the increased blood flow is through cutaneous arteriovenous anastomoses. There is no evidence to suggest that sympathectomy improves nutrient blood flow; rather, it is attended by redistribution of blood flow to the distal cutaneous circulation. There are also some data to suggest that sympathectomy may alter perception of pain by decreasing tissue levels of noradrenaline and reducing central spinal cord transmission of painful stimuli.

From the foregoing, it can be stated that sympathectomy is not indicated in patients with claudication. It may be helpful for relief of ischaemic rest pain in patients who are not candidates for vascular reconstruction, particularly if a resting level of vasoconstriction can be demonstrated. In general, results are best when ischaemia is not profound (i.e. ankle:brachial ratio above 0.3)[2]. Sympathectomy is also useful in patients with causalgia, severe vasospasm and hyperhidrosis, although these are all encountered rather uncommonly in clinical practice.

Preoperative

Assessment and preparation

Several techniques have been used to select patients for lumbar sympathectomy. Non-invasive studies should be performed, because the results of sympathectomy are poor if the ankle:brachial ratio is below 0.3[2]. Because the results of a bypass are generally superior to those of sympathectomy, full angiography with run-off is indicated to evaluate the possibility of vascular reconstruction.

A percutaneous sympathetic block may be helpful in identifying patients with residual vasoconstriction.

Evidence of a clinical response to the block and objective measures, such as an increase in skin temperature, help to identify patients in whom sympathectomy may be beneficial. None of these measures, however, is an absolutely reliable predictor of response.

Once a patient is selected for sympathectomy, no special preparation is required. Repeated sympathetic blocks are generally not as effective as surgical removal of the sympathetic chain. Chemical sympathectomy with phenol or an equivalent solution carries some risk and may make subsequent surgical sympathectomy more difficult if it is required.

Operation

In general, an anterior retroperitoneal approach is adequate for the removal of the L2–L4 sympathetic ganglia.

Position of patient and incision

1 The patient is placed supine. A small sandbag or rolled towel may be used to elevate the operative side by 15–30°. The incision is slightly curvilinear and begins medially at the lateral border of the rectus abdominis muscle, extending laterally to the tip of the 12th rib. The incision may be extended medially for additional exposure.

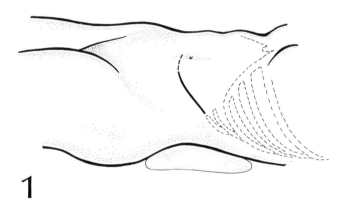

1

Incision of muscles

2a–c The external and internal oblique muscles are incised along the lines of their fibres. The transversus abdominis muscle is then incised parallel to and between the intercostal nerves, which are protected. If additional exposure is necessary, the lateral portion of the anterior and posterior rectus sheath may be incised and the rectus muscle retracted.

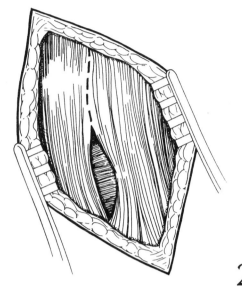

2a

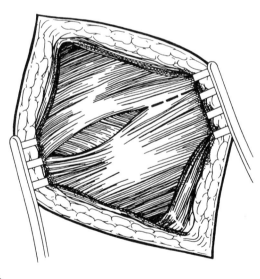

2b

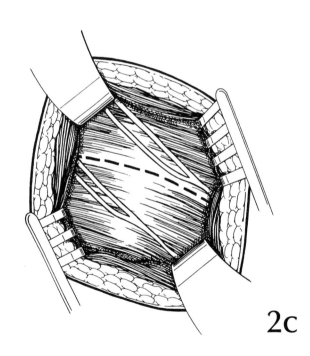

2c

Extraperitoneal dissection

3 The retroperitoneal fat and peritoneal contents are displaced towards the midline using blunt dissection. Retroperitoneal fat should be left posteriorly. Dissection should begin laterally to minimize the possibility of entering the peritoneal cavity. If the peritoneum is inadvertently entered, it may be closed with a running absorbable suture or the peritoneal contents may be packed out of the operative field with a tagged gauze pack. It is important at this point to identify the psoas major muscle and to maintain the plane of dissection anterior to it. This muscle is often more anteriorly located than might be anticipated. As dissection proceeds the genitofemoral nerve is identified on the anterior border of the psoas major, and the ureter is identified and retracted medially with the intraperitoneal contents.

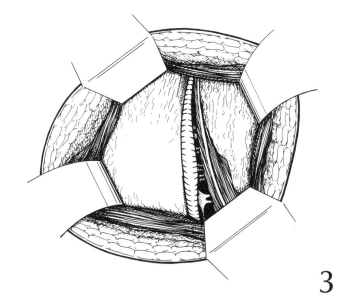

3

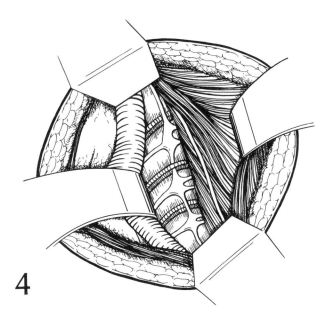

4

Exposure of the sympathetic chain

4 The sympathetic chain is identified on the antero-lateral aspect of the vertebral column. On the left the ganglia lie close to the lateral wall of the aorta, while on the right they are covered by the inferior vena cava. The sympathetic chain is most readily identified by palpation. It is a firm structure, fixed to the vertebral column by the rami communicantes, and the ganglia are readily palpated. The L4 ganglion may be most readily palpable at the sacral promontory. Occasionally two or more of the sympathetic ganglia may be fused, but distal dissection should always proceed to the level of the sacral promontory. Occasionally also the sympathetic ganglion may be confused with retroperitoneal lymph nodes, or more uncommonly with the genitofemoral nerve.

Sympathectomy

5 Once exposed, the sympathetic chain is mobilized with a long nerve hook. The rami communicantes are divided between silver clips, and the sympathetic ganglia are freed. Dissection should proceed cephalad as far as possible and caudad to the pelvic brim. At this point, the dissection will be stopped by the iliac vessels. During mobilization of the sympathetic chain, caution must be exercised to avoid damaging the lumbar veins. Most commonly these pass behind the sympathetic chain, but occasionally, particularly on the right, one or more veins may pass anterior to it. When this occurs, the veins should be divided between clips or the chain threaded out from behind them. Occasionally, the sympathetic chain may be divided in the middle between clamps to facilitate dissection cephalad or caudad. When doubt arises about the identification of the sympathetic trunk, its identity should be confirmed by frozen section before wound closure.

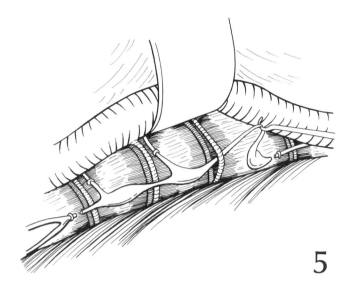

5

Wound closure

Haemostasis is established with particular attention to the lumbar vessels. The wound is then closed in layers using absorbable sutures (2/0 polyglycolic acid). If the rectus sheath has been opened, its anterior and posterior aspects are closed separately with interrupted sutures. The transversus abdominis and oblique muscles are closed separately with a simple running suture. Once again, it is important to protect the intercostal nerves.

Postoperative care

No special measures are usually required in the convalescent period. If the pleura has been entered, a chest radiograph should be obtained in the recovery room. Paralytic ileus, although usually mild, may occur and require gastric decompression. Pain may develop 1–3 weeks after sympathectomy over the lateral thigh and buttock. Often quite discomforting, this pain is best treated with analgesics and will resolve within 2–3 months[3].

Outcome

Sympathectomy is a very effective measure for treating causalgia, with reports of 84% success at 2-year follow-up[4]. In patients treated for rest pain, the best results indicate an 86% long-term improvement in highly selected individuals[5], although most series report response rates of 50–70%.

References

1. Diez J. Un nuevo metodo di simpatectomia periferica para el tratamiento de affecionas trofilas y gangrenosas de los miembros. *Bol Soc Cir Buenos Aires* 1924; 8: 10.

2. Yao JST, Bergan JJ. Predictability of vascular reactivity relative to sympathetic ablation. *Arch Surg* 1973; 107: 676–80.

3. Raskin NH, Levinson SA, Hoffman PM, Pickett JBE, Fields HL. Post-sympathectomy neuralgia: amelioration with diphenylhydantoin and carbamazepine. *Am J Surg* 1974; 128: 75–8.

4. Mockus MB, Rutherford RB, Rosales C, Pearce WH. Sympathectomy for causalgia: patient selection and long term results. *Arch Surg* 1987; 122: 668–72.

5. Persson AV, Anderson LA, Padberg FT Jr. Selection of patients for lumbar sympathectomy. *Surg Clin North Am* 1985; 65: 393–403.

Chemical lumbar sympathectomy

D. M. Justins FRCA
Consultant Anaesthetist and Director, Pain Management Centre, St Thomas' Hospital, London, UK

History

Surgical lumbar sympathectomy was commonly performed on patients with painful obliterative arterial disease. Percutaneous chemical sympathectomy is an alternative to surgery and was described by Mandl in 1926. His approach depended upon the needle contacting the transverse process to gauge depth before being inserted more deeply. Variations of this technique were subsequently described, but it was the introduction of radiographic techniques that allowed identification of landmarks and precise positioning of the needle.

Principles and justification

The lumbar sympathetic trunk is situated in the retroperitoneal connective tissue anterior to the vertebral bodies and the medial margin of the psoas muscle. The genitofemoral nerve lies laterally on the psoas. The aorta and inferior vena cava are anterior; the kidney and ureter are posterolateral. All the sympathetic fibres pass through or synapse at the L2 ganglion, therefore in theory a block at the upper level of L3 should abolish all sympathetic supply to the lower limb. After sympathetic blockade blood flow increases in skin but not muscle. Muscle blood flow may actually decrease. The improvement in rest pain is claimed to follow the improvement in skin blood flow, but pain relief may occur in the absence of any apparent improvement in peripheral circulation. The pain relief may be due to interruption of afferent nociceptive fibres which travel with the sympathetic nerves.

Indications

The indications for chemical sympathectomy in vascular disease are: (1) acute vascular disorders – post-traumatic vasospasm, acute arterial or venous occlusion, and cold injury; (2) chronic vasospastic conditions – Raynaud's disease, acrocyanosis, livedo reticularis; and (3) chronic obliterative disease – thromboangiitis obliterans, atherosclerosis causing rest pain in a limb not amenable to arterial reconstruction or skin ulceration. A sympathetic block may help establish the demarcation of any gangrene. Preoperative lumbar sympathectomy may be used to improve blood flow after surgery. Percutaneous lumbar sympathectomy offers a number of advantages when compared to surgical techniques. Pain relief and improved healing are achieved without the risks of surgery and anaesthesia in an often unfit elderly population of patients. The procedure may be performed as a day case, thereby avoiding 6–10 days as an inpatient after surgery. The duration of the sympathetic blockade is the same as after surgery but the block is easily repeated if necessary. It is also curative in idiopathic hyperhidrosis.

Diagnostic blocks

Diagnostic blocks can be used to determine whether pain is relieved and blood flow increased. An image intensifier is mandatory to confirm precise needle position and the spread of injected solution. Objective signs of sympathetic block should be identified using skin temperature, skin conduction response or tests of sweat production with ninhydrin, cobalt blue or starch iodine. After sympathetic block, dilated veins will become visible in the limb and the increase in blood flow can be measured using a Doppler flow probe or venous plethysmography[1]. When assessing pain relief false-positive results may be because of the spread of solution onto adjacent somatic nerves, the systemic effects of local anaesthetic absorbed from the injection site, or the placebo response. False-negative results may follow an incomplete block or inadequate assessment before or after the injection. Some patients demonstrate unexpected or unusual responses such as contralateral or delayed blocks[2].

Prognostic blocks

These blocks can be used to demonstrate to the patient the effects of the injection on pain and limb temperature. Sometimes the prognostic block will produce an increase in pain or an uncomfortable increase in limb temperature which the patient finds unacceptable. An epidural type catheter can be inserted into the prevertebral area and a continuous sympathetic block maintained by an infusion of local anaesthetic. Some authors recommend that such a block be maintained for up to 5 days before considering neurolytic sympathectomy[1].

Therapeutic blocks

These involve the injection of phenol which is non-selective and destroys all nerve fibre types by protein denaturation. Nerve fibre regeneration will occur eventually and sympathetic control of the limb will be re-established. The strongest possible aqueous solution is 6.6% but higher concentrations can be obtained using an oily base such as a radiographic contrast medium which will also allow the extent of spread of the injected solution to be accurately tracked. Contact of phenol with somatic nerves may cause neuritis.

Opinions differ over where the sympathetic chain should be blocked to produce lower limb sympathectomy. In 1989 Boas examined 500 cases and was unable to demonstrate any difference between single level injection (L2 or L3), double level injection (L2 L3 or L3 L4) or triple level injections (L2 L3 L4)[3]. Other authors have claimed that triple level injection produced the best results[4]. In 1987 Umeda *et al.* studied 19 cadavers

and concluded that the optimal site was either the lower third of the second vertebral body or the upper third of the third vertebral body[5]. A single level injection is certainly safer and faster to perform. The spread of solution can be watched with the image intensifier and if it is insufficient then the injection can be repeated at adjacent levels. An image intensifier capable of biplanar screening is mandatory for chemical lumbar sympathectomy.

Contraindications

Percutaneous chemical sympathectomy is contraindicated in patients taking anticoagulants or those with coagulopathies, in patients with local infection or neoplasm at the injection site and where there are inadequate facilities (especially when there is no image intensifier). Simultaneous bilateral injections should not be performed in patients who would not tolerate any resulting hypotension. Bilateral sympathectomy should not be performed in sexually active males because of the risk of causing failure of ejaculation.

Preoperative

The clinical effect of chemical sympathectomy cannot easily be predicted even with the use of diagnostic or prognostic blocks. This is because of the number of variables in the diseased vascular system which may alter the response in any individual. These influences include 'intravascular steal effects' and the state of any collateral vessels. Multiple vascular lesions and diabetic microvascular disease respond less well to sympathectomy. It has been suggested that chemical sympathectomy is more likely to be successful if ankle systolic pressure is greater than 30 mmHg, if there is no evidence of peripheral neuropathy, and if tissue damage is not too extensive so as to cause only rest pain and digital gangrene. Tests of sympathetic function and of blood flow may be used to provide a baseline for post-injection assessment, but preoperative selection basically remains empirical.

Anaesthesia

Infiltration of local anaesthetic combined with intravenous sedation using short-acting benzodiazepine and opioid is almost always sufficient. General anaesthesia may be indicated in occasional cases. When diagnostic blocks are being performed, intravenous sedatives and analgesics may need to be limited so as to minimize difficulties in the interpretation of the outcome.

Operation

The injection is performed with the patient prone because both the patient and the various anatomical landmarks are more stable in this position, and bilateral blocks can easily be performed. The lateral approach is reserved for patients who are unable to lie prone. Soft support should be provided for painful gangrenous feet or toes. An intravenous cannula should be inserted and patients having bilateral blocks require preloading with intravenous fluids.

1 The image intensifier is used to identify the spine of L3 and a point 7–10 cm lateral to this spine is measured, staying mid-way between the transverse processes of L3 and L4.

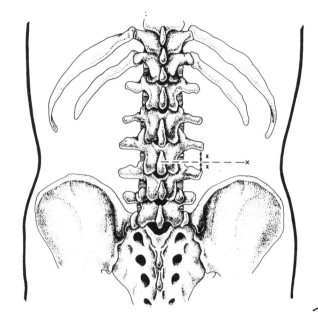

1

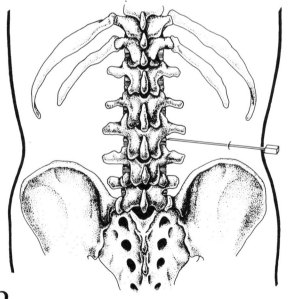

2

2 The skin and deeper tissues are infiltrated with local anaesthetic and a 15-cm 20-gauge needle is inserted at this point and directed towards the side of the L3 vertebral body, taking care to avoid the vertebral foramen. The angle of insertion is approximately 60° to the coronal plane.

3a, b Once contact is made with the vertebral body, lateral radiographs should be used as the needle is gently manoeuvred anteriorly, remaining close to the vertebra, until the point is seen to lie at the anterior edge of the vertebral body. A characteristic click is often felt as the needle passes through the psoas fascia.

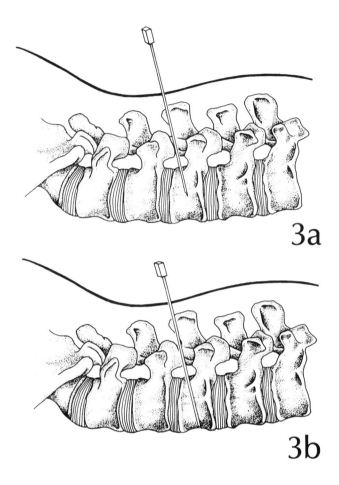

3a

3b

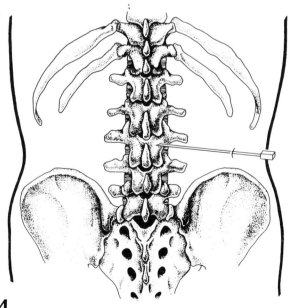

4

4 An anteroposterior radiograph should now show the needle point to be almost midway between the lateral edge of the vertebral body and the spine of the vertebra.

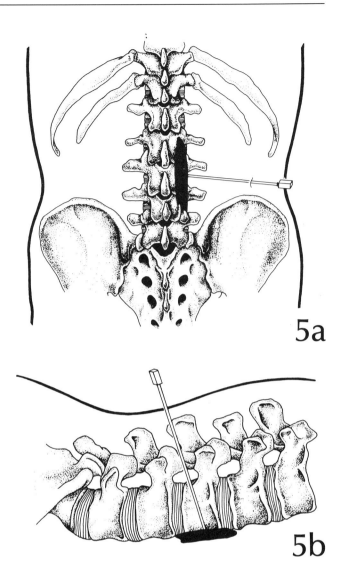

5a, b After a negative aspiration test the injection of 1–2 ml of contrast solution should demonstrate spread in the longitudinal axis without any lateral or posterior extension. This is checked with both anteroposterior and lateral views.

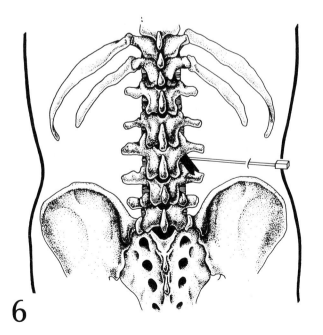

6 Inadvertent injection into psoas muscle produces a characteristic linear pattern which radiates infero-laterally away from the vertebral body. Occasionally the solution will be whisked away in a small vessel even though aspiration tests are negative.

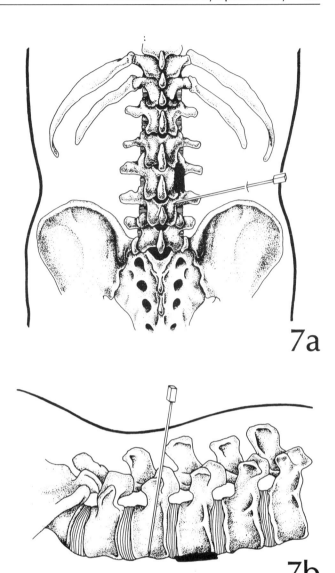

7a, b If the pattern of spread from the single level L3 injection extends up and down in front of the adjacent vertebra, then all of the solution is injected at that site. If the spread is unsatisfactory the same needle is left inserted and is repositioned at L4 using the same sequence of radiographs and contrast injection. The needle will now pass just cephalad to the transverse process of L4 as it approaches the body of that vertebra, whereas for an L3 injection the needle passes just caudad to the transverse process of L3.

Bilateral injections may be performed at the same time in fit patients, or the second side can be blocked after an interval of 2 or 3 days.

Lateral position

The injection can be performed in this position, but the patient is less stable and the operator must ensure that the radiographic views are truly anteroposterior and lateral. Once the patient is well positioned the procedure is basically as for the prone approach.

Choice of solution

A diagnostic block requires a small volume which has been precisely positioned; 2–5 ml of bupivacaine 0.5% at each level should produce a block of sufficient duration. If lignocaine is used for diagnostic purposes then the resulting block may be very brief in duration, so early assessment is necessary. The neurolytic solutions of choice are 6.6% aqueous phenol or a stronger concentration mixed with radiographic contrast solution. A volume of about 2–5 ml is usually sufficient, but recommendations range from 0.1 to 10 ml. The needle should always be flushed with local anaesthetic before withdrawal to avoid leaving a track of phenol through more superficial tissues.

Postoperative care

Routine postoperative observations should be performed in the recovery room. Hypotension is the most frequent problem, and blood pressure should be checked when the patient first stands. Patients may be allowed home with an escort once the blood pressure is stable and recovery from the sedation has occurred. Patients who have had bilateral blocks, or who have cardiovascular disease, should remain under observation until the following day at least. Complications are rarely a problem if radiographic control is used, but the following have been reported.

Complications

Hypotension is the result of peripheral vasodilatation and is most commonly a problem in the elderly or after bilateral blocks. Adequate preloading of the circulation is essential in these cases. The hypotension usually resolves rapidly and responds to conventional therapy, although postural hypotension may persist and patients must be supervised during mobilization after the block.

Direct trauma as a result of needle damage may occur to somatic nerves, blood vessels, the kidney or renal pelvis, or intervertebral discs. Particular care must be taken whenever the needle point is in the vicinity of the vertebral foramen.

Intravascular injection of local anaesthetic or phenol may cause immediate potentially life-threatening reactions. Epidural or intrathecal injection of neurolytic solutions has resulted in permanent paralysis and this risk highlights the need for meticulous radiographic control in every case. Small vertebral vessels may be damaged by phenol, or by the needle, and this may explain some otherwise unaccountable neurological complications. Ureteric strictures have occurred after phenol injection.

Damage to the genitofemoral nerve as it lies on the psoas by the phenol can produce pain and abnormal sensation in the cutaneous distribution of the nerve. In other cases pain and dysaesthesia on the anterior thigh may represent a sympathetic deafferentation syndrome – so-called 'sympathalgia'. Surgical sympathectomy can produce a similar syndrome. Treatment of both genitofemoral neuralgia and sympathalgia involves anticonvulsant medication and transcutaneous electrical nerve stimulation, but it is not always effective and the patient will need reassurance that spontaneous remission will usually occur over a period of 2–7 weeks. Failure of ejaculation is a real risk in males subjected to bilateral neurolytic blocks[6].

The sympathetic blockade may result in dilatation of normally reactive vessels which are proximal or parallel to the diseased vessels and this may cause diminished flow through these compromised vessels and in rare cases may aggravate pain and ischaemia. Blood flow may be diverted from muscle to skin and may theoretically worsen claudication, but this is rarely the case in clinical practice. Ankle systolic blood pressure below 30 mmHg indicates severe vascular disease and may make proximal steal more likely.

Outcome

Neurolytic lumbar sympathetic blocks will relieve rest pain and improve healing of skin ulcers in about 65–75% of patients with atherosclerosis. The procedure is of benefit in a much lower percentage of patients with claudication. A successful block may last for 6–9 months and during this time the patient may develop collateral circulation. The outcome is comparable to that following surgical sympathectomy, but has lower rates of morbidity and mortality. If amputation is necessary then preoperative sympathetic blocks may aid in defining the level of tissue viability and also encourage healing of the stump. There is some evidence to suggest that preoperative sympathetic blocks might diminish the incidence of post-amputation pain syndromes. Established post-amputation pains are occasionally helped by sympathetic blocks, but the management of this condition is often difficult.

References

1. Löfström JB, Cousins MJ. Sympathetic neural blockade of upper and lower extremity. In: Cousins MJ, Bridenbaugh PO, eds. *Neural Blockade in Clinical Anesthesia and Management of Pain*. Philadelphia: Lippincott, 1988: 461–500.

2. Purcell-Jones G, Justins DM, Delayed contralateral sympathetic blockade following chemical sympathectomy – a case history. *Pain* 1988; 34: 61–3.

3. Boas RA. The sympathetic nervous system and pain. In: Swerdlow M, Charlton JE, eds. *Relief of Intractable Pain*, 4th ed. Amsterdam: Elsevier, 1989: 259–79.

4. Walsh JA, Glynn CJ, Cousins MJ, Basedow RW. Blood flow, sympathetic activity and pain relief following lumbar sympathetic blockade or surgical sympathectomy. *Anaesth Intensive Care* 1985; 13: 18–24.

5. Umeda S, Arai T, Hatano Y, Mori K, Hoshino K. Cadaver anatomic analysis of the best site for chemical lumbar sympathectomy. *Anesth Analg* 1987; 66: 643–6.

6. Baxter AD, O'Kafo BA. Ejaculatory failure after chemical sympathectomy. *Anesth Analg* 1984; 63: 770–1.

Upper extremity bypass for hand ischaemia

H. I. Machleder MD
Professor, Department of Surgery, UCLA School of Medicine, Los Angeles, California, USA

Principles and justification

1 The majority of operations to correct hand ischaemia are directed at reconstruction or bypass of the subclavian and axillary arterial segments. The approaches used are the transcervical (supraclavicular), transclavicular and transaxillary routes. The relationships of the major structures in the operative area are shown. In this cadaver dissection the clavicle is reflected laterally to expose the thoracic outlet area.

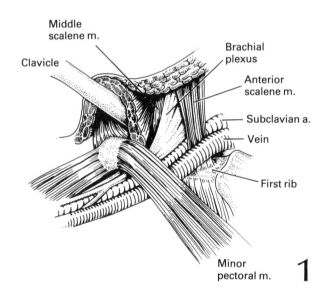

Middle scalene m.

Clavicle

Brachial plexus

Anterior scalene m.

Subclavian a.

Vein

First rib

Minor pectoral m.

1

Indications

Patients with severe hand ischaemia due to occlusion of major arteries should be considered for surgical correction.

2a–d The arteriogram of a patient with severe hand ischaemia secondary to subclavian artery occlusion at the thoracic outlet is shown in *Illustration 2a*. This is repaired via transaxillary first rib resection (to enlarge the thoracic outlet), and vein bypass graft. A traumatic distal subclavian arterial occlusion that is repaired via the transclavicular route with a small interposition graft is shown in *Illustration*

2b. Illustration 2c shows occlusion of the axillary artery at the most lateral aspect of the thoracic outlet, beneath the pectoralis minor tendon insertion, while *Illustration 2d* is an angiogram from a patient with severe hand ischaemia resulting from axillary to brachial arterial occlusion. Repair of this condition requires an additional infraclavicular to axillary incision.

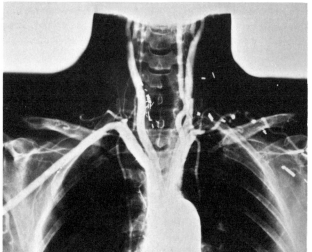

2a

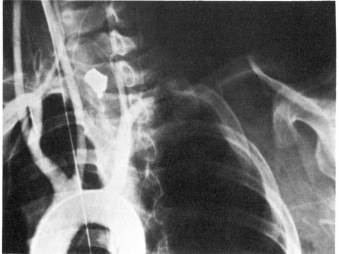

2b

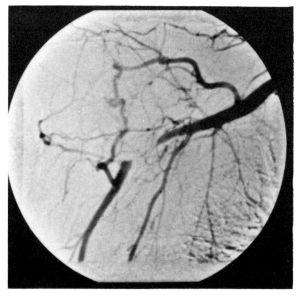

2c

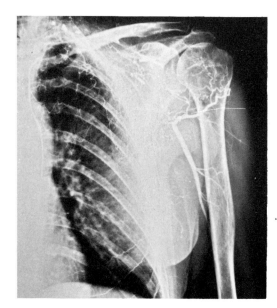

2d

Operations

TRANSAXILLARY APPROACH

Transaxillary first rib resection forms the foundation of our preferred surgical treatment for occlusions in the retroclavicular, costoclavicular and retropectoral spaces of the thoracic outlet. This operative approach may be combined with sympathectomy, transcervical scalenectomy, cervical rib resection, transcervical subclavian artery repair or bypass grafting through the thoracic outlet, as dictated by the specific circumstances.

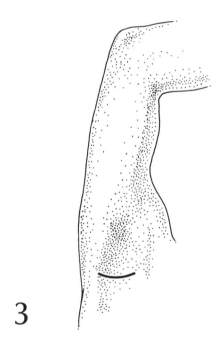

3

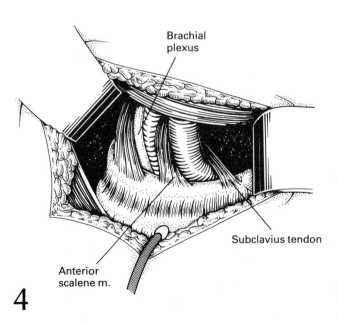

Brachial plexus

Anterior scalene m.

Subclavius tendon

4

Position of patient

The patient is placed in the lateral decubitus position, maintained with a beanbag support. The contralateral axilla and other pressure points are padded and evaluated before preparation and draping. The operation always requires a surgeon, first and second assistant. The surgeon wears a fibreoptic headlight and the first assistant uses a fibreoptic lighted retractor. The second assistant raises the arm using the hammerlock technique described by Roos[1].

Incision

3   A curvilinear incision is made in the axilla at the hairline beneath the axillary fat pad. The incision is carried to the chest wall at the level of the incision, thereby avoiding the axillary lymph nodes and vessels. In this areolar plane at the chest wall the finger is swept up to the apex of the axilla. The positions of the long thoracic and intercostal brachial nerves are noted.

Exposure of first rib

4   The operation is now segregated into several discrete steps of relatively equal time intervals to avoid prolonged retraction of the neurovascular structures. Two retractors are used and are always placed by the surgeon. The first is a Weitlaner self-retaining retractor which holds the skin edges open. The second is a right-angled fibreoptic breast retractor which is placed against the pectoralis major muscle. Before any retraction, and each time the retractor is placed, the tip is visualized and set just posterior to the subclavius tendon. Occasionally the tip can be placed over the axillary vein, but it is never permitted more posterior than the anterior scalene muscle. Retraction further posterior, or any posterior retractor for that matter, is in danger of injuring the brachial plexus.

A small superior thoracic artery and vein will be seen going from the axillary artery and vein to the first intercostal space. These two vessels are ligated with, in general, the only ligatures used during the operation.

A Kutner dissector is swept along the surface of the first rib, identifying each major structure in turn: subclavius tendon, axillosubclavian vein, anterior scalene muscle, axillosubclavian artery, brachial plexus (the T1 root and lower trunk) and the middle scalene muscle. The position of the long thoracic nerve is again noted, along with any anomalies. As the first major step in the operation, the scalene muscle is identified and dissected bluntly (using a small Kutner dissector) on both the venous and arterial sides to visualize a 3-cm segment from the scalene tubercle in a cephalad direction. The muscle is completely separated from the surrounding tissue. Electrocoagulation may be used to control a small branch of the subclavian artery which occasionally traverses the muscle. This concludes the first stage of the operation and the arm retraction is interrupted.

Dissection of rib

5 The second step is division of the anterior scalene muscle over a Lahey type right-angled clamp, leaving a 2–3-cm stump of muscle on the first rib. Transection is performed with Metzenbaum scissors without the use of electrocautery. Using these scissors, the subclavius tendon, costosternal and costoclavicular ligaments are divided, exposing the costochondral junction.

A Cameron Haight periosteal elevator is used to remove the intercostal muscle from the inferior margin of the rib. The parietal pleura is separated from the inner surface of the rib, and the middle scalene muscle is separated from the anterior surface. The T1 nerve root is kept constantly in view. There will be some bleeding from the intercostal muscle and the ends of the middle scalene muscle which is controlled by gently packing the wound with a dry gauze sponge and then relaxing arm retraction.

It is anticipated that there will be 50–60 ml blood loss during the procedure and gentle packing is the only haemostatic manoeuvre used at this stage.

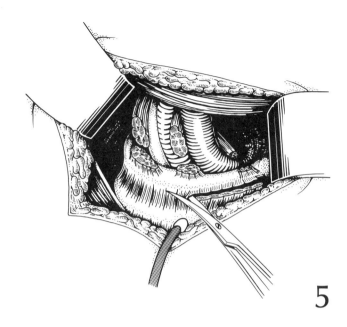

5

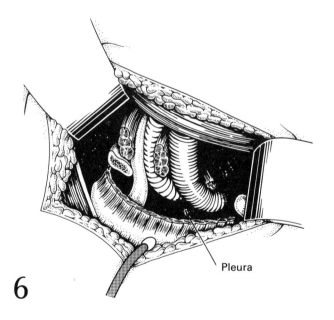

Pleura

6

Transection of rib

6 The third step of the operation is transection of the rib near the transverse process with a Horsley right-angled double-action rib shears, with care taken to protect the T1 nerve root. The rib is grasped with a Kocher clamp and gently distracted from the cut edge. A gauze pack is placed between the rib and the nerve roots, and the rib is disarticulated from the costo-chondral junction. Four pledgets of thrombin-soaked Gelfoam are placed: against the cut rib edge, at the transected edge of the middle scalene muscle, at the anterior scalene muscle, and at the chondral junction. The wound is gently packed and the arm relaxed. The anatomy after rib removal is shown.

The posterior rib stump is evaluated, and if more than 2 cm remains or it is in close proximity to the nerve root, a further portion is removed using a double-action Sauerbruch box rongeurs.

Wound closure

The subcutaneous tissue is closed with 3/0 catgut suture and the skin with an absorbable subcuticular suture. A small strip of gauze soaked in collodion is placed over the incision.

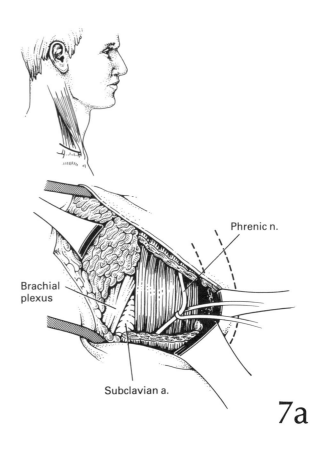

Phrenic n.

Brachial
plexus

Subclavian a.

7a

TRANSCERVICAL APPROACH: SCALENECTOMY

7a, b A transcervical incision is performed just above the clavicle and is carried through the skin, platysma muscle and clavicular head of the sternocleidomastoid muscle. The prescalene fat pad is retracted laterally, exposing the scalene muscle and overlying phrenic nerve. The phrenic nerve is carefully dissected from the surface of the muscle and retracted medially. The scalene muscle is incised, exposing the subclavian artery.

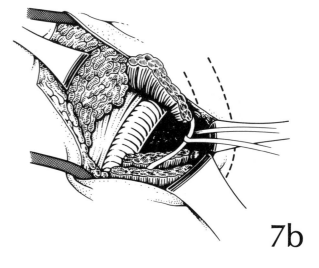

7b

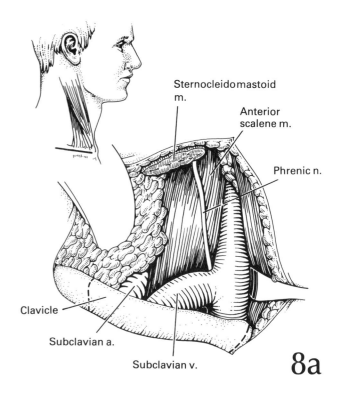

TRANSCLAVICULAR APPROACH

8a, b The transclavicular approach is most commonly used for direct repair of the retroclavicular subclavian artery and is particularly useful when hand ischaemia is a consequence of axillary artery damage from an axillofemoral bypass graft. Repair of a false aneurysm at this site is a good example. The skin incision is made over the clavicle. The clavicle is exposed by subperiosteal dissection and is then resected. The retroclavicular anatomy, with the subclavian artery lying between the vein and the brachial plexus, is shown. This approach provides excellent control and access to the three sections of the subclavian artery. At the completion of the procedure the periosteum is closed without replacing the bone segment.

Repair technique

Vascular bypass is performed with standard grafting and suture techniques. A polytetrafluoroethylene (PTFE) graft is utilized if the repair involves the subclavian or proximal axillary arteries. A vein graft is used for more distal repairs where the graft will be surrounded by brachial plexus elements at the level of the cords.

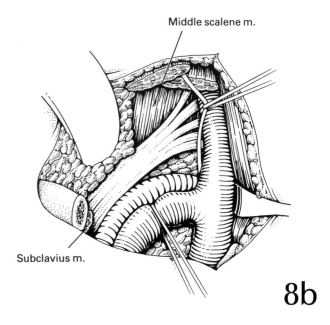

Postoperative care

Complications

Transaxillary approach

Paresis of the anterior serratus muscle from injury to the long thoracic nerve occurs in less than 4% of patients, with half subsequently recovering completely. Although this complication is more likely to occur in reoperations, the defect of scapula winging is described to all patients. The incidence of brachial plexus injury with muscle weakness is estimated to be less than 1% (however, we have not seen this complication in over 400 consecutively treated patients). The patient is advised of the occurrence of this complication as it is recorded in the literature.

Transcervical approach

On the left side, injury to the thoracic duct or major tributary may lead to a lymphocele or lymph fistula. This is avoided by carefully ligating any leaking lymphatic at the time of closure. A thoracic duct leak will usually close if drainage is maintained for about 1 week with a small, closed suction drain system. Transient phrenic nerve palsy can be encountered on either side and merits caution in handling the phrenic nerve during operation. Horner's syndrome can occur and is usually transient.

Pneumothorax is associated with injury to the parietal pleura. It is recognized by a fluttering of the pleura and the fact that the lung is no longer visible, closely applied to the deep aspect of the transparent pleura.

The defect should be enlarged and a suction drain inserted into the pleural space. The anaesthetist inflates the lung as the wound is sutured and suction is then connected. Chest radiography is performed after operation.

Transclavicular approach

The same precautions should be observed as for the transcervical route. This approach should not be performed in the presence of a winged scapula. The clavicle will begin to recalcify after about 1 month.

References

1. Roos DB. Thoracic outlet syndrome. In: Machleder HI, ed. *Vascular Disorders of the Upper Extremity*, 2nd ed. New York: Futura, 1989.

Thoracic outlet compression syndrome: transaxillary approach

J. H. H. Webster MA, MChir, FRCS
Consultant Surgeon, Southampton University Hospitals Trust, Southampton, UK

Principles and justification

Thoracic outlet compression syndrome is a controversial condition occurring mainly in young women, sometimes with a clear history of trauma[1], in whom one or both arms become progressively useless for work above the head or in front because of various combinations of pain, ischaemia, swelling, or discoloration of the hand or forearm. There may also be pain in the shoulder, breast, or neck.

Exhaustive investigations to exclude other causes of neurovascular compression elsewhere in the neck and upper limb may be necessary, but if the symptoms and signs are predominantly arterial, urgent Doppler ultrasonography and arteriography of the subclavian arteries are essential, lest gangrene should rapidly develop.

It is considered by this author and many others that when thoracic outlet compression syndrome has been diagnosed, it is not possible to identify the cause of the compression, e.g. the anterior scalene syndrome, before operation and that the presence of a cervical rib is of no diagnostic significance. A seminal article by Parry[2] describes his progress in the treatment of this condition towards the pioneering demonstration by Roos[3] that the essential operation is removal of the first rib through the axilla. By this operation, which should include removal of an associated cervical rib, all possible sources of thoracic outlet compression syndrome can be identified and eliminated.

Instruments

Several instruments are essential for this operation, which should never be attempted without them.

1 Rib cutters separately and specifically designed for division of the back and front of the first rib are used.

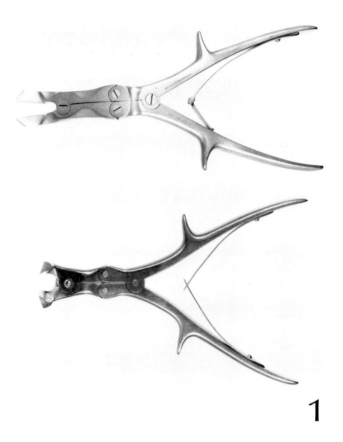

1

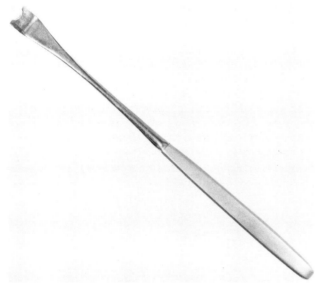

2

2 A recessed rugine that will bite into the back of the rib, and not skate over it, is necessary.

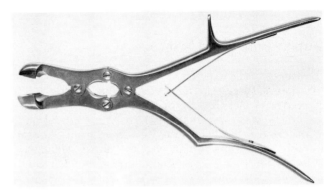

3 A very heavy pair of bone nibblers with long handles is needed to keep the hands clear of the wound and so allow vision.

A headlight for the surgeon is also essential as wound lights get in the way.

3

Operation

Position of patient

The patient, under general anaesthesia, must be positioned very carefully. The affected side is turned exactly halfway into the lateral position, and the accuracy of this is critical. A loose strap over the pelvis, as well as sandbags, are of great help. The assistant who has to hold the arm will need a platform of suitable height to be able to cradle the arm and lift it without undue strain.

Incision

With the arm gently held, a transverse (not angled) incision is made across the axilla, just below the hairline. At the most, the lateral edge of the pectoralis major muscle and the anterior border of the latissimus dorsi muscle should be exposed. The incision seems at this stage to be inadequate. Troublesome bleeding must be controlled, and the dissection must not turn up into the axilla. As it is deepened, the lateral thoracic vessels will need to be divided and ligated. Once the axillary

fascia is divided and the dissection reaches the chest wall, the whole exposure opens up as a layer of loose areolar tissue is entered.

As the arm is raised by the assistant and a retractor is introduced into the wound, finger dissection, aided by a touch with the scissors, lifts the whole of the axillary contents away. The intercostobrachial nerve is seen and felt crossing from medial to lateral. It can usually be gently swept away, but occasionally it 'strings' across the operative field and should be divided, with only minimal sensory loss subsequently in the medial upper arm.

The first rib can now be identified as quite broad, with a sharp medial border and with no rib beyond it. There will be resistance to the finger in the centre of the rib.

When the arm is raised again, the axillary contents are examined. The first structure to be identified is the axillary vein, flapping with respiration. It lies in front of the previously identified band over the rib which comprises the superior intercostal vessels. They should be gently dissected out, divided and tied with a braided ligature. The first rib is now ready to be mobilized.

Mobilization of the first rib

4 Gentle finger dissection across the first rib will press away the soft tissues and define a large part of its medial border, and as the finger moves posteriorly the middle scalene muscle, covering the posterior part of the rib, can be felt. Repeated elevation of the arm allows a clear view of this, and the artery and nerve trunk should now be easily seen and cleaned of their surrounding tissues. In front of the artery the anterior scalene muscle comes clearly into view. At this stage, elevation and lowering of the arm onto the finger allows a clear diagnosis of the cause of the compression.

The anterior scalene muscle is now divided piecemeal with scissors as far from the rib as is convenient. The last few fibres of the muscle can often be broken with the finger. The whole of the medial border of the first rib can now be palpated and confirmed to be clear of the soft tissues.

The lateral border of the rib must now be separated from the second rib. Starting anteriorly the intercostal muscles, which are often thick and fibrous, are incised with scissors. Once the gap is big enough, the pleura can be stripped off the under surface of the first rib with a finger. The pleura may accidentally be opened at this stage. This hazard appears to depend entirely on its thickness and is not related to the age or sex of the patient.

As the intercostal incision is carried posteriorly, it will be seen that elevation of the arm lifts the neurovascular

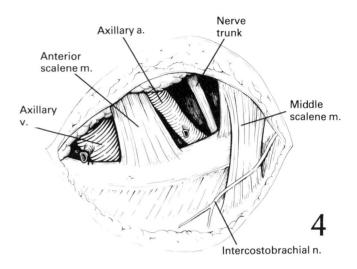

4

bundle well away from the rib. The outer angle of the rib may force the intercostal incision to be extended posteriorly. Further dissection with the finger clears the outer edge and under surface of the rib of its attachments.

All that remains is to remove part of the middle scalene muscle from the upper surface of the back of the rib. With the arm again lifted and the nerve trunk clearly in view, the surface of the middle scalene muscle is incised with scissors. This allows the rugine to bite into the muscle. The muscle must be scraped towards the operator. Only a small piece of the upper surface of the rib needs to be cleared, and the periosteum is not disturbed.

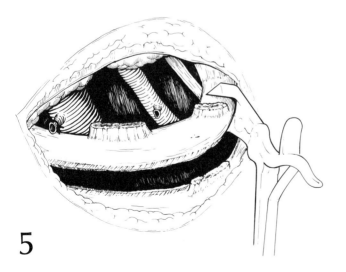

5

Division of the first rib

5 The shears designed for the posterior cut are introduced and are angled carefully across the posterior end of the rib. The nerve trunk will be seen to be lifted away from the rib and correct angulation of the shears pushes it even further away.

After the posterior end of the rib has been cut, the anterior shears cut the rib as close as possible to the costoclavicular ligament and the piece of rib is removed. The arm should again be rested. Heavy bone nibblers are used to smooth off the anterior end of the rib under vision.

The posterior remnant of the rib is now palpated and viewed. The nibblers can be slid over it. Their shape protects the nerve trunk. About 2.5 cm more of the rib can usually be removed until the rib stump is no longer visible and only palpable with difficulty.

Removal of an associated cervical rib

The most usual finding is a very sharp band running from the cervical rib into the medial border of the first rib, across which the nerve trunk is stretched, but occasionally a complete cervical rib articulates with the first rib by a large cartilaginous knob. The artery is often bound to this knob and needs careful dissection to free it.

6 As the posterior end of the first rib is exposed, the gap between it and the cervical rib can gradually be opened so that the back of the first rib is cleaned and can then be divided with the shears. After division of the front of the first rib, the rugine can be used to clean the cervical rib, and the nibblers slid up to divide it. The two ribs can then be removed *en bloc*.

It must be emphasized that the first rib should be divided before the cervical rib. The sequence of cuts for the combined removal of the first and cervical ribs is shown.

After smoothing off all the bone ends, the wound is closed with a simple subcutaneous suture. A suction drain is used if the pleura is intact, and a small chest drain if not.

If the subclavian artery needs to be reconstructed, e.g. for occlusion or aneurysm, an immediate supraclavicular approach will now be found to give remarkably clear and easy access.

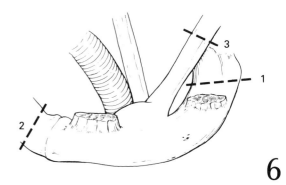

6

Postoperative care

The author has found that a brachial plexus block with local anaesthetic is invaluable in the immediate postoperative management of pain. Gentle exercise should be started as soon as possible, but active physiotherapy, and in particular ultrasound treatment, are detrimental. If pain from the operation persists after about 1 month, non-steroidal anti-inflammatory drugs (if not contraindicated) are of particular value for 1–2 weeks.

Operative complications

In a personal experience of 147 operations on patients aged 12–74 years (male:female, 1:21), the following complications were encountered:

Opening the pleura is of little importance, providing it is recognized and a chest drain is inserted. This drain should not be removed until full expansion of the lung is confirmed by radiography. One patient developed an encysted haemothorax needing formal drainage.

Damage to the neurovascular bundle is likely to be due to inadequate vision, clumsy finger dissection, use of the wrong instruments, or unsupervised prolonged retraction on the arm. One nerve trunk was divided by the use of incorrect shears, and one internal mammary artery was avulsed accidentally. Unless it is clear that such injuries are very easily correctable via the axilla, the approach should be immediately abandoned, the wound packed, and the patient turned into the supine position. The damage can be repaired by appropriate vascular surgery through a supraclavicular incision.

References

1. Sanders RJ, Haug CE. *Thoracic Outlet Syndrome: A Common Sequel of Neck Injuries*. Philadelphia: Lippincott, 1991.

2. Parry E. The thoracic outlet compression syndrome. *Aust NZ J Surg* 1981; 51: 84–91.

3. Roos DB. The place for scalenectomy and first-rib resection in thoracic outlet syndrome. *Surgery* 1982; 92: 1077–85.

Thoracic outlet syndrome: supraclavicular approach

S. W. K. Cheng MD, FRCS
Visiting Assistant Professor, Vascular Division, University of California, San Francisco, USA

W. V. Ellis MD
Department of Neurosurgery, University of California, San Francisco, USA

R. J. Stoney MD
Professor of Surgery, Vascular Division, University of California, San Francisco, USA

History

Controversy has surrounded the aetiology and treatment of choice of the thoracic outlet syndrome. Mechanical compression of the brachial plexus or post-traumatic inflammation has been thought to be the cause. Operative treatment includes scalenotomy or scalenectomy, with or without excision of a cervical and/or first rib, depending on which anatomical structures are regarded by the surgeon to be the cause of compressive symptoms. Four operative approaches are generally adopted: supraclavicular, transaxillary, infraclavicular and posterior parascapular.

In 1861 Coote was the first to excise a cervical rib as the treatment for thoracic outlet syndrome. This was followed by the removal of a normal first rib by Murphy in 1910 to relieve neurological symptoms. Later the technique of anterior scalenotomy was developed as the role of the scalenus anterior muscle in brachial plexus compression was recognized[1]. In the early 1960s Clagett proposed the posterior approach for first or cervical rib resection in thoracic outlet decompression. This was followed by the transaxillary approach to first rib resection described by Roos[2,3], which rapidly became the most popular operation for the thoracic outlet syndrome in the past two decades.

Principles and justification

Pathophysiology

Neurogenic symptoms of pain, paraesthesia and weakness of the upper limb are caused by brachial plexus compression at the thoracic outlet. The clinical progression falls into two general categories: (1) those with an abrupt (usually post-traumatic) onset: they have little, if any, motor disturbances, but suffer severe sensory symptoms similar to early reflex sympathetic dystrophy; and (2) those with a slow, progressive course over years with the gradual evolution of disabling symptoms.

The predisposing factors are primarily anatomical, including osseous anomalies like cervical ribs or an abnormally long transverse process of the C7 vertebra. Congenital fibrous bands, scalene muscle hypertrophy or aberrant interdigitation constitute another source of brachial plexus irritation. The symptoms are frequently precipitated by neck trauma.

The initial injury, whether gross (usually hyperextension injury to the neck) or from repetitive microtrauma, produces a local perineural inflammation. In certain individuals, this sensitizes the local neural net to produce trophic and inflammatory factors (e.g. substance P) which in turn evoke an organizing extracellular response and scar formation. This perineural fibrosis and consequent local vasoconstriction of the vasa nervorum produces local ischaemia and neurogenic thoracic outlet symptoms. These same factors also stimulate type I muscle growth and local muscular hypertrophy. The ischaemia, whether neurogenic or from mechanical irritation, perpetuates the abnormal sensitivity of the perineural network and creates a pathological positive feedback, which eventually results in the surgically correctable condition we know as thoracic outlet syndrome.

Indications for operation

Most patients have some improvement with a period of conservative physical therapy and analgesics. The results of conservative management are usually better if the symptoms are of recent onset. Surgical decompression of the thoracic inlet should be offered if symptoms do not improve or worsen after several months of conservative treatment, or if the patient is severely disabled. A concomitant cervical sympathectomy may be offered if the patient shows severe digital ischaemia or complains of reflex sympathetic dystrophy.

Supraclavicular approach

The transaxillary approach for thoracic outlet decompression was originally adopted in this unit, but was later modified to combine supraclavicular scalenectomy with transaxillary rib resection[4] because a significant proportion of patients had persistent or recurrent symptoms after transaxillary first rib resection alone. Supraclavicular reoperation in these patients disclosed reattachment of the anterior scalene muscle to the scarred first rib bed, and symptoms improved after scalenectomy. Most importantly, the supraclavicular approach allows direct visualization of the anatomy of the thoracic outlet, and permits simultaneous treatment of anomalies of the scalene muscles themselves, so that every source of compression of the brachial plexus can be removed. This approach also gives excellent exposure of the neck of the first rib and the courses of T1 and C8 roots. With careful dissection of the neurovascular structures in the supraclavicular fossa, extraperiosteal mobilization and excision of the first rib is possible via the supraclavicular route alone. We abandoned the transaxillary operation completely in 1983 and have reported a 90% success rate with supraclavicular scalenectomy and first rib resection[5].

With increasing experience with supraclavicular decompression, we began to question the necessity of routine first rib resection. The supraclavicular approach enables accurate identification of the offending struc-

tures. They are usually soft tissue anomalies such as muscular interdigitation or fascial bands and scars. Osseous abnormalities are rare, and the first rib seldom has actual mechanical contact with the brachial plexus. The prevalence of symptoms occurring after trauma and consistent reports of scalene muscle pathology[6] focused our attention on the role of this muscle in symptom production. Frequently after scalenectomy and a complete neurolysis, the brachial plexus runs a free, unobstructed course through the thoracic outlet. Resection of the first rib in these instances is unnecessary and poses additional problems of increased postoperative pain and morbidity, and a higher risk of pleural damage. Moreover, the bed of the resected first rib is often a site of excessive scarring and contributes to the recurrence of symptoms. Since early 1990 we have performed 34 thoracic outlet decompressions by anterior and middle scalenectomy and neurolysis of the brachial plexus using a supraclavicular approach without resecting the first rib. The results were no different from those of supraclavicular scalenectomy and rib resection.

Preoperative

The diagnosis of thoracic outlet syndrome is mainly clinical. A thorough physical examination of the musculoskeletal system of the neck, shoulders and upper extremity must be undertaken to exclude other pathology. Radiography of the cervical spine should be performed for all patients. Osseous anomalies such as cervical ribs or old fractures may be readily diagnosed. Computed tomography or magnetic resonance imaging of the neck are mainly used to rule out degenerative cervical spinal conditions and are not specific for thoracic outlet syndrome. Electromyography and nerve conduction studies are often normal and are only helpful in excluding nerve entrapments like carpal tunnel syndrome. In patients with vascular symptoms, an arteriogram or venogram is mandatory and may be supplemented by non-invasive vascular laboratory studies.

The patient is admitted a day before or on the day of surgery and no special preparation is necessary.

Anaesthesia

The operation is carried out under general anaesthesia with endotracheal intubation. The patient is placed in a semi-recumbent (Fowler) position on the operating table with the head turned away from the side of operation. The arm of the involved side is held parallel to the body with the hand exposed.

Operation

Incision

1 A curvilinear incision is made at the base of the
neck, two fingerbreadths above the clavicle,
beginning over the clavicular head of the sternocleidomastoid muscle, and curving laterally and posteriorly for
about 10 cm. The platysma is incised and subplatysmal
flaps are raised superiorly to the level of the cricoid and
inferiorly to the level of the clavicle. The sternocleidomastoid muscle is retracted medially and its clavicular
head divided if necessary.

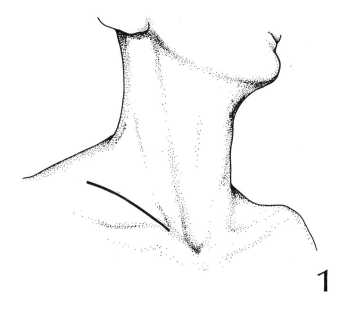

1

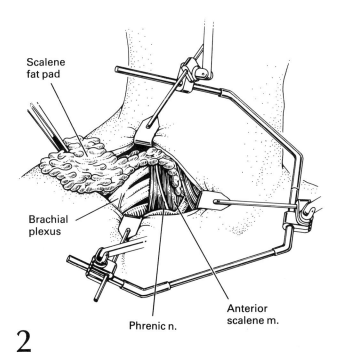

Scalene
fat pad

Brachial
plexus

Phrenic n.

Anterior
scalene m.

2

Mobilization of scalene fat pad

2 The lateral border of the internal jugular vein is
identified and mobilization of the scalene fat pad is
begun at this point. The mobilization proceeds laterally
onto the anterior surface of the anterior scalene muscle
and inferiorly along the clavicle. The omohyoid muscle
is divided. The phrenic nerve, which runs obliquely
from lateral to medial across the anterior scalene
muscle, is identified and gently dissected free. The
scalene fat pad is then reflected on a laterally based
pedicle.

Anterior scalenectomy

3 The phrenic nerve is retracted medially, and the anterior scalene muscle is mobilized down to its attachment to the first rib, taking care to preserve the subclavian artery and the trunks of the brachial plexus posteriorly. Branches of the thyrocervical artery may be encountered running across the anterior scalene muscle and may have to be divided. The muscle is detached flush with the rib and reflected superiorly. This allows optimal visualization of the plexus and the artery. Any muscle fibres which interdigitate with the middle scalene muscle between the trunks of the plexus or which encircle the subclavian artery are now divided. This process proceeds proximally until the origins of the anterior scalene muscle are exposed from the transverse processes of the upper cervical vertebrae; they are then divided and the anterior scalene muscle is removed.

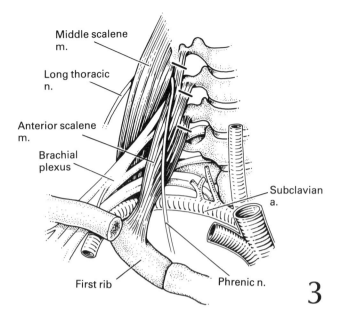

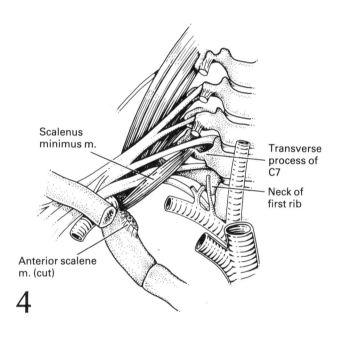

Middle scalenectomy

4 Thorough mobilization of the roots and trunks of the brachial plexus is now performed, until gentle anterior displacement of these structures is possible. This is facilitated by elevating the shoulder to relieve tension on the nerve trunks, allowing further mobilization of the trunks from the anterior surface of the middle scalene muscle. The lateral border of the middle scalene is explored until the point of emergence of the long thoracic nerve is determined. The middle scalene muscle is mobilized completely by gently displacing the trunks of the brachial plexus. Any interdigitating muscle fibres or anomalous bands passing between or compressing the nerve roots or trunks are removed.

5 As this dissection progresses towards the posterior surface of the middle scalene, the first rib will be easily felt behind the muscle. The middle scalene muscle is then transected on a line parallel to and inferior to the course of the long thoracic nerve down to the anterior aspect of the neck of the first rib. The muscle insertion, together with the periosteum, is removed from the rib entirely. This leaves a clean bony surface on the first rib with no muscle adjacent to the brachial plexus.

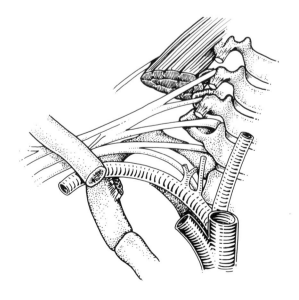

Brachial plexus neurolysis

The brachial plexus is now carefully inspected and each root traced from its interforaminal origin to the level of the clavicle. Any scar tissue and residual muscle fibres are removed by a complete neurolysis until the nerves are skeletonized.

6a–d
A prominent transverse process of the C7 vertebra may be shortened with a rongeur or cut with a pair of heavy scissors. If the medial neck of the first rib is impinging on the course of the T1 root of the plexus, a bone rongeur is used to remove a small rim of the medial border, allowing a free course of the root on its way through the thoracic outlet. The first rib does not cause actual compression of the plexus and is not disturbed.

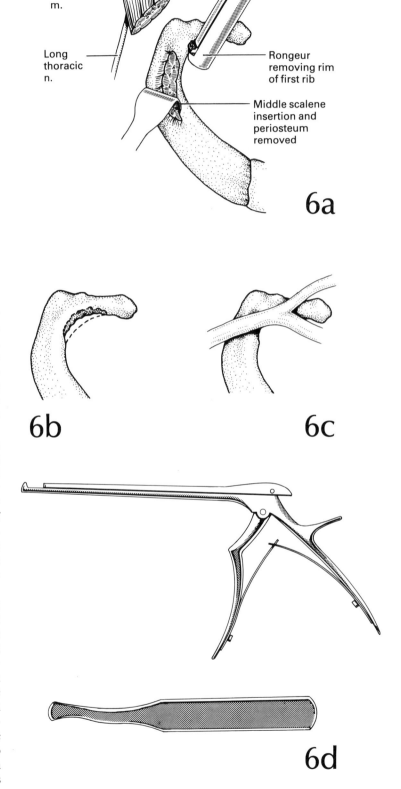

Middle scalene m.

Long thoracic n.

Rongeur removing rim of first rib

Middle scalene insertion and periosteum removed

6a

6b

6c

6d

Intraoperative monitoring

The effectiveness of surgical decompression of the brachial plexus can be monitored during surgery. This involves imaging the pattern of infrared heat emission from the hand on the operated side and observing the pattern of change during the operation. Previous experience in intraoperative monitoring during laminectomy and discectomy has validated the usefulness of this technique in determining the completeness of surgical decompression of the nerve roots.

Using an on-line infrared camera processed by a colourizer, we have monitored over 60 cases during surgery through a draped tunnel, with no physical contact with the patient. The initial thermal asymmetry as determined before operation is characterized by asymmetrical cooling of, principally, the ulnar aspect of the dorsum of the hand and involves multiple dermatomes, unlike disc disease in which only one dermatome is affected. This image is displayed on a small video terminal and is monitored continuously during the operation.

Consistently, we have observed a decrease in heat emission in the dermatome of the cervical nerve root being retracted or manipulated. Conversely, the atraumatic perineural dissection of scar tissue results in increased heat emission in the dermatome corresponding to that nerve. This increase in heat emission is seen when myofascial anomalies and osseous deformities are removed. Interestingly, this heat increase is often dramatic when perineural fibrosis is removed, suggesting that this may be important in plexus irritation. The sensitivity of the brachial plexus roots and trunks to continued irritation directs further surgical exploration and decompression of affected roots. Without this information, an incomplete decompression would result in nearly one-third of patients.

Closure

Haemostasis is carefully secured and the wound inspected for any chylous or lymphatic leakage. The lung is inflated and the pleura examined for any disruption. If a pleural defect is detected, a small catheter is placed through a pleurotomy into the thoracic cavity and the air evacuated by aspiration before closure. The catheter is later withdrawn from the closed wound. A smaller tear in the pleura can be closed directly with absorbable sutures. The mobilized pre-scalene fat pad is positioned loosely over the trunks of the brachial plexus. This provides a soft insulating pad to help protect the nerves. The platysma is reapproximated and the skin closed with a subcuticular suture around a suction drain. An epidural catheter placed through a stab wound and positioned along the course of the proximal root of the brachial plexus can be used for instillation of topical anaesthetic agents for post-operative pain relief or steroids to reduce scar tissue formation in patients undergoing reoperation.

Operative concerns and hazards

The supraclavicular fossa is the seat of many vital neurovascular structures and a thorough understanding of the anatomy is essential to the success of the operation. The surgeon should also bear in mind that diverse anatomical variations and anomalies exist in this region. The anterior and middle scalene muscles may be hypertrophied or have abnormally broad insertions into the first rib. Often, interdigitating bundles from these muscles pass between the roots of the brachial plexus. The plexus may emerge high up in the interscalene space. Frequently, a scalene minimus muscle or a fibrous band will originate from the C7 vertebral body, crossing in front of the lower brachial plexus to insert into the medial border of the first rib, compressing the nerves. Particular attention should be paid during dissection to identify and preserve the following nerves, vessels and lymphatic structures.

Nerves

The roots and trunks of the brachial plexus are prone to damage as they emerge through the intervals between the anterior and middle scalene muscles. In reoperations they may be encased by scar tissue. The T1 root lies close to the neck of the first rib and may be damaged if the rib is resected.

The phrenic nerve, which runs from lateral to medial across the surface of the anterior scalene muscle, must be identified and protected before the muscle is resected. Excessive traction on the nerve should be avoided.

The long thoracic nerve emerges on the lateral border of the middle scalene muscle. Its identification serves as a landmark for the division of this muscle. It may have two roots which join to form the main nerve.

The vagus nerve and its recurrent branch on the right side may be subjected to damage as it courses in front of the subclavian artery.

The cervical sympathetic chain and the stellate ganglion lie behind the common carotid artery and in front of the prevertebral fascia. Damage to the ganglion will result in a Horner's syndrome.

Vessels

The internal jugular vein joins the subclavian vein behind the medial end of the clavicle and runs in front of the anterior scalene muscle.

The subclavian artery lies behind the anterior scalene muscle as it emerges from the thoracic outlet. Any abnormal bands compressing the artery should be freed and the artery protected when the muscle is excised.

Lymphatic structures

Chylous and lymphatic structures, especially the thoracic duct on the left side when it turns laterally at the level of the transverse process of C7 and runs in front of the subclavian artery to drain into the innominate vein, should be preserved.

Postoperative care

The drains are usually removed within 48 h and the patient discharged on the third or fourth postoperative day. Passive arm motion is allowed immediately and a physical therapy programme is started to allow gradual recovery of the range of motion of the shoulder and neck and normal muscle function.

Complications

Wound collection

A collection of serous fluid or lymph under the supraclavicular wound poses an occasional problem. The swelling usually subsides with needle aspiration and antibiotics. In rare cases it becomes encapsulated and operative removal together with ligation of the leaking lymphatic ducts is necessary.

Pleural complications

A small tear in the pleura is the most common complication in our experience. The patient can usually be adequately treated by aspiration with a catheter. Postoperative pneumothorax is rare and may be observed if it is small.

If a major lymphatic duct is damaged, a continuous chylous leak from the drain or wound will result. This may lead to a chylothorax and compromise respiration. Treatment by chest tube drainage followed by re-exploration of the neck and ligation of the leaking lymphatic is essential.

Haemothorax is a rare occurrence and can be avoided by careful haemostasis before closure.

Neuropraxia

Operative irritation or traction can cause neuropraxia of the phrenic or long thoracic nerves and occasionally the brachial plexus. Transient elevation of the diaphragm, winging of the scapula, or weakness of the arm or hand in the brachial plexus distribution will result. A permanent nerve palsy is uncommon.

Accelerated healing

In a few patients excessive scar formation around the brachial plexus can result in early recurrence of pain, tightness, muscle spasm and limited motion. Vigorous physical therapy, steroids and interferon have been tried to alleviate these symptoms without much success. Reoperation to remove the scar tissue may be necessary if the symptoms become too severe. Postoperative magnetic resonance image scan is useful to assess scar development.

Pain syndrome

After a successful thoracic outlet decompression some patients report burning pain and increased sympathetic tone in the upper extremity. These are exaggerated by compressing 'trigger zones' in the supraclavicular area. Neuromas, nerve entrapment by scars and reflex sympathetic dystrophy have been advocated as the cause. Stellate ganglion blocks, trigger point injections and physical therapy including ultrasound and hot packs can provide temporary relief, but the problem is often protracted.

Outcome

From January 1983 to September 1991 we have performed 225 thoracic outlet decompressions using the supraclavicular approach on 196 patients (36 men

and 160 women). More than half (58.7%) of the patients gave a history of trauma to the neck or shoulders. The majority (188) were primary operations and 37 patients were operated upon for recurrence of symptoms after a previous decompression elsewhere.

Of the 188 primary operations, 128 were combined scalenectomy and first rib resections, 26 were scalenectomy and excision of a cervical rib, and 34 were scalenectomy and neurolysis with sparing of the first rib. Anatomical anomalies were frequent operative findings (*Table 1*), and many patients had more than one abnormality.

Table 1 Number of anomalies detected in primary operations

Osseous anomalies	
Cervical rib	26
Abnormal first rib	5
C7 transverse process	24
Soft tissue anomalies	
Anterior/middle scalene	108
Scalenus minimus	52
Fibrous bands	76
Scar	56

Pleural damage occurred during operation in 40–60% of operations. Most were small tears and could be managed adequately with catheter aspiration alone. Postoperative complications are listed in *Table 2*. Most were minor and were treated conservatively. Nine patients underwent re-exploration, of whom seven had chylous leaks and two suffered from haemorrhage.

Table 2 Complications of supraclavicular thoracic outlet decompression (total 225 procedures)

Pulmonary	
Pleura injury	123 (54.6%)
Pneumothorax	21 (9.3%)
Pleural effusion	21 (9.3%)
Nerve injury	
Phrenic nerve	11 (4.9%)
Long thoracic nerve	8 (3.6%)
Brachial plexus	3 (1.3%)
Recurrent laryngeal nerve	2 (0.9%)
Lymphatic injury	13 (5.8%)
Haemorrhage	5 (2.2%)

All patients were examined after operation with a mean follow-up time of 12 months. The assessment of the results of surgery was based on the percentage improvement of preoperative symptoms, and less than 50% were regarded as unchanged. A cure or partial cure was achieved in nearly 90% of primary operations. The results of reoperation were less favourable, with an overall success rate of 76.5%.

References

1. Naffziger HC, Grant WT. Neuritis of the brachial plexus mechanical in origin: the scalenus syndrome. *Surg Gynecol Obstet* 1938; 67: 722–30.

2. Roos DB. Transaxillary approach for first rib resection to relieve thoracic outlet syndrome. *Ann Surg* 1966; 163: 354–8.

3. Roos DB, Owens JC. Thoracic outlet syndrome. *Arch Surg* 1966; 93: 71–4.

4. Qvarfordt PG, Ehrenfeld WK, Stoney RJ. Supraclavicular radical scalenectomy and transaxillary first rib resection for the thoracic outlet syndrome. A combined approach. *Am J Surg* 1984; 148: 111–16.

5. Reilly L, Stoney RJ. Supraclavicular approach for thoracic outlet decompression. *J Vasc Surg* 1988; 8: 329–34.

6. Machleder HI, Moll F, Verity A. The anterior scalene muscle in thoracic outlet compression syndrome: histochemical and morphometric studies. *Arch Surg* 1986; 121: 1141–4.

Further reading

Sanders RJ, Haug CE. *Thoracic Outlet Syndrome. A Common Sequel of Neck Injuries.* Philadelphia: Lippincott, 1991.

Sympathectomy of the upper extremity

R. M. Green MD, FACS
Associate Professor of Surgery and Chief, Section of Vascular Surgery, University of Rochester School of Medicine, Rochester, New York, USA

C. G. Rob MChir, FRCS, FACS
Professor of Surgery, Uniformed Services University of the Health Sciences, F. Edward Hebert School of Medicine, Bethesda, Maryland, USA

Principles and justification

Sympathetic denervation of the upper extremity and most of the axilla can be achieved by removal of the lower portion of the stellate or inferior cervical ganglion and the second and third thoracic ganglia. This portion of the sympathetic chain may be approached by one of seven routes: cervical[1]; transaxillary through the bed of the resected first rib[2]; transaxillary via the third interspace[3]; anterior thoracic[4]; posterior[5]; and recently the thoracoscopic[6] and percutaneous approaches[7]. The cervical approach is the one most commonly used today. It is well tolerated and safe when performed by a surgeon familiar with the complex anatomical relationships in this area. The transaxillary and axillary approach via the third interspace may be preferred when the ganglionectomy should be taken below the level of the third thoracic ganglion, as in hyperhidrosis. The anterior thoracic approach provides excellent exposure but means a thoracotomy. The posterior approach has been largely abandoned. The thoracoscopic approach has recently reappeared and, with recent improvements in video technology and instrumentation, has many advantages.

Anatomy of the sympathetic chain

The cervical sympathetic outflow is composed of a superior cervical ganglion from the fused C1–C4 ganglia, a middle cervical ganglion from C5 and C6, and an inferior cervical ganglion from C7 and C8. The inferior cervical and the first thoracic ganglia fuse to form the stellate ganglion. Sympathetic outflow to the upper extremity comes from spinal segments T2–T9, but in 10% of cases fibres from T1 contribute to arm innervation. There may also be a direct connection between the second and third thoracic ganglia and the brachial plexus, called the nerve of Kuntz.

Recurrence of symptoms after operation

The recurrence of symptoms after upper extremity sympathectomy remains an unresolved problem. The anatomical variation of the sympathetic supply is one of the important explanations of this phenomenon. The nerve of Kuntz passing through the brachial plexus may be relevant in such failures. Regeneration of preganglionic fibres is another explanation, as autonomic fibres do regenerate though ganglion cells do not, making the re-establishment of functional sympathetic pathways most unlikely. Finally, and most likely, progression of an ongoing disease process may also account for the return of symptoms.

Indications

Upper extremity sympathectomy has been recommended for a number of conditions when the disability is sufficiently severe and non-operative methods have failed. Results have been mixed, often because of poor patient selection. Sympathetic denervation is recommended much less often than in the past as the result of a combination of factors, such as advances in the primary repair of arterial injuries and occlusive disease and improvements in vasoactive drugs. Currently, the indications for upper extremity sympathectomy are:

true causalgia; sympathetic dystrophy; inoperable arterial occlusions; refractory Raynaud's and Buerger's (thromboangiitis obliterans) diseases; hyperhidrosis; and the idiopathic 'long QT syndrome'[8]. The potential benefit of an upper extremity sympathectomy can be determined by a diagnostic small volume (10 ml or less) stellate ganglion nerve block.

The best long-term results with upper extremity sympathectomy are obtained in patients with true causalgia and other autonomic nerve dystrophies. Patients with hyperhidrosis also do well, although they may have excessive body sweating after sympathectomy. Successful medical treatment of this condition with a combination of ergotamine tartrate, belladonna and phenobarbitone has eliminated many of these patients as operative candidates. Results in patients with digital artery occlusion from embolism, thrombosis, or frostbite, and with thromboangiitis obliterans, depend on the degree of arterial occlusion and the amount of tissue destruction. If vasospasm is a significant aspect of the problem, a satisfactory result can be obtained. Vasospastic phenomena must be demonstrable by objective criteria such as digital plethysmography.

The greatest controversy in terms of operative indications comes in patients with Raynaud's phenomenon. Because this is a broad diagnostic grouping of a great many diseases, patients must be carefully screened before operation. Patients with primary Raynaud's disease and with symptoms of pure vasospasm should get relief for a prolonged period, but these patients usually respond to medical management and are not often candidates for surgery. Many patients with severe vasospasm refractory to drug therapy will eventually develop collagen vascular disorders. These patients do poorly after operation. Occasionally, surgery will be required to heal finger tip ulcerations.

The long QT syndrome is a familial disorder associated with prolongation of the QT segment on electrocardiography, syncope and fatal ventricular arrhythmias. Treatment consists of β-blockers and pacemakers, and when the condition is refractory to these measures, a left cervical sympathectomy is indicated.

Operations

CERVICAL APPROACH

Position of patient

The patient is placed in the supine position with the head of the operating table elevated to prevent venous engorgement. The patient's head is rotated to the opposite side, and the arms are placed by the side of the body.

Incision

1 The incision is made in a skin crease a finger-breadth above the clavicle. It begins medially at the anterior border of the sternocleidomastoid muscle and extends laterally about 7.5 cm to the external jugular vein. The incision is carried down through the platysma muscle with the cautery tip.

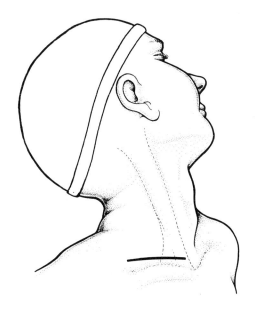

1

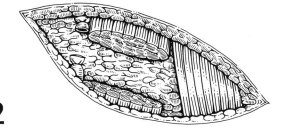

2

Partial division of the sternocleidomastoid muscle

2 The external jugular vein is divided between suture ligatures, sparing the supraclavicular nerves when possible. The sternocleidomastoid muscle is exposed and its lateral border identified. Only the clavicular head is divided with a specially designed, right-angled electrocautery tip (PLP Inc., Colmar, Pennsylvania, USA). Care must be taken to avoid the internal jugular vein which lies under the muscle.

Exposure of the anterior scalene muscle

3 The dissection is carried down through the scalene fat pad, which is dissected from the lateral border of the internal jugular vein and moved laterally. The thoracic duct comes into view on the left side when this is done and should be ligated. There are times when no specific structure can be identified as duct, but lymph oozes around the vein. This area can be oversewn with 6/0 polypropylene sutures to control further leakage. Occasionally, lymphatic leakage occurs on the right side and can be handled in a similar fashion. The fat pad is then swept off the underlying scalene muscle. The transverse cervical artery and vein require division. The phrenic nerve crosses anteriorly and should be dissected away from the scalene muscle over its entire cervical length and gently moved medially with the jugular vein. During this and other parts of the dissection it is important not to retract structures laterally as this might inadvertently injure the upper trunks of the brachial plexus.

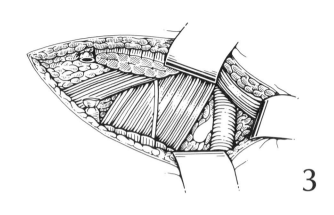

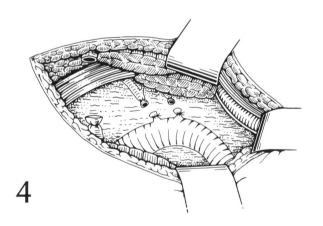

Exposure of the subclavian artery

4 The scalene muscle is mobilized for a distance of 2–3 cm and is then divided, a few fibres at a time. This protects any nerves traversing the muscle and the subclavian artery, which may lie directly under the muscle although it is usually caudad. The medial aspect of the brachial plexus is identified but not manipulated. It is usually found just beneath the already divided external jugular vein which serves as a landmark for the lateral extent of the dissection. The subclavian artery is palpated, dissected free from surrounding structures and controlled with a vessel loop. Division of one or two small ascending branches is necessary for sufficient mobilization of the artery.

Mobilization of the pleura

5 Once the subclavian artery is retracted downwards the suprapleural membrane (Sibson's fascia) is encountered. Division of this membrane is the key to the operation and is best done with the operator's finger. The suprapleural membrane is divided on the inner side of the triangle bounded by the brachial plexus, subclavian artery and internal jugular vein by pushing downwards against the vertebral column with the finger. When Sibson's fascia is penetrated, the operator's finger falls into the retropleural space and the pleura can be stripped from the vertebral column. Small malleable retractors are useful to keep the pleura and subclavian artery out of the way. At this point in the operation, lighting is best achieved with a headlamp on the operator.

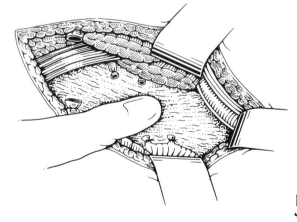

Identification of the sympathetic chain

6 The stellate ganglion is initially identified by palpation against the vertebral column at the base of the first rib. Once the ganglion is localized in this manner, a dissecting swab can be used to expose the chain and its identity can be confirmed visually. A nerve hook is passed around the chain just distal to the stellate ganglion and further dissection is performed. Several intercostal veins will cross the trunk and should be controlled with small haemoclips.

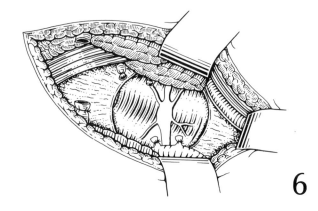

6

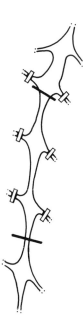

7

Sympathectomy

7 Removal of the stellate ganglion results in sympathetic denervation of the face and eye, resulting in permanent Horner's syndrome, and should be avoided. It is only necessary to remove the fibres from the T1 segment and leave the cervical fibres intact. The authors' preference therefore is to divide the stellate ganglion in its lower third where the rami communicantes from the first thoracic nerve enter. Once divided, the distal end of the chain is clamped and traction is applied to facilitate the remainder of the dissection. Rami should also be clipped. The chain is divided below the third ganglion and removed.

Closure

The lung should be inflated before closure, and if a pneumothorax is present a small catheter should be inserted into the opening in the pleural space and removed after the incision is completely closed with the lung inflated. The divided sternocleidomastoid muscle is repaired. The platysma muscle and skin are closed with absorbable sutures. No drains are necessary.

TRANSAXILLARY APPROACH (AFTER FIRST RIB RESECTION)

Position of patient

The patient is positioned on the operating table by the surgeon before scrubbing. A standard thoracotomy position is used with padding between the knees and under the dependent axilla. Wide adhesive tape placed across the uppermost hip and sandbags placed parallel to the trunk help secure the patient in the proper position. The ipsilateral arm, chest, back and shoulder are prepared and the arm is placed in a sterile stockinette. An elastic wrap is placed around the elbow to keep the stockinette in place during retraction of the arm.

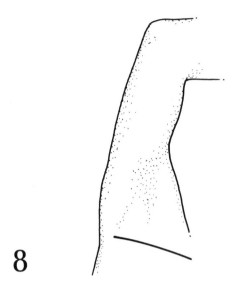

8

Incision

8 The incision is made just beneath the axillary hairline between the latissimus dorsi and pectoralis major muscles.

Resection of the first rib

9 The skin incision is carried down to the chest wall and then with finger dissection into the axilla. The intercostobrachial nerve may require division for proper exposure. There is often an arterial branch from the axillary artery that must be transected between haemoclips before the first rib can be visualized. The superior surface of the first rib is exposed and the anterior scalene muscle divided.

A periosteal elevator is used to strip away the medial scalene and intercostal fibres from the rib. The pleura is gently pushed away from the undersurface of the rib with the operator's finger. The rib is then removed and the ends smoothed with a rongeur.

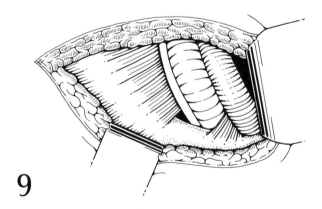

9

Exposure of the sympathetic chain

10 Once the rib is removed the dome of the pleura is exposed and this must be further dissected away from the lateral mediastinum. The sympathetic chain is identified once again by palpation between the T1 nerve root and the subclavian artery. A nerve hook is then passed around the chain and the operation proceeds as described above.

Closure

The wound is filled with saline and the lung inflated. If there is a pneumothorax present a 24-Fr chest tube is inserted through a small stab wound below the skin incision. This is connected to a standard pleural suction device and removed in the recovery room once the chest radiograph shows a fully expanded lung. If there is no pneumothorax, the wound is closed in two layers without drainage. Subcuticular sutures are used to close the skin.

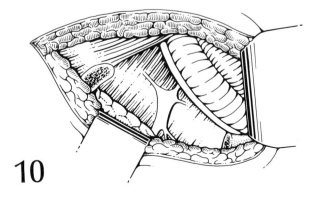

10

TRANSAXILLARY APPROACH (THIRD INTERSPACE)

This is a transpleural operation and is therefore contraindicated if there is evidence that the patient has many adhesions between the visceral and parietal pleura in the region of the apex of the lung. The patient is positioned as for a first rib resection but the arm need not be in the operative field.

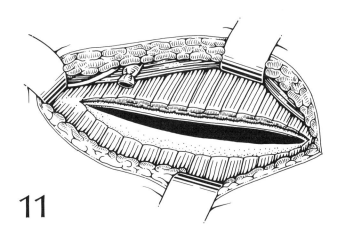

11

Incision

The incision is made in the axilla and follows the line of the third rib. It passes downwards and forwards across the thoracic wall of the axilla from the posterior to the anterior axillary fold and is usually about 15 cm long. In women the incision should stop at least 2.5 cm before the anterior axillary fold is reached, because a major reason for using this approach is the production of a less obvious scar.

Exposure of the third rib

11 The skin incision is carried down to the periosteum of the third rib. The pectoral muscles and breast are retracted well forward and the latissimus dorsi, teres major and subscapularis muscles backwards. The long thoracic nerve is identified and placed under the posterior retractor. The lateral thoracic artery is divided. The third rib is exposed by incising the overlying fibrofatty tissue of the axilla and removing the serratus anterior from its attachment to this bone. The periosteum on the rib is incised with cautery and then separated from the rib.

Exposure of the sympathetic chain

12 The pleura is opened through the periosteum in the upper part of the bed of the third rib, thus avoiding damage to the intercostal vessels and nerve; this upper zone is relatively avascular. A rib spreader is inserted and the thorax is opened to a width of about 10 cm. This usually provides sufficient exposure, but if not the rib above may be divided and a small segment resected. A large gauze pack is placed in the chest and the lung retracted downwards. This exposes the dome of the pleura and the upper part of the mediastinal pleura covering the bodies of the upper five thoracic vertebrae and the posterior portions of the corresponding ribs. The sympathetic chain can easily be seen beneath the pleura as it lies on the heads and necks of these ribs. The parietal pleura is opened and the chain is mobilized and resected as above.

Wound closure

The wound is closed with a chest tube connected to suction.

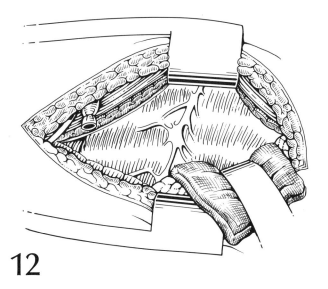

12

THORACOSCOPIC SYMPATHECTOMY

This is described in the chapter on pp. 491–493.

Postoperative care

Complications

The complications of upper extremity sympathectomy are in part related to the choice of incision. Haemorrhage, pneumothorax, lymph fistula, brachial plexus injury and incomplete operation are more common with the supraclavicular approach. Postoperative pain is more severe with the transthoracic transpleural operations.

Horner's syndrome

This condition follows division of the rami from the first thoracic nerve to the stellate ganglion and results in denervation of the ipsilateral face and eye. If the upper two-thirds of the stellate ganglion are left intact the syndrome is usually transient and mild, but it is not unavoidable. The syndrome consists of ptosis of the upper eyelid, enophthalmia and miosis, dryness of the nasal mucosa and loss of facial sweating. The problem must be discussed with the patient before the operation.

References

1. Telford ED. The technique of sympathectomy. *Br J Surg* 1935; 23: 448–50.

2. Roos DB. Transaxillary extrapleural thoracic sympathectomy. In: Bergan JJ, Yao JST, eds. *Operative Techniques in Vascular Surgery*. New York: Grune and Stratton, 1980: 115–16.

3. Atkins HJB. Sympathectomy by the axillary approach. *Lancet* 1954; i: 538–9.

4. Palumbo LT. Anterior transthoracic approach for upper extremity thoracic sympathectomy. *Arch Surg* 1956; 72: 659.

5. Smithwick RH. Modified dorsal sympathectomy for vascular spasm (Raynaud's disease) of the upper extremity. *Ann Surg* 1936; 104: 339–50.

6. Byrne J, Walsh TN, Hederman WP. Endoscopic transthoracic electrocautery of the sympathetic chain for palmar and axillary hyperhidrosis. *Br J Surg* 1990; 77: 1046–9.

7. Wilkinson H. Radiofrequency percutaneous upper thoracic sympathectomy: technique and review of indications. *N Engl J Med* 1984; 311: 34–6.

8. Moss AJ, Schwartz PJ, Crampton RS, Tzivoni D, Locati EH, MacCluer J. The long QT syndrome: prospective longitudinal study of 328 families. *Circulation* 1991; 84: 1136–44.

Illustrations by Mark Iley

Endoscopic upper thoracic sympathectomy

W. P. Hederman MCh, FRCSI, FRCS(Glas), FRCS(Ed)
Consultant Surgeon, Mater Misericordiae Hospital, Dublin, Eire

History

It has long been recognized that sympathectomy is the best treatment for excessive localized sweating from the palms of the hands or the axillae. Operative sympathectomy has been carried out through several different approaches, all reasonably difficult, with a considerable incidence of postoperative morbidity and discomfort and with scars which are not fully acceptable to some patients.

In 1978, Kux[1] described a minimally invasive procedure in which the upper six dorsal ganglia were excised through a thoracoscope.

Principles and justification

This operation should be considered for those patients whose excessive sweating is localized to the palms of the hands and/or the axillae. It should be severe enough to have caused interference with the patient's occupation or lifestyle, or have caused severe social embarrassment or damage to the patient's clothing, and should have proved resistant to other measures. Patients should be investigated for other causes of hyperhidrosis, and those with generalized excessive sweating should normally be excluded. Adolescent patients should be observed for some time as they sometimes improve spontaneously. The possibility of some compensatory postoperative hyperhidrosis from the waist, the back or the head should be explained to the patient.

Preoperative

Normally a chest radiograph should be performed to discover any lesions that might cause adhesions, and thyroid function tests and careful psychological assessment are carried out.

Anaesthesia

General anaesthesia with a double-lumen endotracheal tube is administered.

Operation

The patient is placed supine with each arm abducted to a right angle. A suitably wide intercostal space is identified with the tip of the finger in the anterior part of the axilla just behind the pectoralis major muscle. This will usually be either the third or fourth space. The ipsilateral portion of the double-lumen endotracheal tube is disconnected from the anaesthetic machine. A Verres' needle is inserted into the identified intercostal space and carbon dioxide is insufflated from a Semm pneumoperitoneum apparatus. The pressure recorded on the apparatus should be less than 10 mmHg, and should fluctuate slightly with respiration to confirm that the needle tip is free in the pleural cavity. After 0.5 litres of gas have been insufflated, the needle is replaced by a 7.0 mm trocar and cannula with side stopcock through a small stab incision at the same site.

1 A Hopkins forward-oblique 6.5 mm telescope is introduced through the cannula. Preliminary inspection is carried out to confirm the correct placement of the instrument and a check is made for adhesions, especially at the apex.

More gas is insufflated and the lung apex is pushed downwards with the telescope. The amount of gas needed will vary according to the size of the patient and the ease with which the lung can be retracted. The patient is monitored for development of bradycardia and for any significant alteration in blood gas values. Usually 2 litres is sufficient, but more may be required.

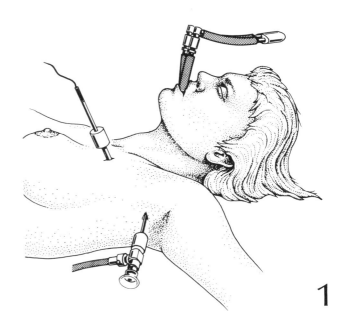

1

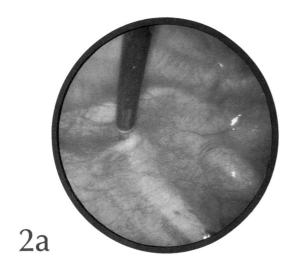

2a

2a, b The sympathetic chain can be seen running downwards over the necks of the upper ribs, providing that the pleura is thin enough and there is not too much subpleural fat. The stellate ganglion cannot be seen as it is covered by a characteristic yellow pad of fat which should be identified in the dome of the pleural cavity.

A unipolar coagulating electrode is next inserted through a 6.5-mm insulated cannula passed through a small stab incision in the third intercostal space in the midclavicular line. If the sympathetic chain was not easily seen on the preliminary inspection, it can be identified by stroking the tip of the electrode along the necks of the second or third ribs. The chain will be seen and felt slipping out from under the probe in the same way that it is felt with the index finger during an operative sympathectomy.

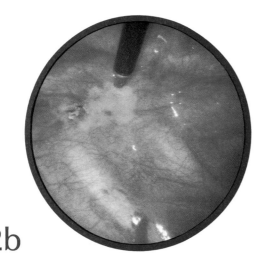

2b

3 When the chain is properly identified, the pleura over it is incised with diathermy, and the second and third upper dorsal ganglia and the intervening chain are fulgurated precisely until destroyed. Tributaries of the azygos vein on the right side can be mobilized carefully and diathermy applied to the chain beneath them.

Thin, flimsy adhesions can be cut with diathermy scissors without difficulty if access to the sympathetic chain is required. However, extensive division of dense adhesions, while possible, is unrewarding because it leaves a bloodstained field in which it is difficult to identify the sympathetic chain.

Minor bleeding from small vessels can be controlled simply by pressure from the probe or by further precise diathermy. We have a clip applicator available should more major bleeding occur, but we have not yet had to use it.

The lung is reinflated by the anaesthetist while the surgeon allows the gas to escape from the pleural cavity through the two cannulae, checking progress through the telescope. When the lung is fully expanded, the cannulae are removed and the small stab incisions closed, each with one stitch. Drainage is not required.

The procedure is repeated straight away on the opposite side in a similar manner. We have observed no disturbances of blood gases or other untoward effects as a result of doing both sides at the same time.

Originally, we used to perform a more extensive sympathectomy, down to the fourth or fifth ganglia for palmar sweating. We have now shown that it is sufficient to deal with only the second and third ganglia; this also reduces the incidence of postoperative compensatory hyperhidrosis.

In cases of isolated axillary hyperhidrosis without palmar sweating, only the fourth and fifth ganglia are coagulated.

At the end of the operation the skin over the treated areas should be warm and dry.

Postoperative care

A routine postoperative chest radiograph is carried out in the recovery room. It usually shows a small apical pneumothorax which can be ignored. Complications are rare. One patient in our series had a pneumothorax sufficiently large to require a chest drain. Minor degrees of surgical emphysema in the root of the neck may occur rarely but are not of significance in the absence of any systemic signs.

Postoperative pain is minimal and opiate analgesia is not usually required.

Most patients are discharged from hospital on the day after operation.

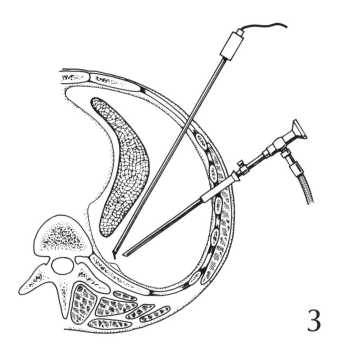

3

Outcome

The immediate results are uniformly good, with abolition of sweating in the treated areas. On long-term follow up, about 6% of patients report some recurrence of sweating. This has been treated with further successful endoscopic electrocoagulation without difficulty.

Some compensatory hyperhidrosis occurred in up to two-thirds of patients when more extensive sympathectomy was used. It faded with time in most. The incidence is much less when only the second and third ganglia are coagulated.

Three transient cases of Horner's syndrome were noted early in the series.

A total of 250 patients have undergone operation since 1980 and the author is happy that this method of treating a distressing symptom is safe, relatively painless, requires only a short hospital stay and can be learned by anybody with a good knowledge of the anatomy of the area and who is familiar with endoscopic techniques.

It is, of course, possible to carry out the procedure using a double-lumen operating laparoscope and thus avoid the necessity for a second incision. However, with the instruments currently available this means using an 11-mm cannula. We have found that a cannula of this size is frequently a very tight fit in the intercostal spaces of younger women, and frequently leads to postoperative discomfort from pressure on the intercostal nerves.

Reference

1. Kux M. Thoracic endoscopic sympathectomy in palmar and axillary hyperhidrosis. *Arch Surg* 1978; 113: 264–6.

Vascular access

Carl H. Andrus MD
Clinical Associate Professor of Surgery, University of Rochester Medical Center, Rochester, New York, USA

History

Vascular access may be defined as any technique that allows removal from and delivery of fluids into the circulatory system at a rate of 200 ml/min or more for lengthy intervals.

The demonstration by Wilhelm Kolff[1] that chronic intermittent haemodialysis could prolong life gave impetus to the development of useful techniques and materials for vascular access. At first, segments of artery and vein were sacrificed for each treatment. Then Quinton et al.[2], using biocompatible polytetrafluoro-ethylene (PTFE, Teflon) cannulae and Silastic tubing, found that one operation could establish useful vascular access for months and sometimes for years. The arterial and venous tubes were connected while the shunt was not in use, so that the constant flow of blood prevented clotting in the device. Thus, it could be used repeatedly for haemodialysis.

In 1966 Brescia et al.[3] reported their experience with the radiocephalic arteriovenous fistula constructed subcutaneously at the wrist. This procedure ensured that the cephalic vein would be kept distended even though blood was continuously and rapidly withdrawn from the vein. The blood was then passed through the dialyser and returned to the proximal segment of the same arterialized vein or to another vein. The advantages of the 'Brescia–Cimino fistula' over the 'Scribner shunt' were the absence of perpetual defects in the skin through which infection could more easily enter and the absence of implanted prosthetic materials. The disadvantage was its common need for time to mature before use, and therefore its unsuitability for emergency use.

Because the Scribner shunt could be used immediately, it became the device of choice for emergency vascular access. Venous catheters designed for percutaneous insertion, however, have made the Scribner shunt obsolete. These catheters are usually inserted through a subclavian vein into the superior vena cava or right atrium. They do not interfere at all with the patient's activity and are available in two types. Stiff catheters are designed for short-term use (weeks) and for percutaneous placement via the subclavian or femoral vein using the Seldinger technique. They may be used while an internal fistula matures or for dialysis support of acute renal failure. Soft, flexible catheters are designed for permanent use (months) and for placement via the subclavian or internal jugular vein using split sheath technology. Percutaneous catheterization of the femoral vein is less satisfactory because it is more difficult to maintain sterility in the groin, because of the more severe consequences of iliofemoral venous thrombosis, and because of the limitations the device imposes on walking and sitting.

Principles and justification

There are many choices of device or technique for achieving permanent, internal vascular access. The simplest one that offers reasonable success should be used. For example, the radiocephalic arteriovenous fistula should always be chosen before a brachio-cephalic fistula, a basilic vein transposition fistula or a prosthetic interposition graft fistula. The last three techniques should be considered successive back-up procedures to be used in case construction of a simpler fistula is not possible. Only after these possibilities have been exhausted should a prosthetic, interposition graft be considered.

To select the best location for construction of an arteriovenous fistula for vascular access, the surgeon must be sure that the vein to be used is adequate to promote success of the fistula and that the arterial supply remaining is adequate to ensure satisfactory perfusion of the limb. Often patients who need vascular access have had a chronic illness and have required repeated phlebotomy and intravenous infusions, which

may have caused thrombosis of many superficial veins. The venous lumen must be patent at the anastomosis and proximally. This can be determined by application of a tourniquet high on the arm and inspection and palpation of the vein. If necessary, phlebography can be used to determine the anatomy and examine suspected areas of stenosis. To ensure adequate arterial supply to the limb after construction of a fistula the surgeon must make sure the following conditions are fulfilled:

1. An alternative arterial supply is available, i.e. in the upper extremity the Allen test should be negative.
2. The artery is not interrupted, i.e. a side-to-side anastomosis is constructed.
3. The anastomosis should be made as peripheral as possible or, if a more central location between larger vessels such as the brachial artery and cephalic vein is required, the anastomosis should be made small enough to avoid a steal syndrome.

Operations

PERCUTANEOUS CATHETERIZATION OF THE SUBCLAVIAN VEIN

Position of patient

1 The patient is positioned supine in bed in the Trendelenburg position with a folded towel along the thoracic spine in order to allow the shoulders to fall back.

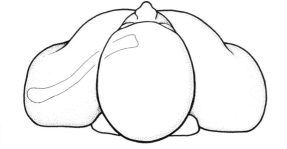

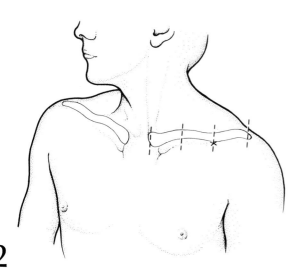

Preparation

2 The shoulder and adjacent parts of the neck, chest and arm are prepared antiseptically and draped to expose the clavicular region. An area of skin just below the junction of the middle and distal thirds of the clavicle is anaesthetized.

Catheter insertion

3 A long hypodermic 18-G needle with syringe attached is passed through the skin, then placed horizontally and inserted towards the suprasternal notch while suction is applied. This should result in the tip of the needle entering the subclavian vein, at which point venous blood will flow easily into the syringe.

Without moving the needle further, the syringe is removed and a wire is inserted into the needle, flexible end first. The wire is advanced until it is well into the superior vena cava. It should advance easily and should never be forced. It is often helpful and occasionally necessary to check the position of the wire fluoroscopically.

The needle is then withdrawn over the wire which is held stationary. The catheter is passed over the wire into the superior vena cava and finally the wire is removed, leaving the catheter in the desired position. If a soft catheter with split-sheath introducer is to be used, the skin is incised at the guidewire, the catheter is laid out in position on prepared skin with its tip just below the angle of Louis and the exit site positioned just beyond the Dacron felt cuff. The skin is anaesthetized and the exit site made as a stab wound. The catheter is drawn through a subcutaneous tunnel from the exit site to the infraclavicular incision and positioned with the cuff 1 cm above the exit site. The dilator and introducer

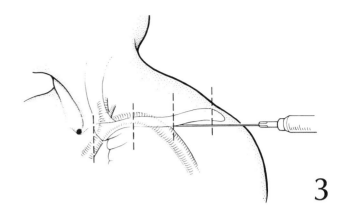

3

are passed together over the wire before the wire is removed. The dilator is then withdrawn, the catheter is passed centrally, and the introducer split and removed, leaving the catheter in the desired position. The incision is closed.

The catheter should be filled with heparin, 1000 units/ml, but not overfilled to avoid a systemic effect and the attendant increased risk of bleeding. A chest radiograph should be obtained as soon as catheterization is completed to detect any air or fluid in the pleural space and to document the position of the catheter.

The catheter should be securely sutured to the skin and a sterile dressing applied to the exit site.

RADIOCEPHALIC FISTULA

Incision

4 A transverse incision is made, and proximal and distal skin flaps are developed to allow exposure of adequate lengths of vessels.

Exposure

5 To expose the artery the deep fascia is incised longitudinally along the palpable radial pulse. Branches are tied with silk or cauterized and divided so that the artery can be lifted from its bed.

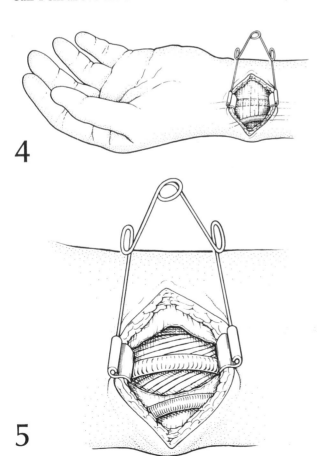

4

5

Isolation of vessels

6 The vein is tied distally, controlled proximally with a vascular clamp, and divided just proximal to the ligature. The isolated segment is dilated gently with a clamp and irrigated with heparinized saline.

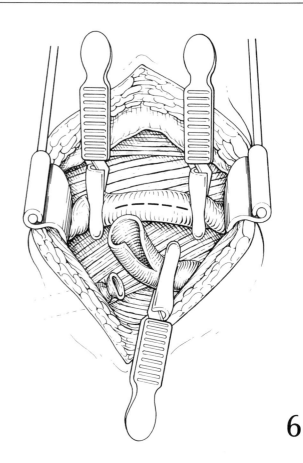

6

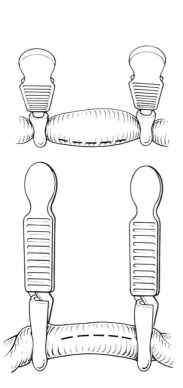

7

Arteriotomy

7 The artery is controlled with vascular clamps applied perpendicularly and is rotated medially to present the lateral aspect of the vessel for anastomosis. A longitudinal arteriotomy 2–3 times the width of the lumen is made and flushed free of blood or clot with heparinized saline.

Anastomosis

8 The cephalic vein end is spatulated to fit the arteriotomy. The anastomosis is constructed with two running 6/0 or 7/0 monofilament polypropylene (Prolene) sutures inserted at the proximal and distal vertices, with the help of lateral and medial stay sutures.

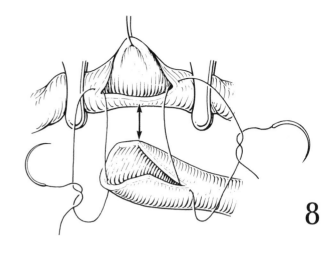

8

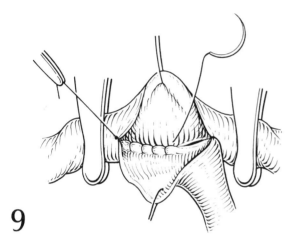

9

9 The posterior anastomosis is constructed through the open anastomosis with the knots tied outside. The vein should describe a gentle curve as it passes from the anastomosis to its native bed and should not be kinked or twisted.

Evaluation

10 When the vascular clamps are removed the vein is checked for filling and for a palpable thrill. Haemostasis is ascertained.

Wound closure

The wound is closed with a single row of continuous vertical mattress sutures of 4/0 monofilament nylon. A loose dressing that is not circumferential is applied to the incision. The patient is advised to make ordinary use of the extremity, to avoid placing it in a dependent position, and not to modify the dressing (except to remove it if wetted).

In men with large veins this sort of fistula can be used for dialysis in 1–2 weeks. In women and children, who tend to have small vessels, a period of maturation of several weeks or months may be desirable before easy use without risk of loss of the fistula.

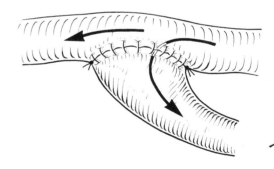

10

BRACHIOCEPHALIC FISTULA

Incision

11 A curved incision is made in the antecubital fossa for exposure of the cephalic or medial cubital vein and the brachial artery.

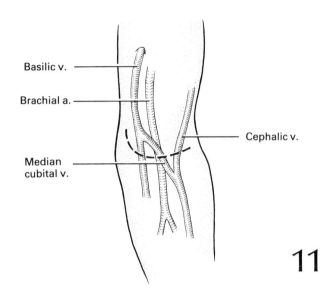

11

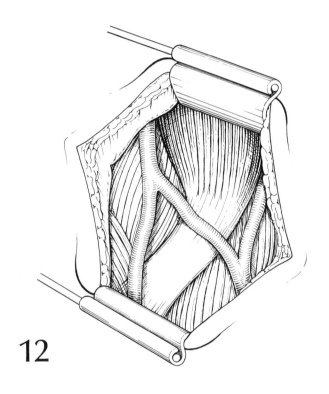

12

Exposure

12 Either vein can be used for the anastomosis, but it is important that only the cephalic vein be arterialized and not the basilic vein, which is too deep in its native position to be useful.

Mobilization

13 The lacertus fibrosis is incised parallel to the course of the brachial artery as it can be felt entering the antecubital fossa. Small branches are divided after ligation in continuity with silk to free 2–2.25 cm of artery. The vein is controlled by ligation at one end and placement of a vascular clamp at the other.

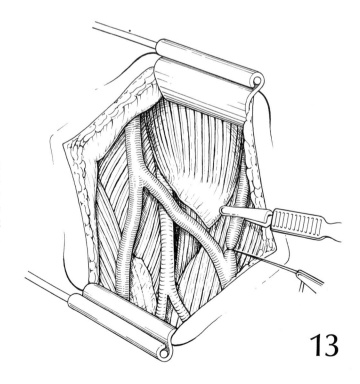

13

14 The brachial artery is controlled proximally and distally with atraumatic clamps as in the construction of a radiocephalic fistula. An arteriotomy is made on its anterolateral surface. To minimize the risk of a steal syndrome and ischaemia of the hand, the length of the arteriotomy should not exceed the diameter of the artery. Both vessels are irrigated with heparinized saline.

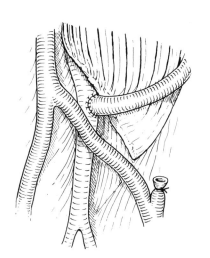

14

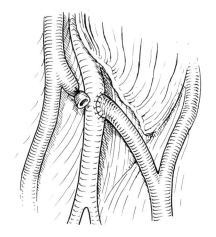

15

15 If the median antecubital vein is used it should be flushed with heparinized saline without a clamp in order to detect valves which might interfere with blood flow. It is occasionally possible to poke out the valves in the forearm portion of the cephalic vein by means of a probe inserted through the medial cubital vein. This will allow arterialization of a longer segment of the cephalic vein. The vein may be dilated gently and spatulated if necessary. A side-to-end anastomosis is performed with a running suture of 6/0 monofilament polypropylene.

The venous clamp is removed. The distal arterial clamp is then released to evacuate any clot into the vein in order to minimize the risk of distal embolization. Lastly, the proximal arterial clamp is removed. The wound is closed with absorbable sutures in the subcutaneous layer and a running monofilament suture in the skin, or by means of a single row of skin sutures. Again, a loose, non-circumferential dressing is applied to the wound, with advice to the patient as before.

BASILIC VEIN TRANSPOSITION FISTULA

16 The basilic vein is exposed through a curvilinear incision passing from the antecubital fossa medially 2 cm anterior to the medial epicondyle of the humerus.

Exposure

17 Care should be taken to avoid injury to the medial cutaneous nerve of the forearm which runs alongside the vein, and the medial nerve which is deep in the antecubital fossa.

Mobilization

18 The vein is followed proximally by extension of the incision high into the axilla. Branches are ligated with silk ties and microhaemoclips and then divided. The basilic vein is freed to its junction with the axillary vein. Occasionally, large branches connect the basilic and brachial veins, and these must be divided and oversewn.

The brachial artery is exposed in the groove medial to the distal belly of the biceps. Small branches are divided after ligation in continuity, and 3 cm of vessel are freed and encircled with vessel loops. A subcuticular tunnel is made from the antecubital portion of the incision, passing along the anteromedial aspect of the biceps muscle and emerging in the axillary portion of the incision. The tunnel should be made wide at the proximal and distal ends.

The distal end of the basilic vein is ligated and divided. A vascular clamp controls the most proximal end of the vein in the axilla. The vein is gently dilated and irrigated with heparinized saline.

Anastomosis

19 The distal end is then drawn through the tunnel, carefully avoiding kinks and twists. It is helpful to close the upper part of the incision temporarily with towel clips to be sure that the course of the tunnel is correct.

The artery is controlled with vascular clamps and an arteriotomy, the length of which should not exceed the diameter of the artery, is made on its anteromedial surface. A side-to-end anastomosis is performed with a running suture of 6/0 monofilament polypropylene with the help of appropriate stay sutures. After completion of the anastomosis the vascular clamps are removed in the order described above.

Wound closure

When haemostasis is ascertained, the wound is closed with a running absorbable suture for the fascia, and non-absorbable sutures or staples for the skin. The dressing should not be circumferential in order to avoid compression of the fistula. The fistula should not be used for at least 2 weeks. Earlier use, before there is obliteration of the tunnel space by healing, will risk a perivenous haematoma.

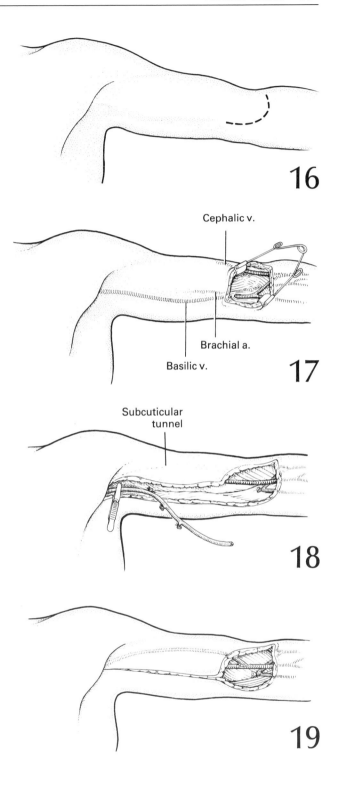

PROSTHETIC INTERPOSITION GRAFT FISTULA

Loop fistula

20 If *in situ* autologous vein is not suitable for fistula construction, a segment of prosthetic graft material (polytetrafluoroethylene (PTFE) is preferred) can be placed in a subcuticular tunnel and anastomosed to artery and vein. Any configuration that will permit placement of a graft of sufficient length to allow for multiple puncture sites can be used. A loop fistula can be constructed by making a curved subcuticular tunnel from the brachial artery down the radial aspect of the forearm, across and up the ulnar aspect of the forearm, to the venous anastomosis at the median cubital or brachial vein.

Attention to certain details of these procedures is important for a successful result. A counter-incision across the course of the tunnel at its distal extremity must be used to allow passage of the graft through the tunnel without a twist. If the graft crosses the elbow joint, it should do so on the medial or lateral aspects of the joint, so that flexion does not cause kinking. This type of fistula should not be used for at least 2 weeks for the reasons given above.

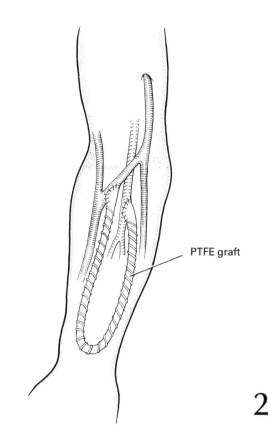

PTFE graft

20

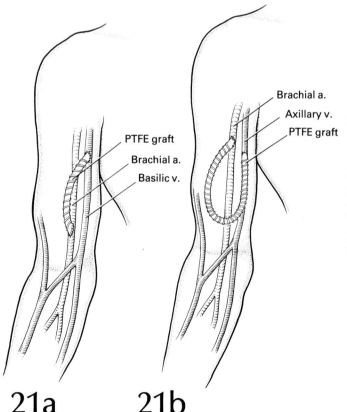

PTFE graft
Brachial a.
Basilic v.

Brachial a.
Axillary v.
PTFE graft

21a   **21b**

Alternative graft configurations

21a, b Prosthetic interposition fistulae can be constructed between the brachial artery proximal to the elbow crease and the proximal basilic or axillary vein in the axilla. The subcuticular tunnel is made along the anteromedial aspect of the biceps. A loop fistula can be constructed in a large arm with anastomosis at the proximal brachial artery and axillary vein.

Postoperative care

Complications of percutaneous catheters

Most percutaneous catheters for vascular access are introduced into the subclavian vein. Because of the proximity of the parietal pleura to the subclavian vein, pneumothorax, haemothorax, or haemopneumothorax can occur. It is therefore essential to obtain chest radiographs after catheterization and before the catheter is used. If there is evidence of such a complication the catheter should be withdrawn and, if necessary, a chest tube should be inserted for control of the pleural space. Because bilateral complications of this kind are extremely hazardous, the contralateral subclavian vein should not be catheterized immediately. If immediate access is necessary after having induced a pneumothorax or haemothorax, then the femoral vein may be catheterized.

If infection of a percutaneous catheter is suspected, it should be used to obtain samples for blood culture, then removed. If signs of infection persist after its removal the patient should be treated with specific antibiotics for endothelial infection. During antibiotic therapy a new venous catheter may be placed at another site, and the sites of catheterization should be changed frequently. As an alternative approach, peritoneal dialysis may be used.

Complications of arteriovenous fistulae

Early complications

Most early complications of arteriovenous fistulae can be avoided by attention to the detail of the surgical procedure. Haemostasis must be satisfactory in order to avoid a perivenous haematoma, which will compress the vein and therefore obstruct blood flow and result in failure of the fistula by clotting. The arteriovenous anastomosis must be made without a twist or kink in the vein, because these interfere with blood flow and result in failure. After the anastomosis has been completed and the wound closed, it is necessary to be sure that blood flow is adequate in order to minimize the chance of an unexpected venous obstruction. The best physical signs of good blood flow are a palpable thrill throughout the vein and an audible bruit. In contrast, a venous pulse is not a reliable sign of good blood flow, e.g. an exaggerated venous pulse may briefly be present distal to or upstream of a complete venous obstruction.

Failure of fistula

This may occur after a fistula has been used successfully for months or years. It often happens as the result of reduction of the blood volume, such as may occur with inadequately replaced surgical blood loss or with excessive haemoconcentration during dialysis. The first sign of this is a lessened turgidity of the arterialized vein; the thrill and bruit then disappear. The fistula can sometimes be salvaged non-operatively in these circumstances if the problem is detected promptly before extensive clotting has developed. If palpation of the vein does not reveal a large thrombus, restoration of the blood volume should be commenced and the offending thrombus, which is usually confined initially to the venous side of the anastomosis, can be dislodged by vigorous massage through to the skin. Lubrication of the skin is of assistance. This manoeuvre has never been followed by symptoms or signs of pulmonary embolus in the author's experience. The technique should not be used when the thrombus is palpable, i.e. large, and it should not be used if the patient is known to have a cardiac septal defect.

Thrombosis of an interposition graft fistula is often reversible. Late occlusion is usually secondary to neointimal hyperplasia, which occurs first at the venous anastomosis but can also occur at the arterial anastomosis. Exposure of both anastomoses, with control of the native vessels, and longitudinal incision across both anastomoses allows open thrombectomy with a balloon catheter. Closure of the anastomotic incisions with an elliptical patch of PTFE preserves the lumen.

Heart failure and distal ischaemia

Heart failure and distal ischaemia may very occasionally be attributable to arteriovenous fistulae constructed for vascular access. These complications always occur in patients who have a particular susceptibility to them. They can usually be successfully treated, but preferably may be prevented by attention to simple technical details during construction of the fistula.

Severe myocardial or valvular disease predisposes the patient to development of high-output heart failure after construction of an arteriovenous fistula, and diabetes mellitus predisposes to development of distal ischaemia. The incidence of both complications can be minimized by using the most distal site for construction of the fistula. This results in a smaller fistulous blood flow, less burden on the heart, and less steal from the distal arterial circulation. If larger proximal vessels must be used, then the anastomosis should be kept small. Furthermore, no more than the vein to be used for dialysis should be arterialized. For example, in the case of a brachiocephalic fistula, it is possible inadvertently to arterialize both the basilic vein and the cephalic vein, if the cephalic vein distal to the median cubital vein is connected to the brachial artery. This can result in an unnecessarily large blood flow through the fistula and congestive heart failure or distal steal ischaemia.

22 If the anastomosis is determined to have been made too large and to be the cause of congestive failure or distal ischaemia, the vein can be 'banded' to limit its blood flow. To do this the venous segment adjacent to the anastomosis is exposed surgically and encircled with a piece of Dacron about 5 mm in width. A mandrel of a diameter equal to the desired narrower lumen is laid beside the vein and within the Dacron strip.

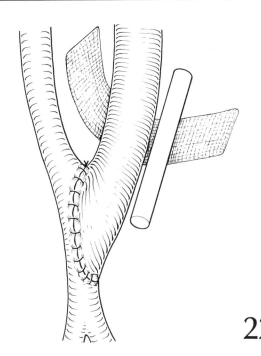

22

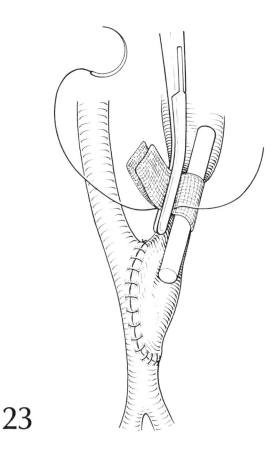

23

23 The patient is heparinized. The Dacron strip is then tightened about the vein and mandrel so as to completely occlude the venous lumen. The Dacron is then clamped with a haemostat and sewn into a closed cuff beneath the haemostat.

24 The haemostat and excess Dacron are removed. The mandrel is then removed to allow the vein to open to the size of the mandrel. The heparin is reversed with protamine sulphate and the wound is closed.

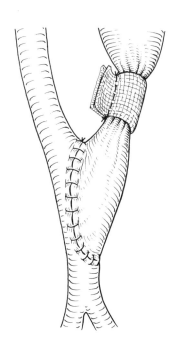

24

Stenosis at the venous outflow

25 Excessive 'recirculation' and inefficient haemo-dialysis can occur when a venous stenosis develops in the vein beyond that part used for access. This may happen with simple arteriovenous fistulae or with fistulae constructed with prosthetic material. With the latter technique the stenosis usually develops at the venous anastomosis.

The stenosis slows blood flow to such an extent that blood, already having passed through the dialysis machine, is recycled through the dialyser several times before it leaves the arterialized vein through the stenosis.

The percentage recirculation can be calculated by means of the formula:

$$\text{Percentage recirculation} = \frac{BUN_P - BUN_A}{BUN_P - BUN_V} \times 100$$

where   BUN = blood urea nitrogen concentration, A = arterial line, V = venous line, P = peripheral venous. Arteriovenous fistula for haemodialysis should not have more than 10% recirculation. Correction of the problem may be achieved surgically by application of a vein or prosthetic patch to widen the stenosis, by reimplantation of the vein or prosthesis, or by use of a 'jump' graft. Vein is the preferred material.

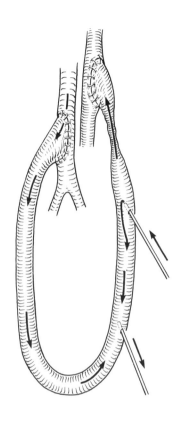

25

Venous hypertension of the hand

This may develop after construction of a radiocephalic fistula. The hand becomes oedematous, uncomfortable and susceptible to infections after minor injuries. The incidence of this problem can be minimized by the use of a side-to-end arteriovenous anastomosis. If sufficiently large collateral veins with incompetent valves develop, however, then symptomatic venous hypertension can occur even with a side-to-end anastomosis. The proper treatment is ligation of the collateral veins.

Conclusion

This consideration of vascular access has not been exhaustive. Many devices have been proposed for the purpose. The author believes that autogenous vein remains by far the best tissue for construction of long-term vascular access.

References

1. Kolff WJ. First clinical experience with the artificial kidney. *Ann Intern Med* 1965; 62: 608–19.

2. Quinton W, Dillar D, Scribner BH. Cannulation of blood vessels for prolonged hemodialysis. *Trans Am Soc Art Intern Organs* 1960; 6: 104–13.

3. Brescia MJ, Cimino JE, Appel K, Hurwich BJ. Chronic hemodialysis using venipuncture and a surgically created arteriovenous fistula. *N Engl J Med* 1966; 275: 1089–92.

Phlebography

The late M. Lea Thomas MA, PhD, FRCP, FRCS, FRCR
Vascular Radiologist, St Thomas' Hospital, London, UK

Despite radiation hazards and the advent of newer non-invasive techniques for demonstration of the venous system, contrast phlebography will retain, for the foreseeable future, an important role in the management of venous problems because of the high image resolution obtainable by the film/screen combination. Contrast phlebography involves injection of an iodinated medium into one of the tributaries of the venous system. As contrast medium is hyperbaric compared with blood, postural manoeuvres are often used to fill parts of the venous system, and catheterization of the venous tributaries or arteriography with follow-through of the contrast medium into the venous phase may be required in certain situations.

By far the most important use of phlebography is in the investigation of diseases of the lower limb. While there are a number of variations of the techniques, those described in this chapter give the required information in the majority of patients[1-5].

Principles and justification

Indications

Lower limb ascending phlebography

The situations in which lower limb phlebography may be of value are as follows:

1. Investigation of deep vein thrombosis: confirmation of diagnosis and information regarding the site, extent and age of the thrombus.
2. Establishing the source of pulmonary embolism and the demonstration of any residual thrombus.
3. Assessment of the deep venous system in cases of incompetent communicating veins before surgery or injection therapy.
4. Demonstration of recurrent varicose veins by direct injection (varicography).
5. Assessment of the state of the deep venous system in patients with post-thrombotic syndrome, including any incompetent communicating veins.
6. Patients with lower limb oedema of unknown cause.
7. Investigation of venous malformations.

Varicography

The indications for varicography are recurrent varicose veins, primary varicose veins at unusual sites, and incompetent communicating veins associated with varicose veins.

Saphenography

Saphenography is indicated to demonstrate the long saphenous vein and assess its suitability for bypass surgery (usually arterial), but is also useful before a saphenofemoral crossover procedure (Palma's operation) for the post-thrombotic limb.

Pelvic phlebography and inferior venacavography

This technique is indicated in patients in whom the iliac veins and inferior vena cava have not been adequately demonstrated by standard ascending phlebography with calf compression.

Descending iliofemoral phlebography

The indications for descending iliofemoral phlebography are to grade deep vein reflux and to assess valvular function, and to show long saphenous vein incompetence.

Upper limb phlebography

This procedure is performed if axillary or subclavian vein thrombosis is suspected.

Superior venacavography

This procedure is indicated for venous thrombosis, the evaluation of mediastinal disease, and congenital anomalies.

Intraosseous phlebography

The main indication is to show the iliac veins and the inferior vena cava when the femoral veins are occluded, although the procedure can be used at many sites when venous access is difficult or impossible by other means.

Digital subtraction phlebography

As a venepuncture is required there is little advantage in digital subtraction techniques except that much less contrast medium is required, reducing the expense. Resolution is not as good as with the film/screen combination and errors in interpretation are frequent[5].

Preoperative

No specific preparation is required. Fasting is no longer necessary as nausea and vomiting are not a feature of injection with low osmolar contrast media. As with all contrast examinations fluids should, if anything, be increased to counteract the dehydrating effect of the contrast medium. Anxious patients may require mild sedation.

Anaesthesia

For most phlebographic examinations no anaesthesia is required. Local anaesthesia is required when deeper vessels such as the femoral vein are punctured. General anaesthesia is rarely required but it may be necessary in children and very anxious adults. Only light anaesthesia is necessary.

Essential equipment

Standard radiographic apparatus is required. A tilting fluoroscopy table with a spot film capability, automatic exposure and television monitoring is sufficient. A rapid serial film changer may be required when demonstrating the large proximal veins (such as the venae cavae) filling collateral veins.

Contrast media

To avoid complications such as pain on injection and postphlebographic thrombosis it is recommended that low osmolar contrast media should be used for phlebography. If, because of financial constraints, conventional hyperosmolar media are used, these should be diluted to bring their osmolarity closer to that of blood. Iopamidol 300 or 370, iohexol 300 or 350, sodium meglumine ioxaglate 180 or 320 or iopromide are suggested media. Ioxaglate, although cheaper, has more generalized side effects. Higher iodine concentrations are needed for the larger proximal veins. The amount of contrast medium needed for a particular examination varies, but as an approximate guide about 50 ml is usually sufficient for ascending phlebography of one leg; however, four times this amount may be required for examination of both legs, for the lower inferior vena cava, or when repeat studies are necessary. The poor quality of phlebograms in the past resulted from an inability to inject sufficient contrast medium because of its toxicity. This constraint does not apply with low osmolar media. It is not necessary to flush the veins with physiological saline to prevent venous thrombosis after phlebography when using low osmolar media.

Techniques

ASCENDING PHLEBOGRAPHY

1 The patient is examined with the foot tilted down 30–40°. Hand grips on the table enable the patient to steady himself and not contract the muscles during the examination, as this tends to obliterate the calf muscle veins. A tourniquet is applied above the ankle to distend the foot veins. A 21-gauge (or smaller) butterfly needle is inserted into a distal vein on the dorsum of the foot. A test injection of contrast medium with fluoroscopy is carried out to confirm that the needle is in the vein. If extravasation is seen, another vein is punctured, leaving the first needle in position to avoid haematoma formation and prevent passage of contrast medium into the tissues when the new vein is injected.

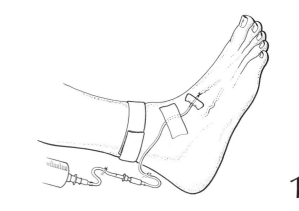

2 When the needle is correctly positioned in the foot vein, a second tourniquet is applied above the knee to delay the flow of contrast medium from the calf veins; this promotes better filling of the deep veins of the calf. Rubber tourniquets about 2.5 cm wide with Velcro fastenings are best as they can be easily adjusted to ensure deep venous filling and not obstruct the arteries. A thin rubber tubing held by forceps should not be used as this can obstruct the arterial flow with serious consequences.

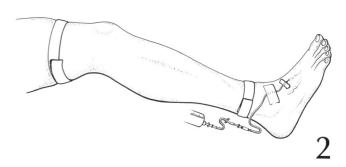

The leg is internally rotated to separate the images of the tibia and fibula. A slow injection by hand is started and the passage of the contrast medium is followed on the fluoroscope from the foot to the lower inferior vena cava.

Films are exposed in the posteroanterior position when there is optimal filling of the deep veins. Three exposures made on a 35 × 35 cm radiograph subdivided into three is a useful format. Brief manual calf compression just before an exposure is helpful to fill the proximal veins.

Difficulties with venepuncture

Difficulties usually occur in the oedematous limb. The medial digital vein of the great toe is not usually affected by oedema of the foot and can often be punctured with a 23-gauge needle. Oedema can be massaged away from a vein on the dorsum of the foot or at the ankle. Hot packs over the feet help to dilate the veins. Although the more distally the vein is injected the better the demonstration of the deep venous system, any vein in the leg (even a varicose vein) can be injected. With a tourniquet applied proximal to the vein and a steeper foot-down table tilt, many of the leg veins below the tourniquet are demonstrated as well as those above.

The examination may have to be postponed for 24 h while the limb is elevated to disperse the oedema.

Rarely nowadays (because alternative methods such as duplex scanning are available), the long saphenous vein can be surgically exposed at its known termination in front of the medial malleolus.

Variations according to clinical need

Deep vein thrombosis

Lateral views of the calf should be taken by rotating the foot externally to display the muscle veins unobscured by bone images. The upper limit of any thrombus or occluded vein must be displayed, if necessary with supplementary injections to the femur or by examining the lower inferior vena cava from the opposite limb.

More than one film must be taken of each segment of the venous tree to confirm any filling defects which are persistent and of constant shape and thus not artifacts.

The tourniquet must not be so tight that the superficial veins are completely obstructed, otherwise superficial vein thrombosis can be missed.

Pulmonary thromboembolism

Both legs should be examined as 50% of clinically normal limbs will also contain thrombus. The feet should be examined as the medial and lateral plantar veins are occasionally the site of venous thrombosis[1].

An attempt should be made to show as much as possible of the foot veins, the deep femoral veins and the internal iliac veins by the use of the Valsalva's manoeuvre when the adjacent main veins are filled with contrast medium.

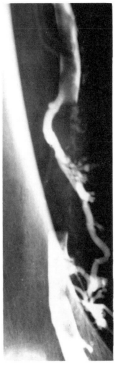

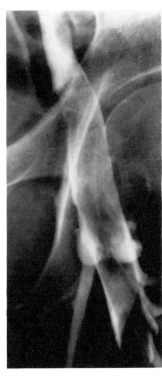

3a

3b

3a, b Thrombus shows as a constant filling defect in an opacified vein which is the same size and shape in at least two films taken with an interval between them. Fresh thrombus has a slightly opalescent appearance and is surrounded by a thin white line of contrast medium. Obliteration of this line indicates adherence of the thrombus to the vein wall. A 'floating tail' at the proximal end of the thrombus is likely to embolize and a straight edge indicates that a part of the thrombus has already embolized.

Post-thrombotic syndrome

4 In addition to showing the deep venous system from the ankle to the lower inferior vena cava, a controlled Valsalva's manoeuvre (as described on page 515) is required to show the venous valves. Post-thrombotic veins are narrowed and irregular, with absent or deformed valves, and have stenosed or occluded segments which are bypassed by collaterals.

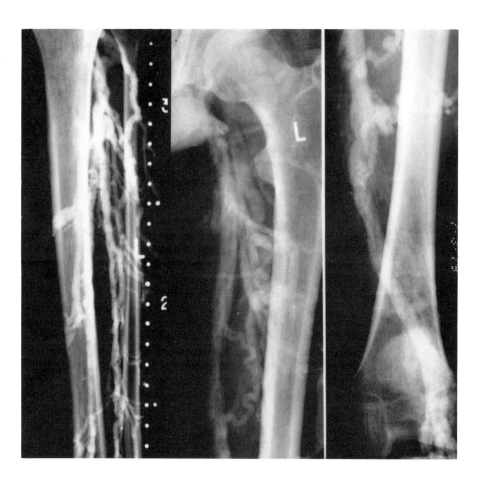

4

Incompetent communicating veins

5   The ankle tourniquet must be sufficiently tight to prevent contrast medium passing into the superficial veins so that the direction of flow from the deep to the superficial veins can be appreciated, indicating incompetence. A ruler with radio-opaque markers at 1-cm intervals placed beneath the leg is helpful in relating the position of incompetent communicating veins to bony landmarks such as the malleoli or knee joint. If a submalleolar communicating vein is suspected, a tourniquet should be placed around the forefoot. If there is ulceration, a tourniquet applied above and below the ulcer helps to isolate a localized incompetent communicating vein.

A typical incompetent communicating vein is dilated (more than 3 mm in diameter) and often connects directly or indirectly with a varicose vein. Communicating veins can also be shown by a direct injection of draining varicose veins (as described on page 508) but incompetence can only be suspected using this technique because the flow of contrast medium is in the normal direction from the superficial to the deep veins.

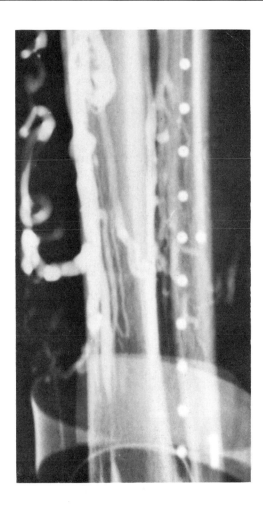

5

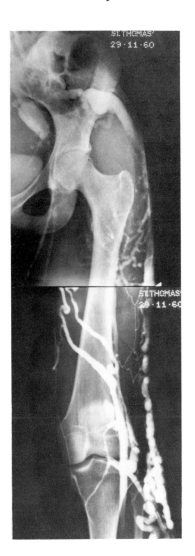

6

Congenital malformations

6   Congenital venous malformations display such a wide clinical spectrum that each case has to be considered separately. If the venous abnormality is localized, a direct injection of contrast medium into the dysplasia to show its size and tributaries may be all that is required. If the complex Klippel–Trenaunay–Weber syndrome is suspected, the whole deep venous system must be examined as aplasia or hypoplasia are common.

VARICOGRAPHY

This involves direct injection of varicose veins with contrast medium.

7 With the patient standing, a varicose vein is punctured. The patient then lies on the fluoroscopy table prone or supine and contrast medium is injected as the table is tilted from a steep foot-down position, through the horizontal, into a steep head-down position. A lateral view around the upper calf and knee is required to show the short saphenous vein.

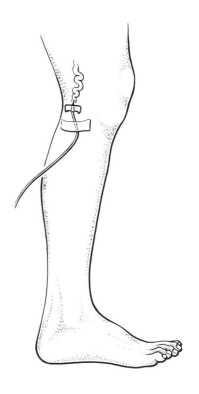

7

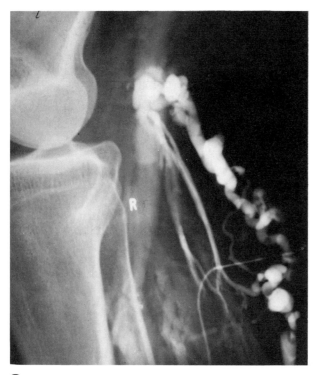

8

8 Because of the complex connections of superficial varicosities, particularly after surgery, multiple injections into different groups of varicose veins may be required and the contrast medium may need to be followed by fluoroscopy in straight, oblique and lateral positions. Because of the hyperbaric nature of contrast medium, prone films are best for showing groin recurrences.

9 Incompetent communicating veins in the mid-thigh region are a common cause of recurrence because of failure of ablation during initial surgery. While these communicating veins usually occur in the adductor canal region, their site is not constant and, although they usually connect with the superficial femoral vein, they may connect with the deep femoral vein. The exact site of such incompetent-looking communicating veins can be related to the knee joint by a ruler with radio-opaque markers placed beneath the leg.

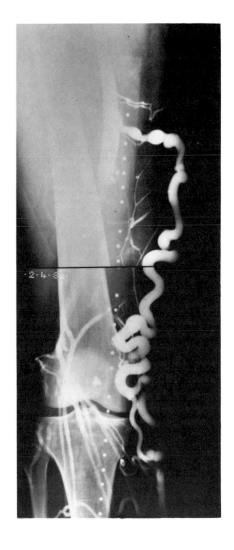

9

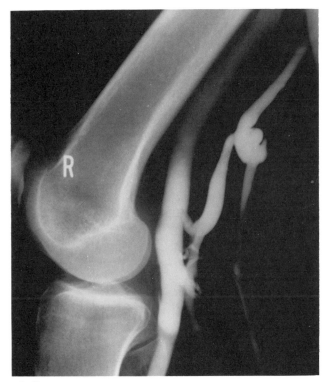

10

10 Other useful information obtained from varicography is knowledge of the presence of multiple long saphenous veins; this is important if surgical stripping is contemplated and to show the termination of the short saphenous vein, which is variable.

Varicography is less useful in the management of primary varicose veins, although varicose veins at unusual sites such as those on the posterolateral aspect of the thigh connecting to the deep femoral venous system may be displayed.

Dilated communicating veins likely to be incompetent can be shown by injection of varicose veins in the calf.

SAPHENOGRAPHY

The long saphenous vein is injected at the ankle and films are taken from the ankle to the groin with the fluoroscopy table tilted from the foot-down to the head-down position. Radio-opaque ballbearings of known size placed on the course of the long saphenous vein enable a more accurate assessment of its diameter to be made. Brief hand compression of the popliteal vein in the popliteal fossa or the femoral vein at the groin before filming directs contrast into the long saphenous vein which may be bypassed by communicating veins.

PELVIC PHLEBOGRAPHY AND INFERIOR VENACAVOGRAPHY

The femoral vein is punctured at the groin. This vein lies medial to the femoral artery at the groin and is identified by palpating the artery at its site of maximum pulsation. After local anaesthesia, a large needle such as an 18-gauge Potts–Cournand needle is useful because it has an obturator which permits threading of the needle into the vein to secure its position. The needle is plunged deeply into the tissues and slowly withdrawn with suction from a syringe with a Tolyvile connection. A Valsalva's manoeuvre is helpful when puncturing the femoral vein because this manoeuvre increases its size by about a one-third. When venous blood is aspirated the needle is threaded into the vein with the obturator and a test injection of contrast medium is then given to confirm its position.

If it is necessary to show the opposite iliac veins and the lower inferior vena cava, a bilateral injection is carried out. Bilateral injections are made by hand using about 50 ml of contrast medium. While a single spot film may be adequate for demonstrating an occlusion, a series of exposures with a serial film changer gives a better display of any altered anatomy and the direction of flow through collaterals.

11 To show the inferior vena cava, bilateral simultaneous injections are made. A tight tourniquet is applied above both knees and 50 ml of contrast medium are injected into veins in both feet. The fluoroscopy table is then tilted slightly head downwards, the tourniquet is removed, the calves are compressed, and a film is taken of the inferior vena cava outlined by the bolus obtained.

Alternatively, a 5-Fr catheter with side holes is introduced into the lower inferior vena cava over a guidewire from a femoral vein and an injection of 50 ml of contrast medium is given, either by hand or by pump injection.

11

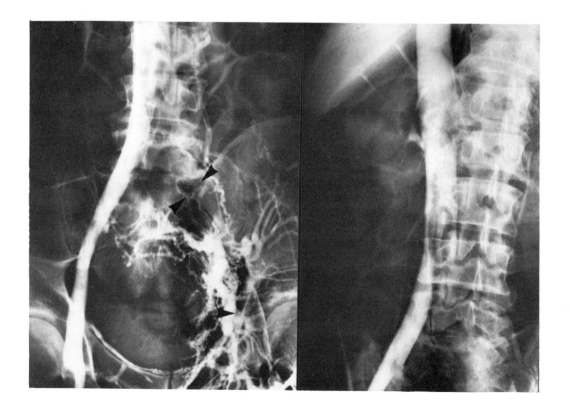

DESCENDING ILIOFEMORAL PHLEBOGRAPHY

12 A Potts–Cournand needle is introduced into the femoral vein as described above. The patient lies supine or with the feet angled slightly downwards on the fluoroscopy table during the injection of contrast medium. A controlled Valsalva's manoeuvre is performed by the patient. This entails maintaining a column of mercury at 40 mm for at least 12 s by blowing into the barrel of a syringe attached to a manometer. The supine position is preferred by patients rather than standing as the standard Valsalva's manoeuvre closes normal valves tightly, thus minimizing the hyperbaric effect of the contrast medium; this avoids false-positive degrees of deep vein reflux. If the patient cannot perform a satisfactory Valsalva's manoeuvre, injection of contrast medium in the semi-erect position is necessary. A bolus of about 15 ml of contrast medium is injected as rapidly as possible and its progress down the limb is followed with the fluoroscope and recorded on films. Deep vein reflux is recorded as a range, from 0 (no reflux) to 4 (reflux to the ankle). It is thought that reflux to below the knee is of clinical significance. Long saphenous vein reflux is not graded but free reflux is always abnormal.

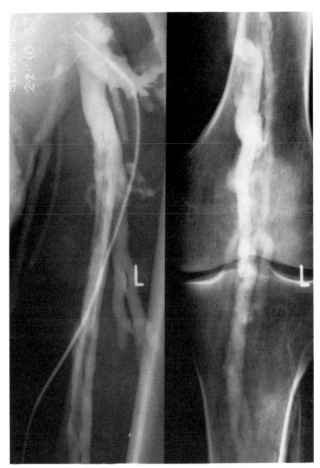

12

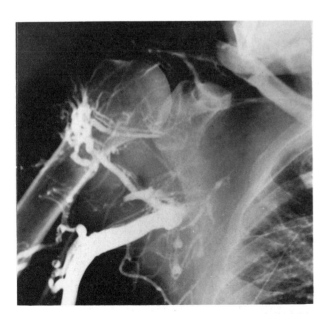

13

UPPER LIMB PHLEBOGRAPHY

13 The axillary and subclavian veins are easily demonstrated by injection of contrast medium through a wide-bore needle placed in the median cubital vein. An injection of 50 ml of contrast medium is performed and films are taken when the veins are shown to be filled on the fluoroscope. If a vein cannot be found at the elbow, any vein of the arm may be injected with a tourniquet above it to direct the contrast medium into the deep veins of the upper arm. If a band of adhesion is suspected, the examination should be performed with the arm at the side and also abducted and externally rotated above the head.

SUPERIOR VENACAVOGRAPHY

Catheters (5-Fr) are passed over guidewires from both basilic veins into the axillary veins. Bilateral simultaneous injections of about 50 ml of contrast medium are made with a pump injector, and films are taken at the rate of about 1 film/s.

INTRAOSSEOUS PHLEBOGRAPHY

This technique is rarely used nowadays, having been largely superseded by selective venous studies and alternative imaging techniques.

As intraosseous phlebography is painful, general anaesthesia is usually necessary.

14 The greater trochanter is palpated by rotating the limb and a 13-gauge drill-tip needle is introduced by penetrating the outer cortex under fluoroscopy. Correct placement of the needle is achieved by aspiration of marrow blood and free clearance of a small test injection of contrast medium from the marrow into the local draining vein. If a second needle is inserted after an unsuccessful puncture, the first is left *in situ* to prevent extravasation along its track.

Both greater trochanters are usually injected simultaneously; each needle is connected to a pump injector and 50 ml of contrast medium are injected at the rate of 10 ml/s. A Y connection is not satisfactory as the contrast medium tends to go into the side offering the least resistance.

Bilateral pertrochanteric iliophlebography shows the upper extent of an occluded inferior vena cava, thus obviating the need to perform retrograde catheterization from the arm.

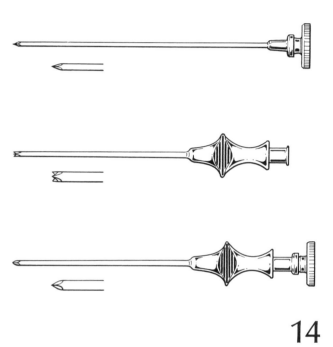

14

Postoperative care

Compression is usually required for a few minutes at the venous puncture site to prevent haematoma formation. If catheter techniques have been used and there is a possibility of vein wall puncture, pulse and blood pressure are monitored for about 2 h. Special care should be taken if patients are taking anticoagulants.

Since the advent of low osmolar non-ionic contrast media there are virtually no contraindications or complications associated with phlebography; the procedure can be regarded as very safe[5].

Sepsis is prevented after intraosseous phlebography by scrupulous aseptic technique. Fat embolism, although rare, represents the most serious complication and may be fatal. The condition can be treated if it is recognized by cerebral symptoms occurring after the procedure[1].

References

1. Lea Thomas M. *Phlebography of the Lower Limb.* Edinburgh: Churchill Livingstone, 1982.

2. Browse NL, Burnand KG, Lea Thomas M. *Diseases of the Veins: Pathology, Diagnosis and Treatment.* London: Edward Arnold, 1988: 103–50.

3. Lea Thomas M. Routine and special phlebography in the evaluation of venous problems. In: Bergan JJ, Yao JST, eds. *Venous Disorders.* Philadelphia: WB Saunders, 1991: 123–36.

4. Walters HL. The venous system. In: Whitehouse GH, Worthington BS, eds. *Techniques in Diagnostic Imaging.* 2nd edn. Oxford: Blackwell, 1990: 156–78.

5. Lea Thomas M. Techniques of phlebography: a review. *Eur J Radiol* 1990; 11: 125–30.

Illustrations by Peter Cox

Venous thrombectomy

Bernard H. Nachbur MD
Professor of Surgery, Department for Thoracic and Cardiovascular Surgery, University of Berne, Berne, Switzerland

History

Successful venous thrombectomy was probably born out of necessity for salvage of a limb threatened by phlegmasia coerulea dolens such as reported by Lenggenhager in 1962. Earliest descriptions date back to 1937. Phlegmasia coerulea dolens is brought on by the total or subtotal obstruction of the venous outflow of an extremity (usually the lower), giving rise to such an increase in interstitial pressure that the critical closure pressure of arterioles is overcome, resulting in progressive ischaemia if adequate treatment is not initiated. Limb salvage is considered a success in these cases, irrespective of long-term venous function. Thereafter, in the 1960s, venous thrombectomy increased rapidly in popularity, being applied to deep venous thrombosis of all ages and aetiologies. Not surprisingly, critical authors soon noted a high percentage of rethrombosis, often more extensive than before operation. As a consequence, venous thrombectomy fell into disrepute, being virtually abandoned or at least not a generally accepted procedure in the USA. It has lived on mainly in Scandinavian and German speaking countries where operative indications have since been defined and from where long-term results comparing conservative with surgical treatment have been reported in recent years[1-3].

Principles and justification

While some superficial leg veins are obviously dispensable in normal limbs and may therefore be harvested for aortocoronary or femorodistal bypass surgery and similar procedures, this is not the case for deep veins which carry the burden of venous return. For this purpose they are equipped with an intricate set of cusps allowing for unidirectional venous flow, which is accelerated by the action of the pedal and calf muscle pump. If deep venous thrombosis (DVT) occurs venous return is immediately impaired to a degree dependent on the extent of the thrombosis. Timely initiation of systemic heparinization followed by long-term (3–6 months) oral anticoagulation will usually prevent further progression or the formation of new thrombosis and also alleviate the initial symptoms of deep venous occlusion, probably by enhancing or increasing the rate and degree of recanalization.

The outlook for patients with DVT treated in this way is no longer as bleak as reported by McDonnell in 1977 and others. In more than 50% of patients, however, valvular function of veins formerly occluded by thrombosis will remain deficient, and varying degrees of postphlebitic syndrome develop as a result of late haemodynamic sequelae of DVT[4]. It is therefore highly desirable and justifiable to aim to restore normal morphology and anatomy and thus the function of deep veins. Moreover, normalization of the anatomy of deep veins is important, bearing in mind the conclusion of the Ad Hoc Committee on Reporting Standards in Venous Disease, which has listed a prior history of lower extremity DVT as the greatest single risk factor for a subsequent episode of DVT[5]. A recurrent episode of DVT, probably due to stagnation, is more likely to occur if the venous outflow is obstructed as the result of earlier DVT. Therefore, an attempt to clear the venous pathway is justified.

Indications

It has never been proved that venous thrombectomy prevents pulmonary embolism, however attractive this approach may appear. It is the author's experience that pulmonary embolism occurs unexpectedly at an early stage of thrombus formation when a clot is loose and friable and before obvious clinical signs of venous obstruction have aroused suspicion of DVT, and also before aggressive methods of clearing the venous pathway are contemplated. Were this not the case, malpractice claims on the grounds of delayed anticoagulant therapy would be numerous considering the number of patients with fatal pulmonary embolism. By the time a leg is swollen or even cyanotic and venous thrombectomy indicated the danger of fatal pulmonary embolism has actually diminished substantially. Therefore it is the author's belief that venous thrombectomy does not prevent pulmonary embolism.

Ideally venous thrombectomy should be performed before the clot has become completely adherent to the endothelial lining, i.e. when small amounts of contrast medium can still be shown to slip past the thrombus in ascending venograms, thus giving rise to a 'railway track' appearance.

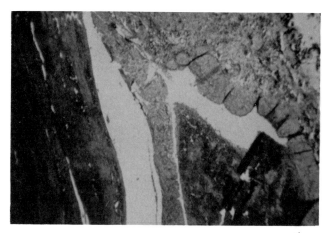

1a

1a, b The success of venous thrombectomy is inversely proportional to the age of the thrombus. It has been convincingly shown by Leu[6] that venous thrombi – if not caused by direct trauma to the endothelium – lie loosely within the lumen of veins for the first 3 days. Thereafter the venous wall reacts and there is infiltration of fibroblasts, heralding the beginning of organization of the thrombus. This may lead to formation of collagen and scar tissue on one hand and to formation of capillaries with consecutive recanalization on the other.

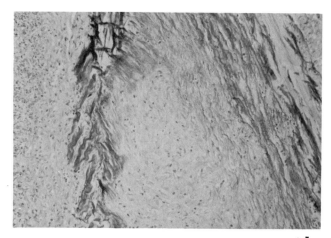

1b

Venous thrombectomy must therefore be performed as soon as possible and before reaction of the endothelium has occurred. It is strictly contraindicated when the process of organization is under way. Rethrombosis, usually to a larger extent than preoperatively, would otherwise occur in these cases, which is the reason why so many failures were reported in earlier days. The best indication for venous thrombectomy is iliofemoral (iliopopliteal) DVT of 1–3 days' duration.

Venous thrombectomy is also indicated in the treatment of phlegmasia coerulea dolens provided this is not the final act of a long series of thrombotic episodes. A good indication might arise, for instance, after childbirth or if acute DVT results from a misplaced caval filter. In many other cases of phlegmasia coerulea dolens, however, the main deep venous pathway has postphlebitic recanalized veins that do not lend themselves to thrombectomy and have to be treated by other means, usually with four-compartment fasciotomy. Phlegmasia coerulea dolens can furthermore occur in the presence of pre-existing low arterial perfusion, acute arterial thrombosis on chronic occlusive arterial disease, and such conservative measures as leg elevation to alleviate the swelling and fasciotomy might not therefore be tolerable. In these cases it is better to plan arterial reconstruction in the first instance. Herein lies the problem with the indiscriminate indication of venous thrombectomy for phlegmasia coerulea dolens. Yet in special cases of bilateral phlegmasia coerulea dolens brought on by bilateral iliofemorocaval thrombosis, venous thrombectomy can be the only way to salvage life and limbs.

Venous thrombectomy not only has the potential to save limbs, or exceptionally a life, but can also restore the function of transplanted kidneys if renal vein outflow is impeded by iliac vein thrombosis. In contrast to native kidneys, renal transplants cannot develop a collateral circulation.

Venous thrombectomy is therefore indicated in cases of venous obstruction in renal transplants and has been successful in all three cases in the author's personal experience.

Contraindications

Venous thrombectomy is contraindicated in patients with a short life expectancy, especially in patients with malignant tumours. The operation is hardly necessary in elderly patients, for instance those who are retired, when the dire consequences of the postphlebitic syndrome can easily be avoided by medical treatment and adaptation to an appropriate lifestyle. Venous thrombectomy will not provide rewarding results if the deep venous system shows postphlebitic changes due to previous episodes of DVT and is contraindicated in these patients.

Preoperative

Assessment and preparation

The rapid onset of swelling and diffuse soft tissue pain is usually the first clinical sign of DVT. Spontaneous pain can occur in the lower back, in the buttock, the groin or the inner side of the thigh. It can be elicited by local pressure in the lower abdomen, the groin, or along the course of the deep femoral vessels. These spontaneous or provoked signs of pain are indicative of iliocaval or iliofemoral thrombophlebitis and suggest inflammatory involvement in the form of mural thrombophlebitis. They are probably of predictive value; during venous thrombectomy a greater degree of mural adhesion of the thrombus is found than in the painless type of venous occlusion. Diagnosis is primarily made by continuous wave Doppler ultrasonography; imaging can be obtained by duplex scanning or ascending phlebography. The diagnostic value of duplex scanning is not inferior to venography; patent veins can be shown to be compressible, while in the presence of thrombosis the vein with its enlarged diameter retains its incom-pressible round shape. Duplex scanning is especially recommended for detecting DVT in pregnancy. For the purpose of documentation, however, ascending venography is still preferable if possible. For precise assessment of thrombosis of pelvic veins or the inferior vena cava, phlebography might also provide more insight than duplex scanning.

At this time the patient will already have commenced treatment with systemic heparin which might have to be discontinued if spinal anaesthesia is envisaged for venous thrombectomy. This is not necessary if the operation is performed under general or local anaesthesia.

As the results of venous thrombectomy depend on the age of the thrombus, it is important to perform the operation as soon as possible. Because a successful operation is usually associated with considerable blood loss, 2–3 units of blood should be cross-matched. Homologous blood transfusions may be avoided by using a cell-saving device for autologous blood retransfusion.

Anaesthesia

General anaesthesia is usual, but some surgeons prefer spinal anaesthesia; in the author's experience local anaesthesia has been found satisfactory. The main advantage of local anaesthesia is that patients can assist in the act of expelling the pelvic clot by performing a Valsalva's manoeuvre. The disadvantage of local anaesthesia is that manual compression of calf and thigh might cause pain.

The anaesthetist should be informed before the start of the operation that during thrombectomy of the iliac segment blood loss in the reverse Trendelenburg position may sometimes be associated with an unexpected drop of blood pressure. Haemocel, plasma, or stored blood should be readily available for this event.

Operations

Vascular anatomy of the groin: general remarks

2   In order to choose the correct incision it is of the utmost importance to be aware that (1) all tributaries of the common femoral vein should be unplugged by thrombectomy in order to increase venous flow; and (2) that these tributaries (medial and lateral circumflex femoral and deep femoral veins) are situated along a longitudinal line in the proximal quarter of the thigh. The junction of the deep and superficial femoral veins is situated at a significantly lower level than the origin of the deep femoral artery. The various important venous tributaries draining the blood from the thigh do much more to increase venous flow than the contribution from the calf veins. By analogy, it is well known from reconstructive arterial surgery that the reflux from the deep femoral artery far outweighs the reflux from the superficial femoral artery. Failure to take the anatomical differences between veins and arteries into account might be one of the reasons why not all surgeons are equally successful when performing venous thrombectomy.

An oblique incision in the inguinal crease gives poor access to the important venous tributaries. It should be remembered that for successful thrombectomy all the tributaries need to be unplugged. Therefore the incision of choice will have to be longitudinal and lateroconvex, in order to avoid and spare the lymphatics which are carefully dissected away medially.

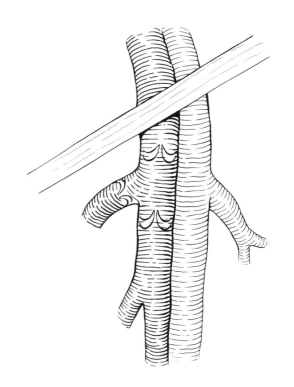

2

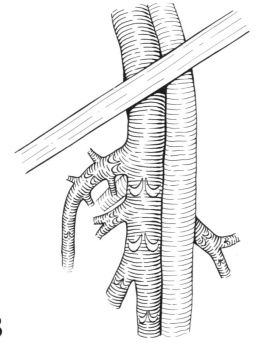

3

3   The major arteries (common femoral, deep femoral, superficial femoral, medial and lateral circumflex femoral) are bunched together. In contrast, the major venous tributaries are aligned longitudinally; the long saphenous vein joins the common femoral vein at the most proximal site, then follow the lateral and medial circumflex veins and finally, distally, the junction of the deep and superficial femoral veins.

Incision

4 A lateroconvex incision crossing the inguinal crease in a lazy S form is chosen to dissect away the inguinal fat pad containing the lymph glands medially. Cutting through the subcutaneous tissue is normally associated with slightly troublesome bleeding from collateral venous circulation. As dissection proceeds to the level of the large vessels there is less bleeding. The common or superficial femoral artery will be narrow in diameter, arterial inflow being impeded by the increased interstitial pressure. In contrast, the common femoral vein is engorged when completely occluded by clot. The long saphenous vein, the common and superficial femoral veins, the circumflex femoral veins and the deep femoral vein are controlled by Silastic slings.

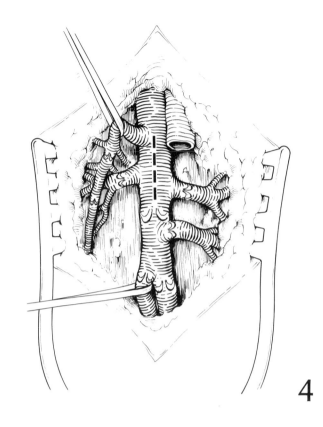

4

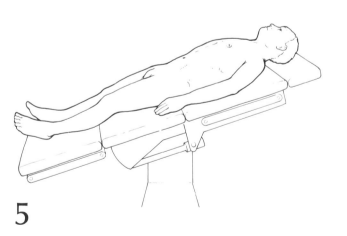

5

ILIAC VENOUS THROMBECTOMY

Position of patient

5 At this point the patient is fully heparinized and placed in a steep reverse Trendelenburg position. This increases the hydrostatic pressure in the veins and ensures that blood flow during iliac thrombectomy will be caudad and not cephalad. When iliac thrombectomy is successful, venous reflux will be copious when the patient performs a Valsalva's manoeuvre because the iliac vein segment is, with very few exceptions, avalvular (without cusps).

Vein incision

6a, b The common femoral vein is incised longitudinally opposite the entrance of the long saphenous vein and the circumflex femoral veins over a distance of about 3 cm. A venous Fogarty balloon catheter with a balloon filling capacity of 40 ml is passed through the clot cephalad into the inferior vena cava, where it is dilated to the caval diameter. The balloon catheter is then pulled downwards while the patient performs a Valsalva's manoeuvre. When passing from the vena cava inferior to the common iliac vein the balloon must be reduced in diameter. Fresh clot will be expelled from the iliac segment followed by blood shooting out from above and swamping the operative field with blood and clots.

If the operation is performed under spinal anaesthesia a Valsalva's manoeuvre cannot be performed, but the surgeon can exert manual pressure from the lower abdomen. Under general anaesthesia the intra-abdominal pressure on the inferior vena cava can be increased by positive end expiratory pressure, i.e. by hyperbaric respiration. Intravenous pressure measurements show clearly that the pressure increase resulting from a Valsalva's manoeuvre under local anaesthesia is considerably greater (up to 70 mmHg) than the increase caused by hyperbaric respiration (30–35 mmHg).

By observing these precautionary measures pulmonary embolism can be safely avoided. Balloon catheterization has to be repeated two or three times and for as long as clots continue to be extracted.

Thrombectomy in right-sided venous thrombosis is generally much easier and sooner accomplished, but left-sided iliofemoral thrombosis is more frequent. The crossing of the right common iliac artery is thought to inflict endothelial damage to the left common iliac vein by chronic intermittent repetitive external compression, which might be the reason for longstanding mural thrombosis at this level, where occasionally a venous spur (as described by May and Turner) will develop.

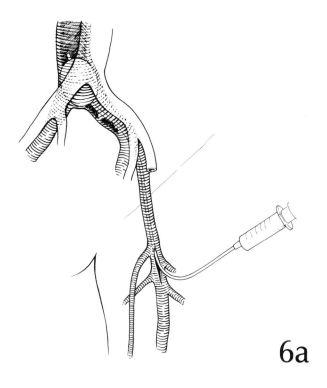

6a

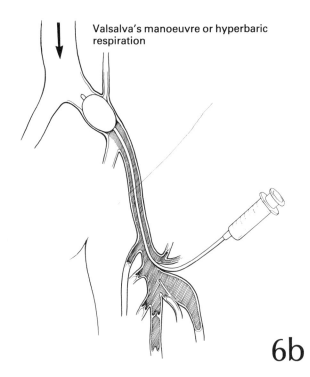

Valsalva's manoeuvre or hyperbaric respiration

6b

Completion angiography of pelvic veins

7a, b Brisk bleeding caused by iliocaval reflux is a reliable sign that patency of the pelvic axis has been achieved. If there is any doubt concerning patency it is advisable to inject contrast medium into the pelvic segment. For this purpose the pelvic vein segment must be closed at both ends. First, a balloon catheter is inflated at the level of the inferior vena cava or at the junction of both common iliac veins. When the iliac veins have emptied into the inguinal wound, a Silastic sling is wrapped twice around the common iliac vein or closed by a tourniquet and then tightened after insertion of a catheter for injection of contrast medium. Good patency is reflected by bright opacification of the pelvic axis, which occasionally reveals an ascending lumbar vein into which the Fogarty catheter has accidentally been inserted. Instead of angiography, inspection of the iliac veins for residual clot can be performed by angioscopy which is probably the best means of assessing complete thrombectomy.

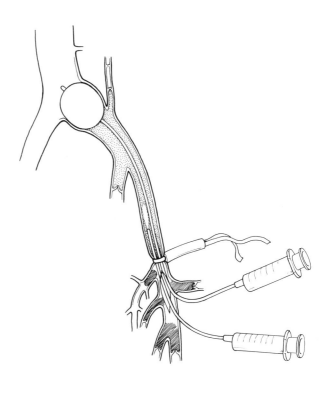

7a

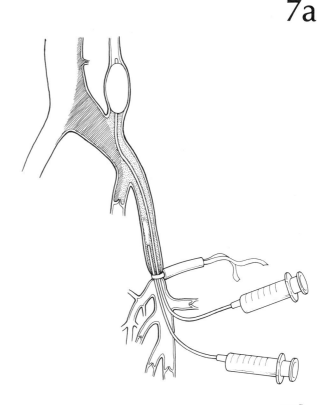

7b

UNPLUGGING OF ORIFICES OF MAJOR TRIBUTARIES TO THE COMMON FEMORAL VEIN

8 A longitudinal incision is chosen for the important reason of removing all clots from the orifices of major tributaries of the common femoral vein. These are the long saphenous vein, the medial and lateral circumflex femoral veins and the deep femoral vein. Sometimes there are other sizeable tributaries. Careful removal of clots from all these tributaries with fine Fogarty catheters or forceps will help to increase flow through the iliac veins. Thus, the chance that the iliofemoral axis will remain open is enhanced. For this part of the operation the patient is placed in a horizontal position.

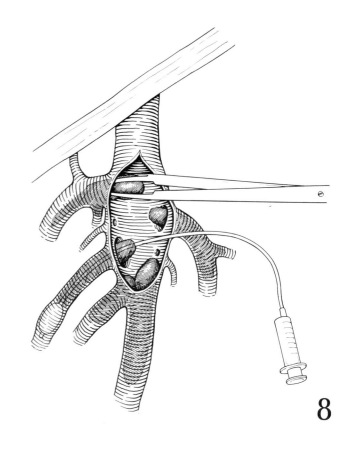

8

THROMBECTOMY OF THE SUPERFICIAL FEMORAL AND POPLITEAL VEINS

9 The patient is placed in the horizontal position. A venous Fogarty catheter (4-ml capacity) is gently introduced down the superficial femoral vein, usually to the middle third of the popliteal vein. It is generally thought that this manoeuvre is not possible because of the cusps that are encountered on the way down. It is not clear whether the valvular leaflets actually remain competent in a superficial vein that is considerably enlarged in diameter if freshly thrombosed. With gentle manipulation and patience the three or four cusps can be passed, thus enabling direct balloon extraction of a long continuous clot. During this procedure the external iliac vein is closed by a Fogarty catheter.

There are two alternatives to this procedure. First, manual compression of the calf and thigh muscles might suffice to expel residual thrombus out of the entire deep venous system. Successful removal of fresh thrombotic material is signalled by brisk efflux of blood from the periphery, which will flush out remaining thrombotic material. Secondly, if the clot in the superficial femoral vein is not easily mobilized an additional infragenicular incision of the distal portion of the popliteal vein can be helpful, either for instilling urokinase, 250 000 units, into the popliteal and superficial femoral veins, in order to loosen the thrombus or for introducing a soft catheter upwards which can be retrieved in the groin where a Fogarty catheter is inserted into the lumen of this slender tube. The catheter is then pushed downwards. Thereafter the Fogarty manoeuvre can be performed in the proper direction without traumatizing the cusps. A combination of these procedures is advisable.

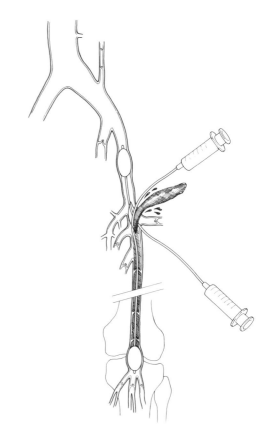

9

MOBILIZATION AND UPWARDS THRUST OF CALF VEIN THROMBI

10 The multiple intermuscular deep veins of the calf are equipped with innumerable cusps that prevent any kind of instrumentation. Because the indication for venous thrombectomy is limited to fresh thrombosis no more than 3 days old, the clots should be readily mobilized manually and moved in a cephalad direction where they can be:

1. Retrieved through the infragenicular incision of the popliteal vein.
2. Harvested by a balloon catheter in the popliteal vein.
3. Expelled through the incision of the common femoral vein.

Largiadèr prefers to cut down the posterior tibial veins at ankle level and to flush out the calf vein thrombi by forceful instillation of a saline solution containing urokinase, 100 000–200 000 units.

TEMPORARY ARTERIOVENOUS FISTULA

It has been mentioned earlier that the key to success is early detection of DVT, establishment of unimpeded patency of the iliac veins and copious flow from the many tributaries to the common iliac vein. It has also been pointed out that acute DVT may occur on pre-existing chronic mural thrombosis of the common iliac vein. When one of the three above-mentioned requisites is not entirely satisfactory it is probably helpful to construct a temporary arteriovenous fistula which will guarantee enhanced flow through the iliac segment.

11a, b The longitudinal incision of the common femoral vein is closed with a running suture. A sufficiently well-developed branch of the long saphenous vein is mobilized and anastomosed end-to-side with the common femoral artery with 6/0 Prolene. The branches of the long saphenous vein are often not suitable and patency of the arteriovenous fistula is therefore very short-lived. In this case it is preferable to use the long saphenous vein itself. It can be demonstrated that the long saphenous vein below will remain patent.

Flow through the pelvic veins will be greatly enhanced. Swelling of the leg has been noted in some cases due to the fistula and will subside as soon as the temporary arteriovenous fistula occludes or is ligated about 6 weeks later. In order to approach the fistula directly at this time it is recommended that some easily detectable non-resorbable material is placed around the loop.

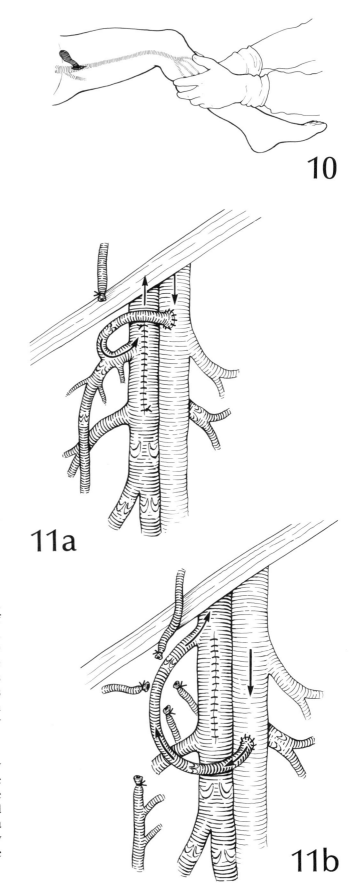

Postoperative care

Following surgical thrombectomy the patient is kept on systemic heparin and mobilized on the second or third day after operation. It may be preferable if the patient's legs are elevated in bed; when mobilized it is important that the patient moves around with compressive stockings or Ace bandages. Sitting passively at the bedside or standing erect and immobile should be strictly avoided. Oral anticoagulation is started on the third or fourth day after operation, overlapping with systemic heparin which will be discontinued when therapeutic levels of prothrombin are reached. If complete success has been obtained following surgical thrombectomy, oral anticoagulation can be discontinued after about 2 months; otherwise it should be continued for 3–6 months or longer, if a haematological disorder such as antithrombin III deficiency is discovered.

Outcome

The short-term and long-term outcome of venous thrombectomy is correctly assessed by follow-up venography, plethysmography, dynamic pressure measurements and duplex ultrasonography. These objective data are supplemented by clinical findings, including dependency on compressive stockings, swelling, eczema or ulceration, hyperpigmentation and dilatation of venous collaterals.

It has been shown by Eklöf *et al.*[1] in a prospective study and by the author in a retrospective comparative study[2] employing the aforementioned clinical and subjective criteria for evaluation that venous thrombectomy can undoubtedly offer highly rewarding results. It is the only means of achieving restoration of function. The key to success for treatment of DVT is early detection and meticulous atraumatic handling of the involved veins. Trauma to the endothelial lining must be avoided at all costs.

Follow-up phlebography

Until the advent of colour-coded duplex ultrasonography the short-term assessment of venous thrombectomy was achieved by ascending phlebography, usually performed before hospital discharge or some weeks or months later. Successful venous thrombectomy is evidenced by restoration of normal anatomy.

12a, b The illustrations show venograms of a man with iliofemoral DVT of the right leg clearly evidenced by collateral circulation before thrombectomy (*Illustration 12a*) and 14 months after surgical thrombectomy (*Illustration 12b*). Note complete restoration of valvular morphology and excellent patency of the iliofemoral axis.

Before　　　　*After*

Before　　　　*After*

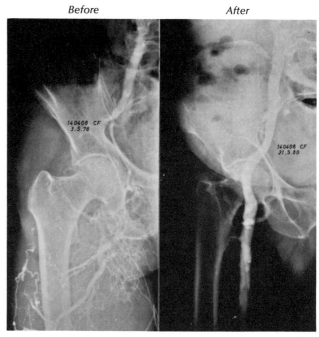

12a

12b

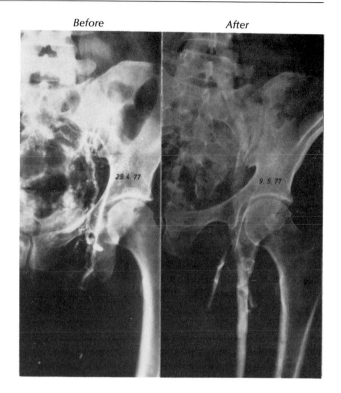

13a

13a, b These are venograms of a 37-year-old woman who was operated on for DVT 3 days after cholecystectomy. *Illustration 13a* (the iliofemoral portion) shows the tell-tale collateral circulation before thrombectomy (left) and the patent iliofemoral axis (right) 5 weeks after thrombectomy with complete anatomical restoration and excellent patency. *Illustration 13b* shows occlusion of the superficial femoral vein before (left) and 5 weeks after thrombectomy with excellent anatomical restoration and patency.

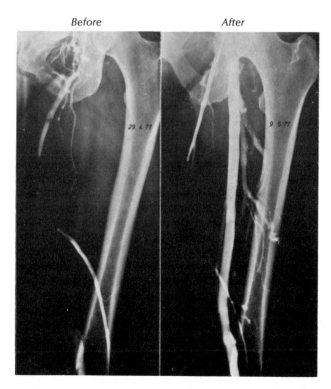

13b

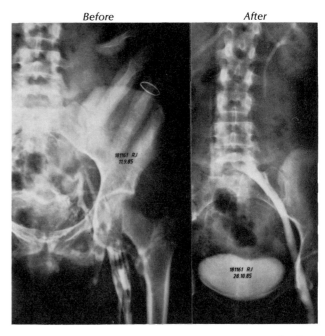

14a

14a, b These are venograms of a 24-year-old woman taking steroids and oral contraceptives with iliofemoral DVT before thrombectomy (left) and 7 weeks after thrombectomy (right). The perfect visualization of a functionally important cusp just adjacent to the trochanter minor following thrombectomy should be noted (*Illustration 14b*, right).

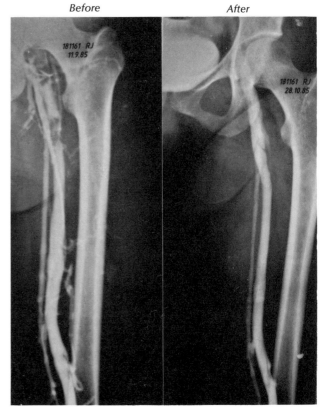

14b

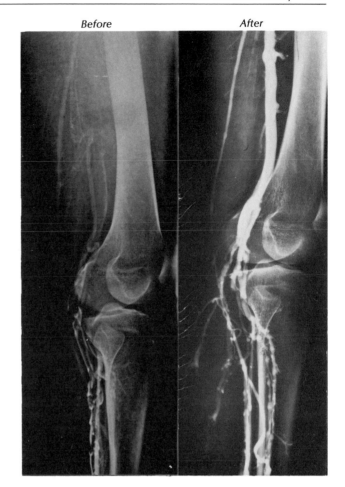

Before   *After*

15 This illustration is presented as proof that normal morphology and patency can also be achieved at the level of the crural and popliteal segments. This 21-year-old woman taking oral contraceptives had four-level DVT. Again, the left half of the illustration shows the near total occlusion of deep veins before thrombectomy and the right half shows near total normalization of venous anatomy after thrombectomy. The normal appearance of the multiple vein cusps should be noted.

Plethysmography

Phlebodynamic pressure measurements are probably the gold standard for assessment of venous function. This invasive investigation can for all practical purposes be replaced by plethysmography. By applying dynamic plethysmography after standardized leg work the volume of blood expelled from the calf can be measured and compared with normal values. In normal subjects the expelled volume is 2–3 ml/100 g soft tissue per minute and may drop to values between 0 and 0.5 ml in patients with occlusive venous disease. For the purpose of assessing venous function it is especially important to compare measurements of one extremity with those of the contralateral leg, as normal values may vary considerably.

15

References

1. Eklöf B, Einarsson E, Plate G. Role of thrombectomy and temporary a–v fistula in acute iliofemoral venous thrombosis. In: Bergan JJ, Yao JST, eds. *Surgery of the Veins*. Orlando, Florida: Grune and Stratton, 1985: 131–45.

2. Gänger KH, Nachbur BH, Ris HB, Zurbrügg H. Surgical thrombectomy versus conservative treatment for deep venous thrombosis: functional comparison of long-term results. *Eur J Surg* 1989; 3: 529–38.

3. Plate G, Akesson H, Einarsson E, Ohlin P, Eklöf B. Long-term results of venous thrombectomy combined with temporary arteriovenous fistula. *Eur J Vasc Surg* 1990; 4: 483–9.

4. Raju S, Fredericks RK. Late hemodynamic sequelae of deep venous thrombosis. *J Vasc Surg* 1986; 4: 73–9.

5. Porter JM, Rutherford RB, Clagett FP *et al*. Ad Hoc Committee on reporting standards in venous disease. *J Vasc Surg* 1988; 8: 172–81.

6. Leu HJ. Histologische Altersbestimmung von arteriellen und venösen Thromben und Emboli. *Vasa* 1973; 2: 265–74.

Bypass of venous obstruction

James S. T. Yao MD, PhD
Mayerstadt Professor of Surgery, Division of Vascular Surgery, Department of Surgery, Northwestern University Medical School, Chicago, Illinois, USA

William H. Pearce MD
Associate Professor of Surgery, Division of Vascular Surgery, Department of Surgery, Northwestern University Medical School, Chicago, Illinois, USA

History

Despite remarkable advances in arterial reconstructive surgery, venous bypass grafting has yet to be established as a standard approach in the treatment of chronic venous insufficiency. In selected instances, however, bypass procedures can help to reduce unrelenting swelling. Procedures commonly used are the crossover vein graft for iliac vein thrombosis and the sapheno-popliteal bypass for femoral vein occlusion. The former was first described by Palma et al. of Montevideo in 1958[1] and was subsequently popularized by Dale of Nashville, Tennessee[2]. Saphenofemoral bypass was first devised by Palma and Warren independently and applied by Husni[3] in the USA and by Gruss[4] and May[5] in Europe. Unlike arterial bypass, venous bypass grafting remains a highly selective surgical procedure.

Principles and justification

Basic techniques in venous bypass

Techniques for venous bypass follow the guidelines of arterial surgery. Several technical points need to be emphasized. These include the construction of vein-to-vein anastomoses, control of the vein for anastomosis, and the construction of panel or spiral grafts.

Anastomosis

1 In end-to-side venovenous anastomoses it is necessary to excise a small portion of the recipient vein in an elliptical fashion to avoid constriction. A similar manoeuvre is also used if a polytetrafluoroethylene (PTFE) graft is used as the conduit.

The saphenous vein or cephalic vein is often too small in size to match with the recipient vein. This is particularly true for vena caval bypass. In this situation a panel graft or spiral vein graft can be constructed and used for bypass.

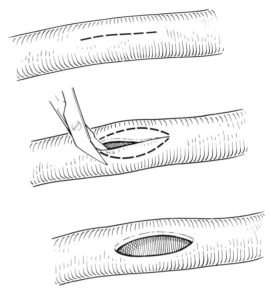

1

Panel graft

2 After the saphenous vein or cephalic vein is removed, it is transected in the middle of the vein. Both segments are then opened longitudinally. A continuous suture technique is used to join these segments along the vein opening.

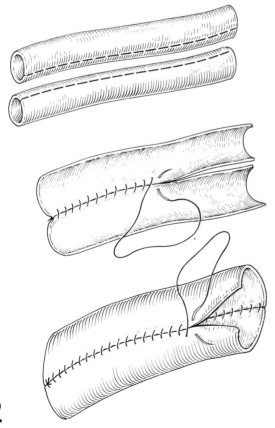

2

Spiral graft

3 After the saphenous vein is removed it is opened
longitudinally. The vein segment is then wrapped
around a large catheter or a small chest tube of the
desired diameter. A continuous 6/0 polypropylene
(Prolene) suture is then started in an oblique manner.

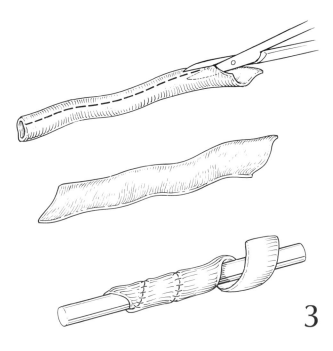

3

Partial occluding clamp

4 Because of dense adhesion of the vein to the
surrounding structures, it may be desirable to avoid
circumferential dissection of the vein, such as may be
used in arterial surgery. The anterior surface of the
recipient vein may be exposed free enough to allow the
use of a partial occluding clamp. This technique avoids
unnecessary blood loss and greatly facilitates the
procedure.

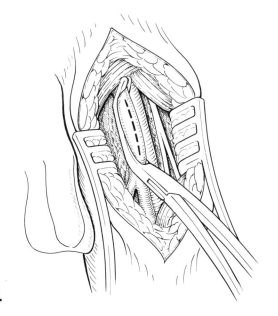

4

Preoperative

Patient selection and evaluation

In general, patients with recent thrombosis (within 1 year) should not be considered for a bypass procedure. With time and intensive compression therapy, most swelling will respond to conservative management. In severe cases, the use of a mechanical pump helps to reduce swelling. Similarly, patients with venous ulcers must first undergo compression therapy together with attention to skin hygiene and avoidance of allergenic medications. Surgery is reserved for those patients who fail to improve despite this treatment. In the majority of cases, compression therapy will be sufficient to relieve the symptoms.

Before surgical correction, patients must undergo venography and non-invasive studies. Several non-invasive techniques are now available to evaluate venous function. These include photoplethysmography, air plethysmography and duplex ultrasonography. In addition, ambulatory venous pressure recording is helpful in providing objective assessment of the function of the venous pump. The availability of autogenous vein as a bypass graft can now be assessed with duplex scanning. Evaluation of the jugular vein by venography is often difficult, but examination of its patency can be established by duplex scanning or by magnetic resonance imaging.

Once a patient is considered a surgical candidate, a complete vein evaluation by contrast venography is mandatory. For lower extremity venous obstruction, visualization of the inferior vena cava is necessary to complete the evaluation. Venography is helpful to determine operability as well as the types of venous reconstruction required.

Operations

VENOUS OCCLUSION OF UPPER EXTREMITIES

Venous bypass is not often needed in patients with isolated occlusion of the subclavian vein, the innominate vein, or the superior vena cava. The rich collateral networks of the upper part of the body usually provide enough decompression, and surgery is reserved for patients with severe obstruction. With increasing use of a central venous catheter for chemotherapy or hyperalimentation, occlusion of the superior vena cava has become a more common problem. One of the interesting problems of upper extremity venous occlusion is the development of subclavian vein thrombosis in patients who have had a functioning arteriovenous fistula constructed for haemodialysis. The presence of a functioning arteriovenous fistula distal to an occluded subclavian or axillary vein invariably causes severe swelling, and a bypass procedure may be necessary. Several authors have reported success in preserving an arteriovenous fistula with a bypass in such patients.

5

Jugular–brachial or axillary vein bypass

5 The internal jugular vein is exposed by placing an incision along the anterior border of the sterno-cleidomastoid muscle. The jugular vein is then dissected free. For distal anastomosis, the axillary vein or the brachial vein is exposed in the upper arm. Once the exposure of these two veins is complete, a tunnel is made subcutaneously underneath the clavicle. The long saphenous vein, if of suitable calibre, is then harvested from the thigh for vein grafting. If the vein is small, a panel graft or spiral graft is constructed and used as the bypass conduit. If vein is not available, a PTFE graft may be used as the bypass conduit. The graft is anastomosed to the jugular vein and the axillary vein in an end-to-side manner using the technique described previously.

Superior vena cava occlusion can be due to tumour compression or to prolonged use of an indwelling catheter for chemotherapy. Marked swelling of the face or the extremity is the common presenting symptom.

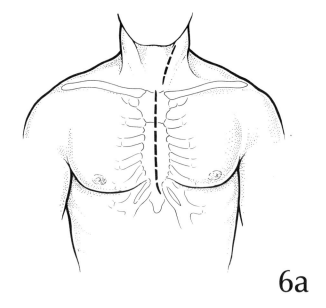

6a

Jugular–atrial graft

6a, b This procedure is used for decompression of superior vena cava occlusion. The right atrium is used as the outflow decompression pathway. The jugular vein is exposed as described previously. The right atrium is approached through a median sternotomy. The choice of graft material depends on the projected longevity of the patient. A spiral vein graft should be used if the prognosis of the patient is favourable; otherwise, a ring-inforced PTFE graft is preferred. After the right atrium and the internal jugular vein are exposed, anastomosis is performed first in the jugular vein in an end-to-end manner. After this is complete, the other end of the graft is anastomosed to the atrium.

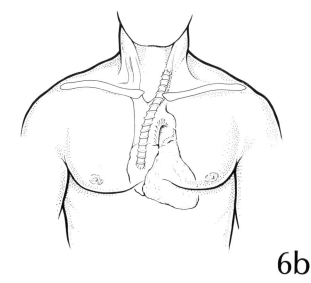

6b

VENOUS OCCLUSION OF THE LOWER EXTREMITIES

Chronic occlusion of the iliac or femoral veins may produce unrelenting swelling requiring surgical decompression. Procedures commonly used are the crossover vein graft and the saphenopopliteal bypass. Both procedures use long saphenous vein as the conduit.

Femorofemoral crossover graft

7a–c The procedure is suitable for unilateral iliac vein occlusion in the presence of a contralateral venous system. On the diseased side, the common femoral vein is exposed by a routine technique using a vertical incision. On the donor (normal) side, the skin incision is extended to the distal thigh for exposure of the long saphenous vein. The femoral vein and saphenofemoral junction are carefully exposed. A subcutaneous tunnel is made over the pubic bone, and the long saphenous vein is dissected free and transected after the desired length is achieved. Because of spasm, gentle manual dilatation of the vein by connecting the distal end of the vein to a syringe filled with heparin–saline solution may be necessary. The graft is then tunnelled over the pubic bone subcutaneously. Care must be taken to ensure that there is no kinking of the saphenofemoral junction of the donor side. The saphenous vein is anastomosed to the femoral vein in an end-to-side manner. No attempt is made to construct a temporary fistula in these patients.

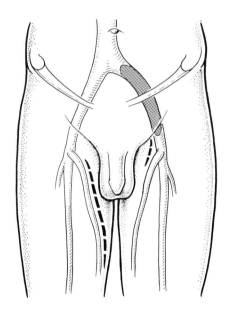

7a

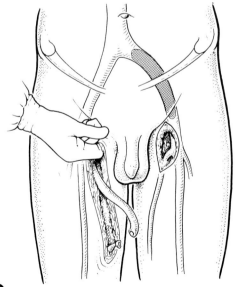

7b

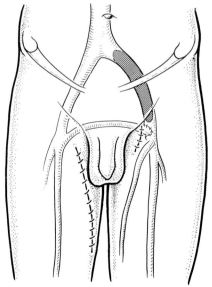

7c

Saphenopopliteal bypass

8a, b Candidates for this procedure must have a patent popliteal vein with an intact long saphenous vein of adequate calibre. A medial skin incision is made in the lower part of the thigh along the course of the long saphenous vein, which is exposed in a manner similar to that for femoropopliteal vein bypass. Following this, the popliteal vein is exposed through a longitudinal incision medially below the knee.

The popliteal vein is dissected free from the popliteal artery. A complete circumferential dissection is often difficult and not needed. For anastomosis, only an adequate portion of the anterior surface of the vein, allowing the placement of a partial occluding clamp, is exposed. The popliteal vein is palpated to ensure that it is patent to act as the origin of a bypass.

Dissection of the long saphenous vein is continued, following the course of the vein above the knee onto the calf wound. Once an adequate length is achieved, the vein is dissected free from the bed and transected. The vein may need gentle dilatation because of spasm during the dissection. The vein is tunnelled through the popliteal space between the heads of the gastrocnemius muscles. Placement of the saphenous vein through the anatomical channel prevents kinking and provides a better angle for the distal anastomosis. After systemic heparinization, a partial occluding clamp is applied to the popliteal vein and the saphenous vein is anastomosed in an end-to-side manner.

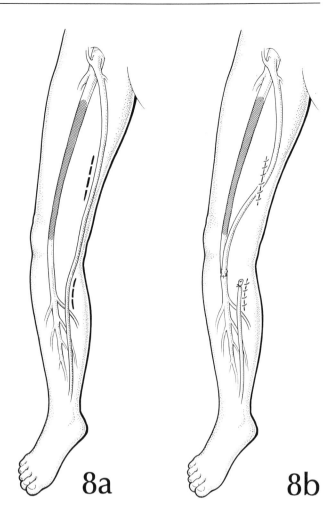

8a

8b

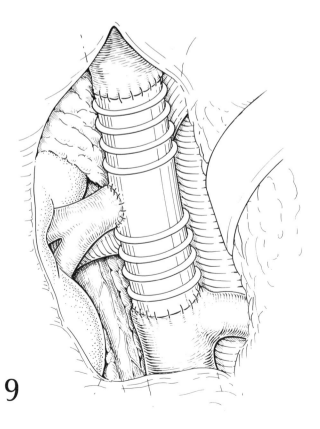

9

Vena caval bypass

Bypass grafting for vena caval occlusion is seldom performed for thrombosis. Vena caval bypass is often needed to restore continuity for tumour invasion of the vena cava by renal cell carcinoma or primary vena caval tumour, such as leiomyosarcoma. Because of the size of the vena cava, prosthetic grafts, e.g. PTFE ring-reinforced grafts, are preferable to autogenous vein grafts

9 The vena cava is best approached by a midline incision. The hepatic flexure of the right colon is dissected free and reflected to the left. By Kocherizing the duodenum medially, the vena cava is now in full view. After the extent of the tumour involvement has been determined, particularly its location in relation to right or left renal vein, it is resected together with the involved vena cava. An external ring-reinforced PTFE graft matching the size of the vena cava is sutured in an end-to-end manner. If one of the renal veins lies in the vicinity of the resection, the renal vein is reattached to the PTFE graft end to side.

VENOUS ANEURYSM SURGERY

Venous aneurysm is uncommon. With the increasing use of duplex ultrasonography in the diagnosis of deep vein thrombosis, there has been an increase in reports of venous aneurysm of the popliteal vein. The venous aneurysm can serve as the source of pulmonary emboli. If uncovered, these aneurysms will require resection.

Resection of venous aneurysm with interposed vein graft

10a, b The technique is simple. Depending on the location shown by venography, the popliteal venous aneurysm can be approached posteriorly. An S-shaped incision is made. The popliteal vein is dissected free from the neurovascular bundle. The aneurysm is resected, and the continuity of the vein is restored with an interposed panel vein graft constructed from the long saphenous vein. The interposed graft is anastomosed end to end.

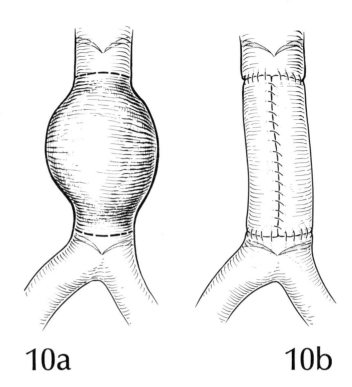

10a **10b**

Postoperative care

Wound haematoma can cause graft occlusion as a result of compression, and postoperative heparin must therefore be given with great caution. Other antithrombotic agents, such as dextran 40, may be preferable. The authors have also found the use of a mechanical compression pump to be helpful, and perhaps this should be considered as part of routine postoperative care. The pump is used until the patient is fully ambulatory. Thereafter, the patient should be fitted for an elastic support stocking with a pressure gradient of 30–40 mmHg. Many patients have a history of venous thrombosis, and therefore long-term warfarin should be instituted during the immediate postoperative period. For evaluation of graft patency the availability of duplex ultrasonography, particularly the colour-encoded imager, has been helpful. Venography is used when the results of duplex scanning are in doubt.

References

1. Palma EC, Riss F, Del Campo F, Tobler H. Tratamiento de los trastornos postflebiticos mediante anastomosis venosa safeno-femoral controlateral. *Bull Soc Surg Uruguay* 1958; 29: 135–45.

2. Dale WA. Chronic iliofemoral venous occlusion including seven cases of crossover vein grafting. *Surgery* 1966; 59: 117–32.

3. Husni EA. Venous reconstruction in postphlebitic disease. *Circulation* 1971; 43(Suppl 1): 147–50.

4. Gruss JD. Venous bypass for chronic venous insufficiency. In: Bergan JJ, Yao JST, eds. *Venous Disorders*. Philadelphia: WB Saunders, 1991: 316–30.

5. May R. Der Femoralisbypass beim prostthrombotischen zustandsbild. *Vasa* 1972; 1: 267.

Venous valve surgery

Robert L. Kistner MD
Department of Vascular Surgery, Straub Clinic and Hospital, Honolulu and Clinical Professor of Surgery, University of Hawaii, USA

History

Internal venous valve repair is illustrated by the original transvalvular technique that was first performed in 1968 and is still practised as the author's choice for primary valve incompetence. This technique was altered by Raju[1] to a supravalvular approach and later by Sottiurai[2] to a supravalvular approach with a vertical limb to the valve sinus.

The external valve repair is illustrated by the external suture method introduced in 1987. Variations of external repair are done by external banding with prosthetic material and by angioscopic guidance of externally placed sutures.

The procedures for treatment of secondary valve incompetence illustrated in this chapter are the transplantation of a valve-containing arm vein segment and the transposition procedure.

Principles and justification

Surgery of the venous valve is used to correct proximal reflux of the deep veins in patients with severe chronic venous insufficiency. The importance of adding treatment of deep vein reflux to established principles of managing saphenous and perforator vein incompetence in these patients has been increasingly recognized. Incompetence of the deep veins is now known to occur in primary and secondary forms; the surgical management of these conditions is quite different and will be addressed in this chapter.

Indications

The candidate for venous valve surgery is the person whose venous insufficiency symptoms prevent a normal way of life and in whom simpler surgical and non-surgical measures are not effective. The limiting symptoms may be aching, swelling, stasis changes or ulceration, or any combination of these. When the full venous examination demonstrates primary or secondary incompetence states that can be surgically improved by direct valve repair or by transposition or transplant techniques, good results can be anticipated in about 70% of patients. The long-term results are better in primary valve incompetence than in the post-thrombotic problems, as judged by current reporting.

Patients with primary valve incompetence have repairable valves that can be managed by direct valvular surgery. The patients with secondary valve incompetence have had previous thrombophlebitis followed by recanalization; the valves are destroyed and cannot be repaired and these patients require transposition or transplantation techniques rather than direct repair to restore proximal competence.

Primary valve incompetence

In patients with primary valve incompetence the normal valve architecture is preserved but the valve function is lost because the upper leading edge of the valve cusp becomes elongated (stretched) and prolapses under stress from above. In some cases the veins appear dilated and have thin, weak walls. Competence can be restored with valvuloplasty techniques. Valvuloplasty can now be performed by one of several internal (inside the vein) or external (outside the vein) techniques that have been described recently.

Secondary valve incompetence

In patients with secondary valve incompetence it is not possible to repair the valves that have been distorted by phlebitis, but proximal reflux can be controlled by transposition of the upper end of the refluxing vein segment into an adjacent segment with a competent valve, or by transplantation of a vein that contains a competent valve from the upper extremity into the area of reflux in the lower extremity.

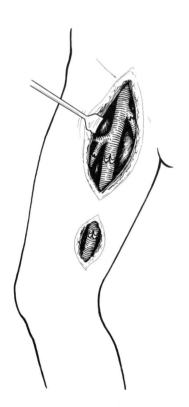

1

Preoperative

The preoperative examination requires a thorough evaluation of the venous history and its physical manifestations. Venous Doppler examination provides an excellent screening mechanism.

Physiological study of the veins is used to identify the dysfunction as a venous problem and helps to differentiate obstruction from incompetence. Differential venous pressures, air plethysmography and photoplethysmographic techniques are the current most helpful tests. Imaging with duplex ultrasonography provides anatomical and functional information about patency and valve function.

Ascending phlebography demonstrates patency of axial veins and the state of competence of the perforator veins in the calf. Descending phlebography is needed to identify accurately proximal valve sites and their state of competence. The descending phlebogram differentiates the leaking valve of primary valve incompetence from the deformed or destroyed valve of the post-thrombotic (secondary valve incompetence) state.

Operations

INTERNAL VALVE REPAIR: TRANSVALVULAR TECHNIQUE

Incision

1 Vertical incisions are used to provide proximal and distal access for control of the vein and for exploration of other areas when the intended valve is not repairable. The usual repair is performed in the highest valve of the superficial femoral vein which requires dissection of the superficial, deep and common femoral veins to provide proximal and distal access. Adjacent repairs in the deep femoral vein or the distal valves of the superficial femoral vein may also be undertaken. When a distal valve in the superficial femoral vein is to be repaired, a vertical thigh incision is made in the appropriate area. The popliteal vein may be exposed for repair by a medial popliteal incision for the high popliteal vein or the patient can be turned prone for an S-shaped incision in the posterior aspect of the popliteal space.

Exposure of valve and placement of marking suture

2 When the vein is exposed, the valve position is identified as a bulbous protrusion. The line of insertion of the valve cusp around the circumference of the vein is identified by careful dissection of the adventitia. This is seen as a white line around the circumference of the vein that leads to the commissures anteriorly and posteriorly. A marking suture is placed in the apex of the commissure on the anterior aspect of the vein. This marking suture is a key step in guiding the line of the venotomy between the valve cusps.

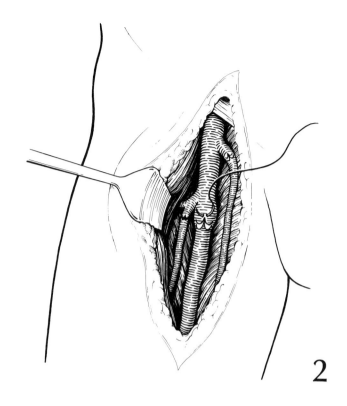

2

Venotomy

3 The venotomy begins 3 cm inferior to and on a direct line with the marking suture at the valve commissure. Traction sutures are placed in the vein wall. Working through the venotomy, the valve cusps are flattened against the side walls by expressing the blood contained in their sinuses, and the venotomy is advanced carefully up to and through the marking suture. The marking suture is cut in the line of the incision and the incision extended proximally into the cephalad portion of the vein for an additional 3 cm. With this technique the vein may be opened directly through the commissure and one may reliably avoid cutting the valve cusp during the venotomy. Traction sutures of 6/0 are placed in the lateral walls above and below the valve cusp to maintain exposure of the valve.

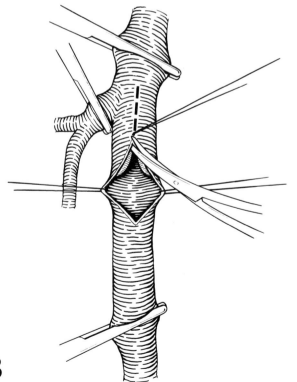

3

Opened vein with floppy valve and first suture

4 With the venotomy complete, the vein is laid open and the valve cusps are inspected. In primary valve incompetence the bicuspid valve is seen to have floppy cusps which usually lie in folds across the opened face of the vein. The cusp itself is gossamer-thin, pliable and shows no evidence of scarring or previous inflammation. When the leading edge of the valve cusp is teased from side to side it will be seen to be redundant and elongated: it is this stretched leading edge that prolapses under load and gives rise to reflux when the patient is erect.

The repair consists of shortening the leading edge of the cusp to the proper length. A 7/0 monofilament suture is introduced from outside to the inside of the vein at the apex of the medial valve commissure.

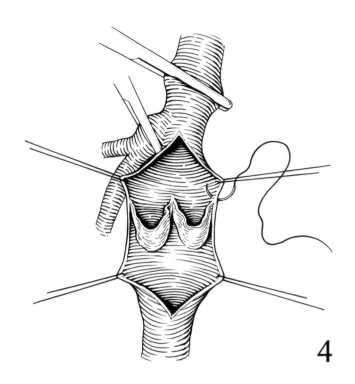

Completing first suture of cusp

5 Once inside the vein, the needle is reversed to engage the leading edge of the cusp 2 mm from its insertion site into the vein wall. This edge is advanced up to the level of the commissure and the needle is passed from the inside to the outside of the vein wall. The suture is tied outside the vein wall. The effect of this suture is to shorten the leading edge of the cusp by 2–3 mm. The repair is performed under magnification.

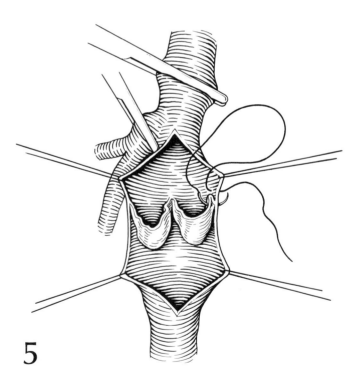

Multiple sutures of cusp

6 Multiple interrupted sutures have been placed in the medial and lateral commissure angles of the open vein to progressively shorten the leading edge of the cusp. Successive sutures may be placed until the leading edge has been sufficiently shortened on each side. In the posterior midline, a single suture introduced at the commissure from outside the vein can engage both valve cusps. Once both cusps have been included in the suture, it is passed from inside the vein to the outside at the upper extent of the commissure and tied outside the vein. The number of sutures that need to be placed at each commissure varies with the individual case but is usually 1–4; the total number of sutures usually required to effect valve repair is 6–10.

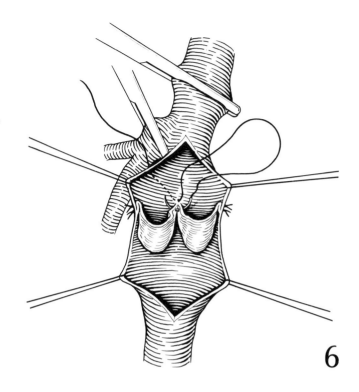

Completion of repair and beginning of closure

7 Interrupted sutures are placed in the commissure angles until the leading edge of the valve cusp lies gently across the face of the vein. The cusp should be free of wrinkles and folds, but it should not be drawn taut. The cusps should be irrigated with heparinized saline to judge the proper degree of shortening of the cusps. It is important that the two cusps lie in the same horizontal plane so that the leading edges of the valve will be level. Closure of the vein begins with a suture that joins the highest point of the medial commissure to the highest point of the lateral commissure. This aligns the valve cusps in the horizontal plane and recreates the anterior commissure.

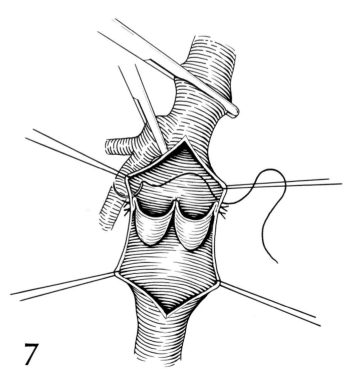

Venotomy closure

8 Closure of the venotomy proceeds from the newly closed anterior commissure cephalad and from the newly closed commissure caudad, using continuous running 6/0 monofilament suture.

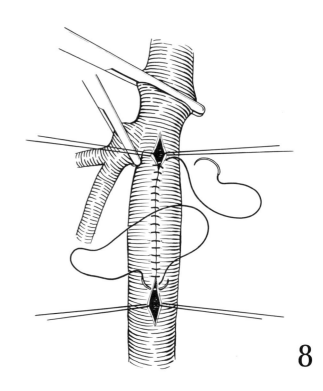

8

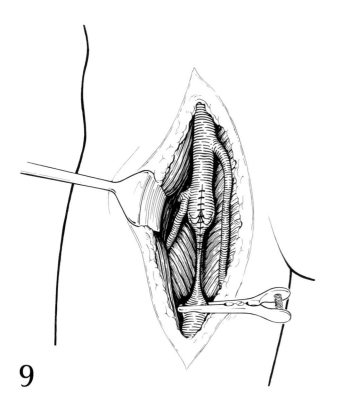

9

Strip test to demonstrate competent valve

9 After closure of the venotomy, valve competence is accurately assessed by clamping the distal vein and stripping the blood up through the valve. With the clamps removed from the proximal vein, competence of the valve is proven when the blood fills the valve cusps but does not reflux back though the valve. Pressure may be applied from above to test the totality of valve competence. In a successful repair the valve will not allow reflux even when strong pressure is manually applied from above.

EXTERNAL VALVE REPAIR

The restoration of valve competence by techniques on the outside of the vein has been termed external repair. This can be achieved by placing materials around the leaking valve and compressing the vein until it becomes competent, as in the case of the Silastic 'venocuff' devised by Lane. An external suture method has been developed that will reliably produce valve competence, and is described below. External methods do not require anticoagulation of the patient, they are quicker than internal repair, and require less dissection of the vein. However, they do not provide precise anatomical repair of the valve cusp defect causing the incompetence.

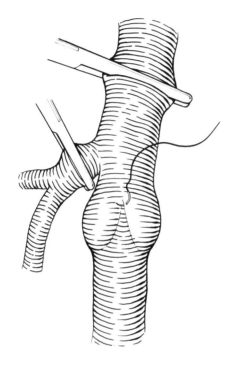

10

Exposure of valve and first suture

10 The skin incision to provide exposure for external repair is similar to that for internal repair. With the vein valve exposed, it is necessary to clear the adventitia and fully expose the line of valve cusp insertion leading up to the commissures on both the front and back of the vein.

Valve competence may be restored by placing a series of sutures along the lines of insertion of the valve cusp as these lines diverge from the apex of the commissure. The first suture is placed just below the commissure. This suture grasps each cusp margin separately and invaginates the vein wall tissue between the margins. The repair is effected by a series of interrupted sutures or an over-and-over running suture, using 6/0 monofilament material.

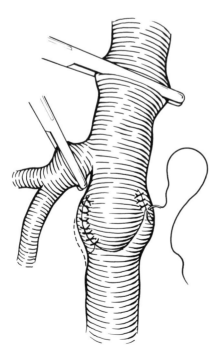

11

Suture of anterior and posterior commissures

11 Sutures are placed in both the anterior and posterior commissures and carried down the vein until the valve becomes competent by the strip test. This usually requires 6–8 interrupted sutures along each commissure. The strip test is performed repeatedly as the sutures are placed until the valve becomes competent.

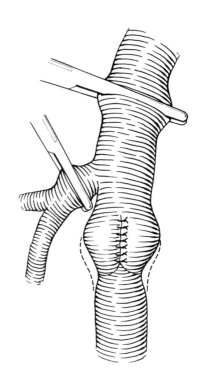

Completion of repair

12 The effect is a mild narrowing (20–30%) of the vein circumference at the bottom of the suture line, which is not a haemodynamically significant stenosis.

12

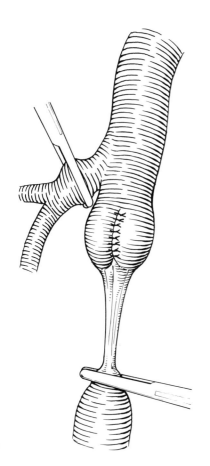

13 The result of the external technique is a fully competent valve, as demonstrated by the strip test.

13

TRANSPLANTATION OF VALVED VEIN SEGMENT

Incision and harvest of arm vein

14a, b Transplantation of vein segments containing a competent valve is used in secondary valve incompetence where the phlebitis has destroyed the lower extremity vein valves. The axillary brachial vein is a good donor site for the valved vein segment because it is readily accessible and can be removed without causing disability in the arm. The axillary vein is harvested through a longitudinal incision in the upper arm on its medial aspect. The valve should be checked for competence with the strip test before the segment is harvested. The vein transplant is placed in the leg in the superficial femoral vein or the popliteal vein. The leg incision is vertical in the upper thigh for the superficial femoral vein, or in the lower medial thigh if the vein segment is to be placed in the upper popliteal vein. An alternative is to place the transplant into the lower popliteal vein through a posterior popliteal approach by way of an S-shaped incision in the popliteal space with the patient prone.

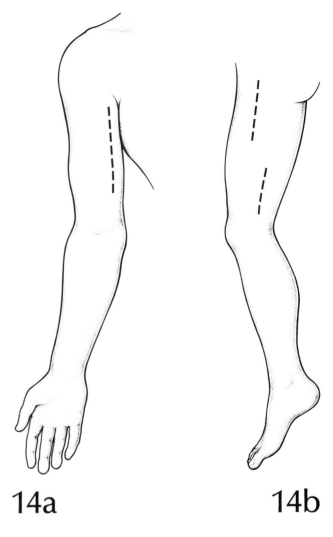

14a   **14b**

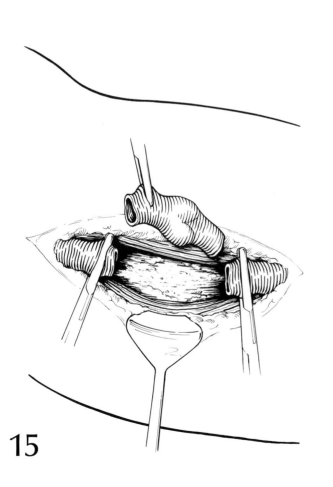

15

Valve insertion

15 The transected recanalized leg vein is carefully inspected to choose the correct lumen because its vein may be occupied by longitudinal septae and have more than one apparent lumen at the site of transection. Exploration of the proximal vein with an uninflated balloon catheter may help to determine which lumen to use for the anastomosis.

Proximal anastomosis

16 The transplanted segment must be sewn in without tension; interrupted sutures of 6/0 monofilament provide optimal lumen size. The proximal anastomosis is performed first so that the surgeon can check the valve function immediately by releasing the proximal clamp.

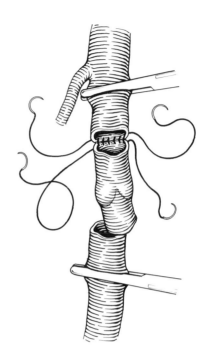

16

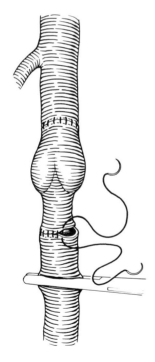

17

Distal anastomosis

17 The distal anastomosis is performed with interrupted sutures. Particular attention to proper length of the segment is necessary to avoid both tension and redundancy in the transplanted segment. Rotational orientation of the distal anastomosis is aided by distension of the proximal vein by release of proximal clamps after the proximal anastomosis is completed.

The tendency for these valved transplants to dilate and become incompetent has led some surgeons to place a wrap of polytetrafluoroethylene or Dacron around the transplant segment.

Wound closure

The wound may be closed with suction drainage.

TRANSPOSITION OPERATION

A transposition operation is useful for patients with post-thrombotic destruction of the valves of the superficial femoral veins but who have a competent valve in adjacent deep femoral or long saphenous vein segments.

Incision

18 The incision is a longitudinal upper thigh approach which provides exposure of the common, superficial and deep femoral veins and the upper long saphenous vein.

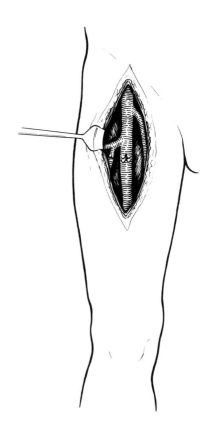

18

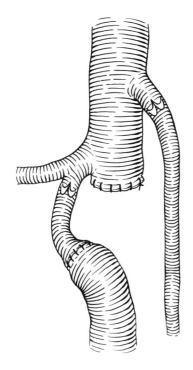

19

End-to-end transposition of superficial and deep femoral veins

19 The recanalized superficial femoral vein segment is transected at its junction with the common femoral vein and the transected cephalad end is oversewn flush with the common femoral vein. The distal superficial femoral vein may then be joined end-to-end to the normally valved deep femoral or long saphenous vein to provide proximal valve competence. Interrupted suture using 6/0 monofilament is advisable.

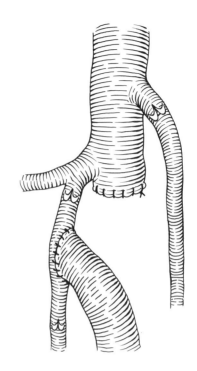

End-to-side transposition of superficial and deep femoral veins

20 When the deep femoral vein has competent proximal and distal valves, an end-to-side anastomosis may be used to place the end of the diseased incompetent superficial femoral vein into the side of the deep femoral vein. The advantage of this technique is that the distal deep femoral vein does not need to be ligated and may be left in its normal anatomic position.

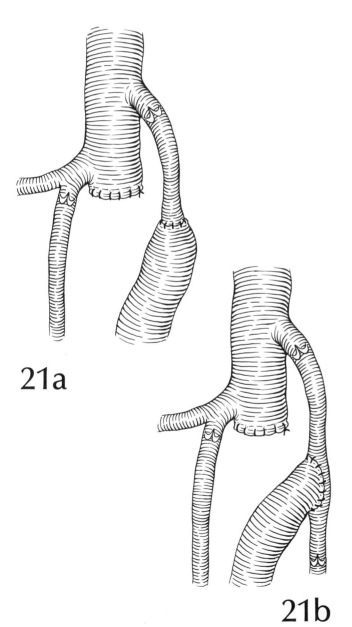

21a

21b

Transposition of superficial femoral and long saphenous veins

21a, b The superficial femoral vein may be placed end-to-end or end-to-side to the long saphenous vein if it has a better valve than in the deep femoral vein. However, late valve fatigue is more common in the long saphenous vein than in the deep femoral vein, and for this reason transposition to the latter is preferred

Transposition of deep femoral to long saphenous vein

22 Occasionally the superficial femoral vein is occluded and the deep femoral vein has severe reflux that communicates via large collaterals into the popliteal vein. In this case, if there is a competent valve in the long saphenous vein, the deep femoral vein may be transposed into the proximal long saphenous vein.

Postoperative care

Transvalvular technique

The operation is performed under heparin anticoagulation and a conservative intravenous heparin regimen is continued for the first 48 h after surgery, followed by dextran, 500 ml daily, for 3 days. After 3 days the anticoagulant is ceased in patients with primary valve incompetence; in those with an element of post-thrombotic disease of the distal vein, treatment with warfarin is continued for 3 months. With this regimen, postoperative thrombophlebitis is a very rare complication. Any haematoma is promptly evacuated in the operating theatre.

Patients are encouraged to walk on the second postoperative day and to leave hospital on the fifth day, unless wound healing becomes a problem. The ulcers and pain usually heal rapidly. On discharge from hospital patients are instructed to wear elastic support to the knee.

Transplantation

Anticoagulants are continued postoperatively in the form of heparin for 48–72 h and coumadin for 3 months, because these patients are prone to deep vein thrombosis. Ambulation is begun on the second postoperative day. Wound haematomas may occur in the anticoagulated patient and should be aggressively treated by evacuation as soon as they are found.

Transposition procedure

Heparin anticoagulation is continued for 48 h, during which time the patient is regulated on warfarin and warfarin treatment is maintained for 3 months. If this degree of anticoagulation results in wound haematomas they should be evacuated immediately. The closure of the wound with suction drainage may help to minimize postoperative bleeding.

Although the potential for later development of recurrent thrombophlebitis is a constant danger in patients with post-thrombotic valve destruction, the incidence of postoperative thrombophlebitis has been low.

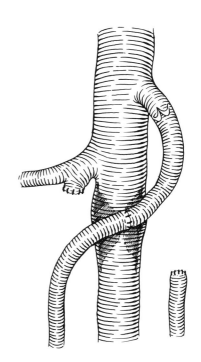

22

Outcome

Transvalvular technique

Long-term results at 4 years and beyond are good to excellent in 70% of patients. About 30% of patients are able to discard their elastic support stocking even at full activity, and have remained asymptomatic for long-term follow-up beyond 10 years.

External repair

This technique gives excellent early results but the long-term effects at 4 years and beyond are not known because it was first performed only in 1987. As this technique is not an anatomical repair there may be a greater chance for recurrence than with the internal repair. The external repair technique can be used to reinforce an internal repair or as an adjunctive repair on additional valves after internal repair of the first valve by those who do not feel secure in using it as the first choice for valve repair.

A newly described technique of external repair by an angioscopically directed external suture makes it possible to perform an anatomical repair of the valve without opening the vein. The results of this method in long-term follow-up are awaited.

Transplantation

Early healing of ulceration and reversal of chronic venous insufficiency may be anticipated in appropriately selected patients. Late recurrence may occur in 30–60% of patients, but many of these are due to new collateral and perforator problems and can be treated by simple secondary procedures. Long-term primary control of chronic venous insufficiency can be expected in 40% of cases, and subsequent peripheral perforator or superficial interruptions will correct recurrences in an additional 25% of cases.

Transposition

Early clinical results are often dramatic with rapid healing of the distal ulcerations and relief of the aching, swelling and stasis changes in the lower leg. The results at 4 years and beyond show a 40–60% incidence of recurrence and ulceration with the passage of time. This may be due to recurrent valve incompetence or to the appearance of perforator or collateral vein reflux in the extremity. In patients who develop recurrence a careful assessment will often define a peripheral interruption that will restore a good result for an additional significant period of time.

References

1. Raju S. Valvuloplasty and valve transfer. *Inter Angio* 1985; 4: 419–24.

2. Sottiurai VS. Technique in direct venous valvuloplasty. *J Vasc Surg* 1988; 8: 646–8.

Further reading

Eriksson I, Almgren B. Influence of the profunda femoris vein on venous hemodynamics of the limb: experience from thirty-one deep vein valve reconstructions. *J Vasc Surg* 1986; 4: 390–5.

Ferris EB, Kistner RL. Femoral vein reconstruction in the management of chronic venous insufficiency: a 14 year experience. *Arch Surg* 1982; 117: 1571–9.

Gloviczki P, Merrell SW, Bower TC. Femoral vein valve repair under direct vision without venotomy: a modified technique with use of angioscopy. *J Vasc Surg* 1991; 14: 645–8.

Jessup G, Lane RJ. Repair of incompetent venous valves: a new technique. *J Vasc Surg* 1988; 8: 569–75.

Kistner R. Surgical technique of external venous valve repair. *The Straub Foundation Proceedings* 1990; 55: 15–16.

Kistner RL, Ferris EB. Technique of surgical reconstruction of femoral vein valves. In: Bergan JJ, Yao JST, eds. *Operative Techniques in Vascular Surgery*. New York: Grune and Stratton, 1980: 291–300.

Nicolaides AN, Christopaulos DC. Methods of quantitation of chronic venous insufficiency. In: Bergan JJ, Yao JST, eds. *Venous Disorders*. Philadelphia: WB Saunders, 1991: 77–91.

O'Donnell TF. Popliteal vein valve transplantation for deep venous valvular reflux: rationale, method, and long-term clinical, hemodynamic, and anatomic results. In: Bergan JJ, Yao JST, eds. *Venous Disorders*. Philadelphia: WB Saunders, 1991: 273–95.

Raju S, Fredricks R. Valve reconstruction procedures for non-obstructive venous insufficiency: rationale, techniques, and results in 107 procedures with two-to-eight year follow-up. *J Vasc Surg* 1988; 7: 301–10.

Taheri SA, Pendergast DR, Lazar E *et al*. Vein valve transposition. *Am J Surg* 1985; 150: 201–2.

Valve reconstruction for primary valve insufficiency. In: Bergan JJ, Kistner RL, eds. *Atlas of Venous Surgery*. Philadelphia: WB Saunders, 1992: 125–33.

Operations for varicose veins

C. V. Ruckley MB, ChM, FRCS(Ed), FRCPE
Professor of Vascular Surgery, University of Edinburgh, and Consultant Surgeon, Vascular Surgery Unit, Royal Infirmary, Edinburgh, UK

Principles and justification

Pathology of venous disease

1a, b Approximately 20% of the adult population have chronic venous disease. Primary varicose veins constitute the great majority and these are mainly of the 'stem' type, the principal incompetent channel being the long or short saphenous vein, or both. In the face of proximal valvular incompetence the thin-walled tributaries draining into these stems form typical variceal patterns. They have a familial tendency and usually become conspicuous in early adult life or even earlier. The valvular dysfunction is believed to be secondary to structural deficiencies in the vein walls.

A variety of pathological processes may either damage valves or obstruct venous outflow and thereby promote the development of secondary varicose veins. Most are due to deep vein thrombosis, but other conditions include pelvic masses, enlarged lymph nodes, bony displacements and tricuspid incompetence.

The pattern of post-thrombotic secondary varicose veins is determined by the site and extent of the original thrombosis and the relative predominance of obstruction or valve imcompetence. Secondary varicose veins, however, tend to be associated with deep vein reflux, incompetent perforators and the skin changes of chronic venous insufficiency, whereas only a minority of patients with primary varicose veins progresses to chronic venous insufficiency.

Chronic venous insufficiency is the syndrome resulting from continuous venous hypertension in the erect posture, whether stationary or exercising, in contrast to the normal individual in whom the superficial venous pressure falls with contraction of the calf muscles. Chronic venous insufficiency consists of postural discomfort, swelling, varicose veins and the changes in skin and subcutaneous tissues collectively known as lipodermatosclerosis: pigmentation, inflammation, induration, eczema and ulceration.

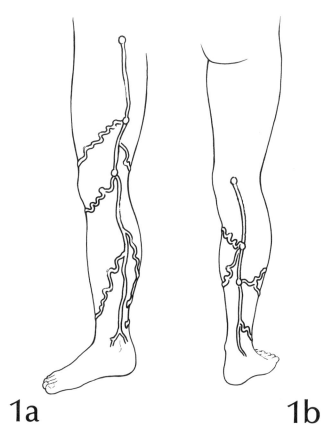

1a　　　　　　　　　　　　　　**1b**

About one-third of patients with chronic venous insufficiency have incompetence of the superficial veins with or without perforator incompetence, a further one-third have added incompetence of the deep system, and one-third have evidence of previous deep vein thrombosis rendering the deep veins obliterated, or incompetent, or both. The term post-thrombotic syndrome should be reserved for the last group.

2   Varices of atypical distribution may be a feature of congenital venous anomalies, the best known of which are the Klippel–Trenaunay syndrome (varicose veins, cutaneous naevus, soft tissue and bone hypertrophy) and the Parkes–Weber syndrome, in which the varices and overgrowth are due to multiple, diffuse arteriovenous fistulae.

Venous flares or spider naevi are common, particularly in women, but are not a suitable subject for surgery. The same applies to the unusually conspicuous but non-varicose veins, the so-called athlete's veins, which sometimes worry young, lean, well-muscled men who have very little subcutaneous fat.

3   Vulval and perineal varices occur in women associated with pregnancy and pelvic inflammatory disease. They may cause discomfort before menstruation or during coitus. They commonly diminish after pregnancy. These varices, which drain into the internal iliac or gonadal systems, extend as multiple channels down the medial aspect of the thigh from the perineum.

Management of varicose veins

Varicose veins are a condition of progressive deterioration. Nevertheless, the high proportions of patients with recurrent or residual varicose veins after operation and of patients who, despite treatment, progress to chronic venous insufficiency and recurrent ulcers, testify to the deficiencies in management of chronic venous disease in general and of varicose veins in particular. This is partly a reflection of poor-quality care and partly due to the fact that the condition is too common and the workload too great for effective care to be provided for all who need it under a state-funded health care system.

Varicose veins should be treated by experienced surgeons who are fully conversant with the anatomical variations so common in the venous system, and who are willing and able to allocate the time and care necessary to achieve satisfactory, long-lasting results.

The first essential is careful preoperative assessment, employing vascular laboratory techniques and radiology in the more complex cases. The surgery must be thorough and must deal with all sites of major reflux from deep to superficial systems in the groin, thigh and calf. Treatment does not end with the operation. Despite careful surgery a proportion of patients will have residual varices or will develop new sites of incompetence. They should therefore be followed up, and any persisting or recurring veins dealt with by sclerotherapy.

Follow-up sclerotherapy should be regarded as an intrinsic part of the surgical treatment of varices, and patients should be clearly informed of this before operation.

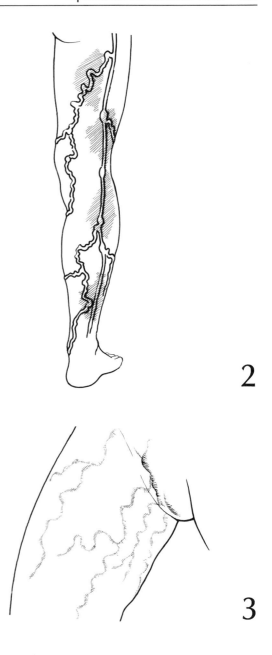

2

3

Indications

Varicose surgery is performed: (1) to relieve symptoms; (2) for cosmetic reasons; (3) for prophylaxis; and (4) to reverse skin changes and effect ulcer healing.

Many varicose vein operations are quite justifiably performed on cosmetic grounds. It is unusual for varices to give rise to distinct pain, although tiredness, heaviness and swelling in the leg are common, as is an aching discomfort in distended veins. An important factor in the minds of many surgeons is prevention, as the natural history is one of progressive deterioration, progressing in a minority of cases to the skin manifestations of chronic venous insufficiency. Varicose veins also predispose to phlebitis, deep vein thrombosis and bleeding in the event of trauma.

Preoperative

Assessment

Preoperative assessment is crucial to the success of varicose vein surgery, and so should be done by the surgeon who is to perform the operation. Some patients with uncomplicated primary varices who are lean and in whom the variceal pattern is easily traced do not require any special investigations, other than those required to assess general fitness for surgery and suitability for day care. Recurrent or residual varicose veins, however, are often the result of saphenofemoral and/or saphenopopliteal incompetence being missed at the original preoperative assessment. Logically, the more frequent deployment of additional investigations should promote more effective surgery and fewer recurrences.

Examination

4 The limb is examined in a good light, with the patient standing on a cloth-covered elevated platform in a warm room, a few minutes being allowed for the veins to distend fully. The leg being examined should be slightly flexed at hip and knee to allow superficial venous filling. Common sites of superficial valvular incompetence give rise to typical distributions of varices. Knowledge of these, verified by palpation and percussion along the line of the vein, allows the varicose venous tree to be fully marked without any further tests in the great majority of cases.

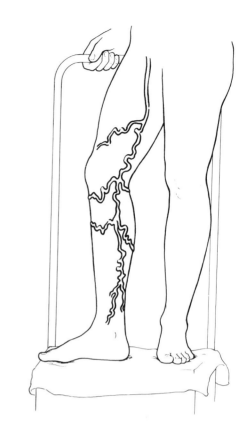

4

Testing for reflux

5a–c Levels of deep-to-superficial reflux can also be verified by the application of venous tourniquets, applied with the patient supine and the leg elevated. On standing it becomes evident whether the tourniquet is controlling reflux or not, and by repeating the test with the tourniquet moved up or down the levels can be precisely identified. In a simpler form of this test, preferred by the author, suspected points of incompetence are controlled by the finger tips.

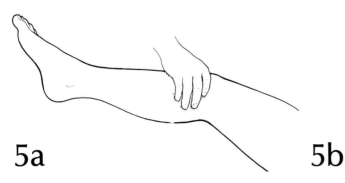

5a

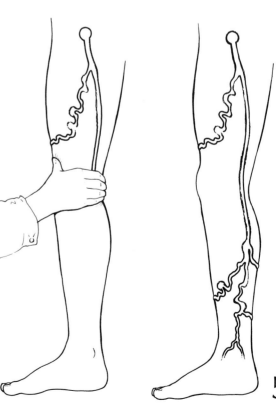

5b　　5c

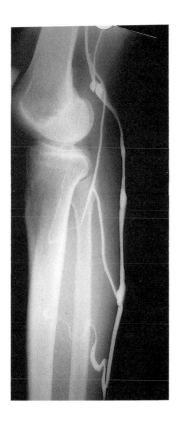

6

Short saphenous incompetence

6 In patients with short saphenous incompetence it is important, in view of the high frequency of anatomical variations in the area, to detect accurately the point at which the saphenous vein turns inwards to join the deep vein. In thin individuals this may be relatively obvious, and the use of Doppler ultrasonography may assist, but in many patients it is advisable to define the junction preoperatively with either duplex scanning or varicography.

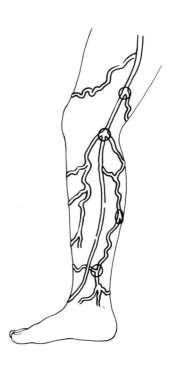

7

7 All varices in the thigh and calf are mapped out as parallel lines with an indelible marker, with specific marks for the sites of incompetent perforators and blow-outs. It is a useful precaution to ask the patient, before completing the marking, whether he or she is aware of any varices that have been missed.

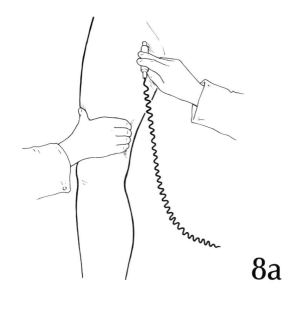

8a

8a, b The continuous wave hand-held Doppler ultrasonographic device will give useful information as to whether reflux is occurring in the region of the saphenofemoral or saphenopopliteal junctions and at suspected sites of perforators.

It is important to be aware, however, that although continuous wave Doppler ultrasonography will demonstrate the presence of reflux, it may not always be clear whether this is occurring in the deep or the superficial veins. Where there is remaining doubt as to the existence of saphenofemoral or saphenopopliteal incompetence, or where it is difficult to distinguish between varices feeding from thigh perforators and incompetence in the groin or perineum, duplex colour-coded scanning and/or varicography become essential.

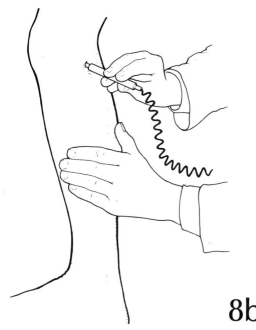

8b

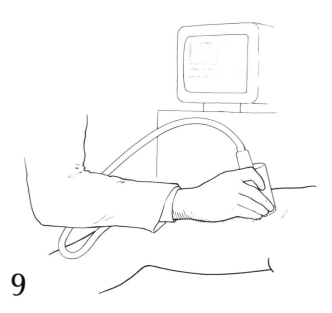

9

9 Colour-coded duplex scanning may be taken as the reference standard for delineating venous anatomy and function at the present time and should be frequently deployed as a guide to accurate varicose vein surgery.

The particular place of varicography is in the investigation of recurrent varices, where it has the advantage of displaying the anatomy as a guide to dissection in the operating theatre.

Operations

SAPHENOFEMORAL LIGATION

This is not an operation for the inexperienced, unsupervised surgeon, for two principal reasons. First, the recurrence of varices due to inadequately performed saphenofemoral ligation is very common. Secondly, the risk of damage to the femoral artery or vein in the groin, with serious consequences for the patient and medicolegal consequences for the surgeon, is considerable.

Anaesthesia and position of patient

10 The operation is performed under epidural anaesthesia, and unless only the short saphenous system requires attention, it begins with the patient supine and in the Trendelenburg position.

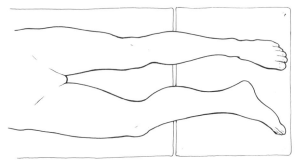

10

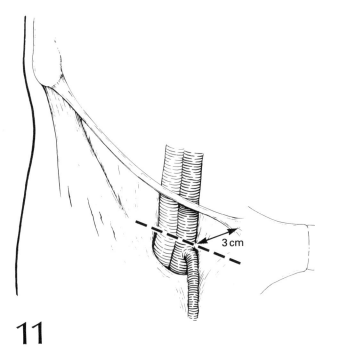

11

Incision

11 The knee is slightly flexed and rotated externally. The surface marking of the saphenofemoral junction is 3–4 cm below and lateral to the pubic tubercle. The incision is centred on this point and is made about 6–8 cm in length, in the skin crease below the inguinal ligament. As these incisions usually heal with a virtually invisible scar, a small incision is no advantage, and indeed is positively conducive to an unsatisfactory operation for reasons made clear below.

The incision is deepened through the membranous layer of the superficial fascia, until the long saphenous vein is encountered. A Travers self-retaining retractor is inserted.

Identification of the long saphenous vein

12 As anatomical variants are common and as in thin or heavily muscled individuals the femoral vein and artery may be close to the surface, the long saphenous vein is not divided until it has been unequivocally identified by sufficient dissection to ascertain the locations of the femoral artery and vein and to identify the saphenofemoral junction.

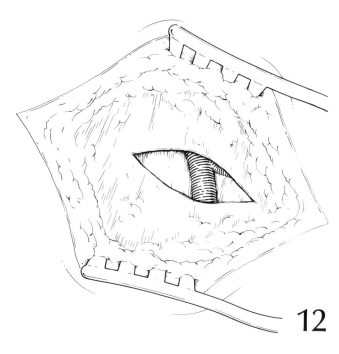

12

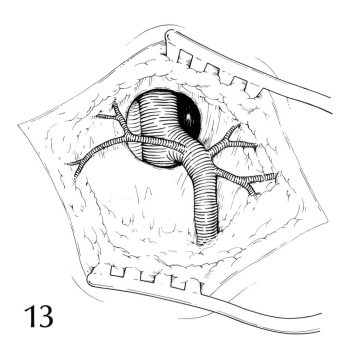

13

Saphenous tributaries

13 Expected tributaries are the superficial external pudenal, the superficial external iliac and superficial inferior epigastric veins, although variations are common. Each of these, when dissected out 2–3 cm from the point of junction with the saphenous vein, will be found to divide into two or more tributaries.

14 These subdivisions are individually ligated with 3/0 absorbable polyglactin (Vicryl) ligature or sealed by diathermy distally. If this dissection is not done and the tributaries are simply ligated where they join the long saphenous vein, there remains a network of superficial veins connecting the veins of the thigh with those of the perineum, the lower abdominal wall and the iliac region, thus promoting recurrence of varices.

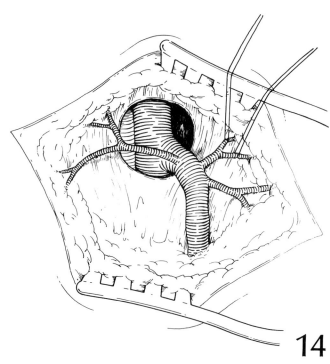

14

Dissection of the saphenofemoral junction

15a–c The long saphenous vein is divided and the upper end lifted up on Mayo's artery forceps, this manoeuvre greatly facilitating mobilization of tributaries and definition of the saphenofemoral junction. The upper end of the vein is mobilized with a pledget mounted on a haemostat, and the investing fascia is cleared from the vein with a DeBakey arterial dissecting forceps, great care being taken not to traumatize tributaries such as the deep external pudendal vein, which joins the femoral vein or the long saphenous vein itself on the medial side of the junction. The deep external pudendal vein is tied by passing a ligature round it. This must be done with care, as avulsion of this vessel followed by efforts to control the bleeding is a potential cause of femoral vein damage.

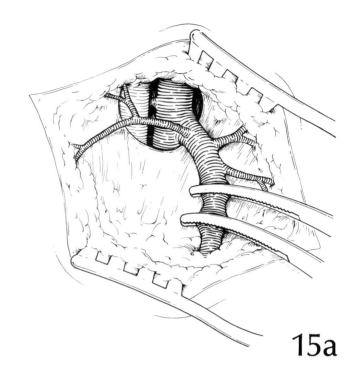

15a

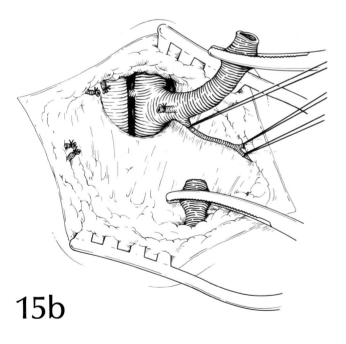

15b

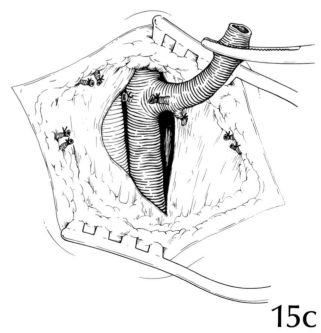

15c

16 To visualize the femoral vein below the junction it is usually necessary to divide the superficial external pudendal artery which crosses below the junction in the lower rim of the foramen ovale. At the end of this manoeuvre the junction plus 2–3 cm of the proximal and distal femoral vein should be clearly seen.

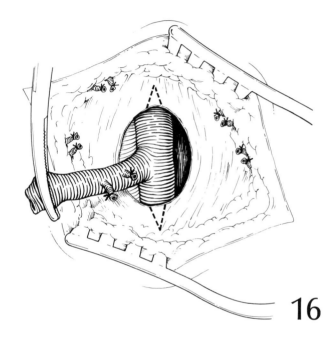

16

Anatomical variants

17a–c Common anatomical variants include: (*a*) double saphenous veins; (*b*) major thigh tributaries joining near the saphenofemoral junction and therefore readily mistaken for the main veins; and (*c*) major tributaries which, instead of joining the long saphenous vein, join the superficial external iliac or the superficial external pudendal veins.

These are all common causes of surgical error and must be sought. They are some of the reasons why a small incision is inappropriate for this part of the operation.

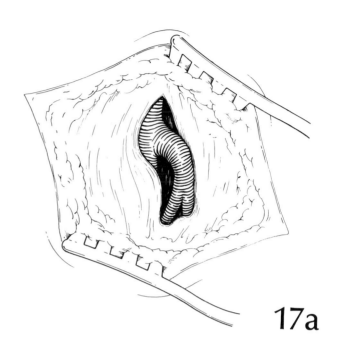

17a

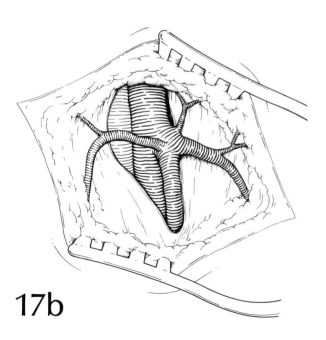

17b

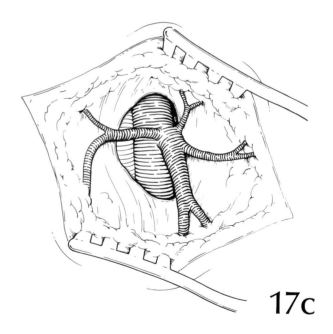

17c

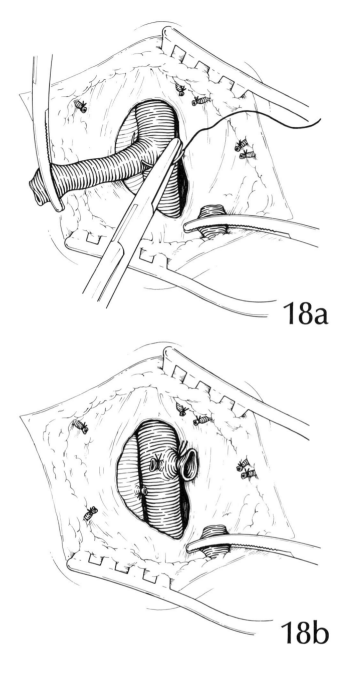

18a

18b

Flush ligation

18a, b The long saphenous vein is transfixed with a 3/0 polyglactin suture almost flush with the femoral vein, care being taken neither to tent up the latter nor to leave a blind sac. It is divided, the lower end being held in a haemostat.

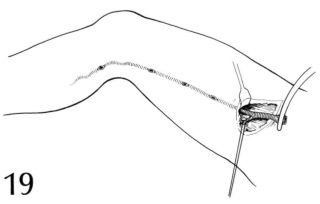

19

Upper thigh tributaries

19 The next step is to ligate the upper thigh tributaries. The self-retaining retractor is removed, the lower edge of the wound elevated by the assistant and the knee flexed. Traction is put on the saphenous vein, which is then mobilized down the thigh by finger dissection. By this means the posteromedial tributary and occasionally other tributaries can be reached through the groin incision. They are ligated with 2/0 polyglactin.

Removal of the thigh portion of long saphenous vein

In order to minimize the likelihood of recurrence, extirpation of the thigh portion of the long saphenous vein is advocated. It may be advisable to conserve the saphenous vein if the patient has risk factors for arterial disease, such as a strong family history of arterial disease, hypercholesterolaemia, diabetes, or smoking. As a generalization, however, the population of patients with varicose veins and the population prone to obliterative arterial disease tend to be two different groups.

Full-length stripping of the long saphenous vein has been abandoned in favour of thigh stripping, as no benefit is derived from stripping the calf portion and saphenous nerve damage in the calf has often been reported.

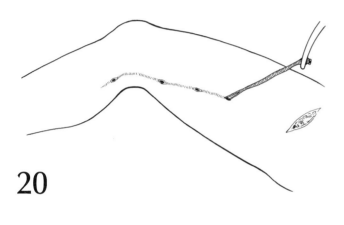

20

20 The author's practice is to remove the long saphenous vein from the groin to the main trifurcation, about 3–4 cm below the knee joint. This may be done without a stripper, through a series of small incisions about 10 cm apart through which the saphenous vein is extracted and the tributaries individually ligated. This method minimizes haematoma formation, allows the groin wound to be closed early and facilitates the performance of the remainder of the operation under tourniquet. It also avoids the not uncommon difficulty encountered in passing the stripper.

Traction on the saphenous vein from above allows it to be readily palpable through the skin. A 5–10-mm incision is made 10 cm below the groin and the vein hooked out. With care any local tributaries can be pulled to the surface and ligated. Serial incisions are made at intervals down to the upper calf and the steps repeated. At the 'goose's foot' trifurcation below the knee, the long saphenous vein is ligated and divided.

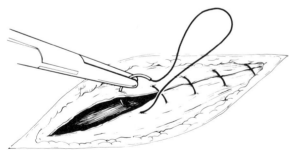

21a

Closure of thigh wounds

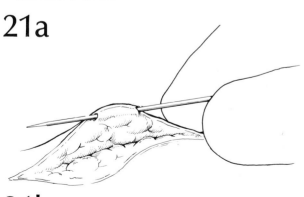

21b

21a, b At this stage all thigh wounds are closed. The groin wound is closed with subcutaneous and subcuticular synthetic absorbable sutures and the lower wounds can usually be closed simply with wound tapes. If any sutures are needed, 4/0 subcuticular polyglactin is employed. The remainder of the operation is conducted under tourniquet.

Phlebectomy

22 The removal of varices through multiple incisions (phlebectomy) is performed under tourniquet. The leg is elevated and exsanguinated by means of a pneumatic exsanguinator or a sterile Esmarch bandage, and a tourniquet is applied around the mid-thigh. This remains in place for the remainder of the operation and is only removed after the final bandage has been applied. The illustration shows a Lofqvist pneumatic tourniquet which is held in position by means of a small rubber wedge.

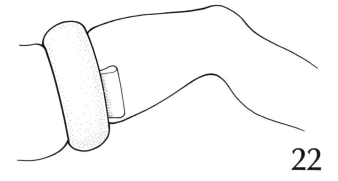

22

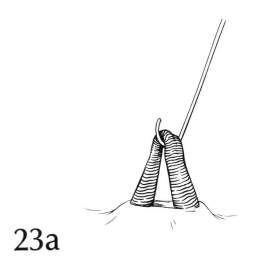

23a

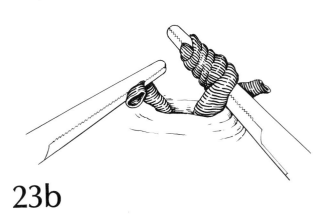

23b

23a, b Varices are removed through 5-mm incisions. These are placed at intervals of 5–10 cm along the lines of the veins, the aim being total removal of the underlying varices. As they are very tiny they can be either longitudinal or transverse. At each incision the vein is mobilized with a combination of fine instruments including a small phlebectomy hook and mosquito forceps and brought to the surface, freed from subcutaneous tissues and avulsed.

Perforators

A medial ankle venous flare or lipodermatosclerosis in the classical gaiter distribution are two signs that incompetent perforators are present and should be intercepted.

24a, b Perforators are approached through slightly larger incisions, sufficient to admit the tip of the little finger to palpate the point of passage of the perforator through the deep fascia where it is ligated flush.

Perforators embedded in areas of indurated lipodermatosclerosis cannot be dissected out and are dealt with by a subfascial approach as described below.

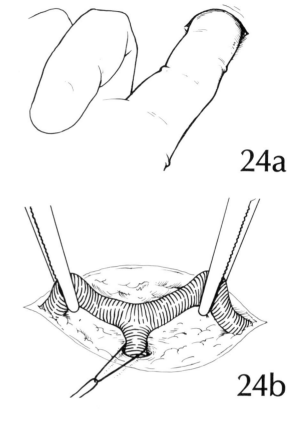

24a

24b

Wound closure

25 The majority of the wounds do not require any formal closure other than wound tapes. Larger ones are closed with subcuticular 4/0 synthetic absorbable sutures.

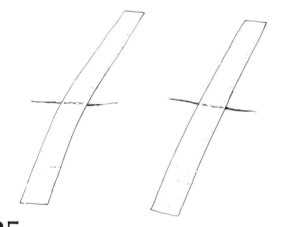

25

Bandaging

26 The leg is bandaged with a cohesive elastic bandage using a figure-of-eight technique over a layer of orthopaedic wool, before the tourniquet is released. The bandage begins at the base of the toes and is continued to the upper thigh. The foot is positioned at a right angle and the turns of the bandage are fashioned so as to allow flexion at the knee and ankle.

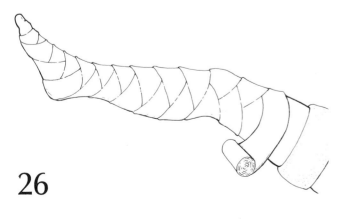

26

SHORT SAPHENOUS LIGATION

Position of patient

If no surgery to the long saphenous system is required, the patient is positioned prone after a tourniquet has been applied to the thigh. If it is part of a more extensive vein operation which is begun with the patient in the supine position, then it is the author's policy to close the thigh wounds, leave the tourniquet in position and turn and redrape the patient for the posterior approach. Some surgeons prefer to position the patient on one side, with the leg to be operated on uppermost and the other knee flexed. This, however, limits access if varices need to be followed onto the medial aspect.

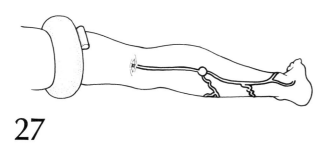

27

Incision

27 It is vital that the saphenopopliteal junction should have been accurately mapped out beforehand and incisions placed appropriately. If the junction is in its normal location 2–3 cm above the transverse skin crease, a transverse 3-cm incision placed in the crease is satisfactory. In about one-third of cases the junction is several centimetres higher, and in 15% of cases the short saphenous vein does not end in the popliteal vein at all but passes medially to join the long saphenous vein.

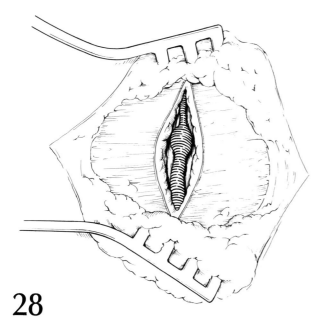

28

Exposure of the junction

28 The deep fascia is opened vertically, which allows the veins to be followed some distance in either direction should it become necessary. The short saphenous vein is identified and carefully mobilized. It usually only has one significant superficial tributary, a median vein running down the back of the thigh. This may connect above with the posteromedial thigh vein or sometimes it is large and connects via perforating veins to the deep femoral vein. It is divided and ligated.

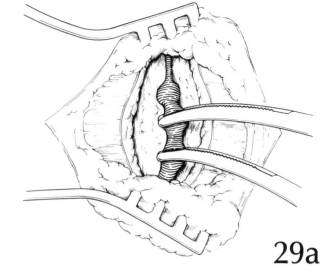

29a

29a, b The short saphenous vein is freed by blunt dissection from the sural nerve and popliteal fat. Once it has been identified with certainty, it is divided between haemostats and the proximal end mobilized.

Mobilization must be done with care. Nerve damage is not uncommon in short saphenous vein surgery. The common peroneal nerve runs down the lateral side of the popliteal fossa adjacent to the medial edge of the biceps femoris, becoming quite superficial as it crosses the back of the biceps tendon and winds around the head and neck of the fibula. The tibial nerve is less likely to be damaged being deep to the popliteal vessels.

The saphenopopliteal junction is less distinct than the saphenofemoral junction, and the popliteal vein may be quite mobile. Care must therefore be taken not to tent up and damage the popliteal vein.

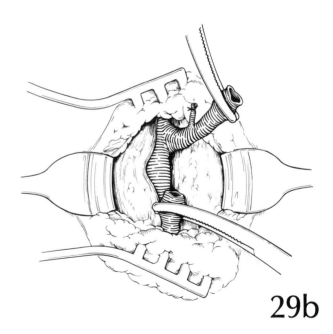

29b

Flush ligation

30 The short saphenous vein is transfixed and flush ligated with 3/0 polyglactin. Gastrocnemius veins sometimes join the short saphenous vein rather than the popliteal vein direct. They should not be ligated, as this can give rise to troublesome discomfort on standing and even venous claudication in the gastrocnemius muscles. When these veins join the short saphenous vein the latter is ligated peripheral to the junction.

It is seldom necessary to strip the short saphenous vein down to the ankle, particularly as this is liable to cause sural nerve damage. A stripper may, however, be useful as a guide, as it is much more difficult to feel the short saphenous through the skin than the long saphenous vein. The downward passage of a stripper can be helpful in identifying the short saphenous vein distally where incisions are placed to intercept tributaries.

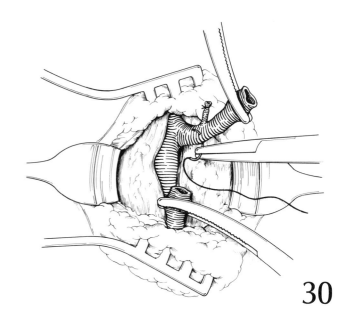

30

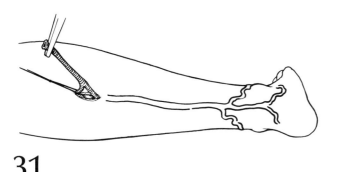

31

31 Tributaries are dealt with through small incisions. In particular there is often a large blow-out at mid-calf, which may connect with the long saphenous system. In dealing with the short saphenous system at all levels great care must be taken not to damage the sural nerve.

Wound closure

Wound closure and bandaging are the same as described above, except that the bandaging is only taken to the level of the tibial tuberosity.

RECURRENT VARICOSE VEINS

It may be difficult to decipher the sources of deep-to-superficial reflux in patients with recurrent veins by clinical examination alone. Hand-held Doppler ultrasonographic probes can be useful, but this technique has limitations in distinguishing between deep and superficial reflux and also between reflux arising at the saphenofemoral junction and thigh varices that are filled from perforators.

Colour-coded duplex scanning is very helpful in examining the venous anatomy and carries the advantage of allowing the reflux to be visualized, but it is not a substitute for the 'road map' guide to surgery provided by varicography.

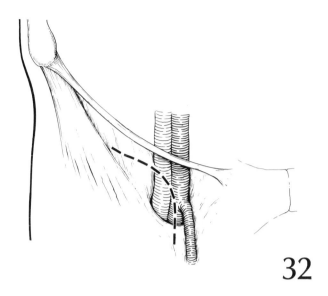

32

Approach to the saphenofemoral junction

Assuming that a groin scar indicates a previous attempt at saphenofemoral ligation, the aim of the approach is to avoid the mass of vascular scar tissue that usually overlies the junction.

32 A 'hockey-stick' incision is centred over the saphenofemoral junction, beginning in the groin skin crease laterally and turning down along the line of the saphenous vein medially.

Exposure of the femoral artery

33a, b The incision is deepened to expose the femoral artery. Dissection is then carried medially to expose the saphenofemoral junction. This will usually be found to be patent. The long saphenous vein at the junction is mobilized and divided between clamps. The stump is transfixed and flush ligated with a 3/0 polyglactin suture.

The more difficult part is to eradicate the tributaries converging on the scar tissue overlying the saphenofemoral junction. It can most easily be achieved by a block removal of the scar tissue, but this carries the possibility of lymphatic damage with subsequent leg swelling or even lymph fistula. Therefore, the alternative course adopted by the author is to dissect around the perimeter, intercepting with ligation or diathermy all converging veins.

The remainder of the operation is conducted as described for primary varicose veins.

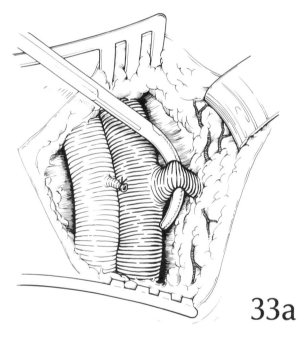

33a

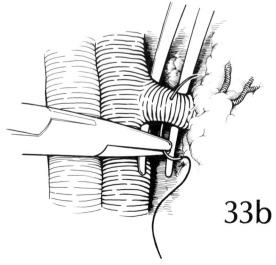

33b

SUBFASCIAL LIGATION

The dense scar tissue of chronic lipodermatosclerosis may render the dissection of perforators outside the deep fascia almost impossible, so that a more radical approach is required. Patients should receive prophylaxis such as subcutaneous heparin against deep vein thrombosis, as slow healing may necessitate several days of bed rest and these patients often constitute a high-risk group.

Subfascial ligation is not usually a 'stand-alone' operation, but requires all proximal sites of deep-to-superficial incompetence also to be dealt with.

Incision

34 The positioning of the skin incision depends on the location of the incompetent perforators and the extent of the skin changes. In the vast majority of patients the important perforators are in the gaiter area on the medial side of the calf at the anterior border of the soleus muscle.

35 If the skin changes are not extensive, the perforators can be approached through a short (4–8-cm) longitudinal incision placed medially.

36 The author's preference, however, particularly if there are also lateral perforators requiring attention, is a posterior 'stocking seam' incision. The operation is performed under tourniquet.

37 The incision is carried straight down through the deep fascia, resisting all temptation to undermine the skin by dissecting out any superficial veins encountered. The deep fascia is elevated with skin hooks, and the subfascial plane is easily developed to expose all perforators. These are ligated with polyglactin and divided.

The deep fascia is not closed. The skin is closed with fine subcuticular absorbable monofilament sutures and bandaged as described on page 565 before tourniquet release.

Several days of rest and elevation of the leg are essential, because these wounds are prone to delayed healing and early ambulation can be damaging.

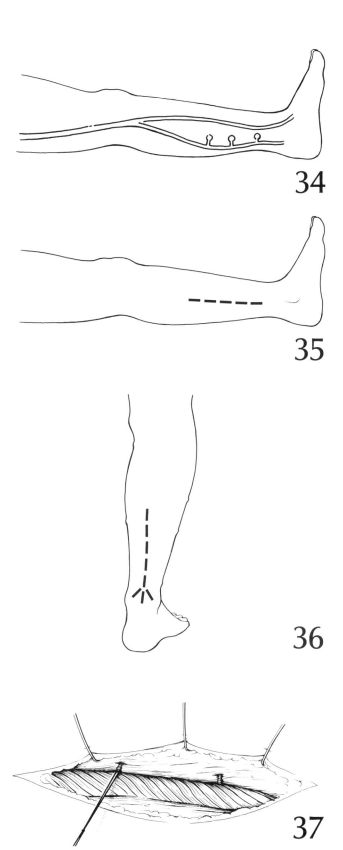

34

35

36

37

SUBFASCIAL ENDOSCOPY

38 An attractive alternative to subfascial ligation is the use of a subfascial endoscope to visualize and intercept the perforators.

The procedure is performed under tourniquet. Proximal sites of incompetence are ligated and varices avulsed.

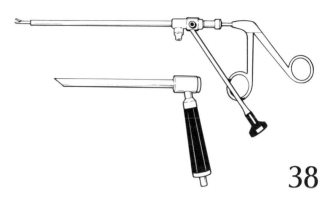

38

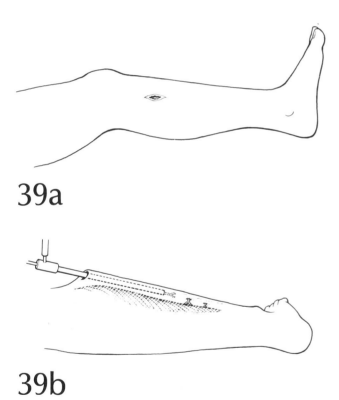

39a

39b

39a, b The endoscope is introduced through a small incision in the upper medial calf. The incision is carried through the deep fascia. The endoscope is then introduced and advanced down the medial border of the tibia.

Dissection can be performed through the endoscope to bring into view the perforators, which can then be clipped, avulsed, or sealed by diathermy.

This procedure allows rapid postoperative recovery and can be incorporated into day surgery practice.

Acknowledgment

Illustration 6 is reproduced from *A Colour Atlas of Surgical Management of Venous Disease*, 1988 with permission of Wolfe Medical Publications.

Ligation of ankle perforating veins

J. H. Scurr BSc, FRCS
Senior Lecturer and Honorary Consultant Surgeon, Department of Surgical Studies, University College and Middlesex School of Medicine, London, UK

Principles and justification

Perforating veins communicate between the deep venous system and the superficial venous system, the two systems being separated by an encircling layer of deep fascia. The presence of these veins has been recognized for a long time, the first description being attributed to von Loder in 1803. Incompetence of the valves in these veins has been implicated in the development of venous ulceration, and this led to the development of operations specifically to ligate them. The original operation for dealing with these veins was described by Linton in 1938, and was modified by Dodd and Cockett[1] in 1956. The operations described involved an extrafascial or subfascial approach, with a long incision extending almost the whole length of the calf, either medially or posteriorly, with a recommendation that any pre-existing ulcer should also be excised. These procedures allowed the fascia to be reflected and the perforating veins to be identified and ligated using absorbable suture material. The operations have been associated with poor wound healing, extensive scarring and reduced ankle mobility.

If the purpose of these operations was to improve venous function and to aid ulcer healing, then recent advances in our understanding of venous physiology and studies looking at ulcer recurrence rates[2] have suggested that there is no improvement in venous function and that ulcer recurrence rates are as high as 55%.

Studies show that between 40% and 60% of venous ulcers are due to superficial venous insufficiency alone[3]. Operations to correct superficial venous insufficiency will therefore result in ulcer healing rates of between 40% and 60%. In those patients in whom the ulcer is due to deep venous insufficiency, the presence or absence of incompetent perforating veins may be irrelevant to long-term ulcer healing.

Anatomical, radiological and more recent duplex ultrasound studies of the perforating veins show that they are present in the normal limb. They range from less than 1 mm in diameter to 10 mm or more. Only the larger veins seem to have valves, but not all valves direct flow from the superficial to the deep system. In 25 studies on fresh post-mortem specimens, Hadfield[4] found no valves in smaller perforating veins and only rudimentary ones in the larger veins. Nicolaides[5] has suggested that outward flow in medial calf perforating veins can only occur if there is axial deep vein incompetence. The importance of incompetent medial calf perforating veins in venous ulceration has not been established and makes the extensive surgical procedures of Linton, Dodd and Cockett unacceptable.

Indications

The indications for surgery are by no means precise and await further clarification. Large perforating veins, contributing significantly to superficial venous insufficiency, should be managed surgically. The common perforating veins include the saphenofemoral junction, the saphenopopliteal junction, a mid-thigh Hunterian perforator, and medial and lateral calf perforating veins. Ligation of the saphenofemoral junction and removal of the long saphenous vein will interrupt most perforating veins in the distribution of the long saphenous system. The presence of duplex long saphenous veins and anatomical variations can result in missed communications between the deep and superficial system. With persisting superficial venous insufficiency, progressive skin changes – lipodermatosclerosis – leading to frank ulceration, may occur. The best results from surgery are obtained when intervention takes place before these changes occur.

Preoperative

Assessment

1 All patients should undergo a formal non-invasive venous assessment. The use of Doppler ultrasound, photoplethysmography and strain gauge plethysmography provides a useful screening mechanism to separate out those patients with superficial venous insufficiency, those with deep venous insufficiency, and those with a combination. A further assessment with B-mode duplex ultrasound will allow direct visualization of the veins, a demonstration of reflux and an opportunity to visualize perforating veins and to determine whether the flow is inward or outward. In most patients with significant superficial venous insufficiency, surgery should be undertaken.

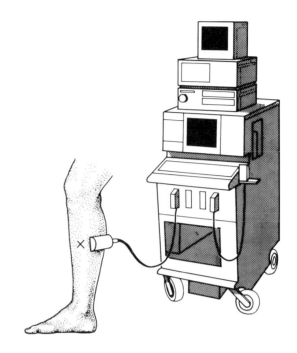

Marking

2 All patients with skin changes, a history of venous ulceration or recurrent varicose veins should be accurately assessed and marked before surgery using either venography or ultrasonographic imaging. With the patient's leg dependent but non-weightbearing, the veins of the superficial system are marked. By applying calf and then foot compression, the presence of perforating veins can be identified and the direction of flow noted. In those patients with large perforating veins with outward flow, a small mark can be placed on the skin to identify the site.

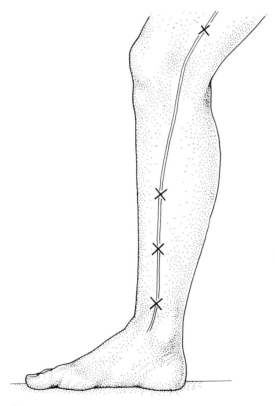

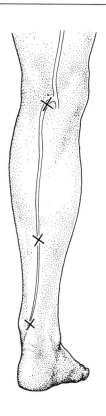

3 A systematic check of the whole leg should be undertaken, starting at the groin and moving down the medial side of the leg, returning then to the posterior aspect of the leg to identify the origin of the short saphenous vein, moving down the short saphenous vein before returning to the lateral border of the leg. In practice, only significant perforating veins are marked and these tend to be in excess of 4 mm, with obvious outward flow.

3

Operation

Position of patient

The patient is placed supine on the operating table under general anaesthesia (local anaesthesia can be used for a small number of perforating veins). The legs are elevated, the skin is prepared, and the patient is draped.

If there are significant posterior perforating veins, including the short saphenous vein, the operation is best started in the prone position, the patient being turned during the course of the procedure.

Incisions

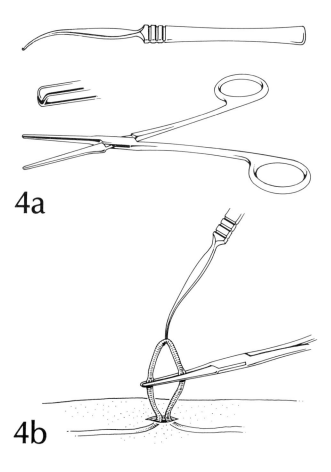

4a

4b

4a, b Small incisions ranging from 1.5 to 3 mm are used over the site of the perforating vein. Even with the leg elevated, bleeding can be quite profuse. The perforating vein is then brought to the surface with a micro-Halstead or an Oesch hook. Gentle traction is applied and a very significant portion of superficial vein, with its connection to the perforating vein, is then removed. Digital pressure is applied to control bleeding.

This operation is repeated until all the perforating veins have been interrupted. The wounds are dressed with small plasters; no sutures are required. Once the skin has been cleaned, a high compression (35–45 mmHg) stocking is applied to the limb.

Postoperative care

The patient is returned to the ward with 15° of foot elevation. This is maintained for 12 h, after which the patient is encouraged to walk maximally and told to rest on the bed or a settee with the feet up if not walking, and to avoid standing still. The stockings can be removed for washing and the patient can shower.

Complications

There are relatively few postoperative complications, but all patients should be warned that they will have considerable bruising, they may have small areas of numbness, and that these areas of numbness may be associated with quite intense tingling pain. Cutaneous nerve damage occurs in an unpredictable manner and may cause the patient considerable distress unless prior warning is given.

Postoperative venous thrombosis is a rare event. Deep vein thrombosis prophylaxis should be administered to those patients with a past history of venous thrombosis, those patients who are relatively elderly, or who are likely to remain immobile.

Superficial thrombophlebitis and cellulitis can occur after these procedures. With adequate compression this is an unusual occurrence, but when it does occur it is associated with considerable pain. This can be managed with non-steroidal anti-inflammatory drugs, rest and compression.

Editors' note

The editors would agree that there is little formal haemodynamic evidence to justify extensive perforator vein ligation and that identification with duplex scanning has proved very valuable, as has varicography (as described on page 506). Many surgeons would prefer to ligate all significant perforating veins formally via a slightly longer incision rather than rely upon avulsion with Oesch hooks. The varices are traced deeply through a 2–3 cm longitudinal incision to the site at which the perforating vein penetrates the deep fascia. The vein is divided between ligatures at this point and thereby formally ligated.

References

1. Dodd H, Cockett FB. *Pathology and Surgery of the Veins of the Lower Limb*. 2nd edn, Edinburgh: Churchill Livingstone, 1976.

2. Burnand K, Lea Thomas M, O'Donnell T, Browse NL. Relation between postphlebitic changes in the deep veins and the results of surgical treatment of venous ulcers. *Lancet* 1976; i: 936–8.

3. Coleridge-Smith P. Noninvasive venous investigations. *Vasc Med Rev* 1991; 1: 139–66.

4. Hadfield JH. *The Anatomy of the Perforating Vein of the Leg in the Treatment of Varicose Veins by Injection and Compression*. Stoke: Manubus and Bergen, 1991: 4–11.

5. Zukowski AJ, Nicolaides AN, Szendro G, Irvine A, Lewis R, Malouf GM *et al.* Haemodynamic significance of incompetent calf perforating veins. *Br J Surg* 1991; 78: 625–9.

Treatment of venous ulcers

C. W. Jamieson MS, FRCS
Consultant Surgeon, St Thomas' Hospital, London, UK

Principles and justification

Venous ulcers represent a common and debilitating condition. Many are associated with pure superficial venous incompetence and varicose veins[1], but a large number, varying from 49%[2] to 87%[3], are due to either deep venous obstruction or deep venous valvular incompetence[2]. In the assessment of any apparent venous ulcer, it is most important that the state of the arterial circulation should be investigated with Doppler ultrasound and, if necessary, angiography if a diminished ankle systolic blood pressure is found[3]. The possibility of squamous neoplastic change in a venous ulcer must also be borne in mind (Marjolin's ulcer), and a biopsy of the ulcer rim should be taken if there is any evidence to suggest that it might be neoplastic. A squamous carcinoma developing in an ulcer usually causes piling up and prominence of an otherwise shelving rim and multiple biopsies of the suspicious areas make the diagnosis, although the disorganized epithelium at the healing edge of an ulcer can confuse the histologist in making a categorical diagnosis of squamous carcinoma and the biopsy must, therefore, be generous. If evidence of squamous carcinoma is found, the prognosis is poor and treatment must involve wide radical excision of the ulcer and a search for associated metastatic nodes in the groin. If present, these should be treated by formal block dissection. Involvement of bone is not uncommon, in which case the only definitive treatment is amputation.

Evidence of associated arterial insufficiency should indicate the need for arterial reconstruction, which may in itself heal the ulcer although there is a venous component in its aetiology and occult arterial disease is common. Routine ankle blood pressure recording should be included in the assessment of all 'venous' ulcers[4].

The basic treatment of venous ulcers consists of local measures to improve the venous circulation and control the oedema, together with treatment of the primary venous cause. The treatment of the primary venous cause is covered in the chapters describing the management of varicose veins, perforator vein ligation and deep venous reconstruction on pp. 530–537, pp. 538–551 and pp. 552–571.

Local treatment of venous ulcers

Local antibiotics and complex antiseptics should be avoided as these patients have a strong risk of allergy to any complex molecule. Indeed, a superimposed hypersensitivity reaction should be considered in every case of venous ulceration; the patient may be sensitive to the rubber in elastic bandages, to their stockings, to detergents or any lotion, and exposure to such immune stimulants must be avoided. Obvious necrotic tissue should be treated by debridement under general anaesthesia. The ulcer should be cleaned regularly with normal saline, swabs taken and specific pathogens treated with the appropriate antibiotics if culture is positive. Some form of firm supporting bandage or stocking should be applied from the forefoot to the knee or to the upper thigh if there is oedema of the whole lower limb. The types of support available are legion, but excellent results have been claimed for the double-bandaging technique advocated by Charing Cross Hospital[5]. Their technique comprises an inner layer of orthopaedic wool (Velband) to absorb exudate and equilibrate compression pressure. Over this is applied a standard crepe bandage, followed by a compression bandage and finally a lightweight elasticated Cohesive bandage. All the layers of bandage are applied at mid-stretch, so that compression is achieved by elasticity rather than tension.

Care must be observed in the use of stockings and bandages on the legs of patients with arterial disease in whom further arterial thrombosis or skin necrosis may be precipitated[6, 7]. Failure to diagnose arterial disease is indefensible and emphasizes the need for routine ankle blood pressure recording in patients with ulcers.

Patients with severe deep venous obstruction may find firm bandages intolerable as they increase the pressure that accompanies exercise in the deep compartments of the limb. Indeed, this symptom is a good indicator of deep venous obstruction. Tight bandages must also be avoided in patients with associated arterial insufficiency as they may cause cutaneous necrosis and even loss of the limb.

After the ulcer has healed, the patient should continue to wear a graded compression stocking exerting a force of between 40 and 60 mmHg. The foot of the bed should be elevated by approximately 10 cm to encourage reduction of oedema at night, and the patient may benefit from the use of a rhythmic compression pneumatic boot such as the Flotron pump which helps to control the oedema and is particularly useful in patients living in a hot climate where a supporting stocking is intolerable.

Surgical treatment of venous ulcers

Venous ulcers develop in areas of dermatoliposclerosis in which there is increased fibrosis and vascularity[8, 9], with a diffusion barrier in the capillary walls because of leakage of fibrin through the capillaries. It is thought that this diffusion barrier is the main factor in their aetiology. Appropriate treatment of the cause of venous hypertension may help to reverse this vicious circle, but in many instances the damage has progressed to such an extent locally that the area of skin is unstable.

Preoperative

Any pathogens cultured from the ulcer are treated with appropriate antibiotics for at least 2 days before operation and the antibiotics are continued for 5 days afterwards. The whole limb is prepared using an aqueous antiseptic and towelled.

Operation

Excision of venous ulcer

1 The limb is elevated through 45° by reverse breaking the operating table to reduce venous pressure.

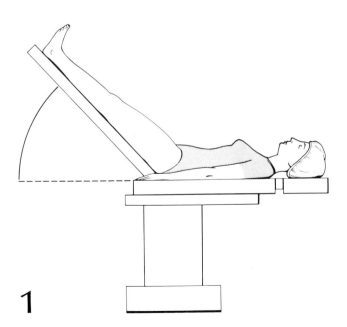

1

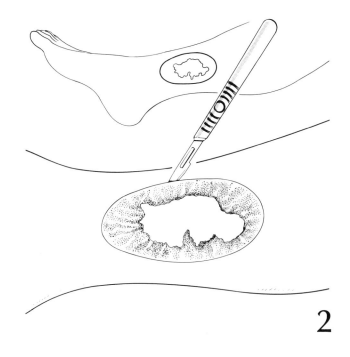

2 The whole area of liposclerosis, including the ulcer, is excised down to the deep fascia.

2

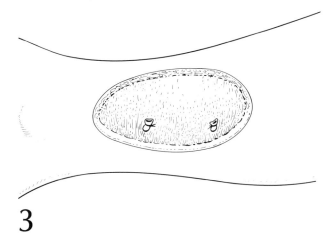

3

3 Large perforating veins are usually found penetrating the fascia and these are oversewn with fine absorbable sutures.

4 A thin split skin graft is taken from the ipsilateral thigh, meshed and applied to the defect after immaculate haemostasis. This graft is held in position by circumferential interrupted sutures. The graft is covered with paraffin gauze and then with a pad of proflavine wool and a gentle crepe bandage over cotton wool. Great care must be taken when applying the crepe bandage not to twist the dressing and dislodge the graft from its correct position.

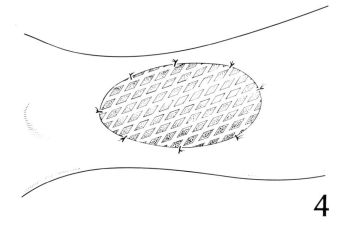

4

Postoperative care

Excess split skin taken at the time of grafting is retained in normal saline in a refrigerator. The dressing is removed after 5 days and areas of graft which have not taken are regrafted using this skin. The wound is then exposed whenever possible, but covered at night to prevent damage. The graft should mature within 9 days.

This operation does not deal with the primary cause of venous hypertension and the patient must still be diligent in protecting the limb with elevation and the use of an elastic stocking or pneumatic compression to prevent recurrence of ulceration.

References

1. Sethia KK, Darke SG. Long saphenous incompetence as a cause of venous ulceration. *Br J Surg* 1984; 71: 754–5.

2. Cornwall JV, Doré CJ, Lewis JD. Leg ulcers: epidemiology and aetiology. *Br J Surg* 1986; 73: 693–6.

3. McEnroe CS, O'Donnel TF, Mackey WC. Correlation of clinical findings with venous hemodynamics in 368 patients with chronic venous insufficiency. *Am J Surg* 1988; 156: 148–52.

4. Callam MJ, Harper DR, Dale JJ, Ruckley CV. Arterial disease in chronic leg ulceration: an underestimated hazard. Lothian and Forth Valley leg ulcer study. *BMJ* 1987; 294: 929–31.

5. Blair SD, Wright DDI, Blackhouse CM, Riddle E, McCollum CM. Sustained compression and healing of chronic venous ulcers. *BMJ* 1988; 297: 1159–61.

6. Heath DI, Kent SJS, Johns DJ, Young TW. Arterial thrombosis associated with graduated pressure antiembolic stockings. *BMJ* 1987; 295: 580.

7. Callam MJ, Ruckley CV, Dale JJ, Harper DR. Hazards of compression treatment of the leg: an estimate from Scottish surgeons. *BMJ* 1987; 295: 1382.

8. Burnand KG, Whimster I, Naidoo A, Browse NL. Pericapillary fibrin in the ulcer bearing skin of the leg: the cause of lipodermatosclerosis and venous ulceration. *BMJ* 1982; 285: 1071.

9. Hopkins NFG, Spinks TJ, Rhodes CG, Ranicar ASO, Jamieson CW. Positron emission tomography in venous ulceration: a study of regional tissue perfusion. *BMJ* 1983; 286: 333.

Illustrations by Mark Iley

Injection treatment of varicose veins

J. T. Hobbs MD, FRCS
Formerly Consultant Surgeon, St Mary's Hospital and St George's Hospital, London and Honorary Senior Lecturer in Surgery, University of London, UK

History

During the past century the treatment of varicose veins by injection became established and was in widespread use. There were many complications and the results were not consistently good. Surgery evolved rapidly and injection treatment fell into disrepute. Outspoken and influential surgeons failed in their dogmatism to differentiate between good and bad methods of sclerotherapy.

Principles and justification

In the past, ineffective sclerosants have been injected with the patient standing and minimal application of pressure. This has resulted in large painful thrombi with surrounding inflammation; the vein often reopened, sometimes with additional valve damage, and pigmentation was frequent. However, sclerotherapy has continued to be practised in Europe during the past 60 years, often to the exclusion of surgery. Fegan established a large clinic in Dublin 30 years ago and the success of his enthusiastic but careful approach resulted in a revival of sclerotherapy. The importance of adequate compression for a sufficient period of time is now well established. Having demonstrated that varicose veins can be eliminated by effective sclerotherapy, several clinical trials have been undertaken to compare surgery and sclerotherapy in the treatment of varicose veins. The late results of these trials have produced three clear conclusions:

1. In the presence of proximal incompetence of the long and/or short saphenous veins surgery is indicated; sclerotherapy is effective for eliminating dilated superficial veins and incompetent lower leg perforating veins.
2. When proximal incompetence is present, it should be eliminated first by surgery as subsequent injection treatment is simpler and often confined to the lower leg.
3. Trials have shown that stripping the incompetent long saphenous vein to the knee is preferable to a combination of proximal ligation plus injection or proximal ligation plus phlebectomies because a rapid and gross recurrence may occur if a large vein is left *in situ*.

Treatment of varicose veins

No treatment

Patients with minor vein problems and symptoms from other causes can be reassured that the veins may not become worse or cause complications.

Elastic stockings

Patients with minor problems for which curative treatment is not indicated or desired can be made symptom-free by wearing elastic stockings.

Surgery

This is described in the chapter on pp. 552–571.

Sclerotherapy

If the veins are to be eliminated, either sclerotherapy or surgery must be used. There is a place for both methods and good results will be consistently obtained only when there is proper assessment, careful planning of treatment and precise execution. This requires the surgeon to be competent and equally enthusiastic for both methods of treatment.

Principles of sclerotherapy

The aim of treatment is to inject a small volume of an effective sclerosant into the vein lumen, which is then compressed to avoid thrombus formation. Compression must be maintained until permanent fibrosis has obliterated the lumen. Good results depend on careful technique. Important aspects of treatment include consideration of where to inject, how to inject and how to bandage.

1 Treatment can be planned according to the flow diagram illustrated.

Sclerosants

It has been established that the most effective sclerosant for eliminating large veins is 3% sodium tetradecyl sulphate (Sotradecol in USA, STD in UK, and Trombovar in France), which is effective in small volumes but must be placed in the vein lumen. If accidentally placed in the skin or subcutaneous tissue necrosis will occur. Allergic reactions are rare but increase if STD is used repeatedly. For smaller veins, such as reticular or dilated superficial veins, it has been recommended that the sodium tetradecyl sulphate solution is diluted, but there is still a risk of skin necrosis. Polidocanol (Aethoxysklerol in Germany, Sclerovein in Switzerland) is preferable for the smaller veins but less effective for large veins. It is painless and available in a range of concentrations from 0.5% to 5%. A 2% preparation is normally effective for small veins, with 3% for larger veins, but this is less effective than 3% STD for the largest veins. The weaker concentrations (0.5% and 1%) have been recommended for the smallest veins and dilated venules, but may cause necrosis with ulceration. Here Scleremo (1.1% sodium chromate in glycerine) is preferable, being the most effective and safest.

Plan of treatment

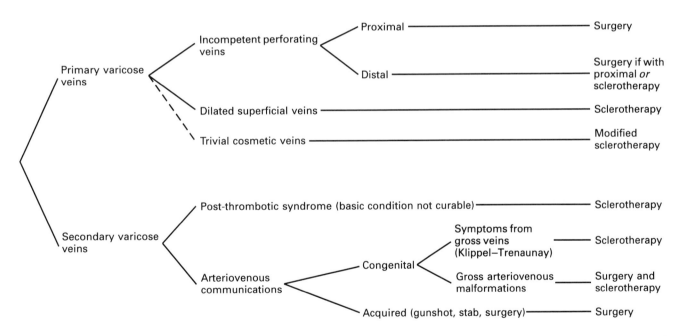

1

Preoperative or pretreatment assessment

Varicose veins are common; it has recently been estimated that 27% of the adult population of the USA have lower extremity venous abnormalities, with 2–3% having clinical manifestations of deep or superficial insufficiency. Veins and their associated problems are usually seen in general surgical or vascular clinics where the potentially serious conditions rightly deserve most attention. Less severe vein problems are often seen and treated by an unsupervised junior team member. A dedicated clinic which is properly equipped and staffed by competent doctors and nurses with adequate secretarial support, so allowing large numbers of patients to be effectively treated, is important.

Record card

2a, b The patient's details are recorded on a specially designed record card for easy reference.

Once the history is complete, the patient is examined after standing on an appropriate stool with hand support for several minutes. Dilatation of the veins will be seen to extend progressively up the leg over a 5-min period and cannot be properly assessed by a cursory inspection. The pattern of veins is drawn on the reverse side of the record card and other relevant notes added.

It is essential that all significant incompetent perforating veins are located. Involvement of the long and short saphenous veins is usually obvious, but proximal incompetence may not be apparent when the patient first stands, particularly in obese legs. The proximal short saphenous vein is obscured when the leg is fully extended. Veins on the lateral aspect of the thighs suggest the possibility of an incompetent lateral thigh perforator, or may arise from the saphenofemoral junction via the anterolateral or posterolateral tributary. Veins on the upper medial aspect of the thigh may not arise from the saphenofemoral junction but pass behind the adductor tendon to communicate with the pelvis via the posterior vulval area (internal pudendal and obturator veins). Significant incompetent perforating veins on the medial aspect of the leg include the mid- and low-thigh perforators above the knee, and below the knee the Boyd's perforator as it joins the medial gastrocnemius vein. On the lower leg the posterior arch vein joins the important ankle perforating veins. Other significant perforating veins are the mid-calf joining the gastrocnemius vein, and a perforator on the lower lateral calf joining the soleal vein.

The points of control are located by sliding the fingers along the vein to empty them and noting the sites of refilling. These points are presumed to include the sites of incompetent perforating veins. Hand-held Doppler instruments will confirm the presence of reflux but cannot always locate the source. At the back of the knee it is not possible to differentiate between the deep veins, gastrocnemius veins, short saphenous vein and vein of the popliteal fossa (sometimes referred to as an accessory short saphenous vein).

When the exact site of incompetence is in doubt and when the state of the deep veins requires assessment, the patient should be referred to a vascular laboratory for further studies. Non-invasive investigations include duplex ultrasonography with or without colour imaging. Invasive studies include measurement of venous pressure and venography (ascending or descending varicography). When proximal incompetence is demonstrated, surgical treatment is preferred and on-table venography can be used if there is doubt about the level and pattern of the proximal incompetence.

If surgical treatment is not indicated the veins can be eliminated by injection compression although, in the presence of proximal incompetence, recurrence will occur progressively after several years. However, the treatment can easily be repeated.

When there is no proximal incompetence and adequate compression can be maintained, injection compression is effective. This is particularly so below the knee where the bandages are less likely to move.

A burst bleeding vein is easily controlled by injecting the adjacent feeding vein and sometimes ulcers which are healing slowly can be rapidly improved by injecting the adjacent veins.

Materials

A suitable stool is required for the patient to stand on, so allowing the doctor to sit comfortably to examine and mark the legs, and a hand rail must be available to support the patient (this may be fixed to the wall). A couch is required for the patient to lie horizontally during treatment (the head may be elevated for comfort so that the patient can sit comfortably while being bandaged). A trolley provides the required materials for treatment. These include: 2-ml plastic disposable syringes fitted with 16-mm, 25-gauge or 27-gauge needles having a transparent hub and each loaded with 1 ml of 3% sodium tetradecyl sulphate; cotton wool balls; 1-inch (2.5-cm) hypoallergenic tape (Micropore or Dermicel); Tubipad (large), inverted, cut in 1-foot (30-cm) lengths; 3-inch (7.5-cm) limited stretch bandages (elastocrepe or STD export); 4-inch (10-cm) limited stretch bandages (elastocrepe or STD export); Tubigrip, flesh coloured, size D; applicators for Tubigrip; plastic tape for fixing bandages; and scissors. Resuscitation equipment must be immediately available.

Clinic No.	**St. Mary's Hospital** London, W.2.	Vein Clinic Mr John T. Hobbs		Hospital No.

Surname	Christian name	M S W D	DOB	SEX M F	First seen Age Date	Referred by	Cosmetic Primary Recurrent

Address		Occupation	G.P.

Telephone:		Posture	

Symptoms	R	L	Past treatment	R	L	Family history
Pain			Support			
			Other			
Prominent veins — Thigh			Injection			
Calf						Pregnancies
Dilated venules						
Pigmentation			Surgery			
Eczema			Groin tie			Thrombophlebitis
Ulceration			LSV strip			Superficial L R
Oedema			Local ties			
Night cramps			Subfascial			DVT { Calf / Proximal
Restless legs			SSV tie			Pulm. embolus
Liposclerosis			SSV strip			Allergy Skin Other
Bleeding			Skin graft			

General health	Past illness	Photos
		Venogram

Smoking No/Yes		Isotope venogram
Weight range		Ultrasound

Skeletal		Haemorrhoids		Venous pressure
Back		Constipation		Impedance plethy.
Hip/Knee		Menopause		Photoplethysmography
Feet		Hormones		
Medication	BP	Weight	Height	

2a

Physical examination

Right
Left

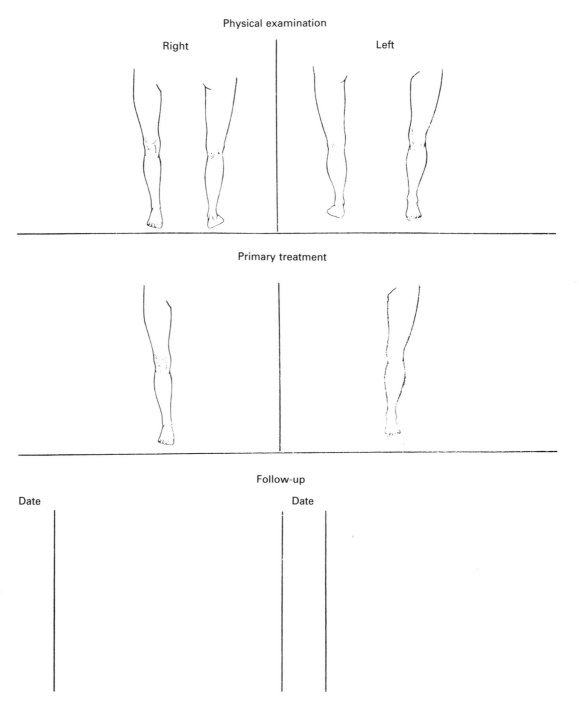

Primary treatment

Follow-up

Date
Date

2b

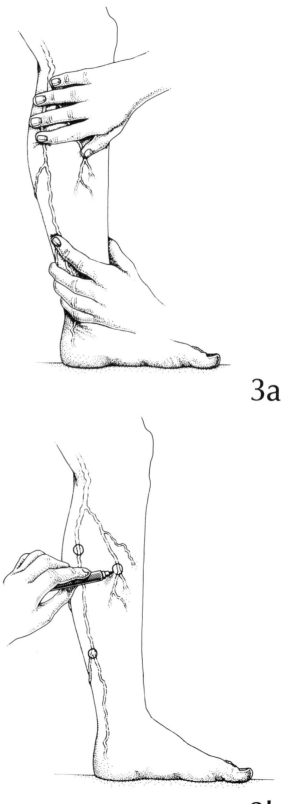

Marking the leg

3a, b   With the patient standing, the vein pattern is drawn on the record card and the leg is then carefully assessed by palpation and the sliding finger method to determine points of control. These are intended to include all sites of incompetent perforating veins. Fascial defects are sometimes easily palpable on the medial aspect of the lower leg and pain is felt when the fingertip is pressed in these defects. However, some so-called defects are nothing more than the site of an emptied varix in the subcutaneous tissue. The sites where sections of the vein can be controlled and kept empty are circled with an indelible marker (Pentel N-50, bullet tip). The convention is to use red circles for injection sites and blue outlines for the veins before surgery.

3a

3b

Placement of needle in vein

4 The patient then lies on the couch, either face down or on the back as appropriate. Using a 2-ml syringe containing 1 ml of 3% sodium tetradecyl sulphate, a 25-G needle is placed obliquely into the vein at the marked site, having previously checked easy movement of the plunger and patency of the needle.

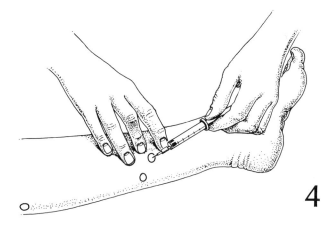

4

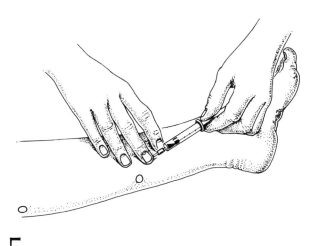

5

Monitoring injection

5 The segment of vein being injected is isolated between the index and ring fingers of the other hand. These fingers are then moved apart to empty the vein being injected. The middle finger is placed over the needle to monitor the injection. Blood is then drawn into the hub of the needle to check its correct placement. If the needle is in an artery, pulsation will be seen on careful observation and the needle must be withdrawn immediately.

Injection of sclerosant

When it is certain that the needle is in the vein lumen, a small volume of sclerosant, 0.25 or 0.5 ml (rarely, 0.75 ml in very large veins) is injected smoothly and rapidly (slow injection allows dilution) into the vein lumen. The feel of the plunger and palpation over the needle are monitored with both hands. Any perivenous leak must be prevented and if there is doubt the injection must be stopped.

Local pressure

6 As the needle is removed a pad of cotton wool is placed over the injection site and held in place with a suitable length of non-allergic adhesive tape. Cotton wool balls are ideal, being conveniently and economically supplied in bags of 250 or 500. When grossly dilated veins are injected, the leg should be elevated onto the operator's arm or shoulder to empty the veins and so ensure an adequate concentration of sclerosant at the injection site.

Sorbo rubber pads are unnecessary and less practical but are useful when bandaging superficial thrombophlebitis. Shaped rubber pads are helpful over ulcers.

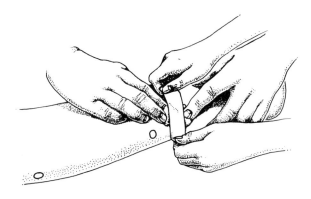

6

Bandaging

Once all the injections are complete (up to ten sites with a maximum of 6 ml of 3% sodium tetradecyl sulphate), the legs are firmly bandaged from the foot to well above the highest injection.

7 A 3-inch (7.5-cm) limited stretch, strong cotton bandage is applied from the head of the metatarsals up to the mid-calf with the leg elevated. The application of the bandage is most important and must be smooth, with steadily reducing pressure on the leg and no constricting turns. This is achieved by using one hand to feel the tension; the active hand is moved to maintain the correct tension at each edge of the bandage. The operator's wrist is abducted or adducted to adjust the tension at the bandage edges.

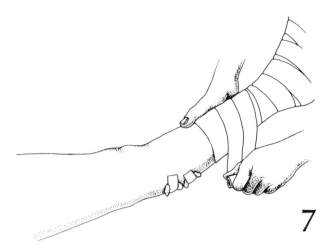

7

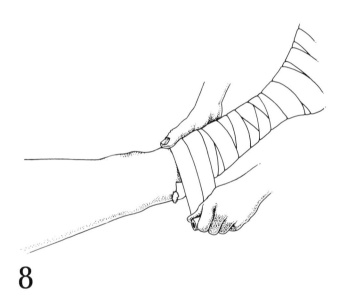

8

8 After the first bandage has been fixed in place, a 4-inch (10-cm) bandage is then placed over it and continued up to just below the knee, taking the same care with its application. The bandage is cut when sufficient has been applied. The bandages must be firm and remain in place to be effective.

Application of Tubigrip

9a, b Finally, the bandages are covered by a length of flesh-coloured elasticized tubular bandage (Tubigrip size D). The Tubigrip is easily applied by means of an applicator and is finished by folding the ends inside which leaves a smooth and neat appearance, holding the bandage in place.

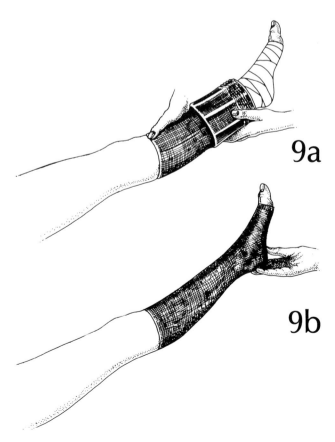

9a

9b

Bandaging above knee

When the veins which have been injected continue across the knee and when injections are made above the knee, then the whole leg must be bandaged to prevent thrombophlebitis developing in the thigh.

10 A length of tubular elastic bandage with a wide foam strip (Tubipad, large size) is first placed over the knee joint to prevent the bandages cutting into the back of the knee. It should be inverted before application so that the foam is not in direct contact with the skin.

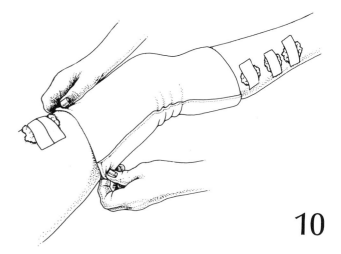

10

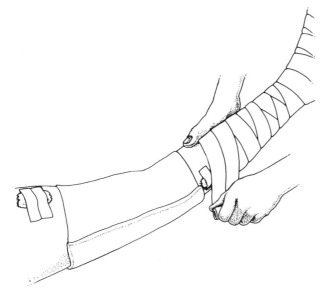

11

11 The 3- and 4-inch bandages are then applied as before, continuing the 4-inch bandage up the thigh to above the highest injection site.

Sometimes, when there are no veins crossing the knee and there are no injections at this level, it is advantageous to apply the 3-inch bandage up to the knee and the 4-inch bandage above the knee, so avoiding bandages over the knee joints.

In obese legs, when it is apparent that the bandages will move, a self-adherent (Cohepress) bandage can be placed over the upper part of the bandage.

12a–c Flesh-coloured tubular elastic bandage is then applied over the bandages.

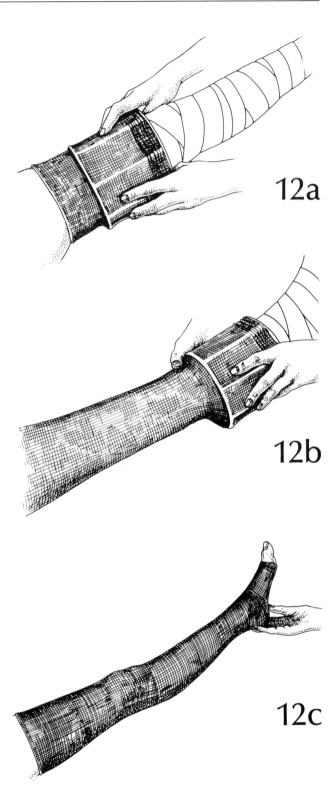

12a

12b

12c

Post-treatment management

Immediate care

The patient will have been resting quietly for up to 30 min during treatment and it has been shown that there is no movement of sclerosant from the injected superficial veins until walking is resumed. This allows sufficient time for the sclerosant to have permanently damaged the intima at the injection site. When treatment is complete the patient should walk to the waiting room and rest there for half an hour, taking gentle strolls. This observation period is important to ensure that no allergic or anaphylactic reaction will occur after leaving the clinic. During this time the nurses and secretary should be watching the treated patient to detect the first signs of reaction since prompt treatment is essential.

On sitting or lying, when the bandages feel tight, the patient is instructed to plantarflex and dorsiflex the ankle joint alternately.

The patient is then told to walk whenever there is any discomfort and to include two half-hour walks in each day's routine. If the legs are inactive, swelling will cause the bandages to be uncomfortable.

Bandages below the knee remain in place because of the shape of the leg, but if the upper calf is obese, the bandages should be continued over the knee to avoid a sharp edge. Bandages continued over the knee and on the thigh will roll down unless supported. Suspenders must therefore be worn and fixed to the outer tubular bandage. For patients with overweight legs, a panty girdle is preferable as support.

Some people find the bandages very uncomfortable when worn in bed and this discomfort and subsequent difficulty in sleeping can be relieved by taking promethazine hydrochloride (Phenergan) 25 mg in the evening (available over the counter).

Long-term care

After injection of large veins, the patient returns for review after 3 weeks. The bandages and all dressings are removed and the leg is inspected.

Intravascular haematoma

Occasionally a clot is found in the vein at the injection site. This collection forms because of inadequate compression resulting from bandage movement after a large vein has been injected. If left it will cause local pain, may result in skin staining, and eventually may allow the vein to recanalize by preventing obliteration of the lumen. However, if the clot is promptly evacuated there is no disadvantage, pain is immediately relieved and complications averted. The haematoma is pricked with a 19-G 50-mm disposable hypodermic needle and manually evacuated.

Further bandaging

When large veins are injected in the lower leg, the bandages are reapplied for a further period of 2–3 weeks. Often it is only necessary to rebandage the lower leg. When dealing with the prevention of recurrent leg ulcers in post-thrombotic limbs, it may be necessary to wear the bandages for more than 6 weeks. If the compression is removed too early, the leg is more painful, and bandaging for too long a period is preferable to too short a period.

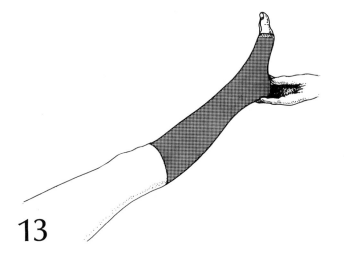

13 After discarding the bandages, class III elastic stockings (thigh or below-knee length as indicated) are then provided and worn during the day for a further 4 weeks. For the first 2 weeks this is all day, every day, and for the second period the stockings may be removed in the evening and for social occasions.

When smaller dilated superficial veins are treated the bandages can be removed at 2 weeks and elastic stockings then worn for 2–4 weeks depending on the degree of resolution of the treated veins.

Providing injection therapy is carefully applied, consistently good results can be obtained and during treatment patients can continue their normal occupation with minimal discomfort.

Complications

Complications rarely occur when the method is correctly performed. However, there are occasional problems, particularly during the initial period of learning while the technique is being perfected. The complications range from trivial skin staining to unexpected sudden death. In general the complications are less serious and less common than those associated with surgical treatment, much of which is unsupervised.

Immediate complications

Vasovagal collapse
This is the most common complication and may be dramatic and without warning. Recovery is rapid on elevation of the legs.

Allergic reaction
Patients with a history of asthma and other allergic phenomena must be treated with extra care. Early signs are urticarial blisters and red blotches spreading from the area surrounding the injection sites. When these signs are recognized injection should be stopped. Chlorpheniramine maleate (Piriton, 10 mg) should be given intravenously and followed by 4 mg orally. The oral dose of 4 mg three times a day can be continued for 24–48 h as necessary.

Anaphylaxis
This is rare, but is dramatic and immediately life-threatening. When treating veins by injection, the operator must always be aware of this so that it is immediately recognized and promptly treated. The early warning signs are the sudden onset of a persistent dry cough and the patient will complain of tightness in the chest and increasing breathing difficulties. Once recognized, treatment should be stopped immediately and 10 mg of antihistamine administered intravenously. If there is a marked reaction with urticaria, wheezing, coughing and anxiety, adrenaline should be given subcutaneously as 0.2–0.5 ml of 1:1000 solution. If the patient collapses without detectable pulse and blood pressure, adrenaline should be given intravenously, 1 ml of 1:10 000. Corticosteroids have no place in the emergency situation but will prevent recurrence several hours later. An intravenous infusion of 0.9% saline should be set up and the patient admitted to hospital. Resuscitation equipment must be immediately available in the treatment room, including airways, ventilation bags and oxygen.

Incorrect placement
If any sclerosant is injected into the subcutaneous tissue, there will be immediate pain and later an area of inflammation will persist and will often resemble an area of lipodermatosclerosis. If near or in the skin, ulceration will occur.

Intra-arterial injection
Accidental injection into an artery is a serious complication which must always be guarded against. The possibility of intra-arterial injection is minimized by using a careful injection technique. If there is the slightest doubt then the injection must be stopped. Most cases of this complication have involved the posterior tibial artery which is close to the skin in an area where significant incompetent perforating veins are found, and injection into this artery will result in some tissue loss in the foot. In thin legs, when attempting injection of the long saphenous vein, the superficial femoral artery has been accidentally injected, resulting in amputation.

Intra-arterial injections cause immediate and persistent severe pain. A sludge forms in the vessels and occludes the microcirculation. There is intense vasospasm. This always results in acute ischaemia, proceeding to gangrene and tissue loss.

Treatment is immediate administration of heparin, vasodilators and analgesics. The limb should be cooled and procaine injected around the artery at the site of injection.

Ocular disturbances
Rarely, patients have described flashing lights, blurred vision or partial visual field loss within 30 min of starting sclerotherapy. This has always recovered spontaneously within hours. In migraine sufferers, an acute episode may be precipitated by the stress of the treatment and should be treated in the usual way.

Early complications

Toxic overdose
This is preventable because excessive volumes of sclerosant should not be administered. There is a wide safety margin because large volumes have been administered without any adverse long-term effects.

Intravenous haematoma
If a large vein is not emptied by leg elevation when the injection is performed, and if the bandages fail to maintain adequate compression, a clot may develop. This should be evacuated and pressure maintained to avoid pain, skin staining and recurrence.

Ascending thrombophlebitis
If the vein is not fully compressed throughout its length, the reaction at an injection site may spread above the bandages. This is most often seen above the bandage in a fat thigh or in the long saphenous vein above the knee when bandaging is only applied below the knee. It responds to adequate compression helped by aspirin or non-steroidal anti-inflammatory drugs.

Thromboembolic phenomena

These are extremely rare when the legs are adequately bandaged and the patient fully mobilized. Occasionally they can happen without obvious reason but usually follows injection into a large vein, such as the proximal part of the long or short saphenous vein.

Problems of bandaging

The most common complication of injection treatment is trouble with the necessary bandaging. This is frequently seen during the learning period of the first year until the method has been mastered. It is also seen when poor quality bandages are used. Most problems relate to bandaging above the knee because of the shape of the leg. Self-adherent bandages (Cohepress) are helpful in this situation, as is the use of a panty girdle. Fat thighs are not suitable for this form of treatment.

Late complications

Injection ulcer

This results from extravenous injection of sclerosant, causing necrosis of subcutaneous tissue and skin. It is slow to heal and only painful during the initial period when there is inflammation. The final result is similar to a vaccination mark without excessive scarring.

Persisting local pain

This is caused by extravenous injection or leakage resulting in inflammatory necrosis of the subcutaneous tissue deep to an intact skin. It is slow to recover and resembles lipodermatosclerosis. It may respond to non-steroidal anti-inflammatory drugs.

Skin staining

If there is longstanding intravenous haematoma or perivenous blood, the skin may be discoloured and this disfigurement can be permanent, because of the deposition of haemosiderin and some melanin. Treatment is not effective and so skin staining must be avoided by careful injection of small volumes of sclerosant followed by adequate compression.

Telangiectatic matting

The appearance of new very fine red vessels is occasionally seen after sclerotherapy, as after surgery. It may be associated with the injection of excessive volumes of sclerosant under pressure in small superficial vessels and the lack of adequate compression. It is seen more often after injection with hypertonic saline. Its appearance cannot always be explained but it is difficult to treat, though it does usually show some resolution with time. Presumably small vertical feeding veins persist.

Illustrations by Raymond Evans

Operative and non-operative interruption of the inferior vena cava

Enrique Criado MD, RVT
Assistant Professor of Surgery, Vascular Surgery Section, University of North Carolina at Chapel Hill, Chapel Hill, North Carolina, USA

George Johnson Jr MD
Roscoe B.G. Cowper Professor of Surgery, University of North Carolina at Chapel Hill, Chapel Hill, North Carolina, USA

History

Deep vein ligation for the prevention of pulmonary emboli arising from the lower extremities was first described by Homans in 1934. Early experience with ligation of the inferior vena cava showed the severe haemodynamic effects of its acute obstruction, which led to death in some cases and to lower extremity chronic venous insufficiency in many of the survivors. During the 1950s inferior vena caval plication procedures were designed to prevent the acute and chronic morbidity of caval ligation. Extraluminal caval clips became popular in the 1960s in an effort to reduce the thrombogenicity of transmural suturing and to simplify the interruption procedure.

Transluminal techniques for partial or total interruption of the inferior vena cava were developed during the late 1960s and early 1970s, and led to the liberalization of indications for caval interruption. Several devices in the shape of umbrellas, balloons and metallic filters were initially placed with the goal of filtering or occluding the inferior vena cava. During the 1980s, filters that would preserve caval patency while effectively trapping emboli of significant size became the most popular form of caval interruption. For years, however, the carriers and sheaths used to deploy these filters transluminally were of large calibre and required significant skill for their safe placement. Recently, new filters and small-calibre delivery systems (7–12 Fr) have contributed to the safety and ease of the transluminal approach.

Principles and justification

Although the current approach to the prophylaxis, diagnosis, and treatment of deep venous thrombosis has effectively reduced the incidence of pulmonary embolism, some patients remain at high risk of death from pulmonary embolism. In general, indications for vena caval interruption are restricted to those patients in whom anticoagulation therapy has failed to prevent pulmonary embolism or is contraindicated[1]. The following are currently acceptable indications for inferior vena caval interruption: (1) documented recurrent pulmonary embolism originating in the lower extremities or pelvic veins, occurring in spite of adequate systemic anticoagulation; (2) in patients with documented acute deep venous thrombosis, with or without pulmonary embolism, in whom the risk of haemorrhage during heparin administration is very high because of the presence of intracranial, gastrointestinal, haematological, systemic or other disorders, and in those who are prone to bleeding, or those undergoing major surgical procedures; (3) in patients with acute lower extremity deep venous thrombosis, with or without pulmonary embolism, with a history of heparin-induced thrombocytopenia or antithrombin III deficiency; (4) in patients undergoing pulmonary embolectomy; and (5) in patients with large non-adherent iliofemoral thrombi in whom surgical thrombectomy has not been performed.

When the indication for inferior vena caval interruption is based on the diagnosis of pulmonary embolism, this should be confirmed with a pulmonary angiogram. Exceptionally, when the critical condition of the patient precludes pulmonary angiography, a high-probability ventilation–perfusion lung scan can be used to support the diagnosis.

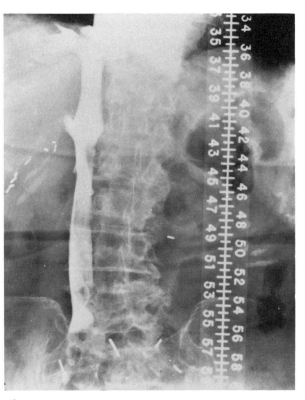

1

Preoperative

Assessment and preparation

1 Once the diagnosis of lower extremity deep venous thrombosis has been established, systemic heparin administration at therapeutic levels should be continued until the inferior vena caval interruption has been completed, unless there is a contraindication for short-term heparin administration.

Before surgical interruption or transluminal placement of inferior vena caval filters, an inferior venacavogram should be obtained to delineate the extent of iliac and caval thrombosis, determine the level of the renal veins, confirm the size of the vena cava to ensure that the filter has an adequate span to securely attach to the caval walls, and to recognize the presence of anatomical variations, such as duplicated or left-sided inferior vena cava[2].

Ideally, the filter should be implanted during the performance of the cavogram. A metallic marker is secured on the left anterior abdomen of the patient to guide the positioning of the filter below the renal veins.

Anaesthesia

Transluminal (percutaneous or operative) inferior vena caval partial interruption through either the femoral or jugular approach is performed under local anaesthesia. Systemic sedation facilitates the comfort and cooperation of the patient. Surgical interruption can be done under general anaesthesia or regional anaesthesia in thin patients.

Filter selection

2 The most important characteristic of an ideal caval filter is its capability to trap large and small emboli without producing significant resistance to blood flow, therefore preserving long-term caval patency. The filter should be able to be securely fixed to the caval wall and remain in a stable position without significant tilting or migration, which would decrease the filtering capability. For this reason, the maximum diameter of the filter must be larger than the caval diameter to prevent tilting and migration. The insertion mechanism should be rapid, safe, and associated with minimal morbidity. Ideally, the filter should be non-ferromagnetic to avoid interference with magnetic resonance or computed tomographic imaging. It should also be cheap and retrievable. Although none of the currently available filters meets all these criteria, the FDA-approved caval filters have good safety records, with fairly low recurrence of emboli[3,4]. However, the incidence of long-term inferior vena caval thrombosis after inserting these devices is not well established.

When selecting a caval interruption filter the physician should choose the one with which he or she is most familiar. Given that new filters are periodically introduced into the market, the physician should seek appropriate documentation of good filtering efficiency, low morbidity, and high long-term caval patency before using a new product.

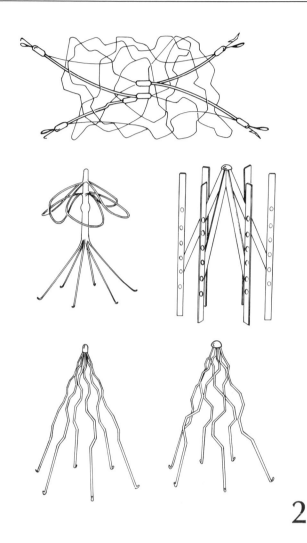

2

Selection of insertion technique and route

Because of its safety and expeditiousness, operative or percutaneous transluminal placement of inferior vena caval filters has become the procedure of choice for partial caval interruption[5]. Direct operative inferior vena caval ligation or plication is currently rarely indicated and should be reserved for those situations in which the transluminal technique has failed or is not feasible or available. Surgical ligation of the inferior vena cava is indicated in cases of septic pulmonary emboli arising from the lower extremities and pelvic veins.

The transluminal approach can be made through the internal jugular vein at the base of the neck or through the common femoral veins in the groin. In patients with a history of right upper extremity or facial swelling, or who previously had central lines placed, a duplex ultrasonographic scan should be performed to assess luminal compromise of the central veins. When the internal jugular or superior vena cava patency is questionable, the femoral approach is preferred. How-

ever, the femoral route should not be used when the venogram or ultrasonographic scan reveals thrombus in the inferior vena cava, iliac and/or femoral veins. Alternatively, some currently available filters that use small carriers (7 Fr) can be introduced through the antecubital or external jugular veins.

The right internal jugular vein offers the straightest route to the inferior vena cava. It requires, however, negotiation of the eustachian valve and avoidance of the hepatic and renal veins when placing the guidewire in the inferior vena cava. The femoral vein approach offers the advantage of less discomfort to the patient and avoids the risk of pneumothorax or arterial injury during percutaneous venous puncture, or air emboliz- ation during the insertion process. When a large carrier device is used, femoral vein thrombosis is a common complication of the femoral approach, because it frequently requires the insertion of vein dilators or sheaths in the femoroiliac system.

Operations

TRANSLUMINAL PARTIAL CAVAL INTERRUPTION

The transluminal approach to insertion of inferior vena caval filters is carried out through the internal jugular vein at the base of the neck or through the common femoral vein in the groin. The selection of percutaneous or operative access to the jugular or femoral vein depends on the operator's experience and the patient's characteristics. In patients with bleeding diathesis operative exposure of the vein allows surgical closure of the venotomy which facilitates haemostasis. With the use of smaller introduction devices, the percutaneous technique has become easy and quite safe in most patients. The principles of percutaneous cannulation of the jugular or femoral vein are exactly the same as those required for central line placement for any other purpose.

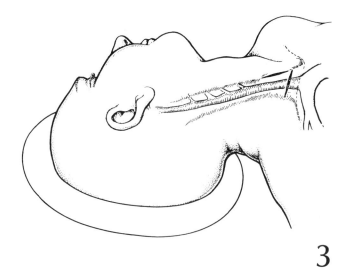

Incision

3 When operative access is selected, the right internal jugular vein is easily exposed through a short horizontal incision placed one fingerbreadth above the medial aspect of the clavicle, between both heads of the sternocleidomastoid muscle. Alternatively, a short vertical incision is made over the anterior border of the sternocleidomastoid muscle.

When the operative femoral approach is chosen, exposure of the femoral vein is performed through a vertical incision just distal to the inguinal ligament and placed one fingerbreadth medial to the femoral pulse.

Vein exposure

4 The platysma is divided and the internal jugular vein is easily located by deep dissection, posterior to the sternal head of the sternocleidomastoid muscle. To minimize blood loss, elastic vessel loops are placed proximally and distally to the venotomy site. With the patient in a slight Trendelenburg position, a longitudinal venotomy is placed on the anterior aspect of the vein and a pigtail catheter introduced into the inferior vena cava under fluoroscopic guidance. Once the procedure is completed the venotomy is closed with 5/0 or 6/0 monofilament non-absorbable suture.

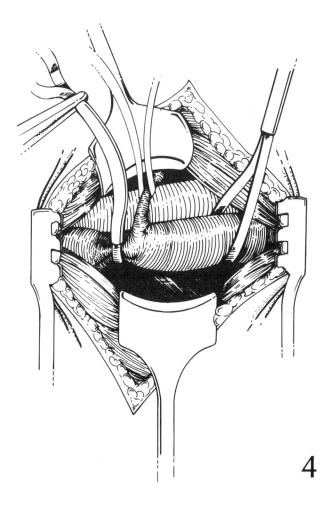

Placement of the filter

The principles of inferior caval filter placement are identical, regardless of whether the vein is accessed percutaneously or through operative exposure[6]. Since there are multiple inferior vena cava filters available with significantly different insertion devices, the operator should be familiar with the manufacturer's insertion instructions. It is beyond the scope of this chapter to describe in detail the use of the different filters available; only the general principles of placement are described herein.

5a–c A pigtail catheter is inserted into the inferior vena cava through the femoral or jugular vein. An inferior venacavogram is obtained and the filter is selected in accordance with the caval diameter. A guidewire is inserted through the pigtail catheter into the inferior vena cava, and the pigtail catheter is withdrawn. When a large (24 Fr) carrier is used, the vein access site may need to be dilated, either with dilators or with an angioplasty balloon up to 8 mm in diameter. Once the vein insertion site is dilated appropriately, a sheath adequate for the passage of the filter carrier is introduced into the vein. The carrier is then introduced over the guidewire, through the sheath, and deployed. Extreme attention should be given to placing the apex of the filter just distal to the renal veins. This prevents the formation of a potentially thrombogenic cul de sac below the renal veins in case of caval thrombosis distal to the filter. Most delivery systems are equipped with irrigating ports that should be frequently flushed with heparinized solution to prevent thrombus formation inside the carrier that may prevent expansion of the filter.

Finally, the carrier, sheath and guidewire are withdrawn and the final position of the filter is assessed with fluoroscopy or hard-copy radiography. When the cavogram has been done at a different time or the metal markers have been moved or are not available, the level of filter deployment is determined by the relationship of the renal veins to the lumbar vertebrae.

If the diameter of the inferior vena cava is larger than the largest available filter, two filters can be placed in both common iliac veins. If there is significant thrombus involving the inferior vena cava up to the level of the renal veins, the filter can be positioned just proximal to the renal veins.

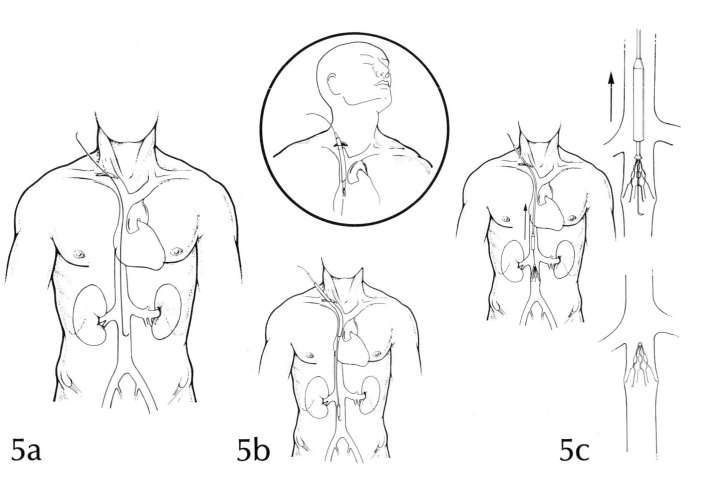

5a   **5b**   **5c**

OPERATIVE INTERRUPTION OF THE INFERIOR VENA CAVA

The inferior vena cava is exposed through a right extraperitoneal approach. In situations where the retroperitoneal route is contraindicated, transperitoneal exposure can be obtained by medial mobilization of the right colon.

Position of patient and incision

6 The patient is placed with the right side slightly elevated by placing a small roll under the right flank. This position improves exposure of the right lateral abdomen and slightly increases the distance between the inferior costal margin and the iliac crest. A transverse incision is made, one fingerbreadth cephalad and three fingerbreadths lateral to the umbilicus on the right side of the abdomen, and extended to the mid-axillary line. Alternatively, the mid-point between the costal margin and the right iliac crest can be used as a landmark, with medial extension into the lateral edge of the right rectus muscle.

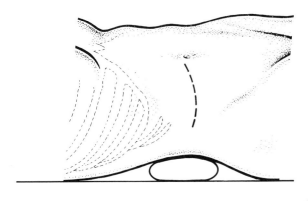

6

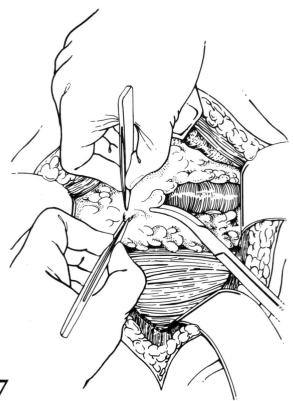

7

Exposure of the inferior vena cava

7 The incision is continued through the three oblique abdominal muscles, which are cut in the direction of the skin incision. The lateral half of the anterior and posterior aspect of the rectus sheath is also transected. The rectus muscle is left intact. The transversalis fascia is divided in the direction of the incision. The peritoneum and its contents are swept medially, superiorly, and inferiorly, and the right psoas muscle is exposed, serving as a major anatomical landmark just lateral to the inferior vena cava. The ureter should be identified and left attached to the peritoneum and its contents, and retracted medially. The genitofemoral and ilioinguinal nerves are identified along the anterior aspects of the psoas and need not be disturbed.

The use of mechanical self-retaining retractors facilitates the exposure and minimizes the number of assistants needed. The areolar tissue overlying the inferior vena cava is longitudinally divided anteriorly.

Placement of the caval clip

8a, b The inferior vena cava should be clipped at a point proximal to the thrombus. In the absence of caval thrombus on the venogram, the inferior vena cava is dissected circumferentially at a mid-point between the iliac bifurcation and the renal veins, with extreme care to avoid lumbar vein injury. A large blunt-nose right-angle clamp is passed behind the vena cava and a Silastic tube holding the tip of the caval clip is drawn around into the posterior aspect of the cava. The tubing is removed and the clip is tied, completing the procedure. The retractors are then removed, the peritoneum and its contents allowed to regain their position, and the wound closed in layers using absorbable sutures.

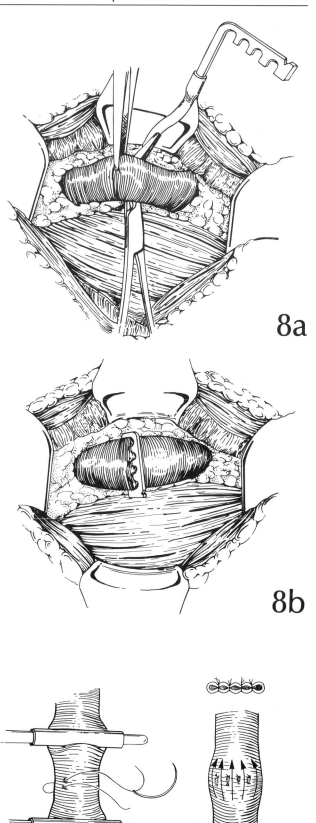

8a

8b

9

Alternative operative methods of caval interruption

9 Alternatively, if a caval clip is not available, the inferior vena cava can be plicated by using longitudinal U-shaped sutures applied along the long axis of the vena cava, grasping both anterior and posterior walls of the vein with the stitches. For this purpose, the vena cava is controlled proximally and distally to the plication sites with soft vascular clamps or vessel loops and the stitches placed and tied without tension.

When the indication for operative inferior vena cava interruption is septic pulmonary embolization, complete caval ligation is indicated. The inferior vena cava is ligated in continuity with two contiguous non-absorbable monofilament ligatures cephalad to the most proximal thrombus. There is no advantage in dividing the inferior vena cava for this purpose. Occasionally, the vena cava needs to be opened and thrombus evacuated to allow ligation without dislodging clot.

Postoperative care

Venous thrombosis at the femoral or jugular vein occurs frequently with the use of large 24-Fr filter carriers. Although no data are available, with the new smaller carrier systems the incidence of venous thrombosis at the insertion site should decrease.

Following transluminal caval interruption, systemic anticoagulation with therapeutic heparin, if not contra-indicated, should be continued for 24–48 h to prevent thrombosis of the veins used for access. Following surgical caval interruption, however, anticoagulation is contraindicated. The position of the filter should be reassessed with a plain abdominal radiograph during the first few postoperative days. If recurrent pulmonary embolism occurs, migration or tilting of the filter should be suspected; 30–60% of inferior vena caval filters will migrate up to several centimetres caudally or distally in the inferior vena cava. However, this generally does not reduce their filtering capability. When the filter has been misplaced into the renal, hepatic or iliac vein it does not protect the patient adequately from pulmonary embolism, and another filter should be placed.

Major complications of transluminal placement include caval perforation with or without arteriocaval fistula and migration of the filter into the heart. In the latter situation, because of the risk of severe arrhythmia, valvular dysfunction, or ventricular perforation, the filter should be removed immediately. Fortunately, major complications from transluminal placement of inferior vena caval filters are unusual.

References

1. Rohrer MJ, Scheidler MG, Wheeler HB, Cutler BS. Extended indications for placement of an inferior vena cava filter. *J Vasc Surg* 1989; 10: 44–50.

2. Martin KD, Kempczinski RF, Fowl RJ. Are routine inferior vena cavagrams necessary before Greenfield filter placement? *Surgery* 1989; 106: 647–51.

3. Grassi CJ. Inferior vena caval filters: analysis of five currently available devices. *AJR* 1991; 156: 813–21.

4. Katsamouris AA, Waltman AC, Delichatsios MA, Athanasoulis CA. Inferior vena cava filters: in vitro comparison of clot trapping and flow dynamics. *Radiology* 1988; 166: 361–6.

5. Greenfield LJ, Cho KJ, Proctor M, *et al.* Results of a multicenter study of the modified hook-titanium Greenfield filter. *J Vasc Surg* 1991; 14: 253–7.

6. Pais SO, Tobin KD. Percutaneous insertion of the Greenfield filter. *AJR* 1989; 152: 933–8.

Illustrations by Peter Cox

Shunt operations to relieve portal hypertension

Kaj Johansen MD, PhD
Professor, Department of Surgery, University of Washington School of Medicine, Seattle, Washington, USA

W. Scott Helton MD
Assistant Professor, Department of Surgery, University of Washington School of Medicine, Seattle, Washington, USA

History

Shunt operations to decompress the portal circulation into a systemic vein – usually the inferior vena cava or a branch thereof – have been performed for more than a century. Since 1945, portacaval shunts have been widely used to treat the haemorrhagic complications of portal hypertension induced by hepatic cirrhosis, but it soon became clear that, although portosystemic shunts may be highly effective in treating portal hypertension, they frequently do so at the cost of accelerated liver failure and a disabling neuropsychiatric dysfunction called portosystemic encephalopathy. Early prospective randomized trials suggested that portosystemic shunts did not prolong survival in patients with bleeding varices but only changed the cause of their demise.

Development of the fibreoptic endoscope and the rediscovery of variceal sclerotherapy has, more recently, led to the utilization of this non-operative approach for the acute control and, especially in compliant patients, for chronic palliation of bleeding. Two other recent developments – the advent of liver transplantation as a definitive therapy for the underlying chronic hepatic dysfunction, and the use of percutaneous angiographic stented shunts between the intrahepatic portal and hepatic veins – may have a significant role in certain patients with advanced hepatocellular degeneration and uncontrollable variceal haemorrhage. For those patients still requiring operative portal decompression, modifications of the traditional portosystemic shunt show promise in obtaining reliable portal decompression yet minimizing the previously certain major complications of the procedure

601

Principles and justification

Bleeding must be controlled as soon as possible in a patient with variceal haemorrhage for these metabolically and nutritionally compromised patients tolerate major or prolonged blood loss poorly. Acute endoscopic therapy by an experienced operator will generally control the bleeding temporarily; gastro-oesophageal balloon tamponade should control those whose bleeding does not stop with this approach.

The patient should be assessed as soon as possible for suitability as a candidate for liver transplantation. If not disqualified by advanced age, hepatitis B seropositivity, significant medical comorbidity or active alcoholism, the patient's portal hypertension should be palliated by persistent aggressive endoscopic therapy or, if appropriate expertise is available, angiographic intrahepatic shunt (transjugular intrahepatic portosystemic shunt: TIPS).

Patients for whom liver transplantation is not possible but who require definitive management of their portal hypertension must be considered for various non-transplantation options. Compliant patients (usually those with non-alcoholic causes for hepatic dysfunction), especially those who live near the hospital, may be candidates for repeated endoscopic therapy. TIPS may be used in such patients, although definitive demonstration that the stented intrahepatic tract produced by balloon dilatation between the portal and hepatic veins will remain open in the long term has not been presented.

A substantial population of patients with variceal bleeding remains in whom operative portal decompression should be considered. These include undependable or non-compliant patients, those who live far from a major medical centre, patients with recurrent or uncontrollable variceal haemorrhage despite best non-operative efforts at control, and those bleeding from gastric varices. Such patients will require one of the operative portal decompressive procedures described in this chapter.

Preoperative

The two major determinants of outcome following operative portal decompression are the urgency with which the procedure is performed and the patient's physiological status (specifically, the degree of hepatocellular dysfunction). Accordingly, if at all possible surgery should be performed once the bleeding has been controlled and the blood volume restored to normal, including attempts to improve nutritional status and clotting capabilities. Child's classification accurately predicts outcome following portosystemic shunt; Child's grade C patients (those with unrecoverable cachexia, intractable ascites, marked jaundice and spontaneous portosystemic encephalopathy) have a high risk of operative mortality and should be seriously considered for TIPS and/or liver transplantation. Child's grade A and B patients may enjoy significantly prolonged survival if (particularly in alcoholic patients) alcohol is avoided assiduously in the postoperative period.

Choice of operation

When operative portosystemic decompression is contemplated, the choice of operation may be significantly dependent upon the data available from physical examination and laboratory findings. For example, portacaval shunt will be successful only if the portal vein is patent, and duplex ultrasonography (or another imaging technique such as splanchnic angiography or magnetic resonance imaging) must be performed to confirm that this vessel is open.

Patients in whom liver transplantation may be a later option should undergo a portal decompressive procedure that avoids the right upper quadrant; mesocaval or distal splenorenal shunt may be a better option in such individuals. Patients in whom distal splenorenal anastomosis is contemplated generally do poorly if the procedure is performed on an emergency basis, in the presence of intractable ascites, or when the splenic or left renal veins are diminutive or anatomically distant from one another; preoperative angiography is mandatory in such patients.

Anaesthesia

Patients with portal hypertension as a result of hepatic dysfunction generally have a significantly disordered coagulation status and are thus not considered for regional anaesthetic techniques. Natural portosystemic shunting is found systemically in cirrhosis, and these patients demonstrate a chronic hypoxaemia due to intrapulmonary shunting. A prolonged effect of anaesthetic agents administered during an operation may be noted postoperatively because many anaesthetic agents are metabolized in the liver. Bleeding during surgery can be significant because of the splanchnic venous hypertension of these patients and their concurrent coagulopathies and thrombocytopenia; administration of intravenous vasopressin may significantly reduce perioperative bleeding, but this may be associated with coronary vasoconstriction and should not be used in patients with known coronary insufficiency.

Operations

PORTACAVAL SHUNT

Position of patient

1 The patient is placed in a 45° left lateral decubitus position with the right arm on an 'airplane' splint and a pillow placed between the knees. The patient is positioned on the operating table so that the 'kidney break' is beneath a point equidistant from the costal margin and the iliac crest; the 'kidney break' is raised to flex the patient at this point. The patient is then placed in a moderate head-down (Trendelenburg) position. This position permits opening up of the intrahepatic space, allows the liver to fall cephalad, away from the operative site, and places the two vessels of major interest – the inferior vena cava and the portal vein – side by side from the perspective of the operating surgeon, rather than overlying one another as they do in a supine position.

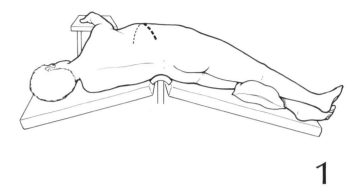

1

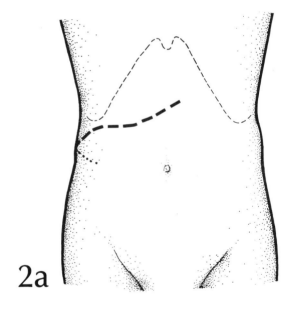

2a

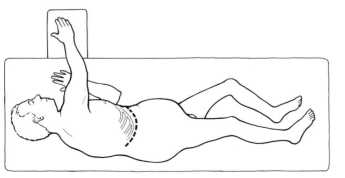

2b

Incision

2a, b An extended right subcostal incision is made with the scalpel from the midline to the mid axillary line, finishing two finger breadths below the costal margin. Electrocautery is used to carry the incision down to the subcutaneous tissue and muscle layers because of the sometimes extensive abdominal wall venous collaterals found in patients with portal hypertension. The falciform ligament and its (occasionally substantial) umbilical vein should act as the medial limit of the incision and should be preserved because this vein remains a valuable portosystemic collateral while the operation is being performed.

Initial dissection of right upper quadrant

3 Ascites should be aspirated assiduously, including from within the pelvis, to prevent its draining into the operative site throughout the procedure. The abdominal cavity and its contents should be explored carefully to discern further potential problems such as colonic cancer, stones in the gallbladder and hepatoma. A Kocher manoeuvre should be conducted to retract the duodenum and pancreas medially. One of several varieties of self-retaining abdominal retractors should be installed and various malleable or right-angled blade retractors used to retract the cirrhotic liver and gallbladder cephalad, the duodenum and stomach medially, and the right colon caudad. The right kidney will be palpable and attention should be directed to the area just inferior to the lower border of the liver, medial to the right kidney.

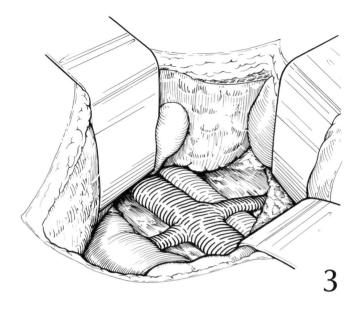

3

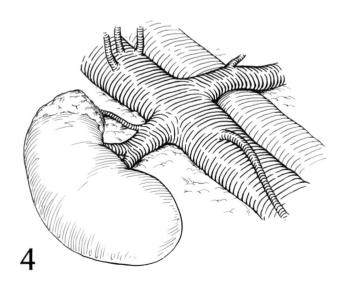

4

Exposure of inferior vena cava

4 Dissection dorsal and medial to the right kidney will encounter the inferior vena cava: often initiating the dissection by incising the peritoneum just inferior to the liver will identify this structure. A dissection straight inferiorly from this point using the electrocautery will reveal the ventral surface of the inferior vena cava; this incision should be carried to a point inferior to the renal veins, at least to the level at which a prominent ventral vena caval branch (the right gonadal vein) can be seen. A complete dissection of the entire infrahepatic vena cava should then be conducted. This dissection is assisted by the absence of lumbar veins cephalad to the renal veins; the only significant branches include the fragile right adrenal vein, which may enter at any point on the rightward aspect of the vena cava (or even the upper border of the right renal vein), and several branches exiting the caudate lobe superiorly and entering perpendicularly into the ventral surface of the inferior vena cava. The adrenal and caudate lobe veins should be divided between ligatures. Both renal veins should be dissected. This dissection of the infrahepatic vena cava is crucial for the performance of the subsequent portacaval anastomosis; about 80% of the mobilization required to bring the inferior vena cava and the portal vein together must come from the former structure.

Exposure of portal vein

5a, b If necessary, the uppermost retractor is moved slightly to retract the gallbladder superiorly and slightly medially. Attention is then turned to the hepatoduodenal ligament, specifically its lateral aspects. The portal vein is found posterolaterally in the hepatoduodenal ligament, and can be located either by incising the peritoneum near the hepatic hilum and carrying this incision straight caudad, or dissecting and excising a large 'sentinel' lymph node found ventrally in the hepatoduodenal ligament. Removal of this node frequently demonstrates the portal vein in the depths of the dense fibrofatty and lymphatic tissue of the hepatoduodenal ligament. Dissection should be carefully directed laterally in order to avoid potential damage to the medially placed common bile duct.

Large venous collaterals within the hepatoduodenal ligament should be ligated and divided. In approximately 10% of patients a replaced right hepatic artery runs along the most lateral aspect of the hepatoduodenal ligament; the tissue in this area should be palpated for an arterial pulse before dissecting it, because inadvertent division of the right hepatic artery could be catastrophic. The portal vein should be dissected carefully from the fibrofatty tissue of the hepatoduodenal ligament, and from the underside of the common bile duct. Retraction of the latter structure with a vein retractor or Gil–Vernet retractor facilitates this dissection. One or more coronary vein branches can be identified, and should be ligated and divided with care. Posteroinferiorly a constant large venous branch entering the head of the pancreas is also identified and ligated.

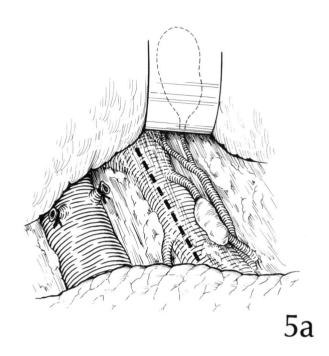

5a

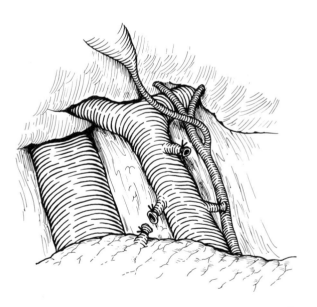

5b

Portacaval anastomosis

6a–d   Primary side-to-side portacaval anastomosis is possible if the inferior vena cava and portal vein can be apposed with only minimal tension. Temporary placement of partially occluding (Satinsky) vascular clamps and drawing the two veins towards one another will permit the surgeon to define the degree of tension required for this manoeuvre. Most of the mobility comes from the inferior vena cava: even the well dissected portal vein will move laterally only about 1 cm. The partially occluding clamps are placed, anteromedially on the vena cava and posterolaterally on the portal vein, and axial venotomies are made. A totally decompressing shunt should have a diameter of at least 2.5 cm: if partial portal decompression is intended the venotomy should be approximately 12–15 mm in length. Stay sutures are placed in the ventral lips of both venotomies. A 4/0 or 5/0 double-needled monofilament vascular suture is introduced inwards from the outside at the superior aspect of the caval incision, and is then used to suture the posterior lips of the anastomosis from within. No effort is made to draw the two veins together until the entire posterior wall is sutured; the two vascular clamps holding the inferior vena cava and the portal vein are then withdrawn in opposite directions to pull them together, while pulling the posterior wall suture tight. Using the second end of the suture the anterior lips of the anastomosis are sutured, taking care not to pick up the back wall of the anastomosis.

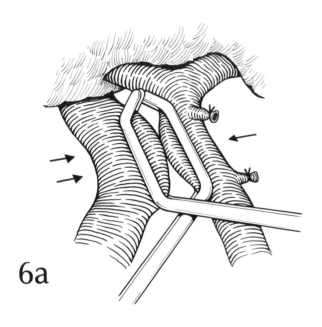

6a

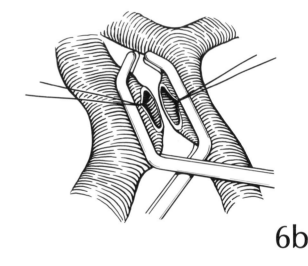

6b

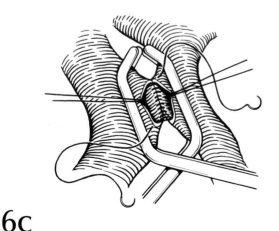

6c

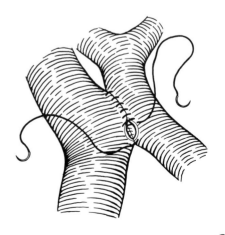

6d

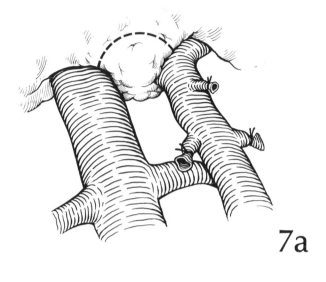

Inability to appose inferior vena cava and portal vein

7a, b If relatively easy apposition of the inferior vena cava and portal vein cannot be accomplished, it is always because of hypertrophy of the caudate lobe of the cirrhotic liver.

In most circumstances the caudate lobe can simply be excised, using knife, transfixion sutures, and electrocautery, in order to permit the two vessels to be brought together without tension. If excision of the caudate lobe cannot be accomplished, or if doing so still does not permit a tension-free apposition of the two vessels, three options exist: (1) end-to-side portacaval anastomosis; (2) portarenal anastomosis; or (3) prosthetic H-graft interposition.

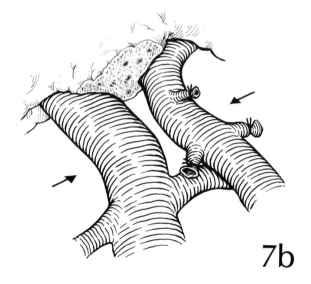

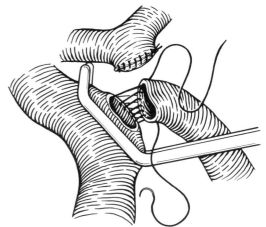

8a

8a–c For end-to-side portacaval anastomosis, the portal vein is divided between clamps as close as possible to the hepatic hilum, and the distal (hepatic) end is ligated with a running 4/0 monofilament vascular suture. The proximal (splanchnic) end of the portal vein is usually easily brought to the side of the inferior vena cava where end-to-side anastomosis is accomplished as previously described. This approach is not favoured by the authors because, although it is an effective means of splanchnic venous decompression, the hepatic sinusoids remain hypertensive and intractable ascites may result.

Portarenal anastomosis has the advantage of relative ease and only a single suture line. The left renal vein is dissected to the left, out at least to where it crosses the aorta. At this point it is divided and the renal end is oversewn using a 3/0 or 4/0 vascular suture. The caval end of the left renal vein is then brought cephalad and anastomosed end-to-side to the portal vein.

Prosthetic H-graft portacaval shunts have become popular recently. Partially occluding clamps are placed on the portal vein and the inferior vena cava, and 8-mm, 10-mm or 12-mm externally supported polytetrafluoroethylene (PTFE) graft, usually 3–5 cm in length, is anastomosed to appropriately sized venotomies in the portal vein and the inferior vena cava using 5/0 vascular suture.

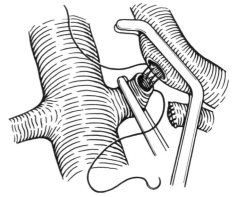

8b

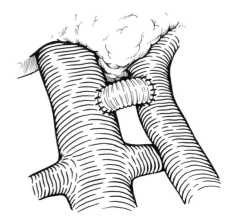

8c

Completion of procedure

9 Shunt patency is suggested by palpation of a thrill in the posterolateral wall of the inferior vena cava opposite the shunt, once the clamps have been removed. Measurement of pressure in the portal vein and the inferior vena cava should demonstrate a pressure difference between the two vessels of less than 15 mmHg; a totally decompressing shunt should have a 'shunt gradient' of less than 5 mmHg. A liver biopsy should always be performed, either using a biopsy needle or wedging out a small segment of the anterior border of this cirrhotic liver. If stones have been palpable in the gallbladder, cholecystectomy may be performed at this time; the decompression of the portal system makes bleeding from the gallbladder bed much less troublesome.

Wound closure

Great care must be taken with closure of the incision to prevent a postoperative ascitic leak. The wound is closed with multiple fascial layers of running absorbable 0 or 1 sutures and a running subcutaneous suture of 2/0 or 3/0 absorbable sutures. The skin edges may be apposed with skin staples or a running nylon suture.

MESOCAVAL SHUNT

10a, b The patient is operated upon in a supine position; coeliotomy is performed and ascites is aspirated.

A leftward visceral rotation of the right colon is performed by dividing the lateral peritoneal attachments, and the right colon and the duodenum are retracted to the left to expose the right kidney and inferior vena cava. After the inferior vena cava has been exposed and mobilized (taking care not to avulse lumbar veins either medially or laterally) the right colon is allowed to fall back to its natural position.

Exposure of superior mesenteric vein

To expose the superior mesenteric vein the transverse colon is retracted cephalad, and a T-shaped incision is made over the superior mesenteric vessels. The superior mesenteric vein is identified and branches entering it from the right side are ligated. The middle colic vein is preserved.

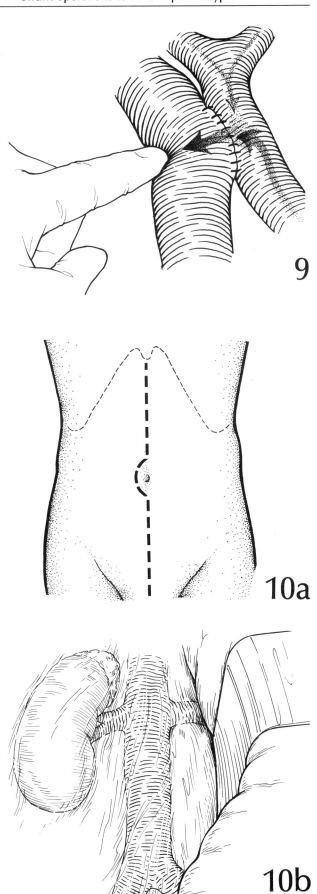

11a–c

An externally reinforced polytetrafluoroethylene graft of 8 or 10 mm is anastomosed to the anteromedial inferior vena cava as close as possible to the inferior border of the second portion of the duodenum using 5/0 or 6/0 monofilament vascular suture; the inferior vena cava is partially occluded using a Satinsky clamp. A tunnel is bluntly formed through the base of the great mesentery into the site of exposure of the superior mesenteric vein. Clamps are placed on the superior mesenteric vein and it is rotated to the left. A right posterolateral axial venotomy is made appropriate to the size of the reinforced vascular graft, and another anastomosis made with a running monofilament vascular suture.

Alternatively, an appropriate length of internal jugular vein may be harvested through a longitudinal neck incision and interposed as an autogenous interposition mesocaval graft. Twisting or extrinsic compression threaten this graft.

Wound closure

Liver biopsy and, if necessary, cholecystectomy are performed. The coeliotomy incision is closed with (if possible) a running absorbable suture for the peritoneum, a running permanent suture for the linea alba, a running subcutaneous absorbable suture of 2/0 or 3/0, and staples or running nylon to appose the skin edges.

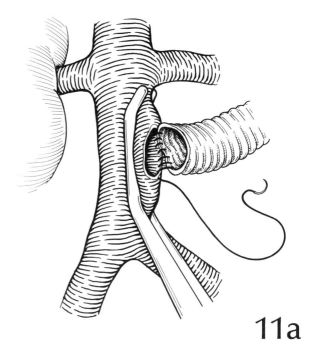

11a

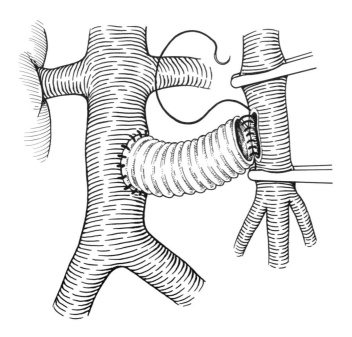

11b

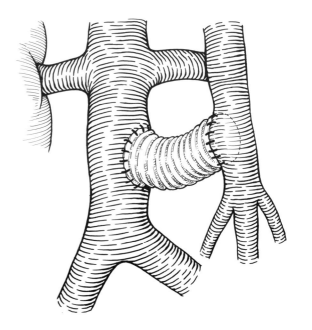

11c

DISTAL SPLENORENAL SHUNT

Incision

12a–c The patient is positioned supine. Exposure is through a left subcostal incision carried slightly across the midline. The left renal vein is approached by retracting the transverse colon cephalad and the intestines to the right; the peritoneum is incised over the aorta, and this incision is carried superiorly until the left renal vein is identified (alternatively, the left renal vein may be identified following dissection of the splenic vein). The left renal vein is dissected from the inferior vena cava to the renal hilum: adrenal, gonadal, and lumbar branches are ligated and divided.

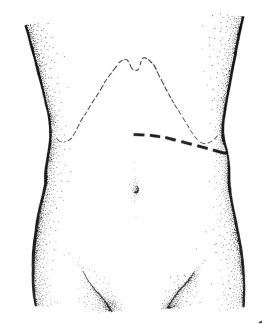

12a

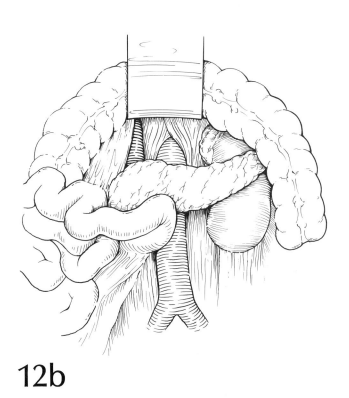

12b

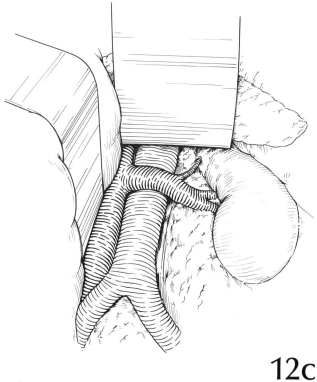

12c

Dissection of the splenic vein

13a, b The lesser sac is entered between the lower border of the stomach and the transverse colon. The splenic vein is located posterior to and usually near the inferior border of the pancreas. The pancreas may be retracted inferiorly and the splenic vein identified near the splenic hilum and dissected medially or, more commonly, following superior and dorsal retraction of the inferior aspect of the pancreas, using sponge sticks. The peritoneum is incised over the splenic vein, and is carefully dissected free from its bed in the pancreas, taking special care to transfix, with fine vascular sutures, multiple short, fragile branches between the splenic vein and the pancreas.

The frequent loss of 'selectivity' of the distal splenorenal shunt (its maintenance of prograde flow in the portal vein) has been ascribed to the development of communications between the persistently hypertensive portomesenteric circulation and the splenorenal shunt, through residual pancreatic venous branches into the splenic vein. Complete 'splenopancreatic dissociation' has been recommended to diminish the likelihood of this. Accordingly, if this is to be pursued, the entire splenic vein from the hilum of the spleen to its confluence with the superior mesenteric vein must be dissected away from the pancreas.

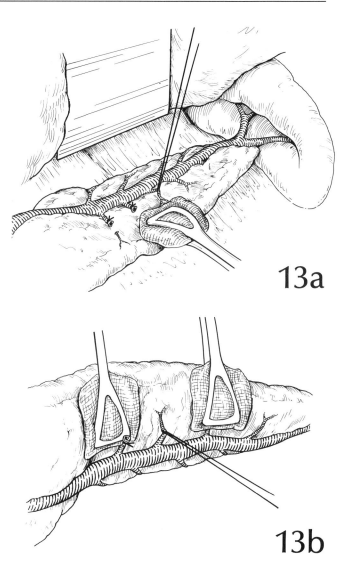

13a

13b

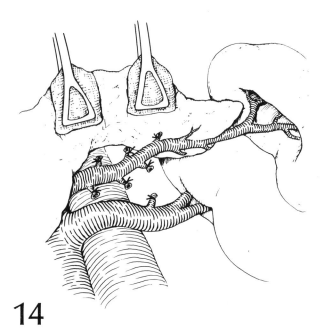

14

14 Once the splenic vein is dissected completely it is divided near its confluence with the superior mesenteric vein, and the portal end of the splenic vein is oversewn using a 4/0 or 5/0 monofilament vascular suture. If the left renal vein has not already been identified and dissected, it may be found dorsally and inferiorly from the site of dissection of the splenic vein through the sac exposure. The left renal vein is dissected free from the left renal hilum all the way to its confluence with the inferior vena cava. Mobilization of the left renal vein is facilitated by ligating and dividing various branches of the left renal vein, including the left adrenal, left gonadal and lumbar branches.

Splenorenal anastomosis

15a, b A partially occluding clamp is placed anterosuperiorly on the left renal vein, and an axial incision approximately 15–20 mm in length made in the vein. It is held open with a stay suture, and the splenic vein is brought into proximity with this venotomy. End-to-side anastomosis of the divided splenic vein is made in tension-free fashion to the left renal venotomy.

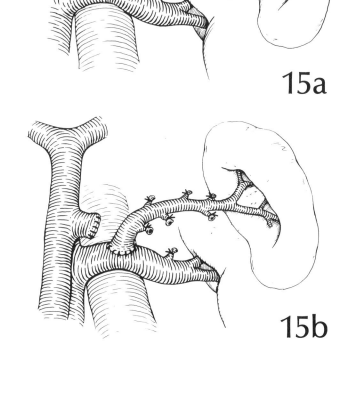

15a

15b

Collateral ligation

16 Ligation of potential future collateral pathways between the portomesenteric and the gastro-splenic venous circulations is a crucial part of this operation. Ligation of the coronary vein, readily found entering the hepatoduodenal ligament from a retrogastric position near the gastro-oesophageal junction, is readily performed; similarly, ligation of the right and left gastroepiploic veins is considered important.

Wound closure

Liver biopsy and, if necessary, cholecystectomy may be performed, although the latter would probably require rightward extension of the incision. The wound is closed with fascial layers of 0 or 1 absorbable suture, and the subcutaneous tissues are closed with a running 3/0 absorbable suture. Skin edges are apposed with staples or running nylon sutures.

16

Postoperative care

All patients should be admitted initially to the intensive care unit. Fluid shifts may be significant, especially if a substantial amount of ascites was aspirated during the operation. Appropriate administration of colloid, blood and blood elements should take place as required. Vigorous pulmonary therapy may forestall atelectasis or pneumonia. If gastrointestinal bleeding was a significant part of the immediate preoperative course, the bowel should be cleansed; magnesium citrate and lactulose are excellent for this purpose. Assessment of shunt patency by duplex ultrasonography or contrast angiography (the latter enabling measurement of pressure gradients across the shunt) are appropriate. The development of ascites, especially in those procedures which only partially decompress the portal system, is common and should be treated by administration of appropriate diuretics.

Outcome

Portosystemic shunt is an extremely effective procedure, providing reliable decompression of the portal system and prevention of further variceal haemorrhage. The recent rebirth of the concept of partial portal decompression may provide a means by which necessary reduction of portal pressure can take place while reducing the risk of development of accelerated liver failure or hepatic encephalopathy. While data still hint, at best, at only moderately improved survival in variceal bleeding treated with operative shunt, there is no doubt that this technique markedly reduces the utilization of homologous blood by these patients.

Lymphography

John H. N. Wolfe MS, FRCS
Consultant Vascular Surgeon, St Mary's Hospital, and Honorary Senior Lecturer, Royal Postgraduate Medical School, Hammersmith Hospital, London, UK

History

Clinical lymphography was introduced by Kinmonth[1] in 1952. The indications are now limited with the advent of less demanding techniques. Isotope lymphography may be used to elucidate the cause of leg oedema and can differentiate between the various types of primary lymphoedema. When clinical assessment is combined with lymphography an accurate prognosis may be obtained in many patients[2] and once the exact anatomical lymphatic abnormality is defined, appropriate operations may be carried out.

Lymphography may also identify the specific leak causing a chylothorax or chylous ascites. Lymphadenograms taken 24 h after lymphography show the lymph nodes and can thus display anatomical or pathological abnormalities.

Preoperative

Before investigation the girth of the limb should be reduced by bed rest with the foot of the bed elevated. Intermittent compression with a pneumatic boot is also of considerable assistance[3]. Cellulitis and areas of infection in the foot should be treated before lymphography.

Special equipment and materials

Lipiodol is the contrast agent most widely used; it gives good anatomical detail of lymphatic vessels and nodes. However, being oil-based, it is not cleared rapidly and the quest continues for better contrast solutions. Direct injection into lymphatics can be difficult and it is to be hoped that good anatomical detail will eventually be achieved by subcutaneous injection. Encouraging results using this route have been achieved in animals, using various water-soluble media, but attempts to use them in patients have been disappointing. Radioactive isotopes have been used but their clearance lacks specificity and no detail can be expected with the present compounds and techniques.

Lipiodol lymphography therefore remains the method of choice for obtaining accurate data on the anatomy of the lymphatic system.

Short skin hooks are useful as skin edge retractors and microvascular scissors for the dissection; a dissecting microscope is imperative for difficult cannulations. A fine needle (30 G) on polyvinyl tubing attached to a constant infusion pump with variable speed settings is used for infusion. Castro Viejo needle holders (with the ratchet removed) can be used to hold the needle, and fine Hoskins forceps to hold the perilymphatic tissues.

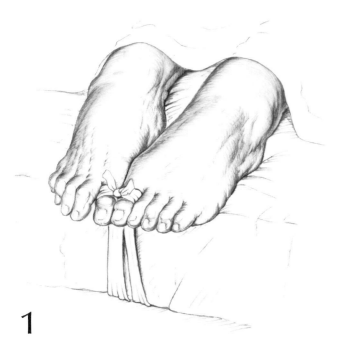

1

Anaesthesia and positioning

1 Cannulation of a normal lymphatic, as in the investigation of lymphoma, is relatively simple and can be performed using local anaesthesia. However, in the lymphoedematous limb, the search may be protracted and uncomfortable. For this reason and because any movement of the patient can dislodge the cannula, lymphography for lymphoedema should be performed under a light general anaesthetic.

It is essential to anchor the foot sufficiently to eliminate movement. A length of ribbon gauze ties the great toes together and is then fixed to the table. This also produces good plantar flexion which helps cannulation of the lymphatics.

Operation

Demonstration of lymphatics

2 Approximately 0.2 ml of 11% Patent Blue Violet dye is injected just beneath the dermis in the web between each toe and also lateral to the fifth toe. Both legs are always investigated. Thus a total of 2 ml of Patent Blue Violet is used. When removing the needle, slight suction avoids spillage of the dye over the skin. A swab is used to massage the injection site and care should be taken not to wipe dye onto the dorsum of the foot.

This highly diffusible dye will, in normal circumstances, be carried rapidly to lymphatic collecting vessels. Normal lymphatics become visible as green-blue lines converging on the dorsum of the foot between the first and third metatarsal heads.

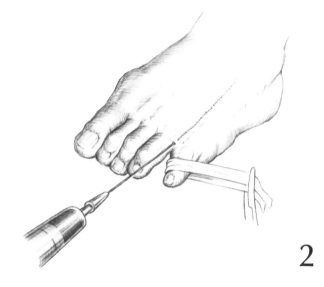

2

Dermal back flow

3 If the collecting vessels are inadequate or obliterated, the dye may diffuse through the dermal plexus of lymphatics and produce a blue marbled appearance in the skin described as dermal back flow. It has been suggested that further lymphography is unnecessary if dermal back flow is present, but this is not a reliable test. Furthermore, identification of pelvic obstruction or hyperplastic lymphatics is of assistance in managing the patient.

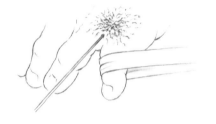

3

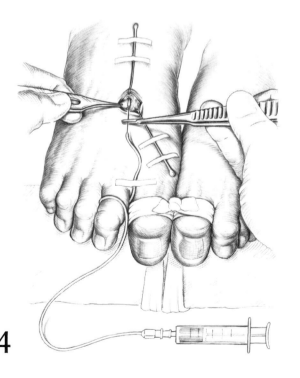

4

Dissection of lymphatics

4 A transverse incision is made over a stained lymphatic. In a lymphoedematous limb, when no lymph vessels can be seen, a transverse incision is made on the dorsum of the foot to dissect the lymphatics lying between the first and third metatarsal heads. These lymphatics eventually pass up the medial side of the leg alongside the long saphenous vein. Lymphatics travelling with the short saphenous vein are found immediately behind the lateral malleolus.

The incision is taken just through the dermis and beneath this the lymphatic collecting vessels are sought. In the lymphoedematous foot, bleeding may impair vision but diathermy should be used sparingly and accurately; bleeding usually stops with pressure.

A small vein can easily be mistaken for a lymphatic. The vein, however, appears thicker walled and a darker grey-blue.

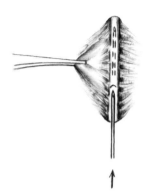

5a

Cannulation of lymphatics

5a–c Once the lymphatic has been located it is teased out of the tissues and should be handled as little as possible (*Illustration 5a*). Only two-thirds of the circumference of the vessel wall should be dissected free since an isolated diseased lymphatic tears easily and the mobility hinders cannulation (*Illustration 5b*). The lymphatic may also go into spasm. This spasm may be relieved by a little 4% procaine in the wound. If only a short length is isolated the cannulating needle disappears beyond the operator's vision and may transfix the vessel (*Illustration 5c*). The cannula should not be tied into the lymphatic. This is unnecessary and may damage the vessel. Occasionally, there is considerable leakage of Lipiodol through the puncture site and a single throw using silk may reduce this.

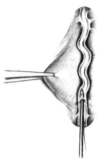

5b

Injection

When the needle is primed with contrast medium a small amount of air should be left in the attached polyvinyl tubing so that an air bubble can be seen passing up the lymphatic when the pump is switched on. Slight extravasation of air into the wall may allow manipulation and subsequent successful injection, but extravasation of Lipiodol ends any further attempts to cannulate that particular lymphatic. An injection pump is necessary and should be set at a rate of 12 ml/h; otherwise, the diseased narrow lymphatic will rupture or there may be extravasation of dye as it passes up the lymphatic. As Lipiodol forms fat emboli in the lungs no more than 7 ml should be injected into each leg, that is 14 ml for a single investigation.

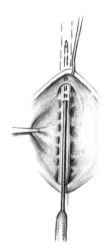

5c

Inguinal node lymphography

6a, b Obliterated lymphatics in the foot may be associated with normal pelvic lymphatics and a good prognosis, or with abnormal and obliterated pelvic lymphatics and a consequent poor prognosis. For this reason, direct injection of inguinal lymph nodes may be valuable where foot lymphography has failed.

A small (2-cm) incision is made over an inguinal lymph node which should be exposed with a minimum of dissection. Once its superficial surface is exposed it can be stabbed with the cannulating needle and lymphography performed. Previous injection of Patent Blue Violet dye into the thigh may allow a lymphatic entering the node to be seen and cannulated, thus producing a better lymphogram.

After injection either into the foot or the inguinal lymph nodes, a radiograph should be taken within a few minutes to ensure that the lymphatics are filled with Lipiodol. If there is any evidence of globules of contrast medium (caviar sign), the injection should be stopped immediately since this is diagnostic of an intravenous infusion. Further lymphangiograms should be taken as required. When the infusion is complete, massage and movement of the leg improves visualization of the thoracic duct which is best shown by a right oblique chest radiograph. Lymphadenograms should be taken 24 h later.

Complications

Anaphylactic reactions to Patent Blue Violet and Lipiodol are rare. However, patients have developed pulmonary oil embolism leading to a pyrexia and diffuse pulmonary infiltration on the chest radiograph. Providing that no more than 14 ml of Lipiodol are used this does not occur. If Lipiodol is seen intravenously then the investigation should be terminated immediately. Lipiodol should not be infused after lung irradiation because cerebral oil embolism may occur in these circumstances.

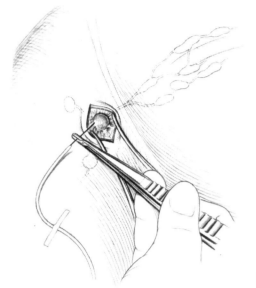

6a

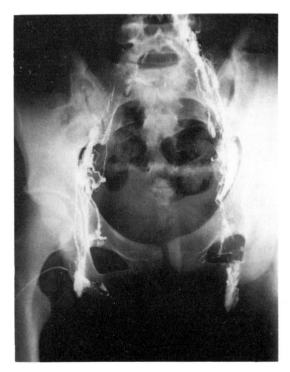

6b

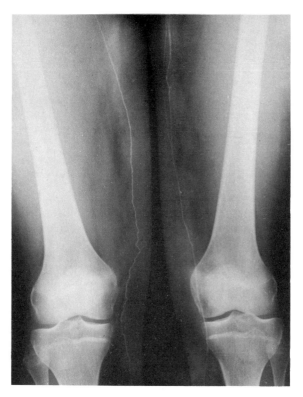

Lymphographic abnormalities

Distal obliteration of primary lymphoedema

7a, b Hypoplastic lymphatics confined to below the groin are illustrated in the right leg and are also demonstrated by the lymphogram in *Illustration 7a*. Normal lymphatic anatomy is outlined in the left leg (*Illustration 7b*). Distal hypoplasia is usually seen in women with bilateral distal oedema. This is the most common form of the disease and is usually mild and non-progressive, responding well to conservative treatment.

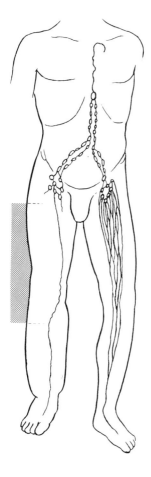

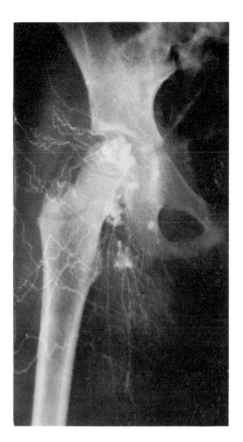

8a

Pelvic obstruction

8a, b This is often found where there is whole leg unilateral oedema; men and women are equally affected. In these patients, the lymphographic abnormality is in the pelvis and is associated with adequate distal lymphatics and a normal thoracic duct. If the patient is treated early in the process a small bowel mesenteric pedicle graft may be successful[4]. However, there is now evidence that delay may make this impossible because of secondary obliteration of distal lymphatics[5]. Some patients have both proximal *and* distal obliteration and a normal thoracic duct.

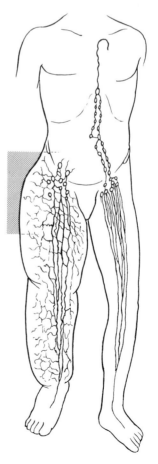

8b

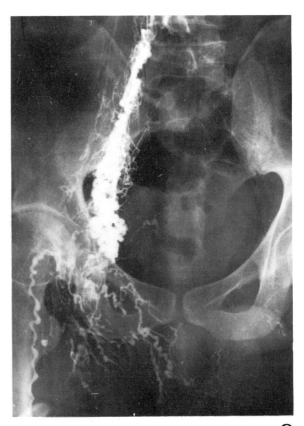

9a

Megalymphatics

$9a, b$ Occasionally, varicose lymphatics may be seen. This abnormality allows reflux of chyle or lymph and may produce vesicles on the limbs or genitalia. It may also produce chylothorax, chylous ascites or chyluria. This type of lymphoedema may be treated by ligation of the lymphatics which have been identified by lymphography[6].

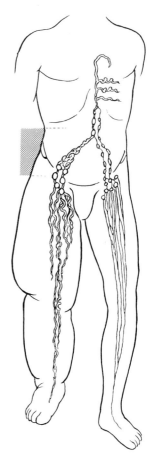

9b

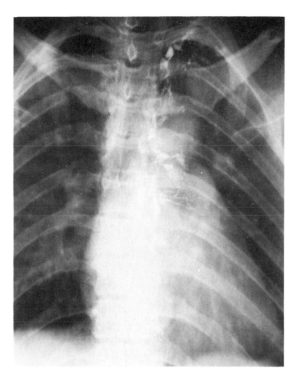

10a

Bilateral hyperplasia of lymph vessels

10a, b Bilateral hyperplasia of lymph vessels is the other form of identifiable primary lymphographic abnormality. In these patients the abnormality appears to be in the thoracic duct with secondary distension, tortuosity and collateral formation in the vessels distal to this. A lymphonodal venous or lymphaticovenous shunt may be helpful in these patients[7,8].

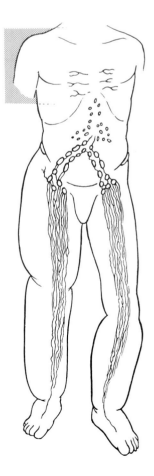

10b

Postoperative care

The wound should be carefully sutured with poly-propylene (Prolene) and great care taken with sterility since wound healing is impaired in these lymphoedematous limbs.

References

1. Kinmonth JB. Lymphangiography in man. A method of outlining lymphatic trunks at operation. *Clin Sci* 1952; 11: 13–20.

2. Wolfe JHN, Kinmonth JB. The prognosis of primary lymphedema of the lower limbs. *Arch Surg* 1981; 116: 1157–60.

3. Zelikovski A, Manoach M, Giler S, Urca I. Lympha-press, a new pneumatic device for the treatment of lymphedema of the limbs. *Lymphology* 1980; 13: 68–73.

4. Kinmonth JB, Hurst PA, Edwards JM, Rutt DL. Relief of lymph obstruction by use of a bridge of mesentery and ileum. *Br J Surg* 1978; 65: 829–33.

5. Fyfe NC, Wolfe JH, Kinmonth JB. 'Die-back' in primary lymphedema – lymphographic and clinical correlations. *Lymphology* 1982; 15: 66–69.

6. Kinmonth JB, *The Lymphatics: Surgery, Lymphography and Diseases of the Chyle and Lymph System*, 2nd ed. London: Arnold, 1982; 227.

7. Nielubowicz J, Olszewski W, Muszynski M, Sawicki Z. Late results of lymphovenous anastomosis. *J Cardiovasc Surg* 1973; Special no. 113–20.

8. O'Brien BMcC, Shafiroff BB. Microlymphaticovenous and resectional surgery in obstructive lymphoedema. *World J Surg* 1979; 3: 3–15.

Direct operations on the lymphatics

Peter Gloviczki MD

Associate Professor of Surgery, Mayo Medical School and Consultant, Division of Vascular Surgery, Mayo Clinic and Foundation, Rochester, Minnesota, USA

History

Progress in microvascular surgical techniques and instrumentation has made direct reconstructions of the lymph vessels possible. Lymphovenous anastomoses to bypass the obstructed lymphatic system have been performed for secondary lymphoedema of the upper or lower extremities for over 20 years. The largest series of patients with long-term follow-up after lymphovenous anastomoses was recently reported by O'Brien et al.[1].

Lymphatic grafting, either as suprapubic lymph vessel bypass for unilateral lower extremity lymphoedema, or as transplantation of leg lymph vessels to the arm for postmastectomy lymphoedema, has been introduced by Baumeister[2]. Significant, well documented experience from other authors with this operation is not available.

Principles and justification

Surgical excision of major lymph nodes, irradiation, infestation with *Wuchereria bancrofti* (filariasis), inflammation, tumour invasion, or trauma are the major causes of obstructive lymphoedema. Obstructive lymphangitis may severely damage or occlude major lymph vessels distal to the site of surgical excision or irradiation, though in many patients the distal lymph vessels stay patent, dilate and drain through the more or less developed collateral lymphatic circulation. Lymphovenous anastomosis or lymphatic grafting with dilated lymph vessels is attractive, and in the early stage of chronic lymphoedema it has the potential to improve lymph drainage of the extremity. In long-standing chronic lymphoedema, however, progressive valvular incompetence, fibrosis of the lymph vessels, loss of intrinsic contractility, decreased interstitial pressure and interstitial fibrosis decrease the chances of effective drainage with lymphatic reconstructions[3]. Patients with early secondary lymphoedema without episodes of cellulitis and lymphangitis, who do not respond to a trial of at least 3 months of correct conservative compression treatment, are potential candidates for lymphatic reconstructions.

Preoperative

Assessment and preparation

In over 90% of patients lymphoedema can be diagnosed from a thorough history and physical examination, complemented with a hand-held Doppler examination of the venous system. Additionally, routine blood analyses, chest radiography and non-invasive venous studies are performed in all patients with lymphoedema who are considered for surgical treatment. Venous outflow obstruction can be assessed by impedance, strain gauge, or air plethysmography. Duplex scanning of the deep veins is performed in patients with clinical signs or symptoms of venous disease, or with evidence of venous outflow obstruction on plethysmography. Contrast venography is performed selectively.

Venous hypertension, caused either by obstruction or by venous valvular incompetence, is a contraindication for lymphovenous anastomoses. An underlying primary, metastatic, or recurrent malignant tumour should be excluded in every patient with lymphoedema. Computed tomography is excellent for this purpose, and this is performed in every adult patient with a recent onset of limb swelling. If arteriovenous malformation or soft tissue tumour is suspected, magnetic resonance imaging is performed.

Contrast lymphangiography for evaluation of patients with lymphoedema has been almost completely replaced by isotope lymphangiography. Although this method does not provide the fine anatomical details of contrast lymphangiography, it is non-invasive, has no side effects, and is well tolerated by patients. Lymphoscintigraphy performed with ^{99m}Tc-labelled antimony trisulphide colloid is an excellent method of confirming the diagnosis of lymphoedema and documenting any delay in lymphatic transport. In the author's experience with 190 examinations, lymphoscintigraphy had a 92% sensitivity and a 100% specificity in the diagnosis of lymphoedema[4].

Before surgery every attempt is made to decrease the volume of the extremity with conservative measures to facilitate dissection. Patients with lower extremity lymphoedema are hospitalized for 48h for bed-rest, elevation of the extremity and forced diuresis. Patients with upper extremity lymphoedema are asked to elevate the extremity and use an intermittent compression pump for several hours during the day before the operation.

Anaesthesia

Because these operations last several hours, in the author's practice general anaesthesia with endotracheal intubation is performed in every patient.

Operations

LYMPHOVENOUS ANASTOMOSES IN THE LOWER EXTREMITY

Incision

1 Depending on the site of lymphatic obstruction, a longitudinal incision is made over the long saphenous vein at the groin or upper calf, or a transverse incision is made at mid-thigh to dissect the large medial superficial lymph vessels and the long saphenous vein and its tributaries.

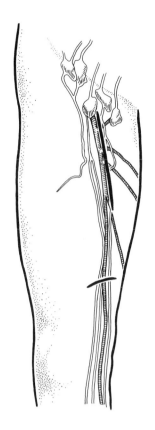

1

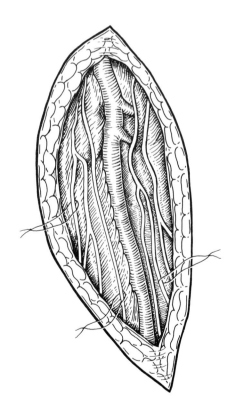

2

Dissection of lymph vessels

2 To visualize the lymph vessels, 5 ml of sulphan blue (or 2–4 ml of brilliant blue FCF dye) is injected subcutaneously into the extremity 15 min before dissection. Half of the amount is injected between the first and second interdigital space of the foot, while the other half is injected at 10–15 cm distal to the site of the incision. Manual massage of the limb helps passage of the dye up to the area of dissection.

In some patients, dye does not advance because of severe lymphatic obstruction. With experience, however, the greyish looking lymph vessels, which measure 0.3–1.5 mm in diameter, can be dissected under the operating microscope even if not stained by dye. Subcutaneous nerves, which may look similar, have a shiny white appearance and show transverse striae. The dissected lymph vessels are marked with 6/0 silk loops. Vessels less than 0.5 mm in diameter are not suitable for anastomosis.

Dissection of veins

3 The long saphenous vein and its tributaries are carefully dissected. The lymph vessels and veins are continuously irrigated throughout the procedure with normal saline containing heparin, 100 000 units/l and papaverine, 150 mg/l, to avoid spasm and drying out of the vessels.

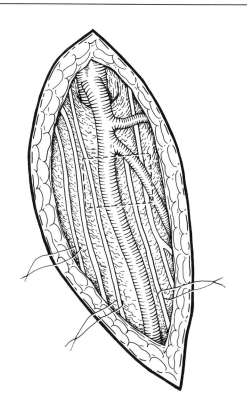

3

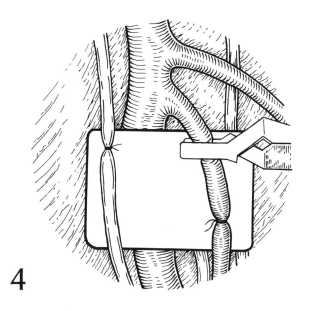

4

Technique of anastomosis

4 The lymph vessel to be used for anastomosis is ligated with 6/0 silk proximally and the vein is ligated distally. A small microvascular clamp is placed on the vein to avoid back-bleeding, but no clamp is placed on the lymph vessel to avoid any trauma. No attempt is made to remove the adventitia from the lymph vessels and only a small amount of adventitial tissue is resected from the end of the vein.

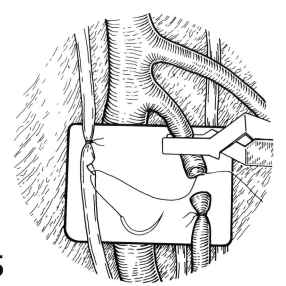

5

5 The lymph vessel is incised, but it is not completely transected to allow better visualization of the lumen. Drainage of lymph can usually be observed from the lymph vessel. The vein is completely transected, leaving sufficient length for a tension-free anastomosis. The field is continuously irrigated with the heparinized papaverine solution. A 10/0 or 11/0 monofilament non-absorbable suture is placed, inserting the needle first through the vein and then through the lumen of the lymph vessel.

6 After placement of the first suture, the lymph vessel is completely transected and the first knot is tied. Additional sutures are placed first into the posterior wall and then into the anterior wall of the vessels.

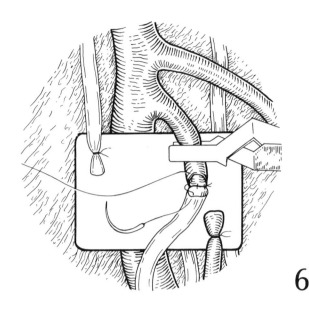

6

7 Four to six interrupted sutures are sufficient to perform the end-to-end anastomosis under the operating microscope, using 4–40 times magnification. Distension of the vein by lymph proximal to the anastomosis should be readily seen under the microscope, confirming patency.

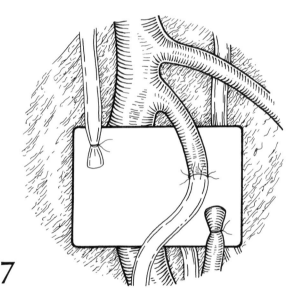

7

8 Multiple anastomoses should be performed with as many lymph vessels as possible. If no more venous tributary is available, an end-to-side anastomosis can be performed with the long saphenous vein using interrupted sutures.

Wound closure

After performing the anastomosis, the wound is irrigated with antibiotic solution, the subcutaneous layer above the anastomoses is closed with interrupted 3/0 polyglactin (Vicryl) sutures and the skin is closed with interrupted 4/0 vertical mattress nylon sutures.

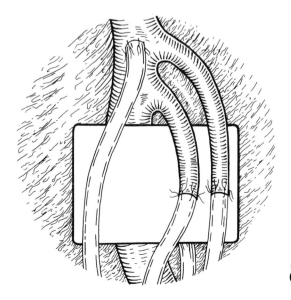

8

SUPRAPUBIC LYMPHATIC GRAFTING FOR UNILATERAL LEG OEDEMA

Incision

9 The skin incision on the proximal thigh of the swollen extremity is the same as for lymphovenous anastomosis. On the donor leg a similar longitudinal incision is made over the long saphenous vein and is extended distally for 20–25 cm to dissect an adequate length of the medial superficial lymphatics for suprapubic grafting.

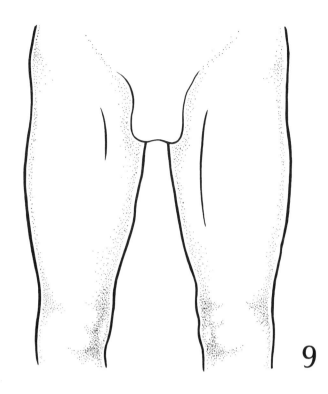

9

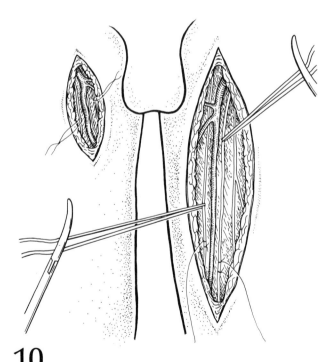

10

Dissection of lymph vessels

10 Dissection of the lymph vessels in the swollen leg is performed under the operating microscope as described previously. The lymphatic grafts are then dissected on the donor side, using loupe magnification. Because lymphatic transport on this side is normal, the dye injected into the interdigital space of the foot is easily visible in the lymphatics 5–15 min after injection. The lymph vessels have few or no side branches in the thigh. A small rubber vessel loop is placed under the lymphatic grafts and, if a satisfactory length of 20–25 cm is freely dissected, two lymph vessels are double ligated in the distal thigh with 6/0 silk and transected.

Tunnelling

11 The lymph vessels are tunnelled subcutaneously to the contralateral groin through a Silastic tube placed subcutaneously above the pubic symphysis. The lymphatic grafts are pulled through the tube with 6/0 silk tied to a guidewire.

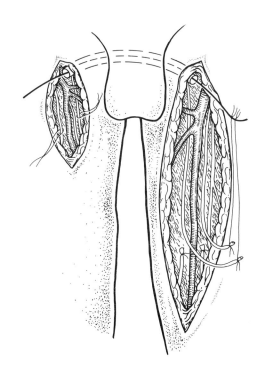

11

Anastomosis

12 The lymphatic grafts are prepared for a tension-free end-to-end anastomosis, performed under the operating microscope with 4–40 times magnification, with the lymph vessels of the lymphoedematous limb.

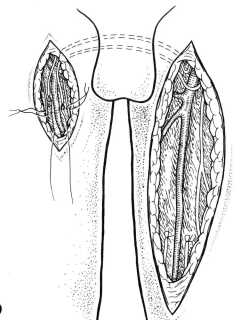

12

13 The lymphatic graft is completely transected while the lymph vessel of the lymphoedematous leg is incised. The technique of anastomosis is similar to that for lymphovenous anastomosis, placing the first suture into the lymphatic graft and then into the lymph vessel; 11/0 monofilament non-absorbable sutures are used.

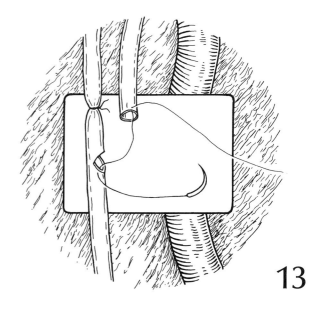

13

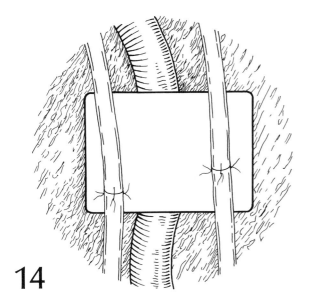

14

14 Depending on the number of lymphatic grafts, two or three end-to-end anastomoses are performed, usually with four interrupted sutures for each anastomosis.

Wound closure

Closure of both sides is performed in two layers with interrupted 3/0 polyglactin for the subcutaneous closure and interrupted 4/0 vertical mattress nylon for the skin. The skin of the normal extremity can be closed with running 4/0 subcuticular polyglactin.

LYMPHOVENOUS ANASTOMOSES IN THE UPPER EXTREMITY

15 The skin incision is longitudinal on the medial aspect of the mid-arm, above the course of the basilic vein. If patent lymph vessels are not found, a more distal skin incision can be made transversely in the antecubital fossa or on the dorsal surface of the arm, just proximal to the wrist. The technique of lymphovenous anastomoses is the same as described in the lower extremities. The basilic and brachial veins and their tributaries can be used for anastomoses.

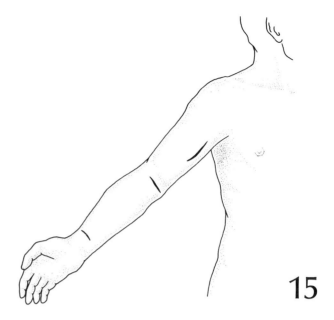

15

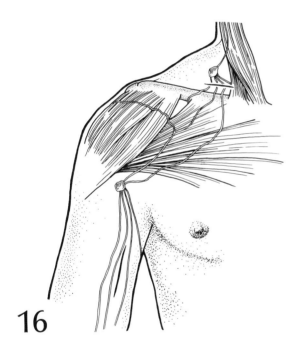

16

LYMPHATIC GRAFTING IN THE UPPER EXTREMITY

16 The lymph vessels for lymphatic grafting are dissected through a longitudinal incision on the medial aspect of the arm. If suitable lymph vessels at this level are found for anastomoses, a transverse neck incision is made one fingerbreadth proximal to the clavicle, just lateral to the lateral edge of the sternocleidomastoid muscle.

17 Descending neck lymphatics are dissected medial to the sternocleidomastoid muscle in the supraclavicular fat pad. All lymphatics are marked with 6/0 silk loops.

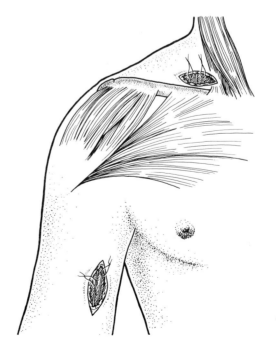

17

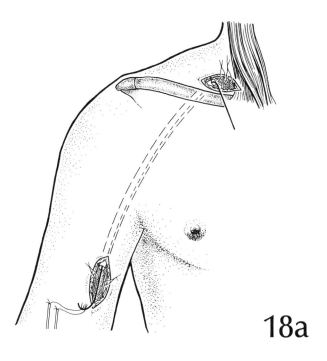

18a, b Two lymphatic grafts are harvested from the thigh with the technique described previously. The lymphatic grafts are tunnelled subcutaneously from the arm up to the supraclavicular fossa through a Silastic tube with a guidewire. The arm anastomoses are performed first in an end-to-end fashion using a technique similar to that described for suprapubic grafting. The neck anastomoses are performed next in an end-to-end fashion between the lymphatic grafts and the descending neck lymphatics in the supraclavicular triangle.

Wound closure

The neck incision is closed with interrupted 3/0 polyglactin sutures for the platysma and running 4/0 subcuticular polyglactin for the skin. The incision at the arm is closed with interrupted 2/0 polyglactin for the subcutaneous layer and interrupted 4/0 vertical mattress nylon for the skin. The incision at the thigh is closed with interrupted 2/0 polyglactin for the subcutaneous layer and running 4/0 subcuticular polyglactin for the skin.

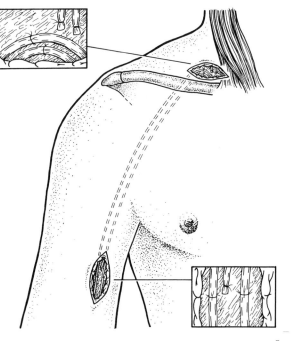

Postoperative care

Elevation of the extremity, elastic compression and intermittent pneumatic compression using low (less than 60 mmHg) pressures to stimulate flow are used. The pneumatic boot or cuff is placed only to the distal extremity remote from the site of operation to avoid disruption of the anastomoses. The use of elastic compression and elevation of the extremity during the night is advised after discharge.

Outcome

Evaluating the long-term effectiveness of lymphatic reconstructions has been difficult. Decrease in circumference or volume of the extremity, decrease in episodes of cellulitis and improvement in lymphatic clearance as measured by lymphoscintigraphy have been used as criteria of success. In the author's review of 18 cases operated on for lymphoedema, four of seven patients with secondary lymphoedema improved after a mean follow-up of 37 months[5]. O'Brien *et al.*[1] reported 52 patients who underwent lymphovenous anastomoses for secondary lymphoedema without additional excisional procedures; the mean follow-up in these patients was 4.3 years. Long-term improvement was documented by volume measurement in 42% of the patients, the oedema was unchanged in 12% and worse in 45%; 83% of the patients discontinued the use of conservative measures after the operation.

Demonstration of patency of lymphovenous anastomoses would be possible with contrast lymphangiography, but this invasive test, which may occasionally worsen lymphoedema[1], has not been used in postoperative evaluation. Patent lymphatic grafts can quite reliably be imaged by lymphoscintigraphy[2,6,7]. Although the patency rate of lymphatic grafting in patients is still unknown, lymphoscintigraphy has shown improved lymphatic transport after grafting in 30 patients with postmastectomy lymphoedema[2]. Volume measurements showed significant improvement in 36 patients with arm lymphoedema, in 16 more than 2 years after surgery. Significant improvement was documented in eight of 12 patients with lower extremity lymphoedema more than 1 year after suprapubic grafting[2].

Direct operations on the lymph vessels continue to be controversial. Controlled randomized studies, which would be the only proof of late effectiveness after lymphatic reconstructions, are not available. Although long-term clinical improvement has been described, objective evidence of long-term patency and function of lymphovenous anastomoses in patients is not at present available. Similarly, results with lymphatic grafting need confirmation by more than one surgical team, and the late patency and function of these grafts need further evaluation. Therefore, it is the opinion of the author that, until further evidence is collected by experienced microsurgical teams, these operations should still be considered experimental.

References

1. O'Brien BM, Mellow CG, Khazanchi RK, Dvir E, Kumar V, Pederson WC. Long-term results after microlymphatico-venous anastomoses for the treatment of obstructive lymphedema. *Plast Reconstr Surg* 1990; 85: 562–72.

2. Baumeister RG, Siuda S. Treatment of lymphedemas by microsurgical lymphatic grafting: what is proved? *Plast Reconstr Surg* 1990; 85: 64–76.

3. Clodius L, Piller NB, Casely-Smith JR. The problems of lymphatic microsurgery for lymphedema. *Lymphology* 1981; 14: 69–76.

4. Gloviczki P, Calcagno D, Schirger A, Pairolero PC, Cherry KJ, Jr, Hallett JW Jr *et al*. Noninvasive evaluation of the swollen extremity: experiences with 190 lymphoscintigraphic examinations. *J Vasc Surg* 1989; 9: 683–90.

5. Gloviczki P, Fisher J, Hollier LH, Pairolero PC, Schirger A, Wahner HW. Microsurgical lymphovenous anastomosis for treatment of lymphedema: a critical review. *J Vasc Surg* 1988; 7: 647–52.

6. Gloviczki P. Microsurgical treatment for chronic lymphedema: an unfulfilled promise? In: Bergan JJ, Yao JST, eds. *Venous Disorders*. Orlando, Florida: WB Saunders, 1991: 344–59.

7. Gloviczki P, Bergman RT. Lymphatic problems and revascularization edema. In: Bernhard VM, Towne JB, eds. *Complications in Vascular Surgery*. St Louis, Missouri: Quality Medical Publishing, 1991: 366–88.

Illustrations by Denise Smith and Timothy C. Hengst

Percutaneous balloon angioplasty for lower extremity arterial occlusive disease

Peter A. Schneider MD
Vascular Laboratory, Saint Joseph Medical Center, Burbank, California, USA

George Andros MD, FRCS(Glas)
Vascular Laboratory, Saint Joseph Medical Center, Burbank, California, USA

Robert W. Harris MD
Vascular Laboratory, Saint Joseph Medical Center, Burbank, California, USA

History

The current clinical application and technique of percutaneous transluminal balloon angioplasty (PTA) are the culmination of work which began in 1964, when Dotter and Jenkins dilated vascular lesions using a rigid coaxial catheter system. Catheters were later modified into tapered tubes by Van Andel and Staple. A balloon catheter was introduced by Porstmann in 1973, and Gruntzig developed the double-lumen, non-elastomeric, polyvinyl balloon catheter in 1974. The Gruntzig device permitted catheter placement over a guidewire and controlled balloon inflation, and it formed the basis for modern PTA techniques.

Principles and justification

PTA has become essential in the therapeutic armamentarium for atherosclerotic occlusive disease of the lower extremities. It permits autologous vascular reconstruction and provides a treatment option that significantly expands the spectrum of patients to whom therapy may be offered. At one end of the spectrum are patients whose symptoms would not traditionally warrant operative intervention, such as those with moderate-to-severe claudication; at the other end are patients who require revascularization but are at excessive risk for surgery.

Revascularization with PTA is not as durable as open surgery. Nevertheless, its low morbidity and the ability to repeat the procedure or proceed to surgery in the event of failure suggest that dilatation should be the initial therapeutic choice when amenable lesions are associated with appropriate clinical indications. Patient selection for PTA is the cornerstone of a successful outcome. This chapter will cover the percutaneous technique for balloon angioplasty, but this approach can be adapted to intraoperative balloon interventions during revascularization surgery.

Preoperative

Assessment and preparation

The surgeon should decide whether to revascularize and how it should be accomplished. The history and physical examination reveal the severity of the ischaemic disease and allow localization of the lesions. Non-invasive studies provide confirmatory assessment and are obtained as a baseline for comparison with postoperative studies.

Renal function and coagulation status are evaluated before operation. The groins are prepared and draped bilaterally. Intravenous antibiotics are given if the patient has prosthetic graft material in place or has gangrenous tissue. A protective lead apron, thyroid shield and leaded gloves and glasses are worn by the surgeon.

Operative strategy

Arteriography is a strategic manoeuvre, not a diagnostic one. Before the availability of non-invasive physiological testing, arteriography was the only confirmatory diagnostic method. As angiographic experience was correlated with clinical syndromes, claudication was usually found to be associated with single stenoses and short occlusions, whereas gangrene was the product of long or tandem lesions. Angiography has become unnecessary for diagnosis, and is meddlesome if there are no therapeutic implications.

Strategies for obtaining arteriographic imaging must complement the intended revascularization procedure. The site for vascular access is selected at the initial patient visit. Occasionally, arteriography has already been performed. If none has been done, abdominal aortography with bilateral run-off is performed through the femoral artery contralateral to the artery to be treated. The arteriographic catheter is intermittently flushed with heparinized saline and left in place for pressure measurements and angiography after the procedure.

Anaesthesia

Anaesthesia standby is desirable and provides monitoring and intravenous sedation resulting in greater patient comfort, compliance and safety. Lack of movement during arterial puncture and catheter manipulation decreases operative time and prevents blurred films.

Operations

Standard equipment

The standard equipment required for PTA (*Table 1*) should be at hand at the start of the procedure.

Guidewires

The straight Bentson guidewire is green and has a 15–20-cm floppy tip. When exchanging this guidewire or inserting a catheter, it must be advanced so that at least 7.5–10 cm of the stiffer portion of the catheter are in the artery. The Wholey wire is stiff and steerable. A plastic handle is locked onto the shaft of the wire, and the tip can be rotated with a 1:1 turning ratio by turning the handle. The Terumo glidewire has a slippery hydrophilic coating when moistened, which enables it to slip through severe, irregular and lengthy stenoses. It must be gripped firmly when wet. The surgeon may mistakenly perceive the glidewire as being advanced when in reality the hand is sliding along it. Long enough guidewires must be selected so that sufficient length will remain outside the patient while catheters are being exchanged.

Angiographic catheters

The current generation of angiographic catheters has been reduced to 5 Fr or less in diameter, and these are useful for performing arteriography and guiding the advancement and placement of guidewires. The tip of each of the catheters determines its usefulness. The straight catheter, with end and side holes, is a standard arteriographic catheter. The tennis racket catheter, similar to the pigtail catheter, allows redirection of the guidewire and also avoids forceful injection of contrast medium from the catheter tip into the aortic wall. The bent tip of the cobra catheter is useful for passing a guidewire over the aortic bifurcation and for selective vessel catheterization, and it can be used to redirect the guidewire tip. The sidewinder catheter is useful for selective cannulation of branch vessels.

Balloon catheters

Balloon catheters have a double lumen: one lumen accommodates a distal port for passage of a guidewire or

Table 1   Standard equipment for PTA

Miscellaneous	Guidewires	Angiographic catheters	Balloon catheters
Scalpel (11 blade)	Bentson 0.035 inch	Straight	Iliac: 6–10-mm diameter
Local anaesthetic	Glidewire (Terumo)	Tennis racket	Femoropopliteal: 3–7-mm
Kelly clamp	Wholey	Cobra	diameter
Gauze pads	Extra-stiff wire (Amplatz or Rosen)	Sidewinder (65-cm length)	(length of balloon 4–10 cm)
Sterile field	(145-cm length)		(length of catheter 95 cm)
Arteriographic contrast medium			
Entry needle (No. 18)			
Sheath introducer			
Heparinized saline			
Inflation device			

injection of contrast medium or drugs such as heparin or papaverine; the other fills and empties the balloon. The balloons are cylindrical and have the manufacturer's recommended inflation and estimated bursting pressures. The balloon portion of the catheter has radio-opaque markers on each end which allow it to be visualized by fluoroscopy. The packaged balloon is wrapped in a counterclockwise manner around the shaft and should not be preinflated.

Catheters may be passed percutaneously or through a sheath introducer. This device provides access for arteriography or medications through a side-arm port, maintains the desired access to the femoral artery and provides a site of introduction for balloon catheters. Indications for the use of a sheath include: a vessel entry point with severe plaque; severe vessel tortuosity; and complex lesions requiring numerous guidewire and catheter exchanges. The use of a sheath should be decided at the beginning of the procedure. The sheath makes a larger arteriotomy and is associated with a higher rate of bleeding complications.

Imaging

Intraprocedural imaging comprises multiformat image intensification (14 × 14, 9 × 9 and 5 × 5 inch), cut film and digital subtraction angiography formats. Classic cut film requires more contrast medium than digital subtraction imaging, but gives the best detail, particularly for the infrainguinal arteries. Digital imaging decreases contrast load by employing digital enhancement and computerized subtractions. Subtractions, however, remove bony landmarks and often give inadequate

resolution to characterize luminal irregularities in patent infrainguinal arteries.

Road mapping is a feature of some digital units, in which a previously obtained arteriographic image is superimposed on a real-time fluoroscopic image. Correct placement of a balloon catheter can be simplified using this technique, because the location of a previously identified lesion is visible on the fluoroscopic image as the balloon catheter is inserted.

Arteriography is usually performed using an automated contrast injector through a straight or tennis-racket 5-Fr catheter. If renal insufficiency is present, arteriography should be limited to selected areas of symptomatic occlusive disease. Arterial pressure proximal and distal to a lesion should be measured by connecting an appropriately placed angiographic catheter to a pressure manometer. If no gradient is present across a suspicious lesion, papaverine, 30 mg (one ampoule) over 30 s, should be injected into the distal circulation. Pharmacologically induced vasodilatation often helps to identify a gradient.

Choice of entry site for catheter introduction

1a, b PTA can usually be performed through a transfemoral approach; iliac PTA is performed through an ipsilateral retrograde approach and femoropopliteal PTA through an antegrade approach. When the ipsilateral femoral artery cannot be used, the contralateral femoral artery is punctured, and a guidewire is passed over the aortic bifurcation. If neither femoral artery is satisfactory, a catheter may be introduced through the left brachial or axillary arteries.

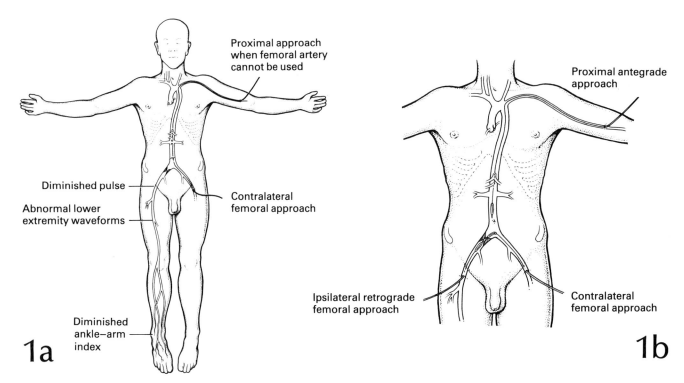

1a

Proximal approach when femoral artery cannot be used

Diminished pulse

Abnormal lower extremity waveforms

Contralateral femoral approach

Diminished ankle–arm index

1b

Proximal antegrade approach

Ipsilateral retrograde femoral approach

Contralateral femoral approach

ILIAC ARTERY BALLOON ANGIOPLASTY

Retrograde femoral puncture

2 The skin and soft tissue over the femoral artery selected for catheter insertion are anaesthetized with 1% lignocaine. A right-handed surgeon stands on the patient's right side. The femoral artery is palpated and immobilized between the second and third fingers of the left hand while other fingers are used to retract surrounding soft tissue. The left hand retains its position until the guidewire is secured within the artery. A small stab wound is made and a straight No. 18, thin-walled entry needle is placed retrogradely through the anterior wall of the common femoral artery.

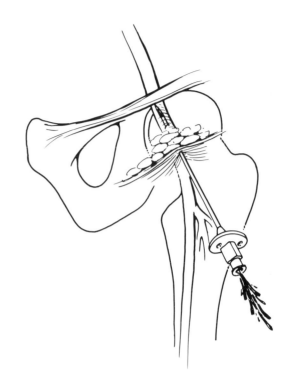

2

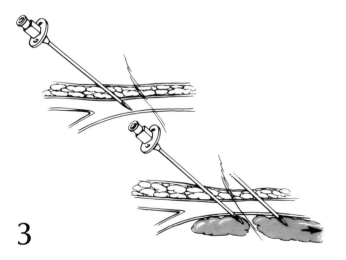

3

Needle entry

3 The needle is angled so that it will puncture the artery just distal to the inguinal ligament. This places the needle entry site 2–4 cm proximal to the femoral bifurcation. Only the anterior wall of the artery should be punctured. Posterior wall punctures may cause bleeding or disrupt a posterior wall plaque.

Techniques of locating the common femoral artery

4 Puncture of a femoral artery with a weak or absent pulse can be accomplished by a variety of techniques.

1. If the artery is palpable or there is a weak pulse present, the vessel can be trapped between the second and third fingers as described above.
2. Digital road mapping can be performed by injecting through a catheter placed in the contralateral femoral artery. Road mapping allows an arteriographic image of the artery to be superimposed on a real-time fluoroscopic image.

3. The artery can be located by using landmarks derived from an arteriogram obtained previously through another approach.
4. The femoral artery usually passes over the medial third of the femoral head. This area can be located and puncture can be guided fluoroscopically.
5. Puncture can be guided by vascular calcification.
6. The pulseless artery can often be palpated, particularly if it is firm. On entering the pulseless artery, the initial impression may be that it is a vein. A small amount of hand-injected contrast viewed under fluoroscopy helps to identify the vessel.

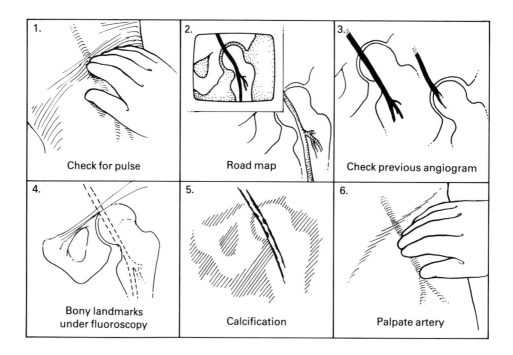

| 1. Check for pulse | 2. Road map | 3. Check previous angiogram |
| 4. Bony landmarks under fluoroscopy | 5. Calcification | 6. Palpate artery |

4

Crossing the lesion

5 The iliac lesion intended for dilatation is localized on the arteriogram and the site of the lesion is marked using bony landmarks or road mapping. A straight Bentson guidewire is placed in the femoral artery and advanced under fluoroscopic guidance. When difficulty is encountered in traversing the stenotic lesion, a Terumo glidewire or a steerable Wholey wire are alternatives. Fluoroscopy should be used to monitor the guidewire encountering the lesion so that it can be redirected if necessary. Force is to be avoided. Angiographic catheters are often useful for redirecting a guidewire across a recalcitrant lesion as the catheter confers stiffness and steerability to the guidewire. The catheter is advanced to within 1–2 cm of the lesion or abutting the lesion, and the tip of the guidewire probes the orifice of the stenosis. Imaging of a lesion that is difficult to cross can often be enhanced by oblique projections. If the lesion cannot be crossed through a retrograde approach, it must be traversed using an antegrade approach from either the contralateral femoral artery or the axillary artery.

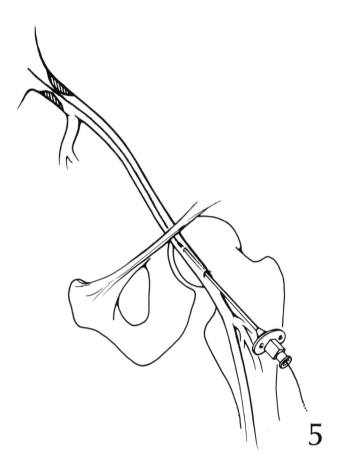

5

6

Balloon selection and placement

6 The balloon catheter is selected after measuring the diameter of the native artery to be dilated and the length of the lesion. The length is usually 4 cm or 10 cm. The radio-opaque balloon markers should extend at least 0.5 cm beyond each end of the lesion. A slight overdilatation of the artery is ensured by a 10–20% magnification of the arterial diameter measured on the plain film arteriogram. Common iliac lesions require balloons 6–10 mm in diameter and external iliac lesions require 5–8-mm balloons. The patient is given intravenous heparin, 75 units/kg. The balloon catheter is placed over the guidewire and inserted with a clockwise rotating motion. If the balloon catheter cannot be advanced across a severe stenosis, a straight angiographic catheter can be used to predilate the lesion. If unsuccessful, other choices include predilatation with a smaller balloon catheter (2.5–3-mm diameter) or a Van Andel tapered 4–7-mm catheter.

Balloon inflation

7 The balloon is filled with a saline–contrast mixture (50/50) which permits visualization of balloon inflation. The balloon luminal pressure at which the atherosclerotic 'waist' opens reflects the degree of hardness of the lesion and is recorded. The balloon is gradually inflated over 5–10 s using the Indeflator to the specified balloon pressure for 1 min. Deflation is allowed for 30 s to permit distal flow, and inflation is then repeated for 1 min. Cut film arteriography with the balloon inflated documents elimination of the waist and compares the balloon size with the adjacent normal artery.

After dilatation, complete aspiration of the balloon is verified under fluoroscopy. If the plaque was particularly difficult to disrupt, a longer inflation time or an additional inflation should be considered. As a rule, intimal hyperplastic lesions are more difficult to dilate than atherosclerotic lesions. The balloon is then withdrawn while turning the catheter in a counterclockwise direction as the wire is maintained in position across the lesion.

Completion arteriography is performed through a straight 5-Fr catheter placed over the ipsilateral guidewire or through a catheter placed more proximally in the aorta. The colour and temperature of the feet and the pedal pulses are evaluated. Following inspection of the clinical and radiographic results after the procedure, the catheter is pulled back and pressure is measured across the lesion to check for gradient. After catheter and guidewire removal, manual pressure is held over the femoral puncture site for 15 min. The last device removed is the guidewire across the dilated segment.

Proximal iliac artery lesions

8 Plaque dilatation at the origin of the common iliac artery may disrupt lesions at the origin of the contralateral iliac artery. PTA is accomplished by protecting the contralateral common iliac artery with a separate balloon of equal size, which is inflated simultaneously (kissing balloons). The contralateral balloon catheter is usually placed through the contralateral femoral artery.

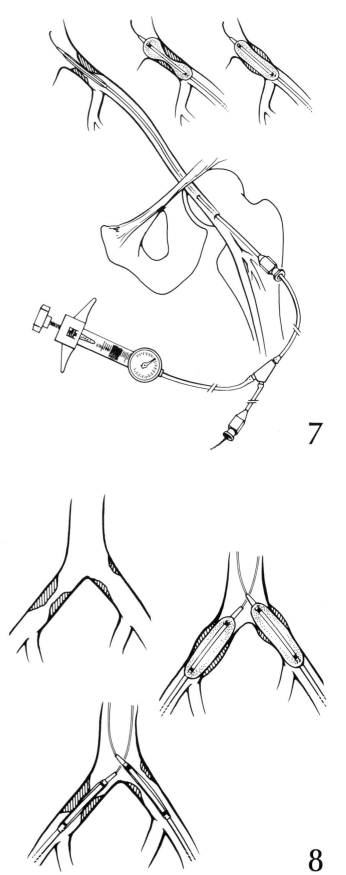

7

8

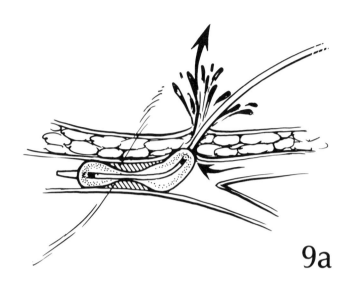

9a

Distal external iliac and proximal common femoral artery lesions

9a, b The working distance between the retrograde femoral puncture site and lesions in the ipsilateral distal external iliac and proximal common femoral arteries is short. The relationship of the balloon to the femoral arterial puncture site is usually unclear, and inflation while it is still in the femoral artery entry site causes major haemorrhage. These lesions are therefore approached through the contralateral femoral artery. A cobra catheter directs the guidewire over the aortic bifurcation and antegradely down the iliac system to the intended angioplasty site.

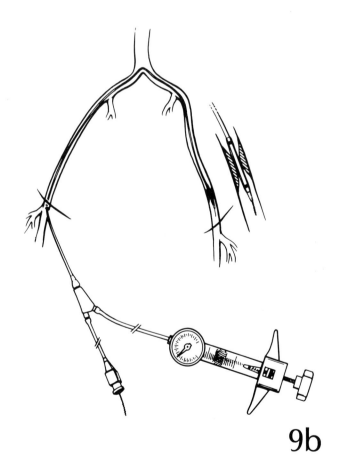

9b

FEMOROPOPLITEAL ARTERY BALLOON ANGIOPLASTY

Antegrade femoral puncture

A right-handed surgeon stands on the patient's left side. Puncture of the proximal common femoral artery at the inguinal ligament allows room to manipulate the guidewire between the puncture site and the femoral bifurcation. The abdominal and groin tissue are retracted superiorly, and the artery is trapped between the second and third fingers of the left hand.

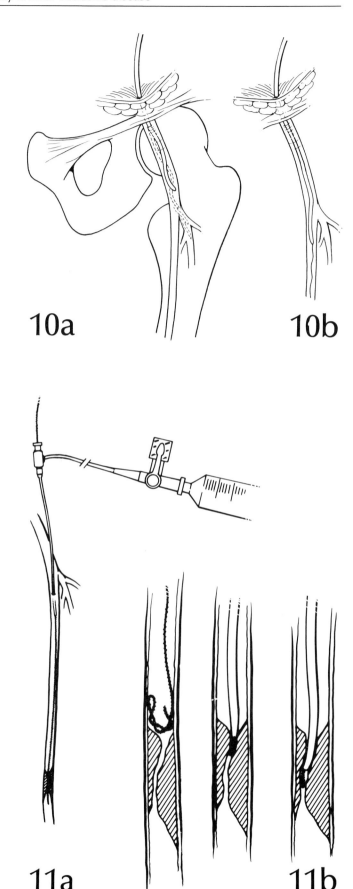

10a   10b

10a, b The needle entry site at the skin level is several centimetres superior to the level of needle entry into the artery. The needle is placed at an angle of 45° or less. Punctures superior to the inguinal ligament may result in retroperitoneal haemorrhage from the external iliac artery, which cannot be manually compressed. A guidewire is passed into the superficial femoral artery under fluoroscopy.

If difficulty occurs in directing the guidewire into the superficial femoral artery (rather than the deep femoral artery), the following steps are taken.

1. The guidewire is left in the deep femoral artery.
2. The needle is removed and the puncture site is dilated with a 5-Fr straight dilator.
3. The dilator is exchanged for a 5-Fr cobra catheter (30-cm length).
4. The cobra catheter is gradually withdrawn while contrast is manually injected.
5. When the femoral bifurcation is visualized, the wire is guided into the superficial femoral artery using the directive tip of the cobra catheter.

Crossing the lesion

11a, b The cobra catheter is exchanged for a straight 5-Fr catheter which is placed in the proximal superficial femoral artery, and femoropopliteal arteriography is performed. The lesion intended for treatment is localized with a radio-opaque ruler (or with road mapping). Heparin, 75 units/kg, is administered through the angiographic catheter.

A Bentson guidewire is inserted through the catheter and is advanced across the lesion. The guidewire sometimes enters a large collateral just proximal to the site of severe stenosis or occlusion. The straight catheter can be used to help guide the wire. Other options include the steerable Wholey wire or the Terumo glidewire for crossing very tight stenoses. If a complex or tandem lesion that will require more than one type of balloon is present, a sheath introducer can be placed in the femoral artery. If a simple femoropopliteal angioplasty involving a single balloon catheter is planned, a sheath introducer is unnecessary.

11a   11b

Balloon placement and inflation

12 The femoral arteriogram is used to measure the desired diameter of the artery and the length of the lesion. The balloon diameters required are 4–7 mm for superficial femoral arteries and 3–5 mm for popliteal arteries. These are available on 5-Fr catheter shafts. Inflation is performed to the manufacturer's specified pressure in the sequence outlined for iliac artery angioplasty (usually 6–10 atmospheres). A radiograph documents full balloon inflation.

Low molecular weight dextran is administered (50 ml bolus followed by 25 ml/h) by constant intravenous infusion for infrainguinal angioplasties. Heparin is not neutralized with protamine. Serial lesions are managed by sequentially dilating the lesions and advancing the catheter from proximal to distal. Long lesions may be dilated by a single balloon (up to 10 cm in length) or by multiple overlapping dilatations using a shorter balloon (4 cm). Completion arteriography is performed, and lower extremity perfusion is evaluated clinically. The balloon catheter is aspirated completely and removed. The last device withdrawn is the guidewire from the angioplasty site. Puncture site haemostasis is obtained with pressure held both above and below the inguinal ligament. Manual pressure must be adequate to control bleeding but not occlude the vessel.

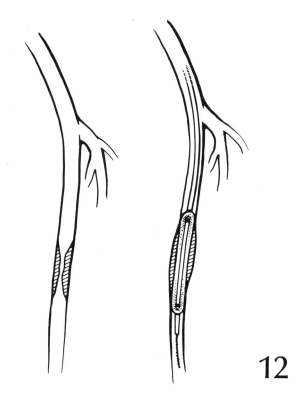

12

Postoperative care

After PTA patients are admitted to hospital and kept in bed overnight. Dextran is continued until the next morning; aspirin, 325 mg/day, is initiated after the operation or may be started before operation. The clinical result of the procedure is noted and ankle/arm indices are determined before discharge.

Complications

Immediate complications of PTA include arterial rupture or dissection leading to occlusion, both of which are rare. Massive intra-abdominal haemorrhage from arterial rupture can be stopped by replacing and reinflating the balloon at the angioplasty site while preparations are made for emergency surgery. Puncture site haemorrhage or haematoma is uncommon if adequate manual compression is maintained at the site. Retroperitoneal haemorrhage from a high femoral or external iliac puncture is often difficult to detect and may not become clinically evident until a few hours after the procedure.

Contrast medium injection may cause allergic reactions and occasionally renal insufficiency. Patients with underlying renal insufficiency are hydrated before the operation and given mannitol, 25 g, immediately before contrast medium injection. The most significant long-term complication of PTA is failure due to recurrent stenosis or progression of disease at another site.

Follow-up

Clinic follow-up is at 1 week, 1 month, every 3 months for the first year and every 6 months thereafter. During follow-up examination, patients should be evaluated for changes in pulse status and bruits of the iliac, femoral, superficial femoral and popliteal arteries.

Outcome and comments

Vascular surgeons should be the central physicians in the management of atherosclerosis with endovascular procedures, because of their clinical knowledge of the disease and the treatment options. The vascular surgeon is responsible for the patient from the initial visit through long-term follow-up.

PTA devices, techniques and results have improved steadily over the past decade. The success of PTA has reinforced the importance of autologous reconstruction. As experience with PTA has grown, so too has knowledge of the pathophysiology of atherosclerotic occlusive disease. For example, what appear to be long lesions on arteriography may actually be short atherosclerotic occlusions with thrombosis of the vessel to the next collateral branch or short lesions with inadequate collaterals that prevent visualization of a patent artery distally. PTA results have shown that several lesions in series may each have differing degrees of haemodynamic significance. Arteriography alone often does not reveal this.

PTA has become the treatment of choice for many patients. The best results are obtained with well localized (short) stenotic lesions in larger proximal arteries, e.g. the common iliac artery, in extremities with good run-off. Early success rates for iliac PTA are 95–100% in most series. At 1 year, 90–95% patency can be expected with 75–80% patent at 3 years. PTA of the superficial femoral and suprageniculate popliteal arteries is followed by a 1-year patency rate of 70–80%.

Acknowledgements

Illustrations 2–9, 11a, 11b and *12* are reproduced with kind permission of Timothy C. Hengst, FAMI.

Further reading

Andros G, Harris RW, Dulawa LB, Oblath RW, Salles-Cunha SX. Balloon angioplasty of iliac, femoral and infrainguinal arteries: percutaneous and intraoperative strategies and techniques. In:Bergan JJ, Yao JST, eds. *Techniques in Arterial Surgery*. Philadelphia: WB Saunders, 1990: 381–98.

Deutsch LS. Techniques of percutaneous balloon angioplasty including aortoiliac and femoropopliteal systems: indications, results and complications. In: Moore WS, Ahn SS, eds. *Endovascular Surgery*. Philadelphia: WB Saunders, 1989: 163–208.

Harris, RW, Dulawa LB, Andros G, Oblath RW, Salles-Cunha SX, Apyan RL. Percutaneous transluminal angioplasty of the lower extremities by the vascular surgeon. *Ann Vasc Surg* 1991; 5: 345–53.

Laser-assisted angioplasty

R. A. White MD
Chief, Vascular Surgery, Harbor-UCLA Medical Center, Torrance, California, and Professor of Surgery, UCLA School of Medicine, California, USA

History

The unique attribute of laser energy for endovascular surgical applications is that it can be delivered over considerable lengths via very small fibreoptic fibres (200–600-μm diameters). This property distinguishes laser angioplasty devices from other angioplasty instruments which are being evaluated. The first feasibility studies evaluating lasers for angioplasty were performed in the early 1980s. Thus, there has been only limited development and evaluation of this technology. The initial studies revealed that tissue ablation was achieved by the intraluminal application of laser energy, but that imprecise delivery and thermal injury caused a high rate of vessel wall perforation. These injuries were related to characteristics of the continuous wave argon and neodymium yttrium aluminium garnet (NdYAG) lasers that were available for initial trials. In an attempt to capture precise tissue ablation but avoid excessive thermal penetration and perforations, an ovoid metal cap was placed on the end of the fibreoptic to confine the thermal effect to the tip and to promote intraluminal recanalization. This 'hot-tip' laser probe developed as a way of controlling tissue ablation with continuous wave lasers[1].

Newer instruments which emit free laser energy demonstrate the feasibility of evolution of this technology if improved guidance methods become available. Pulsed energy systems provide precise non-thermal or limited thermal ablation and have the ability to recanalize more resistant lesions, including those which are calcified. Until devices can be developed which create lumens large enough, the diameter of the laser channel must be enhanced by concomitant balloon angioplasty. For this reason the current method is known as laser-assisted angioplasty. Thus, the procedures are subject to the combined complications of lasers and dilatation devices.

Principles and justification

Initial feasibility studies and successful reports of the use of laser thermal and controlled free energy devices were performed primarily by non-surgeons in cases of stenotic lesions or short occlusions. Patients with favourable lesions were chosen carefully to compare the method with conventional balloon angioplasty and to enable evaluation of the safety and efficacy of the technology in a low-risk patient population. The lesions evaluated initially usually caused neither severe claudication nor limb threat (the surgically accepted criteria for intervention) so that participation in the preliminary studies by surgeons was minimal. Later, when surgeons and radiologists began to use these devices in patients with longer occlusions, the conventional indications for surgery (the incidence of arterial wall perforations, reocclusions and early recurrence of lesions) increased[2–6]. These findings, combined with the rapid evolution of technology, consumer and media interest, multiple subspecialty competition (cardiologists, radiologists and surgeons), differing indications and significant economic incentive for use and development, all make clinical indications for laser-assisted angioplasty a controversial issue.

Indications

In general, the indications for any of the new endovascular surgical devices (lasers, atherectomy, stents) are not established, and extensive studies will be required to determine appropriate use. Definition of indications is further complicated by continual change in the devices to overcome present limitations and modes of failure. Further, the methods are being applied by multiple subspecialties, each with varying criteria for intervention and for determining success. Those who advocate intervention for early lesions feel there is a significant benefit if relief of symptoms improves the quality of life. Treatment requires only a percutaneous procedure with low risk and no worsening of symptoms if the recanalization is unsuccessful. Some of the early data support this contention, while anecdotal reports of compromised clinical status or lost limbs and documentation of persistently high restenosis rates for angioplasties lessen the appeal of this argument. The current need for improved patency and limited liability has reduced the enthusiasm for application of these methods to minimal lesions. The author feels that improvement in clinical results must be accomplished before their use becomes widespread.

Preliminary data do support the use of the new technologies in selected high-risk patients or those who are not good candidates for standard bypass procedures. Seeger et al.[5] reported that this might apply to 10–15% of surgical patients. The author has observed benefit in 20–30% of patients who were spared a major reconstruction or were able to have surgery delayed until an intercurrent illness permitted reconstruction[6]. A review and analysis of the data from cases which have been performed with laser technology suggest that the indications for use of this method may include: (1) arterial stenoses and short occlusions; (2) iliac artery lesions; (3) chronically occluded polytetrafluoro-ethylene grafts; and (4) selected patients who are at a high risk from conventional surgery, and in whom an interval patency may improve the operability at a later date.

At present it is reasonable to state that laser-assisted angioplasty is an investigational method which is undergoing rapid evolution and that current success is inferior to conventional surgical methods, with the exception of a few limited applications. An overall estimate of the utility of laser-assisted angioplasty with regard to length and site of occlusion is presented in Tables 1 and 2. In the author's institution patients are chosen as candidates for laser-assisted angioplasty using conventional surgical indications, with the therapy being administered by an experienced interventionalist. One reason to be conservative when treating minimal disease with the current state-of-the-art devices is that short stenoses or occlusions can be converted to long occlusions if imprecise technique is used or if complications occur.

Table 1 Success rates related to length of lesion*

Length of stenoses and occlusions (cm)	Initial recanalization (%)	One-year follow-up patency (%)
1–3	85–90	60–70
3–7	80	50–60
7–10	70	45
>10	60	20–40

*Values estimated from survey of the available published values. Table reproduced from White and White[2] with permission of the publishers.

Table 2 Success rates related to site of lesion*

Site	Initial recanalization (%)	One-year follow-up patency (%)
Iliac	80	70 (stenoses 80%; occlusions 50%)
Mid SFA	70	60 (stenoses 70%; occlusions 50%)
Diffuse SFA	50–60	40
Distal popliteal and limited run-off	50	20

SFA, superficial femoral artery. *Values estimated from survey of the available published values. Table reproduced from White and White[2] with permission of the publishers.

Preoperative

Assessment and preparation

Preoperative assessment of patients for laser-assisted angioplasty is identical to that for conventional revascularization of limbs by other percutaneous or operative means. Treatment should be based on identification of lesions amenable to the proposed form of therapy, usually by angiography, with clinical symptoms and haemodynamic evidence demonstrating significant improvement consistent with the indications for intervention. The most appropriate parameters are ankle:arm pressure indices and possibly ultrasonic flow or duplex image quantification of the severity of the lesion.

Patients should have conventional screening assessment for cardiovascular disease before the procedure as this group of patients has been identified as having a significant risk of concomitant coronary and carotid disease. Symptomatic patients should undergo aggressive investigations, with some requiring coronary artery angioplasty or bypass surgery or carotid endarterectomy before embarking upon elective peripheral vascular angioplasty. For patients being treated for limb threat, duplex scanning of the limb to evaluate the suitability of the saphenous vein for distal limb bypass is appropriate as some patients may require bypass as an alternative in order to salvage the limb if the angioplasty is unsuccessful or if a complication further threatens limb viability. If bypass is considered as a possible alternative, preparation should include the consent of the patient for possible conversion to general anaesthesia for bypass surgery.

When beginning the procedure, the patient should be positioned and prepared on the operating table to allow access to the entire limb for imaging or for subsequent surgery. A radio-opaque ruler placed under the leg is very helpful for locating the lesion during fluoroscopic examinations and for minimizing the amount of contrast material used during the procedure. Having the lower leg and foot included in the sterile field is essential to permit pulse evaluation and assessment of viability of the limb during and following the intervention.

Before starting the procedure, the patient and all personnel in the interventional suite should wear protective lenses to avert possible eye damage from free laser energy. In addition, all aspects of the procedure should be conducted according to laser safety guidelines adopted by the institution where the procedure is being performed.

Anaesthesia

Anaesthesia may be either local, regional or general. In most cases, local or regional anaesthesia is employed as these are the safest techniques, yet provide comfort for the patient. Some patients experience pain in the extremities when manipulation of the arteries is undertaken during local anaesthesia; thus, regional blocks are frequently desirable. Epidural anaesthesia also has the advantage of helping to prevent the vasospasm of distal arteries that sometimes occurs during instrumentation of vessels. In instances where more extensive surgery is required to treat unsuccessful attempts or complications, both local and regional anaesthesia may be converted to general if the patient has been properly evaluated before surgery.

Operation

Intravascular surgical procedures may be performed by either percutaneous or open incision surgical techniques. Outside the operating room the percutaneous route is used in the majority of procedures, while in the operating room a higher percentage of interventions is done through an open surgical incision (in patients who are not candidates for percutaneous methods) to accommodate the introduction of larger devices, or to combine an intravascular procedure with a conventional operation. Aside from balloon angioplasty catheters, many new intravascular devices are difficult to use percutaneously owing to size limitation. As interventional devices are developed, percutaneous adaptation occurs after miniaturization of the instruments.

Introducer sheaths which have a haemostatic valve at the instrument introduction port and additional ports for infusion of fluids and contrast dyes are extremely useful in reducing the trauma to vessel walls and controlling blood loss. Newer intraluminal access devices for use during both percutaneous and open incision approaches are being developed to decrease vessel trauma, to provide better haemostasis, and to facilitate removal of intravascular material.

Percutaneous procedure

The Seldinger technique

1a–c The percutaneous procedures are limited to those which can be performed with low-profile catheters (less than 8–10-Fr diameter), and to procedures which have a segment of patent vessel available proximal to the interventional site for introduction of the instruments. Introduction of percutaneous devices is usually accomplished with the conventional Seldinger technique. The percutaneous vascular access is performed by inserting a bevelled needle with an inner stylet through both walls of the artery via a small skin incision to facilitate subsequent insertion of larger vessel dilators and instruments. The stylet is removed and the needle is slowly withdrawn until pulsatile arterial blood flow is achieved, signifying that the needle tip is in the arterial lumen. Poor blood flow from the needle indicates that the tip is misplaced or is too close to the arterial wall.

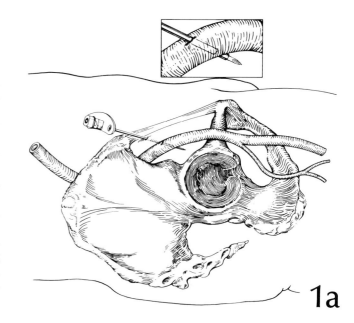

1a

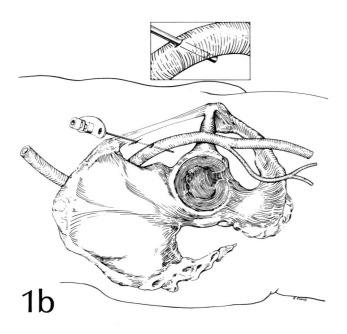

1b

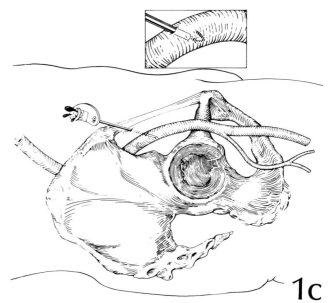

1c

Introduction of guidewire

2a–d A guidewire is then introduced through the lumen of the needle and is positioned using fluoroscopy control. The guidewire is inserted and advanced into the artery. With the guidewire in place, a combined vessel dilator and instrument introducer sheath is advanced as one unit over the guidewire and positioned within the vessel. The dilator is then removed from the sheath, leaving the guidewire in place if it is to be used for introduction of interventional devices.

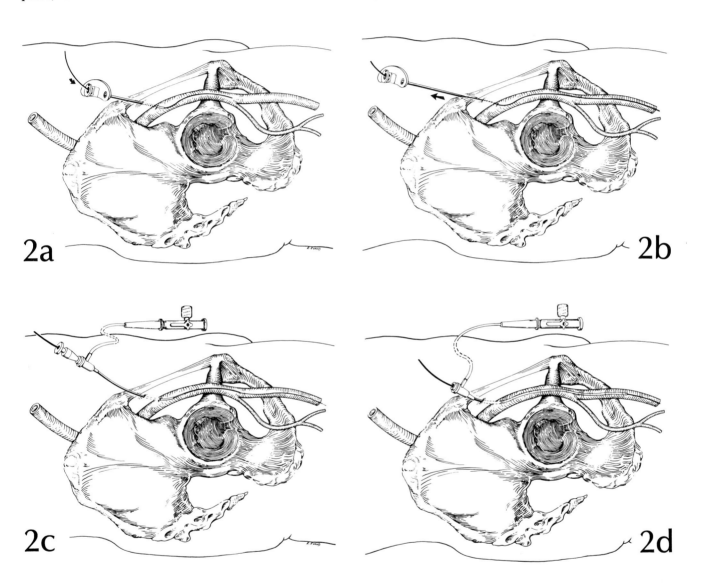

2a

2b

2c

2d

Intraoperative applications of endovascular devices

Intraoperative application of endovascular devices permits use of a larger variety of instruments as either primary therapy or as an adjunct to another vascular procedure. A key factor in accomplishing successful angioplasty in the operating room is adequate radiological imaging. High-resolution images significantly enhance the precision of procedures and are a limiting factor in many institutions. Digital subtraction techniques have increased contrast imaging sensitivity, allowing detection of low levels of iodinated materials. Many digital units have freeze-frame and road mapping features that permit superimposition of a subtracted contrast image of a vessel onto a live fluoroscopic visualization. The quality of equipment available for radiological imaging of procedures varies from conventional C-arm fluoroscopes to sophisticated image intensifiers and televisual monitoring systems. Immediate image replay systems can improve the accuracy of information and enhance the safety of interventions. Recent advances in computerized image processing systems extend the advantages of digital imaging technology to C-arm fluoroscopy by enabling modular addition of contrast enhancement, image holding and road mapping during angiographic procedures using available equipment.

Intraoperative percutaneous use of devices is accomplished by the methods described in the previous section. Many patients have significant vascular occlusive disease near a possible insertion site which precludes safe passage of a percutaneous introducer. In these cases, surgical incisions provide the best access to the vessel. Introduction of intravascular instruments through an open surgical incision has several advantages compared with percutaneous methods, as well as potential risks. Open incisions permit inspection of intravascular anatomy such as the orifices of adjacent branch vessels, and help to decrease the incidence of vessel wall dissection during device introduction. Control of blood flow from collateral vessels by conventional operative methods also expedites angioscopic intraluminal visualization.

Once an arteriotomy has been fashioned, it is advantageous to work through a haemostatic introducer sheath with a sideport similar to ones used for percutaneous procedures to help prevent trauma to the blood vessel wall by repeated introduction and withdrawal of devices, to provide haemostasis at the introduction port and to provide a port for injection of contrast dye. Introducer sheaths must be used very carefully as it is quite easy to injure the luminal surface of the artery during placement of the sheath, particularly when it is introduced for some distance into an artery. If a vessel is too diseased to accommodate an introducer sheath, haemostasis can be maintained with Roumel tourniquets with the endoluminal devices passed carefully through the controlled area.

Surgical incisions also permit continuation of anticoagulation throughout the procedure and after it if the wound is drained. This helps prevent acute thrombosis of difficult recanalizations in comparison with percutaneous procedures where anticoagulation is reversed and pressure is applied to the wound after removal of the intraluminal device to assure haemostasis. An obvious liability of the open incision technique is the risk of wound infection, particularly if a patch material or prosthetic is used in the repair. The incidence of wound infection has been shown to be slightly higher using the open technique during endovascular procedures[6].

Laser-assisted angioplasty technique

Passage of guidewire

3a, b Laser-assisted angioplasty is accomplished by attempting passage of a guidewire through an arterial lesion. If the guidewire is successfully introduced, subsequent devices are introduced over the guidewire.

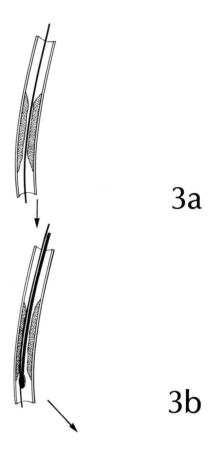

3a

3b

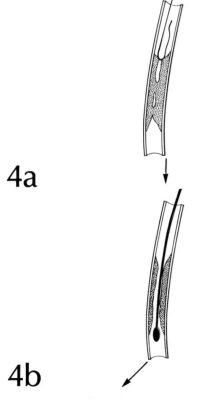

4a

4b

Passage of laser probe

4a, b If the guidewire does not pass easily without resistance, a laser probe is introduced and activated to accomplish the initial vessel recanalization.

Balloon dilatation

5a–c   After recanalization with the laser probe, the lumen is subsequently enlarged either by using larger laser devices or by subsequent balloon dilatation of the lesion. The laser-assisted procedure is monitored throughout using fluoroscopic guidance and possibly angioscopic and/or intravascular ultrasonographic inspection, if these devices are available, to ensure adequate restoration of the lumen.

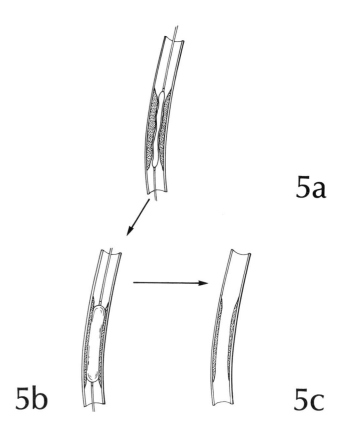

5a

5b

5c

Postoperative care

Postoperative care for laser-assisted angioplasty procedures entails monitoring the patient for potential procedure-related complications such as fluid overload from excessive administration of irrigation fluids for angioscopic examinations and maintenance of access catheter patency, blood loss beyond the amount estimated during the intervention, and kidney dysfunction from radiological contrast. In general, postoperative observation should only include routine haematological and haemodynamic assessment, particularly since patients are usually fully awake after the local or regional anaesthetic required for these procedures.

Limb viability must be carefully observed for possible thromboembolic events. Serial quantitative measurement of pulse pressure and limb perfusion is required to monitor continued patency of the angioplasty. Anticoagulation may be administered to enhance patency of the revascularization and varies from maintaining full heparinization for 24–48 h after the procedure in particularly difficult cases to less aggressive therapy such as dextran. Long-term anticoagulation can be accomplished with warfarin or aspirin, with the level of treatment and length of administration varying depending upon the difficulty of the recanalization, the training of the physician, and other factors.

Outcome

Complications

A variety of introducers is used to provide access to the vascular lumen for guidewires and angioplasty devices. The main complications of the introducers are disruption of the vascular surface producing intimal flaps or embolization, vessel wall injury leading to thrombosis or the development of intimal hyperplasia, and formation of thrombus on the catheter surfaces when they are positioned in low blood flow areas without anticoagulation. Some catheters incorporate anticoagulants in the catheter surface to decrease thrombogenicity, although systemic anticoagulation is required in most instances to prevent thrombosis.

The complications related to introducer sheath placement can be reduced by accurately judging the appropriate diameter and length of the device for the vascular segment being treated. Many diseased vessels have segmental narrowings or friable luminal surfaces which can easily be disrupted. If intimal flaps result, a localized endarterectomy can sometimes be performed, although an otherwise successful angioplasty procedure can be disrupted by introducer complications which frequently require a vascular reconstruction to bypass the segment.

Microembolization of thrombus or atheromatous material is usually of no consequence if it is limited and there is no evidence of distal ischaemia. If larger artery occlusion develops, percutaneous aspiration thrombectomy or open surgical embolectomy is required to restore flow. Intra-arterial infusion of thrombolytic therapy may also be effective in dissolving fresh thrombus. Massive embolization of small (20–200-μm diameter) particles can cause diffuse necrosis of tissues, producing devastating clinical consequences such as a 'trash limb'.

Guidewires are extemely useful for introducing intravascular devices and helping to maintain intra-luminal guidance. Stiffer wires with less flexible tips have a higher tendency to produce intimal lesions, dissections and perforations. Some of the newer flexible tip wires and catheters have hydrophilic polymer coatings which enhance atraumatic passage through stenotic or occluded vessel segments. Although intro-duction of angioplasty devices over guidewires can be used to help prevent complications, the obligatory off-centre positioning of the guidewire through eccen-tric atherosclerotic obstructions prevents complete debulking of lesions without affecting adjacent vessel walls which have minimal or no involvement. Allevi-ation of this problem awaits improved guidance systems to provide concentric alignment of the device within the arterial lumen. Combined intraluminal ultrasono-graphy and angioscopy-guided angioplasty catheter delivery systems are promising in this regard.

The most frequent complication of laser-assisted angioplasty is vessel wall dissection or perforation if the probes are used in lesions where a guidewire cannot be initially passed. In most situations perforations are of no consequence as only a small hole is made tangentially through the lesion in the arterial wall which subse-quently rethromboses. Arteriovenous fistulae usually close readily once anticoagulation is reversed although, rarely, venous trauma may lead to vein thrombosis which requires anticoagulant therapy. Also rarely perforations may continue to bleed, requiring surgical control. The most frequent site where this occurs is in intraperitoneal vessels or with punctures to the external iliac artery done above the inguinal ligament to facilitate antegrade access to the femoral vessels. This approach is associated with a risk of haemorrhage into the retroperitoneum.

False or pseudoaneurysms at the puncture site in the arterial wall are unique to percutaneous introduction sites and the frequency increases with increasing size of the cannulae and endovascular instruments. False aneurysms frequently become apparent at relatively short intervals after procedures and require repair to prevent bleeding or embolization.

Laser-assisted angioplasty has been used widely in its early evolution and accentuates the problems of guidance of endovascular devices. An additional com-plication of laser-assisted angioplasty, which is related to imprecise delivery of energy to normal or minimally diseased arteries, is the development of lesions in previously unaffected sites adjacent to the treated segment. The most evident presentation of this com-plication is apparent when patients who were previous-ly treated for short stenoses or occlusions return with long segments of reoccluded vessels. This limitation emphasizes the importance of treating only well-defined lesions that can be precisely ablated with current devices. It also emphasizes that treatment of minimal disease, such as claudication, should be reserved for interventionalists who have technical excellence, vast experience and optimal systems available to treat these lesions.

Current use and future perspectives

The complication rates of laser-assisted angioplasty are potentially high because many of the new devices are in an early development phase. The indications for some of the instruments have not yet been determined so their use to treat lesions beyond the capabilities of the device increases the potential for adverse outcome.

Complications during the procedure may lead to immediate failure or may compromise the long-term durability of the repair. Even though immediate vessel recanalization may be accomplished, long-term patency is frequently limited by imprecise recanalizations and inadequate removal of lesions. The complications of intravascular interventions are directly affected by the skill and training of the operator. A learning curve is experienced by almost all investigators during the initial procedures, particularly if the interventionalist is inexperienced with endoluminal methods. Other vari-ables, including the quality of ancillary equipment such as fluoroscopy and imaging devices, significantly affect the success of intravascular procedures.

Resolving the current limitations and complications of endovascular surgical procedures and devices must address the problems related to guidance of angioplasty instruments and restenosis subsequent to initial recanal-ization. The guidance issue is particularly relevant since most atherosclerotic lesions are eccentrically pos-itioned within the vessel wall. Many of the failures, including initial perforations and dissections and short-term reocclusion, are because of imprecise guidance of angioplasty devices and inadequate debulk-ing of lesions[7]. For this reason, major emphasis is being directed towards development of improved guidance and ablative methods for endoluminal instruments.

References

1. Sanborn TA, Cumberland DC, Greenfield AJ, Motarjeme A, Schwarten DE, Leachman R. Peripheral laser assisted balloon angioplasty: initial multicenter experience in 219 peripheral arteries. *Arch Surg* 1989; 124: 1099–103.

2. White RA, White GH. Laser thermal probe recanalization of occluded arteries. *J Vasc Surg* 1989; 9: 598–608.

3. Wright JG, Belkin M, Greenfield AJ *et al*. Laser angioplasty for limb salvage: observations on early results. *J Vasc Surg* 1989; 10: 29–38.

4. Perler BA, Osterman FA, White RI, Williams GM. Percutaneous laser probe femoropopliteal angioplasty: a preliminary experience. *J Vasc Surg* 1989; 10: 351–7.

5. Seeger JM, Abela CS, Silverman SH, Jablonski SK. Initial results of laser recanalization in lower extremity arterial reconstruction. *J Vasc Surg* 1989; 9: 10–17.

6. White RA, White G, Mehringer M, Chaing C, Wilson SE. A clinical trial of laser angioplasty in patients with advanced peripheral vascular disease. *Ann Surg* 1990; 212: 257–65.

7. White RA, White GH, Vlasak J, Fujitani RM, Kopchok GE. Histopathology of human laser thermal angioplasty recanalization. *Lasers Surg Med* 1988; 8: 469–76.

Atherectomy

Samuel S. Ahn MD
Assistant Professor, Department of Surgery, UCLA School of Medicine, Los Angeles, California, USA

Principles and justification

Mechanical atherectomy, which removes atheroma from stenotic or occluded vessels, provides an appealing alternative to balloon angioplasty which simply fractures and dilates the arterial lumen. In a similar way to balloon angioplasty, mechanical atherectomy can be performed percutaneously or through a limited surgical exposure. Recent reports have shown that the results of atherectomy are no better than those of balloon angioplasty and may even be worse[1-7]. On the other hand, atherectomy has been shown to enhance immediate results in arteries that are diffusely diseased or have eccentric stenosis, or in hard, calcified, non-distendable arteries[2, 4, 7].

Indications

The current indications for atherectomy thus appear to be arterial stenoses that are not amenable to balloon angioplasty. Specifically, these include:

1. Hard, calcified lesions that cannot be dilated easily with balloon expansion.

2. Ulcerated or polypoid lesions that present with embolic symptoms or have a high embolic potential when dilated by balloon.
3. Markedly eccentric lesions that have a high potential for arterial rupture if dilated.
4. Arteries that abruptly close due to intimal flaps or dissections during balloon angioplasty.

Atherectomy, like balloon angioplasty and standard surgical revascularization, should be reserved for patients with disabling claudication or limb-threatening ischaemia. Immediate and long-term results are not currently satisfactory enough to warrant a relaxation of these well established indications. Like balloon angioplasty, atherectomy achieves better results with shorter lesions (less than 7 cm in length)[3-6]. Longer lesions are better treated by standard bypass procedures. Although atherectomy can be technically successful with these lesions, long-term results are poor and complication rates high[3-6]. Thus, atherectomy for longer lesions should be reserved for those patients who are extremely poor surgical candidates and not suitable for standard bypass or open procedures.

Finally, atherectomy can be used as an adjunct to standard revascularization to improve inflow or outflow for a bypass graft[8].

Preoperative

Assessment and preparation

A standard history and physical examination, with particular emphasis on the vascular examination, should be obtained for all patients. Pulses should be palpated, and the ankle:brachial index should be measured in both lower extremities. In the presence of non-compressible vessels, other non-invasive assessment such as Doppler ultrasonography or digital plethysmography should be performed. Angiography is currently recommended to analyse the anatomical and pathological characteristics of the artery; however, external duplex scanning may provide a better assessment of plaque composition and the characteristics of the lesion. Intravascular ultrasonography is an alternative technique that may enhance visualization of the plaque characteristics.

Duplex scanning and intravascular ultrasonography allow the surgeon to choose the best atherectomy device based on the characteristics of the lesion. For example, atherectomy may be chosen rather than balloon angioplasty in the presence of a hard calcified plaque that is severely ulcerated or polypoid in nature. Furthermore, these studies may allow better assessment of the completeness of the atherectomy procedure by cross-sectional assessment of the lumen and the residual atheroma. Angiography can miss eccentric or posteriorly placed plaques, and thus may not be as accurate in assessing residual luminal stenosis.

As many of these patients will undergo intraoperative angiography, they should be well hydrated before the operation. Furthermore, patients should undergo the usual preoperative preparation for a standard surgical revascularization procedure, as an acute complication or failure of the atherectomy may lead to immediate surgery.

The patient is prepared and draped from the umbilicus to the ankle, in a similar way to the preparation used for a standard femoropopliteal bypass. A patient scheduled for iliac atherectomy should be prepared from the nipple to the knees. If the patient is undergoing both iliac and femoropopliteal artery atherectomy or reconstruction, preparation from the nipple to the foot is required. It is advisable to prepare widely in case the atherectomy procedure fails or leads to a complication that requires standard surgical reconstruction or repair.

Anaesthesia

Atherectomy can be performed under local anaesthesia. It is preferable, however, to perform the procedure under spinal or epidural anaesthesia for several reasons. First, regional anaesthesia induces peripheral vasodilatation and prevents vasospasm induced by arterial trauma during atherectomy. Secondly, the patient is more comfortable and is able to lie still for a longer period of time. Thirdly, the atherectomy procedure can be uncomfortable for the patient because the atherectomy catheter can often be felt coursing inside the artery. Most patients under local anaesthesia feel a severe burning sensation during the actual atherectomy portion of the procedure. Finally, regional anaesthesia avoids the necessity of emergency general anaesthesia if a complication requiring further adjunctive vascular reconstruction or repair occurs.

Operation

Position of patient

The patient is placed in the supine position. The surgeon should make sure that the operating table is radiolucent to allow intraoperative fluoroscopy and angiography. A carbon-fibre table is ideal, but other radiolucent operating tables are available. It must also be ensured that the proposed atherectomy site is not directly over the operating table pedestal, which prevents the X-ray machine from visualizing that site. These points are important to make because most operating rooms currently do not have the optimal carbon-fibre fluoroscopy tables that allow full visualization of the patient's entire body.

The surgeon should stand at the side of the table most convenient for guidewire and catheter manipulation. A right-handed surgeon should stand on the patient's right side if the lesion is to be treated by retrograde access to the iliac artery; however, the surgeon should stand on the patient's left side when performing an antegrade puncture to access the superficial femoral or popliteal artery. The opposite applies for a left-handed surgeon.

Vascular access

Vascular access is required for all atherectomy procedures and may be obtained percutaneously or by an open cut-down of the femoral artery. A cut-down is preferred for patients with unfavourable anatomy, i.e. those who are morbidly obese or have an orifice lesion that requires a local femoral endarterectomy, or in cases where the lesion is in close proximity to the access site. Most other situations allow for the preferable percutaneous method.

Percutaneous approach

It is extremely important to identify the femoral artery by palpation and by reference to the bony landmarks. As the needle should enter the common femoral artery just below the inguinal ligament, this structure should be clearly identified as it courses from the anterior iliac spine to the pubic symphysis. Skin folds should not be relied on as landmarks, because these folds are often inconsistent and inaccurate in identifying the inguinal ligament.

In the presence of a palpable pulse, the longitudinal axis for placement of the needle can easily be determined. The position of the horizontal axis, however, should be carefully calculated based on the inguinal ligament and the patient's body habitus. It should be remembered that the needle has to penetrate a variable amount of subcutaneous tissue before reaching the femoral artery.

Entry of the needle into the external iliac artery above the inguinal ligament should be avoided. Such an entry site makes haemostasis difficult to obtain after the catheter is removed. Any puncture above the ligament can bleed massively into the retroperitoneum. On the other hand, puncture of the superficial or deep femoral artery should be avoided, as these vessels are smaller and may not tolerate a catheter disrupting the artery, leading to acute thrombosis or an intimal flap.

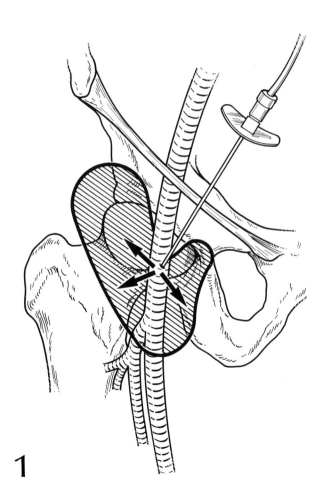

1

1 The skin puncture is started with the needle at a 45° angle to the skin at the site that will lead to a puncture of the common femoral artery just below the ligament. In performing an antegrade puncture, this may require the needle to begin in the lower abdomen above the inguinal ligament so that the angle of the needle and catheter will not be too acute when it enters the common femoral artery.

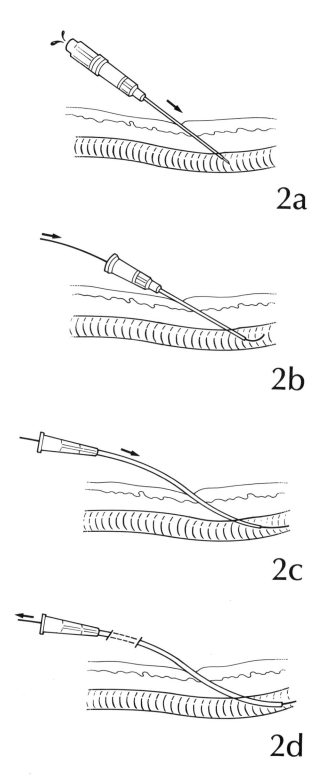

2a

2b

2c

2d

$2a–d$ After identifying the proper anatomical landmarks, the site of the needle puncture and the angle of the needle are determined, and access to the artery is gained using the standard Seldinger method. Briefly, this consists of placing an 18-gauge needle into the artery and observing any back-bleeding. Either a single or a double puncture technique can be used. The author prefers the single puncture so that only one hole is made in the anterior wall of the artery. As soon as bleeding from the needle is observed, the needle is advanced slightly into the lumen while changing the angle slightly to a shallower one. A 0.035-inch (0.89-mm) or 0.036-inch (0.91-mm) guide-wire is then inserted through the 18-gauge needle, which is removed.

A number 11 blade is used to enlarge the skin incision, and a dilator and introducer sheath are introduced over the guidewire under fluoroscopy to ensure satisfactory placement of both the guidewire and the introducer sheath. In placing the introducer sheath and dilator over the guidewire, care must be taken to keep the guidewire steady so that the introducer slides over it rather than moving together with it. Once the introducer sheath is in place, the dilator and guidewire are removed.

The side arm of the introducer is aspirated and then flushed with heparin solution to ensure proper placement in the arterial lumen and to flush away any blood in the catheter. An intraoperative angiogram is now obtained through the side arm to ascertain that the introducer sheath is properly placed in the arterial lumen.

Cut-down approach

The patient is prepared and draped, and the anatomical landmarks are identified as described above. The author prefers a vertical groin incision, although an oblique incision in the groin crease can be performed instead.

3 Proximal and distal control of the common, deep and superficial femoral arteries are achieved as for a standard bypass procedure.

With direct exposure and control of the femoral arteries, the patient is given systemic heparinization (usually 5000–10 000 units). The anterior wall of the common femoral artery is then punctured with an 18-gauge needle and access is gained using the Seldinger technique, as described above.

Occasionally, blood leaks round the introducer sheath. If this occurs, the inflow is temporarily controlled while a purse-string suture is placed in the arterial wall around the catheter to prevent bleeding. Alternatively, a slightly larger introducer sheath can be inserted. The proximal occlusion should be temporary to minimize the risk of thrombosis or ischaemia of the lower extremity.

Generally, an introducer sheath is chosen that is just large enough to allow the atherectomy device to pass. Although balloon angioplasty can be performed through a 5 Fr or 6-Fr sheath, atherectomy often requires a 9-Fr, 10-Fr or even a 12-Fr sheath, depending on the size of the atherectomy catheter. When using the larger introducer sheaths, the open technique may be preferable so that the puncture site can be better controlled and repaired.

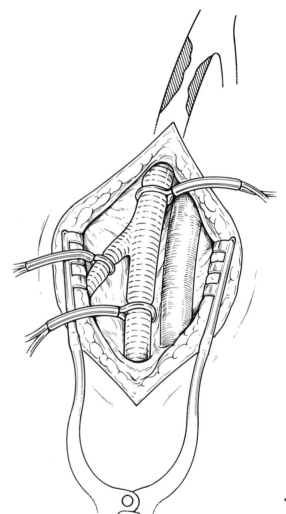

3

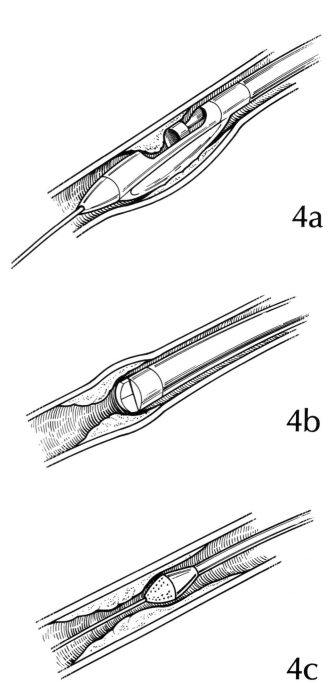

Atherectomy

4a–c Over a dozen atherectomy catheters are currently under development. Only four, however, are approved for commercial use in the USA. Of these, only three have produced any significant results: the Simpson Atherocath (*Illustration 4a*), the Theratek catheter (*Illustration 4b*) and the Auth Rotablator (*Illustration 4c*). Each of these has different mechanisms and requires a different technique. The surgeon should be thoroughly familiar with the device before using it; these devices have been well described in previous publications, to which the reader is referred[1, 2, 5, 8].

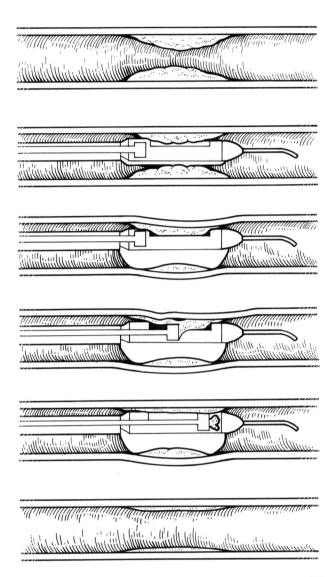

Simpson atherectomy

5 The atherectomy catheter is advanced through the sheath, into the artery and through the stenotic lesion. A 9-Fr atherectomy catheter is usually used. The smaller 7-Fr catheter may be used if the larger catheter is not able to pass readily through the stenosis. The opened side window is positioned against the atheroma and the contralateral balloon is inflated to 70–140 kPa. The motor drive unit is then activated and the cutter is slowly advanced over 5–7 s until it has traversed the whole length of the open housing. The cutter should pass easily with minimal resistance, unless there is heavy calcification. The atheroma is sliced and pushed into the distal collecting chamber.

At this point the cutter is maintained distally against the collecting chamber to prevent any dislodgement and distal emboli of the atheroma. The balloon is deflated, the catheter is rotated and repositioned for another atheroma slice. The balloon is reinflated to 70 kPa, while the inner cutter is retracted back to its proximal position. The balloon is then fully inflated to 70–140 kPa, and the cutting is repeated. This process is repeated up to 20 times, at which point the collecting chamber can no longer hold further atheroma.

The catheter is withdrawn with the cutter securely against the distal collecting chamber to prevent any emboli. The atheroma in the distal collecting chamber is carefully removed and examined. Angiography is performed to assess the results. There should be no more than 25% residual stenosis after the atherectomy procedure. Further atherectomy may be performed if residual stenosis is 30% or more. If repeat atherectomy produces no further atheroma specimen but the residual stenosis remains 25% or more, the balloon can be inflated to a higher pressure of 140–350 kPa to force the opened housing more firmly against the atheroma. In general, as much atheroma as possible should be excised to create a wide lumen, as restenosis occurs more often when the residual stenosis is 30% or more.

5

Theratek Atherocath (Trac–Wright atherectomy device)

6 The device utilizes a curved cam tip rotating at speeds up to 100 000 rpm to recanalize obstructed arterial lumina. An 8-Fr atherectomy system is placed through a 9-Fr introducer sheath and positioned just proximal to the obstructive lesion. Under fluoroscopic guidance the Theratek catheter is advanced while a mixture of radio-opaque contrast medium, dextran, urokinase and heparin is infused under pressure through the catheter. This mixture allows visualization of the atherectomy procedure, prevents aggregation of platelets and induces regional thrombolysis. The catheter is moved gently to and fro, while the rotary cam tip spins at 60 000–90 000 rpm. The catheter follows the path of least resistance, and any resistance should warn the operator to stop. Extravasation of contrast medium through the arterial wall can often be seen, but this should not be interpreted as arterial wall perforation.

The 8-Fr atherectomy catheter creates a 2.8-mm lumen, and adjunctive balloon angioplasty is often necessary to enlarge the lumen to match the diameter of the normal portion of the artery. Thus, in most cases, the Theratek atherectomy catheter allows some debulking but generally acts as a pilot guidewire to allow easier balloon angioplasty. The catheter is then removed and exchanged for the balloon angioplasty catheter, which is used in the standard fashion.

The Theratek catheter should not be used for heavily calcified arteries, particularly at the abductor's canal where calcification is worst, and the perforation rate is extremely high. Embolization has not generally been a problem, perhaps because of the urokinase and heparin that is used in the infusion.

Auth Rotablator

7 Conceptually, rotary atherectomy is simple, but the procedure must be done very carefully, with strict attention to details and gentle advancement of the atherectomy catheter. Depending on the size of the atherectomy burr chosen, a 9-Fr or 12-Fr introducer sheath is inserted. A small atraumatic guidewire is inserted and advanced under fluoroscopic and/or angioscopic guidance through the stenotic lesion. The author prefers a 0.014-inch (0.36-mm) high-torque floppy coronary guidewire to cross the lesion first. Next, a 3-Fr guide catheter is inserted over the guidewire, and the high-torque floppy guidewire is exchanged for the more rigid 0.009-inch (0.23-mm) atherectomy guidewire. The guide catheter is then removed, leaving the atherectomy guidewire in place, and the burr is back-loaded onto the atherectomy guidewire. The burr and the drive shaft are then fed over the guidewire and advanced to the site of the obstructed lesion.

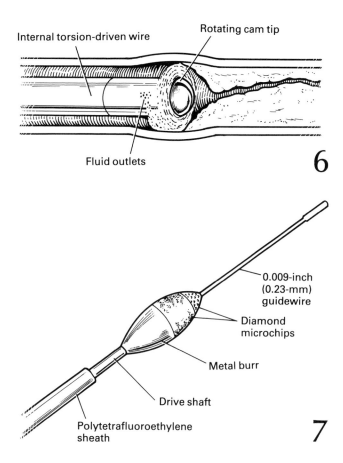

The author generally starts with a burr of approximately half the diameter of the native artery and uses a series of burrs of increasing size until the final lumen size is reached. A 2-mm or 2.5-mm burr is often used, followed by a 3–3.5-mm burr and finally a 4–4.5-mm burr.

With the burr adjacent to the lesion and under fluoroscopic guidance, the burr is advanced as the compressed nitrogen is released to turn the atherectomy turbine. Generally the nitrogen pressure is set at 280–350 kPa, which allows the turbine to rotate at 100 000–175 000 rpm. The compressed nitrogen should be controlled to maintain the rotation at these speeds. Slower rotation will cause the surrounding atheromatous tissue to snag onto the burr. Faster rotation may produce excessive heat, although the fluid around the atherectomy burr quickly dissipates this heat. The burr must be advanced slowly, in a to-and-fro fashion, and delicately, not keeping the burr in one place for too long, but also not advancing too rapidly to avoid meeting significant resistance. A fine darting in-and-out motion of the burr is ideal.

After the burr crosses the lesion, it is retracted and completion angiography is performed. If residual stenosis persists, a larger burr is used to enlarge the opening. This procedure is repeated until the residual luminal stenosis is 25% or less.

Precautions

Atherectomy requires the surgeon to demonstrate extreme patience and a delicate touch. The procedure is tedious and can occasionally be prolonged. The arteries require extremely gentle handling to avoid creating intimal flaps and over-treatment. Oversized catheters should be avoided by choosing a smaller catheter and working up to the larger ones.

When performing atherectomy in conjunction with standard revascularization, the latter should be completed first to avoid prolonged blood stasis in the atherectomized segment while the standard revascularization is proceeding. By completing the standard revascularization first, immediate blood flow through the atherectomized segment can occur. The arterial puncture site should be opened longitudinally to allow the revascularization procedure to accommodate the anastomosis or repair. If adjunctive standard revascularization is not planned, then the arteriotomy and repair is performed transversely.

Postoperative care

Full anticoagulation should be given for 24–48 h following the procedure to avoid thrombosis. The author also routinely uses aspirin before the procedure and dextran afterwards to inhibit platelet aggregation. Vasodilators are also administered after the procedure to inhibit the vasospasm that can occur. Finally, vigorous intravenous hydration should be maintained for 24 h, as the patient receives intravenous contrast medium throughout the procedure.

Complications

Haematomas, pseudoaneurysms and arteriovenous fistulae at the catheter insertion site can occur. The patient should be followed closely for any evidence of thrombosis secondary to dissection or hypercoagulation states. Manifestations of thromboemboli including disseminated intravascular coagulation should be watched for. Cases of haemoglobinuria have been reported following treatment with the Auth Rotablator, secondary to disruption of red blood cells by the rapidly spinning atherectomy burr[7]. If dark amber urine is encountered, the patient should be tested for haemoglobinuria and haemoglobinaemia and treated immediately with vigorous intravenous hydration, alkalinization of the urine and diuretics.

Experience with mechanical atherectomy is currently limited, and long-term results are not yet available. Much refinement of the technology is still required before atherectomy can become a standard routine procedure. Atherectomy should be strictly reserved for the indications described earlier.

References

1. Ahn SS. Peripheral atherectomy. *Semin Vasc Surg* 1989; 2: 143–54.

2. Simpson JB, Selmon MR, Robertson GC, Cipriano PR, Hayden WG, Johnson DE. Transluminal atherectomy for occlusive peripheral vascular disease. *Am J Cardiol* 1988; 61: 96–101G.

3. Von Polnitz A, Nerlich A, Berger H, Höfling B. Percutaneous peripheral atherectomy: angiographic and clinical follow-up of 60 patients. *J Am Coll Cardiol* 1990; 15: 682–8.

4. Graor RA, Whitlow PL. Transluminal atherectomy for occlusive peripheral vascular disease. *J Am Coll Cardiol* 1990; 15: 1551–8.

5. Cull DL, Feinberg RL, Wheeler JR, Snyder SO, Gregory RT, Gayle RG *et al*. Experience with laser-assisted balloon angioplasty and rotary angioplasty instrument: lessons learned. *J Vasc Surg* 1991; 14: 332–9.

6. Desbrosses D, Petit H, Torres E, Barrioneuvo D, Figueroa A, Wenger JJ *et al*. Percutaneous atherectomy with the Kensey catheter: early and midterm results in femoropopliteal occlusions unsuitable for conventional angioplasty. *Ann Vasc Surg* 1990; 4: 550–2.

7. Ahn SS, Eton D, Yeatman LR, Deutsch L-S, Moore WS. Intraoperative peripheral rotary atherectomy: early and late clinical results. *Ann Vasc Surg* 1992; 6: 272–80.

8. Ahn SS, Moore WS. Lesions amenable to mechanical atherectomy: clinical strategies. In: Moore WS, Ahn SS, eds. *Endovascular Surgery*. Philadelphia: WB Saunders, 1989: 299–309.

Index